Professional Issues in Nursing

CHALLENGES AND OPPORTUNITIES

Professional Issues in Nursing

CHALLENGES AND OPPORTUNITIES

Carol J. Huston, RN, MSN, MPA, DPA, FAAN
Emerita Professor, School of Nursing
California State University,
Chico, California

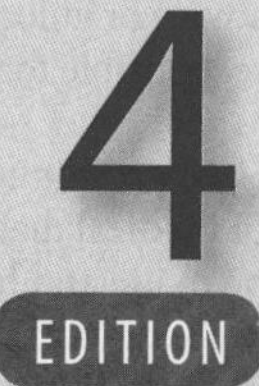

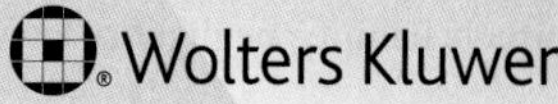

Philadelphia • Baltimore • New York • London
Buenos Aires • Hong Kong • Sydney • Tokyo

Acquisitions Editor: Christina Burns
Product Development Editor: Shana Murph
Production Project Manager: Marian Bellus
Manufacturing Coordinator: Karin Duffield
Design Coordinator: Stephen Druding
Production Services: S4Carlisle Publishing Services

Copyright © 2017 Wolters Kluwer

All rights reserved. This book is protected by copyright. No part of this book may be reproduced or transmitted in any form or by any means, including as photocopies or scanned-in or other electronic copies, or utilized by any information storage and retrieval system without written permission from the copyright owner, except for brief quotations embodied in critical articles and reviews. Materials appearing in this book prepared by individuals as part of their official duties as US government employees are not covered by the above-mentioned copyright. To request permission, please contact Lippincott Williams & Wilkins at Two Commerce Square, 2001 Market Street, Philadelphia, PA 19103, via email at permissions@lww.com, or via website at lww.com (products and services).

9 8 7 6 5 4 3 2 1

Printed in China

Library of Congress Cataloging-in-Publication Data

Huston, Carol Jorgensen, author
Professional issues in nursing: challenges & opportunities/Carol J. Huston—Fourth edition
p.; cm
Includes bibliographical references and index
ISBN 978-1-4963-3439-8 (alk. paper)
I. Title.
[DNLM: 1. Nurse's Role—United States. 2. Nursing—trends—United States. 3. Ethics, Nursing—United States. 4. Nursing—manpower—United States. 5. Professional Competence—United States. WY 16 AA1]
RT82
610.73—dc23

2015033117

This work is provided "as is," and the publisher disclaims any and all warranties, express or implied, including any warranties as to accuracy, comprehensiveness, or currency of the content of this work.

This work is no substitute for individual patient assessment based upon healthcare professionals' examination of each patient and consideration of, among other things, age, weight, gender, current or prior medical conditions, medication history, laboratory data and other factors unique to the patient. The publisher does not provide medical advice or guidance and this work is merely a reference tool. Healthcare professionals, and not the publisher, are solely responsible for the use of this work including all medical judgments and for any resulting diagnosis and treatments.

Given continuous, rapid advances in medical science and health information, independent professional verification of medical diagnoses, indications, appropriate pharmaceutical selections and dosages, and treatment options should be made and healthcare professionals should consult a variety of sources. When prescribing medication, healthcare professionals are advised to consult the product information sheet (the manufacturer's package insert) accompanying each drug to verify, among other things, conditions of use, warnings and side effects and identify any changes in dosage schedule or contraindications, particularly if the medication to be administered is new, infrequently used or has a narrow therapeutic range. To the maximum extent permitted under applicable law, no responsibility is assumed by the publisher for any injury and/or damage to persons or property, as a matter of products liability, negligence law or otherwise, or from any reference to or use by any person of this work.

LWW.com

CCS1215

I dedicate this book to my friend and colleague, Margaret (Peggy) Rowberg. Your passion, energy, tireless work ethic, and friendship inspire me.

Carol J. Huston

Contributors

Sheila A. Burke, DNP, MBA, MSN, RN, NEA-BC
Dean of Nursing
Carrington College
Wheaton, Illinois
(CHAPTER 25)

April M. Clayton, PhD
Postdoctoral Fellow
National Institutes of Health
National Institute of Allergy and Infectious Diseases
Bethesda, Maryland
(CHAPTER 17)

Rebekah Damazo, RN, PNP, MSN
Rural Northern California Clinical Simulation Center Project Coordinator
Certified Pediatric Nurse Practitioner
Emerita Professor
School of Nursing
California State University
Chico, California
(CHAPTER 14)

Cassandra D. Ford, PhD, MSN, MBA, RN, FAHA
Assistant Professor
Capstone College of Nursing
The University of Alabama
Tuscaloosa, Alabama
(CHAPTER 2)

Cynthia Foronda, PhD, RN, CNE, ANEF
Assistant Professor
Department of Acute and Chronic Care
Johns Hopkins University School of Nursing
Baltimore, Maryland
(CHAPTER 17)

Sherry D. Fox, RN, PhD
Emerita Professor
School of Nursing
California State University
Chico, California
(CHAPTER 14)

Lynn Gallagher-Ford, PhD, RN, NE-BC
Director
Center for Transdisciplinary Evidence-Based Practice
Clinical Associate Professor
College of Nursing
Ohio State University
Columbus, Ohio
(CHAPTER 3)

Perry M. Gee, PhD, RN, CPEHR
Lecturer
California State University
Chico, California
(CHAPTER 12)

Charmaine Hockley, PhD, LLB, GDLP, RN, FACON, JP
Charmaine Hockley and Associates
Director
Workplace Relationships Consultant
Strathalbyn, Australia
(CHAPTER 11)

Carol J. Huston, RN, MSN, MPA, DPA, FAAN
Emerita Professor
School of Nursing
California State University
Chico, California
(CHAPTERS 1, 5, 6, 7, 8, 9, 10, 13, 19, 21, 22, 23, 24)

Pamela R. Jeffries, PhD, RN, FAAN, ANEF
Dean and Professor of Nursing
George Washington University
Washington, District of Columbia
(CHAPTER 17)

Deloras Jones, RN, MS
Former Executive Director
California Institute for Nursing and Health Care
Oakland, California
(CHAPTER 16)

Emily L. Jones, MA
Emerging Technologies Manager
Johns Hopkins University School of Nursing
Baltimore, Maryland
(CHAPTER 17)

Jennifer Lillibridge, PhD, RN
Emerita Professor
School of Nursing
California State University
Chico, California
(CHAPTER 20)

Kathy Malloch, PhD, MBA, RN, FAAN
President, KMLS, LLC
Professor of Practice
ASU College of Nursing and Health Innovation
Phoenix, Arizona
Clinical Professor
College of Nursing
Ohio State University
Columbus, Ohio
Clinical Consultant
API Healthcare Inc.
Hartford, Wisconsin
(CHAPTER 3)

Bernadette M. Melnyk, PhD, RN, CPNP/PMHNP, FNAP, FAAN
Associate Vice President for Health Promotion
University Chief Wellness Officer
Dean and Professor
College of Nursing
Professor of Pediatrics and Psychiatry
College of Medicine
Ohio State University
Columbus, Ohio
(CHAPTER 3)

Khadijah A. Mitchell, PhD, MS
CRTA Postdoctoral Fellow
National Cancer Institute
Center for Cancer Research
Laboratory of Human Carcinogenesis
Bethesda, Maryland
(CHAPTER 17)

Donna M. Nickitas, PhD, RN, NEA-BC, CNE
Professor
Hunter College and Executive Officer
The Graduate Center—City University of New York
New York, New York
(CHAPTER 25)

George C. Pittman, MSN
Assistant Professor
School of Nursing
California State University
Chico, California
(CHAPTER 18)

Suzanne S. Prevost, PhD, RN, FAAN
Dean
Capstone College of Nursing
The University of Alabama
Tuscaloosa, Alabama
(CHAPTER 2)

Keith Rischer, RN, MA, CEN, CCRN
Owner KeithRN, Author, Blogger, Critical Care Staff Nurse
Minneapolis, Minnesota
(CHAPTER 15)

Margaret J. Rowberg, DNP, APN
Certified Adult Nurse Practitioner
Director
School of Nursing
California State University
Chico, California
(CHAPTER 4)

Patricia E. Thompson, EdD, RN, FAAN
Chief Executive Officer
Honor Society of Nursing
Sigma Theta Tau International
Indianapolis, Indiana
(CHAPTER 26)

Cynthia Vlasich, MBA, BSN, RN
Director
Global Initiatives
Honor Society of Nursing
Sigma Theta Tau International
Indianapolis, Indiana
(CHAPTER 26)

Nikki West, MPH
Program Director
California Institute for Nursing and Health Care
Oakland, California
(CHAPTER 16)

Reviewers

Cathy H. Abell, PhD, MSN, MS, RN, CNE
Professor
Western Kentucky University
Bowling Green, Kentucky

Kathy Baton, PhD, RN-BC
Instructor
Hinds Community College
Jackson, Mississippi

Lorraine Bormann, PhD, RN, MHA, CPHQ, FACHE
Associate Professor
School of Nursing
Western Kentucky University
Bowling Green, Kentucky

Margaret A. Boyce, MSN, RN, MBA
Assistant Professor of Nursing
Mount Aloysius College
Cresson, Pennsylvania

Beryl K. Broughton, MSN, CRNP, CS, CNE
Instructor of Nursing
ARIA Health School of Nursing
Trevose, Pennsylvania

Michele Bunning, MSN, RN
Associate Professor
Good Samaritan College of Nursing and Health Science
Cincinnati, Ohio

Ruth A. Chaplen, DNP, RN, ACNS-BC, AOCN
Associate Professor
School of Nursing
Rochester College
Rochester Hills, Michigan

Betty B. Daniels, PhD, RN
Associate Professor
Brenau University
School of Nursing
Gainesville, Georgia

Marguerite DeBello, MSN, RN, ACNS-BC, CNE
Assistant Professor
Eastern Michigan University
Ypsilanti, Michigan

Cheryl Dover, DNP, MS, RN, NE-BC
Chair, Professor
Department of Nursing
Prince George's Community College
Largo, Maryland

Kathleen Ducey, MS, APRN-CNS
RN-BSN Program Director and Associate Professor of Nursing
University of Saint Mary
Leavenworth, Kansas

Lori A. Edwards, DrPH, MPH, RN, APHN
Assistant Professor
University of Maryland School of Nursing
Baltimore, Maryland

Shondell Hickson, DNP, APN, ACNS-BC, FNP-BC
Associate Professor
School of Nursing
Austin Peay State University
Clarksville, Tennessee

Tara J. Latto, MS, RN
Nursing Instructor
Morton College
Cicero, Illinois

Rosemary Macy, PhD, RN, CNE, CHSE
Associate Professor
Boise State University
Boise, Idaho

Nancy Overstreet, DNP, GNP-BC, CWOCN, CDP
Director of the Master of Science in Nursing (MSN) Program
Assistant Professor of Nursing
Lynchburg College
Lynchburg, Virginia

Ida L. Slusher, RN, PhD, CNE
Professor, Baccalaureate & Graduate Nursing
Eastern Kentucky University
Richmond, Kentucky

Susan Smith, MSN, PCPNP-BC
Assistant Professor
The University of Oklahoma College of Nursing
Oklahoma City, Oklahoma

Tamara L. Zurakowski, PhD, GNP-BC
Adjunct Associate Professor
University of Pennsylvania
Philadelphia, Pennsylvania

Preface

As a nursing educator for almost 35 years, I have taught many courses dealing with the significant issues that impact the nursing profession. I often felt frustrated that textbooks that were supposed to be devoted to professional issues in the field instead deviated significantly into other areas including nursing research and theory. In addition, while many of the existing professional issues books dealt with the enduring issues of the profession, it was difficult to find a book for my students that incorporated those with the "hot topics" of the time.

The first three editions of *Professional Issues in Nursing: Challenges & Opportunities* were efforts to address both of these needs. The fourth edition maintains this precedent with content updates, the deletion of two chapters and the addition of four new chapters. In addition, the implications of health care reform and the Institute of Medicine (IOM) recommendations noted in *The Future of Nursing: Leading Change, Advancing Health* influenced this edition greatly.

This book continues, however, to be first and foremost a professional issues book. While an effort has been made to integrate research and theory into chapters where it seemed appropriate, these topics in and of themselves are too broad to be fully addressed in a professional issues book. This book is also directed at what I and my expert nursing colleagues have identified as both enduring professional issues and the most pressing contemporary issues facing the profession. It is my hope, then, that this book fills an unmet need in the current professional issues text market. It has an undiluted focus on professional issues in nursing and includes many timely issues not addressed in other professional issues texts. This is an edited book, 13 of whose chapters have been contributed by the primary author, and the remaining 13 chapters by guest contributors with expertise in the specific subject material.

This book has been designed for use at both the baccalaureate and the graduate levels. It is envisioned that this book will be used as a primary textbook or as a supplement for a typical two- to three-unit professional issues course. It would also be appropriate for most RN–BSN bridge courses and may be considered by some faculty as a supplemental reader to a leadership/management course that includes professional issues.

The book can be used in both the traditional classroom and in online courses because the discussion question format works well for both small and large groups onsite as well as in bulletin board and chat room venues.

ORGANIZATION AND FEATURES

The book is divided into six units, representing contemporary and enduring issues in professional nursing. The six sections include Furthering the Profession, Workforce Issues, Workplace Issues, Nursing Education Issues, Legal and Ethical Issues, and Professional Power. Each unit has four to five chapters.

Features

Each chapter begins with **Learning Objectives** and an overview of the professional issue being discussed. Multiple perspectives on each issue are then identified in an effort to reflect the diversity of thought found in the literature as well as espoused by experts in the field and varied professional nursing and health care organizations. **Discussion Points** encourage readers to pause and reflect on specific questions (individually or in groups), and **Consider This** features encourage active learning, critical thinking, and values clarification by the users. In addition, at least one research study is profiled in every chapter in **Research Study Fuels the Controversy**, an effort to promote evidence-based analysis of the issue. Each chapter ends with **Conclusions** about the issues discussed, questions **For Additional Discussion**, and a comprehensive and current reference list. Also included in each chapter are multiple displays, boxes, and tables to help the user visualize important concepts.

NEW TO THIS EDITION

- Chapters on the use of social media in nursing, teaching clinical reasoning, MOOCs and virtual learning spaces, and academic integrity in nursing education.

- New or updated content has been added throughout the book to reflect cutting-edge trends in health care and nursing education including an ever-increasing demand for quality and safety in the workplace for patients as well as workers; workforce projections and changing population demographics; the impact of health care reform; the IOM recommendations put forth in *The Future of Nursing: Leading Change, Advancing Health;* changing nursing education paradigms and increasingly virtual learning environments; and the challenges and opportunities that accompany the provision of nursing care and nursing education in an increasingly global, rapidly changing, technology-driven world.

TEACHING/LEARNING RESOURCES

Professional Issues in Nursing: Challenges and Opportunities, fourth edition, includes additional resources for both instructors and students that are available on the book's companion website at http://thePoint.lww.com/Huston4e.

Instructor Resources

Approved adopting instructors will be given access to the following additional resources:

- Test Generator containing NCLEX-style questions
- PowerPoint Presentations
- Journal Articles
- Answers to Journal Articles Critical Thinking Questions
- Case Studies with Answers
- Internet Resources

Student Resources

Students who have purchased *Professional Issues in Nursing: Challenges and Opportunities*, fourth edition, have access to the following additional resources:

- Case Studies
- Journal Articles with Critical Thinking Questions
- Spanish—English Audio Glossary
- Learning Objectives

In addition, purchasers of the text can access the searchable full text online by going to the *Professional Issues in Nursing: Challenges and Opportunities*, fourth edition, website at http://thePoint.lww.com/Huston4e. See inside the front cover of this text for more details, including the passcode you will need to gain access to the website.

Carol J. Huston, RN, MSN, MPA, DPA, FAAN

Contents

1

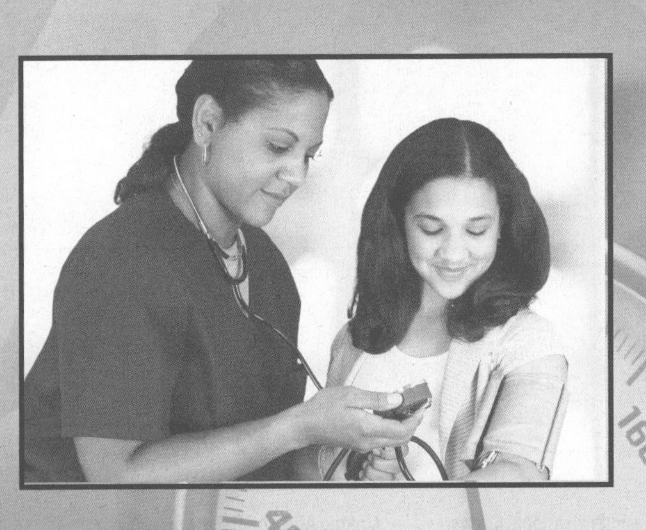

Furthering the Profession

Entry Into Practice
The Debate Rages On

Carol J. Huston

1

ADDITIONAL RESOURCES

Visit thePoint for additional helpful resources
- eBook
- Journal Articles
- WebLinks

CHAPTER OUTLINE

Proliferation of ADN Education
Licensure and Entry Into Practice
Educational Levels and Patient Outcomes
Employers' Views and Preferences
Shifting Health Care Delivery Sites and Required Competencies
Entry Level and Professional Status
The 2-Year ADN Program?
Shortages and Entry-Level Requirements
Professional Organizations, Unions, and Advisory Bodies Speak Out
Grandfathering Entry Levels
Linking ADN and BSN Programs
An International Issue
Conclusions

LEARNING OBJECTIVES

The learner will be able to:

1. Differentiate between technical and professional nurses as outlined in Esther Lucille Brown's classic *Nursing for the Future.*
2. Identify what if any progress has been made on increasing the educational entry level for professional registered nursing since publication of the 1965 position paper of the American Nurses Association on entry into practice.
3. Identify similarities and differences between contemporary associate and baccalaureate degree nursing programs.
4. Describe basic components of associate degree educational programs as outlined by Mildred Montag and compare those with typical associate degree programs in the 21st century.
5. Analyze how having one NCLEX for entry into practice, regardless of educational entry level, impacts the entry-into-practice dilemma.
6. Identify key driving and restraining forces for increasing the educational entry level for professional nursing.
7. Analyze the potential impacts of raising the educational entry level on the current nursing shortage, workforce diversity, and intraprofessional conflict.
8. Examine current research that explores the impact of registered nurse educational level on patient outcomes.
9. Explore how shifting health care delivery sites and increasing registered nursing competency

(continues on page 3)

requirements are impacting employer preferences for hiring a more educated nursing workforce.

10. Compare the nursing profession's educational entry standards with that of the other health care professions.
11. Identify positions taken by specific professional organizations, certifying bodies, and employers regarding the appropriate educational level for entry into practice for professional nursing.
12. Explore personal values, beliefs, and feelings regarding whether the educational entry level in nursing should be increased to a baccalaureate or higher degree.

Few issues have been as long-standing or as contentious in nursing as the entry-into-practice debate. Although the entry-into-practice debate dates back to the 1940s with the publication of Esther Lucille Brown's classic *Nursing for the Future*, the debate came to the forefront with a 1965 position paper by the American Nurses Association (ANA, 1965a, 1965b). This position paper suggested an orderly transition from hospital-based diploma nursing preparation to nursing education in colleges or universities based on the following premises:

- The education of all those who are licensed to practice nursing should take place in institutions of higher education.
- Minimum preparation for beginning professional nursing practice should be baccalaureate education in nursing.
- Minimum preparation for beginning technical practice should be associate degree education in nursing.
- Education for assistants in the health care occupations should be short, intensive, preservice programs in vocational education institutions rather than on-the-job training programs.

In essence, two levels of preparation were suggested for registered nurses (RNs): *technical* and *professional*. Persons interested in technical practice would enroll in junior or community colleges and earn associate degrees in 2-year programs. Those interested in professional nursing would enroll in 4-year programs in colleges or universities. Hospital-based diploma programs were to be phased out.

The curriculums for the two programs were to be very different, as were each program's foci. The 2-year technical degree was to result in an associate degree in nursing (ADN). This degree, as proposed by Mildred Montag (Fig. 1.1) in her dissertation in 1952, with direction and support from R. Louise McManus, would prepare a beginning, technical practitioner who would provide care in acute-care settings, under the supervision of a professional nurse.

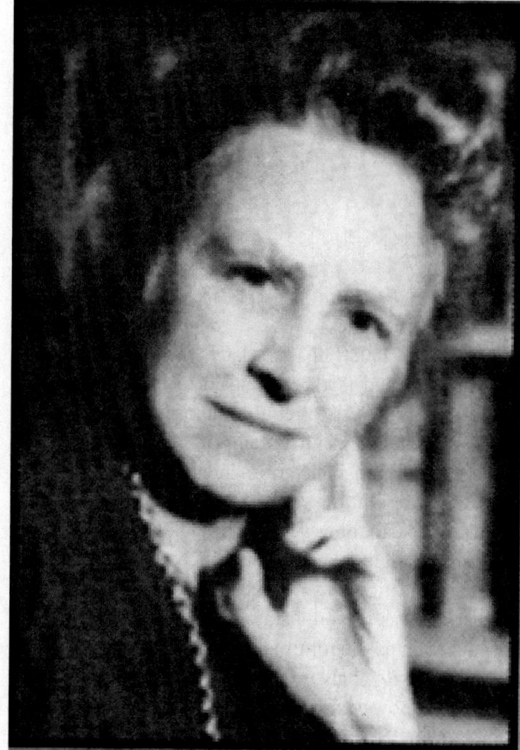

Figure 1.1 Mildred Montag.

In a typical associate degree program, approximately half of the credits would be fulfilled by general education courses such as English, anatomy, physiology, speech, psychology, and sociology and the other half were fulfilled by nursing courses. The 4-year degree would result in a bachelor of science in nursing (BSN) and would encompass coursework taught in ADN programs as well as more in-depth treatment of the physical and social sciences, nursing research, public and community health, nursing management, and the humanities. The additional course work in the BSN was intended to enhance the students' professional development, prepare them for a broader scope of practice, and provide a better understanding of the cultural, political, economic, and social issues affecting patients and health care delivery.

The ANA 1965 position statement was reaffirmed by a resolution at the ANA House of Delegates in 1978, which set forth the requirement that the baccalaureate degree would be the entry level into professional nursing practice by 1985. Associate degree and diploma programs responded strongly to what they viewed as inflammatory terminology and clearly stated that not being considered "professional" was unacceptable. In the end, both ADN and diploma programs refused to compromise title or licensure. Dissension ensued both within and among nursing groups, but little movement occurred to make the position statement a reality.

Consider This Titling (professional vs. technical) was and will be an important consideration before consensus can be reached on the entry-into-practice debate.

Finally, in 2008, 30 years later, the ANA House of Delegates stepped forth once again to pass a resolution supporting initiatives to require diploma- and associate-degree-educated nurses to obtain a BSN within 10 years of license. The responsibility for mandating and implementing this new resolution was passed on to individual states.

Just one state, however, North Dakota, became successful in changing the Nurse Practice Act so that baccalaureate education was necessary for RN licensure. For 15 years, it was the only state to recognize baccalaureate education as the minimal education for professional nursing, despite challenges from opposing groups. Unfortunately, however, North Dakota repealed this act in 2003, bowing to pressure from nurses and some health care organizations, to once again allowing nonbaccalaureate entry into practice.

Other states, however, continue to consider increasing educational entry levels. California, for example, requires a BSN for certification as a public health nurse in that state, and multiple states require a BSN to be a school nurse because that is considered to be a part of public health nursing. In addition, state nursing associations or other nursing coalitions in California, New York, Rhode Island, and New Jersey have, over the past few years, called for initiatives to establish the BSN as the entry level for nursing in their respective state. Other states are pursuing some type of initiative requiring newly graduated RNs to obtain a BSN within a certain time frame in order to maintain their licensure.

The result is that more than 50 years after the initial ANA resolution, entry into practice at the baccalaureate level has not been accomplished. Even the strongest supporters of the BSN for entry into practice cannot deny that, despite almost six decades of efforts, RN entry at the baccalaureate level continues to be an elusive goal.

PROLIFERATION OF ADN EDUCATION

It is doubtful that Mildred Montag had any idea in 1952 that ADN programs would someday become the predominant entry level for nursing practice or that this education model would proliferate like it did in the 1960s—just one decade after she completed her doctoral work. While the overwhelming majority of nurses in the early 1960s were educated in diploma schools of nursing, enrollment in baccalaureate programs was increasing and associate degree programs were just beginning. By the year 2000, diploma education had virtually disappeared, and although BSN education had increased significantly, it was ADN education, which represented nearly two thirds of all nursing school graduates.

Indeed, ADN education continues to be the primary model for initial nursing education in the United States today. As of 2010, 45.4% of nurses initially graduated from associate degree programs, followed by baccalaureate programs (33.7%), and then diploma programs (20.44%) (Health Resources and Services Administration, 2010).

Yet, enrollment in baccalaureate nursing programs is also on the rise with 15 consecutive years of enrollment growth. The American Association of Colleges of Nursing (AACN, 2014a) states that as of 2013, somewhere between 55% and 63% of the RN workforce holds a baccalaureate or graduate degree.

LICENSURE AND ENTRY INTO PRACTICE

Critics of BSN as a requirement for entry into practice argue that there is no need to raise entry levels because passing rates for the National Council Licensure Examination (NCLEX) show only small differences between ADN, diploma, and BSN graduates (Table 1.1). Although some might argue that this suggests similar competencies across the educational spectrum, the more common precept is that the NCLEX is a test that measures minimum technical competencies for safe entry into basic nursing practice and, as such, may not measure performance over time or test for all of the knowledge and skills developed through a BSN program. One must also ask why the nursing profession has not differentiated

TABLE 1.1 2014 NCLEX-RN Passage Rate per Educational Program Type

Program Type	Number of Graduates	NCLEX-RN Passage Rate (%)
Diploma	2,500	84.24
Associate degree	78,176	80.71
Baccalaureate degree	62,316	85.52

Source: National Council of State Boards of Nursing. (2015). *2014: Number of candidates taking NCLEX examination and percent passing, by type of candidate.* Retrieved January 20, 2015, from https://www.ncsbn.org/Table_of_Pass_Rates_2014.pdf

RN licensure testing based on educational preparation for RNs, just as has been done for practical nurses, RNs, and advanced practice nurses.

Discussion Point

Should separate licensing examinations be developed for ADN-, diploma-, and BSN-educated nurses?

Complicating the picture is that both ADN and BSN schools preparing graduates for RN licensure meet similar criteria for state board approval and have roughly the same number of nursing coursework units. All of these factors contribute to confusion about differentiations between ADN- and BSN-prepared nurses and result in an inability to move forward on implementing the BSN as the entry level for professional nursing.

Consider This Critics of BSN entry into practice argue that ADN-, diploma-, and BSN-educated nurses all take the same licensing examination and therefore have earned the title of RN. In addition, nurses prepared at all three levels have successfully worked side by side, under the same scope of practice, for more than 50 years.

Research also suggests that there are differences in the demographics of BSN and ADN graduates with BSN nurses being younger as a cohort than their ADN counterparts. It is also generally believed that ADN graduates represent greater diversity in race, gender, age, and educational experiences than BSN-prepared nurses. Critics of the BSN requirement for entry into professional nursing suggest that greater diversity is needed in nursing, and this may be lost if entry levels are raised. Indeed, recent research by Sabio (2014) supports this concern, suggesting that 37% of ADN students would not have enrolled in a BSN program if the BSN had been the only option for professional nursing practice and up to 89% would not have enrolled in the ADN program. Situational barriers such as the costs of BSN education and home and job responsibilities were of most concern among respondents.

In addition, many employers state that they are unable to differentiate roles for nurses based on education because both ADN- and BSN-prepared nurses hold the same license. Ironically, state boards of nursing have asserted their inability to develop a different licensure system given the fact that employers have not developed different roles.

Furthermore, many employers provide no incentives for BSN education in terms of pay, recognition, or career mobility and are afraid to do so, fearing they may be unable to fill vacant nursing positions. The starting rate of pay for ADN- and BSN-prepared nurses historically has not been significantly different, although this appears to be changing.

Finally, some impassioned supporters of maintaining ADN education as the entry level for nursing practice argue that associate degrees allow students to graduate in a shorter amount of time so that they can support their family and that the cost of baccalaureate education would be cost or time prohibitive to many working students with families (Moltz, 2010).

Discussion Point

Should licensure be equated with professional status?

EDUCATIONAL LEVELS AND PATIENT OUTCOMES

Perhaps the most common argument against raising the entry level in nursing is an emotional one, with ADN-prepared nurses arguing that "caring does not require a baccalaureate degree." Many ADN-educated nurses argue passionately that patients do not know or care what educational degree is held by their nurse as long as they receive high-quality care by the nurse at their bedside. ADN nurses also frequently claim that BSN-prepared nurses are too theoretically oriented and thus are not in touch with real practice. In addition, many ADN nurses suggest that baccalaureate-prepared nurses are deficient in basic skills mastery and conclude that care provided by ADN nurses is at least as good as, if not better than, that provided by their BSN counterparts.

Consider This Most ADN-prepared nurses argue that significant differences exist between their practice and that of a licensed vocational/practical nurse (LVN/LPN), despite there typically being only 12 months' difference in length of educational preparation. Yet, many ADN-educated nurses argue that the additional education that BSN-educated nurses have makes little difference in their practice over that of their ADN counterparts. How can this argument be justified?

An increasing number of studies, however, report differences between the performance levels of ADN- and BSN-prepared nurses. In a landmark 2003 study, Aiken, Clarke, Cheung, Sloane, and Silber at the University of Pennsylvania identified a clear link between higher levels of nursing education and better patient outcomes (AACN, 2014b). This study found that surgical patients have a "substantial survival advantage" if treated in hospitals with higher proportions of nurses educated at the baccalaureate or higher degree level and that a 10% increase in the proportion of nurses holding BSN degrees decreased the risk of patient death and failure to rescue by 5% (AACN, 2014b).

Research by Aiken and colleagues also showed that hospitals with better care environments, the best nurse staffing levels, and the most highly educated nurses had the lowest surgical mortality rates. In fact, the researchers found that every 10% increase in the proportion of BSN nurses on the hospital staff was associated with a 4% decrease in the risk of death (Aiken, Clarke, Sloane, Lake, & Cheney, 2008); see Research Study Fuels the Controversy 1.1.

A more recent study by Yakusheva, Lindrooth, and Weiss (2014) of 8,526 adult medical-surgical patients found similar results with BSN education being associated with lower mortality ($p < 0.01$), lower odds of readmission ($p = 0.04$), and 1.9% shorter length of stay ($p = 0.03$). Economic simulations supported a strong business case for increasing the proportion of BSN-educated nurses in the workforce.

Another recent study by Kutney-Lee and colleagues found that a 10-point increase in the percentage of nurses holding a BSN within a hospital was associated with an average reduction of 2.12 deaths for every 1,000 patients—and for a subset of patients with complications, an average reduction of 7.47 deaths per 1,000 patients (AACN, 2014b). Similarly, Blegen, Goode, Park, Vaughn, and Spetz published findings in 2013 from a cross-sectional study of 21 University Health System Consortium hospitals to analyze the association between RN education and patient outcomes. The researchers found that hospitals with a higher percentage of RNs with baccalaureate or higher degrees had lower congestive heart failure mortality, decubitus ulcers, failure to rescue, and postoperative deep vein thrombosis or pulmonary embolism and shorter length of stay (AACN, 2014b).

Research Study Fuels the Controversy 1.1

Effect of Education on Patient Outcomes

Data from 10,184 nurses and 232,342 surgical patients in 168 Pennsylvania hospitals provided stinging evidence that educational entry level makes a difference in patient outcomes.

Source: Aiken, L., Clarke, S. P., Sloane, D. M., Lake, E. T., & Cheney, T. (2008). Effects of hospital care environment on patient mortality and nurse outcomes. *Journal of Nursing Administration, 38*(5), 223–229.

Study Findings

This study found that patients experienced significantly lower mortality and failure to rescue rates in hospitals where more highly educated nurses were providing direct patient care. Nurses reported more positive job experiences and fewer concerns with care quality, and patients had significantly lower risks of death and failure to rescue in hospitals with better care environments.

As more outcome research becomes available suggesting an empirical link between educational entry level of nurses and patient outcomes, nursing leaders, professional associations, and employers are increasingly speaking out on the need to raise the profession's entry level as a means of improving quality patient care and patient safety. Patricia Benner, director of a recent landmark Carnegie study on nursing, professor emerita at the University of California at San Francisco School of Nursing, and a former graduate of an ADN program, concurs, asserting that "I'm not against community college nursing programs, and this is not a diatribe against community colleges. But something is out of whack when students get a degree that doesn't allow them to go on to advanced practice. It's just not adequate to meet current demands" (Moltz, 2010, para. 6).

EMPLOYERS' VIEWS AND PREFERENCES

Nursing employers are still somewhat divided on the issue of entry into practice. The academic requirements of associate degree, diploma, and baccalaureate programs vary widely, yet health care settings that employ nursing graduates often make no distinction in the scope of practice among nurses who have different levels of preparation.

Employers, however, appear to be increasingly aware of purported differences between BSN and ADN graduates, and this is increasingly being reflected in their hiring preferences. A recent study found that 39% of hospitals across the country required new hires to have a bachelor's degree, up 9 percentage points from the year before (Delgado, 2013). Similarly, AACN reported that 59% of new BSN graduates had jobs at the time of graduation, compared to the national average across all professions of 29.3% and that 89% of new BSN graduates had secured employment in nursing within 4 to 6 months after graduation (New AACN Data, 2014). "One reason is the Magnet Recognition Program, a prestigious designation for hospitals that recognizes quality nursing. One of the chief requirements is that nurse managers and leaders have at least a baccalaureate in nursing" (Delgado, 2013, para. 20). Magnet hospitals are also required to have a higher percentage of nurses educated at the baccalaureate level.

In addition, some employers are now giving preference for clinical placements to students in baccalaureate and higher degree programs over those enrolled in associate degree programs.

Indeed, LaRocco (2014) suggests that

> *while state boards of nursing and legislatures fail to act to change the entry requirements for professional nursing, in many areas of the country the baccalaureate is becoming the de facto requirement. Major medical centers in the Boston area no longer hire nurses with associate's degrees. At least one large, for-profit hospital chain has decreed that their nurses must obtain a baccalaureate within a stipulated period of time, typically 3 to 5 years. Nurses with associate's degrees are limited in both their initial employment and their long-term options.* (p. 11)

Discussion Point

If indeed employers prefer hiring BSN-prepared RNs, why don't more employers offer pay differentials for nurses with BSN degrees?

The Veterans Administration (VA), with its 35,000 nurses on staff, is leading the nation in raising the bar for a higher educational entry hire level in nursing. The VA established the BSN as the minimum education level for new hires and as the minimum preparation its nurses must have for promotion beyond the entry level (AACN, 2014b).

SHIFTING HEALTH CARE DELIVERY SITES AND REQUIRED COMPETENCIES

Although hospitals continue to be the main site of employment for nurses, there is an ongoing shift in health care from acute-care settings to the community and integrated health care settings. This shift will clearly require more highly educated nurses who can function autonomously as caregivers, leaders, managers, and change agents. These are all skills that are emphasized in a baccalaureate nursing curriculum.

Consider This Baccalaureate and graduate-level skills in research, leadership, management, and community health are increasingly needed in nursing as health care extends beyond the acute-care hospital.

In May 2010, the Tri-Council for Nursing, a coalition of four steering organizations for the nursing profession (AACN, ANA, the American Organization of

Nurse Executives [AONE], and the National League for Nursing [NLN]), issued a consensus statement calling for all RNs to advance their education in the interest of enhancing quality and safety across health care settings. The statement suggested that a more highly educated nursing workforce will be critical to meeting the nation's nursing needs and delivering safe, effective patient care and that failure to do so will place the nation's health at further risk (AACN, 2014a).

The recommendations of the IOM (2010) report, *The Future of Nursing*, were even stronger. This landmark report called for increasing the number of baccalaureate-prepared nurses in the workforce from 50% to 80% over the next 10 years and doubling the population of nurses with doctorates to meet the demands of an evolving health care system and changing patient needs.

In addition, in December 2009, Patricia Benner and her team at the Carnegie Foundation for the Advancement of Teaching released a new study titled *Educating Nurses: A Call for Radical Transformation*, which recommended preparing all entry-level RNs at the baccalaureate level and requiring all RNs to earn a master's degree within 10 years of initial licensure (Benner, Sutphen, Leonard, & Day, 2010). The authors found that many of today's new nurses are "undereducated" to meet practice demands across settings. Their strong support for high-quality baccalaureate degree programs as the appropriate pathway for RNs entering the profession is consistent with the views of many leading nursing organizations, including AACN (AACN, 2014b).

Similarly, the National Advisory Council on Nurse Education and Practice (NACNEP) suggests that nursing's role for the future calls for RNs to manage care along a continuum, to work as peers in interdisciplinary teams, and to integrate clinical expertise with knowledge of community resources. This increased complexity of scope of practice will require the capacity to adapt to change; critical thinking and problem-solving skills; a social foundation in a broad range of basic sciences; knowledge of behavioral, social, and management sciences; and the ability to analyze and communicate data (AACN, 2014b). All these are integral components of BSN education. As a result, NACNEP has recommended to Congress that at least two thirds of the nurse workforce hold baccalaureate or higher degrees in nursing (AACN, 2014a,b).

The Council on Physician and Nurse Supply also released a statement in 2007 calling for a national effort to substantially expand baccalaureate nursing programs, citing the growing body of evidence that nursing education impacts both the quality and safety of patient care. Consequently, the group is calling on policy makers to shift federal funding priorities in favor of supporting more baccalaureate-level nursing programs (AACN, 2014b). Some nurse leaders have even suggested that a BSN degree may not be an adequate preparation for these expanded roles and that, instead, master's or doctoral degrees should be required for entry into practice for registered nursing.

Discussion Point

Would raising the entry level to the master's or doctoral degree eliminate the tension between supporters of ADN and BSN as entry levels into nursing, since both educational preparations would be considered inadequate? Is a graduate degree currently feasible as the entry level for professional nursing? If not, what would it take to make it happen?

ENTRY LEVEL AND PROFESSIONAL STATUS

Nurses, consumers, and allied health care professionals are currently questioning why the entry level into professional nursing is so much lower than other health care professions. Does nursing require less skill? Is the knowledge base needed to provide nursing care skill based instead of knowledge based? Should nursing be reclassified as a vocational trade and not a profession? The answer to these questions, of course, is no. Yet clearly, nurses have resisted the normal course of occupational development that other health care professions have pursued. As a result, nurses are now the least educated of the health care professionals, with most health care professions now requiring graduate degrees for entry. Indeed, one must question whether nursing is at risk for losing its designation as a profession because of its failure to maintain educational equity.

Discussion Point

Is nursing in danger of losing its designation as a "profession" if it fails to maintain educational entry levels comparable to those of the other health professions?

The primary identity of any professional group is based on the established education entry level. Attorneys, physicians, social workers, engineers, clergy, and physical therapists, to list a few examples, have in common an essential education at the bachelor's level. Nursing is unique among the health care professions in having multiple educational pathways lead to the same entry level license to practice. In fact, advanced degrees are required in many professions for entry positions at the professional level. Only nursing continues the hypocrisy of pretending that education is unimportant and does not make a difference. Only nursing allows individuals with no college course work, or with limited college study that lacks a well-rounded global college education, to lay claim to the same licensure and identity as that held by nurses having a baccalaureate education.

Indeed, the educational gap between nursing and other health professions continues to grow (Table 1.2). Disciplines such as occupational therapy, physical therapy, speech therapy, and social work all require master's or doctoral degrees. Pharmacy has also raised its educational standards to that of a doctoral degree.

> **Consider This** Unlike the other health care professions which now require master's and doctoral degrees, nursing continues to put forth an argument that educational degree does not matter or that requiring a BSN for entry into practice is elitist.

Failure to maintain educational parity with other health care professions also contributes to nursing being viewed as a "second-class citizen" in the health care arena. It is difficult to justify the profession's argument that nursing should be an equal partner in health care decision making when other professions are so much better educated, suggesting that nurses are either undereducated for the roles they assume or that the nursing role lacks complexity.

> **Consider This** Nursing is the only health care "profession" that does not require at least a bachelor's or higher degree for entry into practice.

Lavizzo-Mourey (2012), a physician as well as President and CEO of the Robert Wood Johnson Foundation, suggests that for nurses to ensure that they maximize their contributions to health and health care, they will need advanced skills and expertise in care management, interdisciplinary teamwork, problem solving, and more... making higher education imperative.

THE 2-YEAR ADN PROGRAM?

Many ADN-prepared nurses also express frustration when discussing the need to raise the entry level in professional nursing because they feel the ADN degree does not appropriately represent the scope of their education or the time they had to put in to earn what is typically considered to be a 2-year degree. ADN nurses argue that the "2-year" ADN program is a myth. Many ADN students follow nontraditional education paths, and almost all ADN programs currently require 3 or more years of education, not 2, with a minimum of 12 to 24 months of prerequisites and a full 2 years of nursing education. Most associate's degrees require approximately 60 semester units or 90 quarter units of coursework although there is a great deal of variance with some programs now requiring more than 70 semester units and over 100 quarter units.

> **Consider This** The 2-year ADN program is a myth.

Indeed, it is almost impossible to graduate from an ADN program in less than 3 years and often 4 or more years are required to complete the general education,

TABLE 1.2 Entry-Level Degrees for the Health Professions

Health Profession	Entry-Level Degree
Medicine	Doctorate
Pharmacy	Doctorate
Social work	Master's
Speech pathology	Master's
Physical therapy	Master's transitioning to doctorate
Occupational therapy	Master's
Nursing	Associate

prerequisite, and nursing requirements. Given that most BSN programs require approximately 120 semester units for graduation, the question must be asked whether requiring so many units at the associate degree level, without granting the upper division credit that could lead to a BSN degree, is an injustice to ADN graduates. Patricia Benner goes so far as to suggest that "if the baccalaureate were made the minimum requirement for entrance into the field, then community college programs would at least have to be more honest about how much time it takes students to get through their programs and how much opportunity cost is there for them" (Moltz, 2010, para. 4).

This addition of units and extension of educational time in ADN programs has generally been attributed to the need to respond to a changing job market; that is, the need to prepare ADNs to work in more diverse environments (nonhospital) and to increasingly assume positions requiring management skills. While Montag clearly intended a differentiation between level of education and level of practice between ADN- and BSN-prepared nurses, many ADN programs have added leadership, management, research, and home health and community health courses to their curriculums in the past two decades.

One must ask then what part of the associate degree curriculum should be cut to add these new experiences. What should the balance be between community and acute-care experiences in ADN programs? How much management content do ADN nurses need and what roles will they be expected to assume? If no content is deleted from the ADN programs to accommodate the new content, how can ADN education reasonably be completed within a 2-year framework?

Montag expressed concern that when ADN programs add content inappropriate for technical practice, appropriate content may have to be deleted to maintain the estimated time for completion. The question that follows then is, If ADN education now incorporates much of what was meant to be BSN content, and if the time needed to complete this education is near that of a bachelor's degree, why are ADN graduates being given associate degrees, which reflect expertise in technical practice, rather than BSN degrees, which reflect achievement of these higher-level competencies?

SHORTAGES AND ENTRY-LEVEL REQUIREMENTS

Whenever there are shortages, legislators and workforce experts suggest a need to reexamine or reduce educational requirements. Indeed, Montag's original project to create ADN education was directed at reducing the workforce shortage of nurses that existed at that time, by reducing the length of the education process to 2 years. Clearly, the immediate short-term threat of raising the entry level to the bachelor's degree may be to exacerbate predicted nursing shortages. Tollick (2013) argues, however, that despite the number of associate degree programs and the numbers of graduates they produce, nursing continually cycles through shortages and in all likelihood will continue to do so.

In addition, raising the entry level may in the long run elevate the public image of nursing and increase recruitment to the field since the best and the brightest may seek professions with greater academic prestige. Raising the entry level may also impact retention rates in nursing. Having more BSN nurses may actually then stabilize the nursing workforce as a result of their higher levels of job satisfaction, a key to nurse retention.

Consider This The impact of raising the entry level in nursing to the baccalaureate level on the current nursing shortage is not known.

The other reality is that a chronic shortage of nursing personnel has persisted despite the proliferation of ADN programs. This negates the argument that the current nursing shortage should be used as an excuse for postponing action to raise educational standards. A nursing shortage existed at the time of the 1965 ANA proposal and has occurred intermittently since that time. Clearly, nursing has been swept along by a host of social, economic, and educational circumstances that have little to do with nursing or the clients we serve. Perhaps, then, the decision to raise the entry-to-practice level in nursing should be made because it is the right and necessary thing to do and not as a result of the influence of external communities of interest.

Consider This Nurses, professional health care and nursing organizations, credentialing programs, and employers are divided on the entry-into-practice issue.

Debate over entry into practice is as varied among professional health care and nursing organizations, credentialing programs, and employers as it is among individual nurses. Getting support for the BSN as the entry-level requirement for nursing will be difficult because the overwhelming majority of nurses are currently ADN prepared and there are inadequate workplace incentives to increase entry requirements to the BSN degree.

PROFESSIONAL ORGANIZATIONS, UNIONS, AND ADVISORY BODIES SPEAK OUT

Not surprisingly, a 2006 position statement issued by the National Organization for Associate Degree Nursing (NOADN) on entry into practice reaffirmed the role and value of associate degree nursing education and practice. The position statement suggested that ADN graduates were essential members of the interdisciplinary health care team, that these nurses were prepared to function in diverse health care settings, and that associate degree education provided a dynamic pathway for entry into professional RN practice. A follow-up position statement issued by the NOADN in 2008 suggested that a BSN should not be required for continued practice beyond initial licensure as an RN and that the choice to pursue further education should remain the choice of each ADN graduate based on his or her personal preferences and professional career goals.

Similarly, the position of the NLN, the national voice for nurse educators in all types of nursing education programs, historically was that the nursing profession should have multiple entry points. As such, the NLN suggested that instead of investing energy debating entry into the profession, the focus should turn toward opportunities for lifelong learning and progression for those who enter the nursing profession through diploma and associate degree programs.

More recently, however, NOADN partnered with the American Association of Community Colleges, the Association of Community College Trustees, AACN, and NLN to author a joint statement acknowledging their full support for the academic progression of every nursing student and nurse. This statement was endorsed by the ANA in January 2014 ("Joint Statement," n.d.). The joint statement suggests that it is only through the collaboration and partnering of organizations that a seamless academic progression of students and nurses will occur.

In addition, the Nurse Alliance of the Service Employees International Union (SEIU) Healthcare, an organization of more than 85,000 RNs, has firmly rejected any bill that would limit entry into or maintenance of practice to the BSN, arguing that this would only exacerbate the current nursing shortage (SEIU, 2014). Instead, they argue that more resources must be made available to support nursing education at all levels, to give academic credit for work experience, to provide workplace support for nurses who wish to return to school, and to develop more online and hybrid programs for nurses who cannot attend traditional on-site classes to advance their education.

An increasing number of professional nursing organizations, however, are now supporting the BSN requirement for entry into professional nursing. The ANA, however, is no longer the standard bearer in this effort. Instead, organizations such as the AACN, the National Association of Neonatal Nurses (NANN), the American Nephrology Nurses' Association, the Association of Operating Room Nurses (AORN), and the AONE have published position statements supporting BSN entry.

For example, the AACN suggests that the primary pathway for entry into professional-level nursing, as compared to technical-level practice, is a 4-year BSN. NANN issued its position statement in 2009, arguing that "the increasing acuity of patients and their more complex needs for care in community and home settings demand a higher level of educational preparation for nurses than was necessary in the past" (National Association of Neonatal Nurses, 2009, para. 1).

AORN has also supported the baccalaureate degree for entry into nursing since 1979. AORN's current position statement on entry into practice reaffirms its belief that there should be one level for entry into nursing practice and that the minimal preparation for future entry into the practice of nursing should be the baccalaureate degree (Association of Operating Room Nurses, 2011). In 2004, the AONE also published guiding principles suggesting that "the educational preparation of the nurse of the future should be at the baccalaureate level."

The National Advisory Council on Nurse Education and Practice (NACNEP), which advises the Secretary of the U.S. Department of Health and Human Services and the U.S. Congress on policy issues related to nurse workforce supply, education, and practice improvement, also urged in 2007 that a minimum of two thirds of working nurses hold baccalaureate or higher degrees in nursing by 2010 (AACN, 2014a). Yet, federal and state regulation of entry into practice has, for the most part, not occurred. In addition, the Tri-Council for Nursing (ANA, AONE, NLN, and AACN) issued a consensus statement in 2010 calling for all RNs to advance their education in the interest of patient safety and enhanced quality of care across all settings (Edwards, 2012).

Funding is also increasingly available to support these efforts. Nine state action coalitions received funding (Academic Progression in Nursing grants) in 2012 to further the IOM's goal of 80% BSN or higher workforce by 2020 (Making Progress Toward BSN Goal, 2013).

GRANDFATHERING ENTRY LEVELS

Traditionally, when a state licensure law is enacted, or when a current law is repealed and a new law enacted, a process called "grandfathering" occurs. Grandfathering allows individuals to continue to practice his or her profession or occupation despite new qualifications having been enacted into law. Should the entry-level requirement for nursing be raised to a bachelor's or higher degree, debate will undoubtedly occur as to how and when grandfathering should be applied.

> **Consider This** "Grandfathering" current ADN nurses as professional nurses would smooth political tensions between current educational entry levels but threaten the essence of the goal.

Several professional organizations have actively advocated that all RNs should be grandfathered if the entry level is raised. Other professional organizations have argued that it should not occur at all. Still others believe that grandfathering should be conditional. For example, all RNs licensed at the time of the law would be allowed to retain their current title for a certain time, but would be required to return to school to increase their educational preparation if it did not meet the new entry level.

LINKING ADN AND BSN PROGRAMS

Returning to school, unfortunately, is not part of the career path for many nurses, which makes the entry level even more important. Intimidation, cost, impact on family, and lack of clarity about the possible gains from additional education deter many nurses from returning to school. Still, only 25% of respondents in a recent study of nurses with less than a baccalaureate degree felt they were already adequately educated (Byrne, Mayo, & Rosner, 2014). Most felt that furthering their education would provide more career opportunities but that returning to school would not be a pleasant experience.

Indeed, there a number of internal and external motivators that encourage or discourage RNs from pursuing higher degrees. Incentives include career and professional advancement; gaining new knowledge; improving social welfare skills; and being a positive model for one's children (Kovner, Brewer, Katigbak, Djukic, & Fatehi, 2012). RNs also identify a desire to achieve personal and job satisfaction and professional achievement as important motivators. Nurses with graduate degrees are more likely to report being extremely satisfied with their jobs, compared with nurses who hold associate's degrees, who more frequently report moderate to extreme dissatisfaction with their jobs.

Yet, research by Byrne et al. (2014) revealed that while 50% of the respondents in their study intended to return to school in the next 12 months, many had a fear of failure. Respondents suggested that more nurses would return to school if their colleagues did and that having the support of a significant person was important in both their decision to return to school and their retention. In addition, positive talk by nurse leaders and educators regarding the importance and value of advancing their education by earning a BSN is often critical to a nurse's decision to return to school. Tuition reimbursement, flexible work hours, and pay for attending classes are also powerful employer-based motivators.

Unfortunately, Haverkamp and Ball (2013) in their survey of members of AORN of central Ohio found that participants stated they valued higher education but were unaware of the need for more BSN nurses and stated they were unaware of the professional and financial effects of obtaining a baccalaureate degree or the resources available to help them earn one. They also suggested that they were relatively unaware of collaborative nursing association partnerships to advocate for higher educational entry-level legislation, suggesting a need for broader communication to RNs about the need for advancing educational entry levels in nursing (Research Study Fuels the Controversy 1.2).

Currently, more than 690 RN-to-BSN programs nationally build on the education provided in diploma and ADN programs, including more than 400 programs that are offered at least partially online (AACN, 2014a). In addition, 400 RN-to-master's degree programs are available, which cover the baccalaureate content missing in the other entry-level programs as well as graduate-level course work (AACN, 2014a). In addition, statewide articulation agreements exist in many states, including Florida, California, Connecticut, Arkansas, Texas, Iowa, Maryland, South Carolina, Idaho, Alabama, and Nevada, to facilitate credit transfer from community colleges to universities with BSN programs.

Indeed, the growth in RN pathways to baccalaureate and graduate degrees has been so rapid in the past decade that some nurse leaders have suggested that this has resulted in a lack of educational standardization and significant variability in expectations and requirements

Research Study Fuels the Controversy 1.2

A focus group of 32 AORN members from central Ohio (approximately half did not have a baccalaureate degree) was asked to deliberate the question "Is there a need to legislate that newly licensed RNs in Ohio obtain a baccalaureate degree within 10 years?"

Source: Haverkamp, J. J., & Ball, K. (2013). BSN in 10: What is your opinion? *AORN Journal, 98*(2), 144–152. doi:10.1016/j.aorn.2013.06.006

Study Findings

Three themes emerged. The first was a lack of knowledge about the effects of nursing education on patient outcomes, health policy news and, in particular, the IOM 2010 report The Future of Nursing, and Ohio's 2015 initiative to require RNs to have their baccalaureate degree within 10 years of initial licensure. The second theme was that the participants perceived many barriers to returning to school including the difficulty of transferring college credits, cost, a lack of geographic accessibility, scheduling conflicts, and the difficulty of balancing work, school, and personal life. The final theme was that participants appeared to value the idea of BSN education in nursing and that if barriers were removed, more nurses would further their education.

among RN-to-BSN programs. McEwen, Pullis, White, and Krawtz (2013) suggest that numerous questions must be answered and concerns addressed to develop strategies to maintain growth, improve access, and remove barriers without sacrificing quality. Only then can the public be assured that RN-to-BSN education prepares graduates for the future health care system and that the outcome is not just a piece of paper (McEwen et al., 2013).

In addition, sometimes there is little integration, standardization, or cooperation between public systems of education. Such integration, standardization, and cooperation will be essential for transition to BSN entry levels. This is why one of the key recommendations in *The Future of Nursing* was that all nursing schools should offer defined academic pathways that promote seamless access for nurses to higher levels of education (Institute of Medicine, 2010). Transition programs or services for non-baccalaureate-prepared nurses must be designed, which facilitate entry into baccalaureate and advanced education and practice programs. In addition, funding must continue to be increased for colleges and universities sponsoring baccalaureate and advanced practice nursing education programs.

Consider This A broad new system, composed of direct transfer, linkage, and partnership programs, is needed between community college and baccalaureate institutions to ensure a smooth transition from ADN to BSN as the entry-level requirement for professional nursing practice. This transition will be costly.

Finally, raising the entry level in professional nursing practice will be costly. University education simply costs more than education at community colleges and significant increases in federal and state funding for baccalaureate and graduate nursing education will need to occur. Given the significant budget deficit currently faced by almost all states, the likelihood of funding increases for nursing education is directly related to the public and legislative understanding of the complexity of roles nurses assume each and every day and the educational level they perceive is needed to accomplish these tasks.

Clearly, barriers for educational reentry must be removed if the educational entry level in nursing is to be raised to a bachelor's or higher degree. Alternative pathways for RN education must be developed to create opportunities for learners who might not otherwise be able to pursue additional nursing education.

Consider This Edwards (2012) suggests that it is unlikely that IOM workforce goals (80% of RNs have BSNs by 2020) will be achieved without legislation requiring new nurses to earn their BSN within a reasonable amount of time.

AN INTERNATIONAL ISSUE

The entry-into-practice debate in nursing is not limited to the United States, although several countries have already established the baccalaureate degree as the minimum entry level and grandfathered all those with a license before that date. For example, since 1982, all the provincial and territorial nurses associations in Canada have advocated the baccalaureate degree as the education entry-to-practice standard and most provincial and territorial regulatory bodies have achieved this goal (all but Quebec). The Canadian Nurses Association (CNA) believes that the knowledge, skills, and personal attributes that today's health system demands of its RNs can be gained only through broad-based bachelor's nursing programs (CNA, 2014).

Similarly, Australia moved toward the adoption of a BSN for entry into nursing during the 1980s, initially encountering resistance by both physicians and by nurses themselves, who feared university education would minimize needed hands-on training. Registered nursing as a university degree, however, was mandated in the 1990s. *Enrolled nurses* (scope of practice similar to LPNs/LVNs in the United States) continue to be educated in diploma programs and work under the supervision of the RN. Postgraduate diplomas provide further vocational training for specialist areas.

Similarly, in South Africa, nurses who complete a 2-year course of study are called *enrolled nurses* or *staff nurses*, whereas those who complete 4 years of study attain *professional nurse* or *sister* status. Enrolled nurses can later complete a 2-year bridging program and become *registered general nurses*.

Wales, Scotland, and Northern Ireland also offer only one entry point for nursing entry and that is a 3-year university degree. Other one entry-point countries include Italy, Norway, and Spain (3-year university degree); Ireland (4-year university degree); and Denmark (3.5-year degree at nursing school in university college sector). Many countries, such as Sweden, Portugal, Brazil, Iceland, Korea, Greece, and the Philippines, already require a 4-year undergraduate degree to practice nursing. All new nurses in England were required to hold a degree-level qualification to enter the profession after 2013. The aim was to increase skills and train a medical workforce capable of operating in a more analytical and independent manner.

Consider This A growing list of countries, states, and provinces now require baccalaureate education in nursing.

Thus, international efforts to advance nursing education appear to be gaining momentum. The 2009 World Health Organization's Global Standards for the Initial Education of Professional Nurses and Midwives, written between 2005 and 2007, with participation from Sigma Theta Tau International, called for all nurses to be educated with a bachelor's degree, recognizing that country-specific standards would be necessary due to differing resources, history, and environments (Edwards, 2012).

In addition, in a 2012 London gathering of advanced practice nurses from around the globe, inconsistency in the entry-level preparation and criteria for taking the licensing exam in the United States were identified as issues that continue to impede nursing's progress toward a better-prepared professional workforce globally (Gyurko & Nardi, 2013). Participants encouraged US nursing leaders to consider adopting a process similar to the *Bologna process* (agreement by 47 European countries that created a standardized 3-cycle system of nursing education; undergraduate, graduate, and doctoral and removed many barriers for return to school) so that the nursing profession can focus on engaging all nurses to practice to the full extent of their training and education (Gyurko & Nardi, 2013).

Conclusions

The entry-into-practice debate in the United States continues to be one of the oldest and hottest professional issues nurses face as we enter the second decade of the 21st century. It appears that limited progress has been made since 1965 in creating a consensus to raise the entry level into professional nursing practice.

Achieving the BSN as the entry degree for professional nursing practice will take the best thinking of our nursing leaders. It will also require courage, as well as a respect for persons not seen in the entry debate, and collaboration of the highest order. It will also require nurses to depersonalize the issue and look at what is best for both the clients they serve and the profession, rather than for them individually.

LaRocco (2014) suggests:

> *While the leaders of 1965 were visionary in their proposal of baccalaureate education as the entry to professional nursing, they were less effective in creating the change that they proposed. Will our current nursing leaders be successful in completing this unfinished business?* (p. 11)

Even the most patient planned-change advocate would agree that more than years is a long time for implementation of a position. Clearly, the driving forces for such a change have not yet overcome the restraining forces, although movement is apparent. The question seems to come down to whether the nursing profession wants to spend another 50 years debating the issue or whether it wants to proactively take the steps necessary to make the goal a reality.

For Additional Discussion

1. What are the greatest driving and restraining forces for increasing entry into practice to a bachelor's or higher level?
2. Are the terms *professional* and *technical* unnecessarily inflammatory in the entry-into-practice debate? Why do these terms elicit such a "personal" response?
3. Is calling the associate degree in nursing a 2-year vocational degree an injustice to its graduates?
4. What is the legitimacy of requiring so many units at the community college level for an ADN degree? Should the current movement by community colleges to award baccalaureate degrees in nursing be encouraged?
5. How does the complexity of nursing roles and responsibilities compare to that of other health professions with higher entry levels?
6. What is the likelihood that nurses and the organizations that represent them will be able to achieve consensus on the entry-into-practice issue?
7. If the entry level is raised, should grandfathering be used? If so, should this grandfathering be conditional?
8. Is the goal of BSN entry a realistic one by 2020? If not, when?

References

Aiken, L. H., Clarke, S. P., Cheung, R. B., Sloane, D. M., & Silber, J. H. (2003). Educational levels of hospital nurses and surgical patient mortality. *JAMA, 290*(12), 1617–1623.

Aiken, L. H., Clarke, S. P., Sloane, D. M., Lake, E. T., & Cheney, T. (2008). Effects of hospital care environment on patient mortality and nurse outcomes. *The Journal of Nursing Administration, 38*(5), 223–229.

American Association of Colleges of Nursing. (2014a). *Fact sheet: Creating a more highly qualified nursing workforce.* Retrieved November 22, 2014, from http://www.aacn.nche.edu/media-relations/NursingWorkforce.pdf

American Association of Colleges of Nursing. (2014b). *Fact sheet: The impact of education on nursing practice.* Retrieved November 23, 2014, from http://www.aacn.nche.edu/media-relations/fact-sheets/impact-of-education

American Nurses Association. (1965a). *A position paper.* New York, NY: Author.

American Nurses Association. (1965b). *Educational preparation for nurse practitioners and assistants to nurses: A position paper.* New York, NY: Author.

Association of Operating Room Nurses. (2011). *AORN Position statement on entry into practice.* Retrieved November 29, 2014, from http://www.aorn.org/Clinical_Practice/Position_Statements/Position_Statements.aspx

Benner, P., Sutphen, M., Leonard, V., & Day, L. (2010). Educating nurses: A call for radical transformation: Preparation for the professions. San Francisco, CA: Jossey-Bass/The Carnegie Foundation for the Advancement of Teaching.

Blegen, M. A., Goode, C. J., Park, S. H., Vaughn, T., & Spetz, J. (2013, February). Baccalaureate education in nursing and patient outcomes. *Journal of Nursing Administration, 43*(2), 89–94. doi:10.1097/NNA.0b013e31827f2028

Byrne, D., Mayo, R., & Rosner, C. (2014). What internal motivators drive RNs to pursue a BSN? *Nursing, 44*(10), 22–24. doi:10.1097/01.NURSE.0000453707.43199.ea

Canadian Nurses Association. (2014). *Education.* Retrieved November 27, 2014, from http://www.cna-aiic.ca/en/becoming-an-rn/education

Carramanica, L., & Thompson, P. A. (2012, January). AONE Survey: Gauging hospitals' use of preferential hiring policies for BSN-prepared nurses. *Voice of Nursing Leadership, 1,* 17,18.

Delgado, J. (2013, May 1). Nurses go back to school to get their bachelor's degree. *Chicago Tribune.* Retrieved November 29, 2014, from http://articles.chicagotribune.com/2013-05-01/health/ct-met-nursing-degrees-20130501_1_nursing-program-nursing-leaders-associate-degree

Edwards, D. S. (2012). An 80% BSN workforce by 2020? *Reflections on Nursing Leadership, 38*(1). Retrieved from http://www.reflectionsonnursingleadership.org/Pages/Vol38_1_Edwards_IOM%20Report.aspx

Gyurko, C. C., & Nardi, D. A. (2013). It's time to end the debate and require a BSN! *Reflections on Nursing Leadership, 39*(3), 1–4.

Haverkamp, J. J., & Ball, K. (2013). BSN in 10: What is your opinion? *AORN Journal, 98*(2), 144–152. doi:10.1016/j.aorn.2013.06.006

Health Resources and Services Administration. (2010, March). *The registered nurse population.* Retrieved November 23, 2014, from http://bhpr.hrsa.gov/healthworkforce/rnsurveys/rnsurveyinitial2008.pdf

Institute of Medicine. (2010, October). *The future of nursing: Leading change, advancing health.* Retrieved January 31, 2015, from http://thefutureofnursing.org/IOM-Report

Joint statement on academic progression for nursing students and graduates. (n.d.). AACC, ACCT, AACN, NLN, NOADN. Retrieved November 24, 2014, from https://www.noadn.org/component/option, com_docman/Itemid,250/task, doc_view/gid,476/

Kovner, C. T., Brewer, C. S., Katigbak, C., Djukic, M., & Fatehi, F. (2012). Charting the course for nurses' achievement of higher education levels. *Journal of Professional Nursing, 28*(6), 333–343. doi:10.1016/j.profnurs.2012.04.021

LaRocco, S. (2014). Where are the visionary nursing leaders of 1965? *American Journal of Nursing, 114*(4), 11. doi:10.1097/01.NAJ.0000445661.74531.b8

Lavizzo-Mourey, R. (2012). The nurse education imperative. *Pediatric Nursing, 38*(2), 61–62.

Making progress toward BSN goal. (2013). *American Nurse,45*(4),4.Retrievedfromhttp://www.theamericannurse.org/index.php/2013/09/03/making-progress-toward-bsn-goal/

McEwen, M., Pullis, B. R., White, M. J., & Krawtz, S. (2013). Eighty percent by 2020: The present and future of RN-to-BSN education. *Journal of Nursing Education, 52*(10), 549–557. doi:10.3928/01484834-20130913-01

Moltz, D. (2010, January 7). *Nursing tug of war.* Retrieved June 16, 2011, from http://www.insidehighered.com/news/2010/01/07/nursing

National Association of Neonatal Nurses. (2009). *Educational preparation for nursing practice roles* [Position statement No. 3048, NANN Board of Directors]. Retrieved February 6, 2011, from http://www.nann.org/pdf/09educational_prep.pdf

National Organization for Associate Degree Nursing. (2014). *Nursing facts.* Retrieved November 22, 2014, from https://www.noadn.org/resources/nursing-facts.html

New AACN data on BSN-prepared hiring. (2014). *American Nurse, 46*(1), 5.

Sabio, C. C. (2014). "Would you have enrolled? Decision factors in baccalaureate-only nursing among associate degree nursing students." Capella University. *CINAHL Plus with Full Text,* EBSCO*host.* Accessed November 23, 2014.

Service Employees International Union. (2014). *Position statement on BSN requirement for RN practice.* Retrieved November 24, 2014 from http://www.seiu.org/a/healthcare/position-statement-on-bsn-requirement-for-rn-practice.php

Tollick, K. (2013). BSN Required. *Nursing News, 37*(1), 4–5.

Yakusheva, O., Lindrooth, R., & Weiss, M. (2014). Economic evaluation of the 80% baccalaureate nurse workforce recommendation: A patient-level analysis. *Medical Care, 52*(10), 864-869. doi:10.1097/MLR.0000000000000189

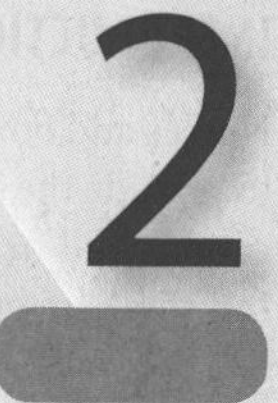

Evidence-Based Practice

Suzanne S. Prevost and Cassandra D. Ford

ADDITIONAL RESOURCES

Visit thePoint for additional helpful resources

- eBook
- Journal Articles
- WebLinks

CHAPTER OUTLINE

Introduction

What Is Evidence-Based Practice?

Why, When, and Where Is Evidence-Based Practice Used?

Why Is Evidence-Based Practice Important?

When and Where Is Evidence-Based Practice Used?

Evidence-Based Practice Around the World

How Do Nurses Determine Evidence-Based Practices?

Finding Evidence to Answer Nursing Questions

Supporting Evidence-Based Practice

Garner Administrative Support

Collaborate With a Research Mentor

Seek Assistance From Professional Librarians

Search Already Reviewed or Summarized Research

Access Resources From Professional Organizations

Benchmark With High-Performing Teams, Units, or Institutions

Challenges and Opportunities: Strategies for Changing Practice

Challenges to Implementing Evidence-Based Practice

Conclusions

LEARNING OBJECTIVES

The learner will be able to:

1. Differentiate between evidence-based practice and best practices.
2. Explain why the identification and implementation of evidence-based practice is important both for ensuring quality of care and in advancing the development of nursing science.
3. Identify personal, professional, and administrative strategies, as well as support systems, that promote the identification and implementation of evidence-based practice.
4. Describe the types of knowledge and education that nurses need to prepare them for conducting research and leading best practice initiatives.
5. Recognize the need to ask critical questions in the spirit of looking for opportunities to improve nursing practice and patient outcomes.
6. Delineate research and nonresearch sources of evidence for answering clinical questions.
7. Describe and compare practices that have evolved in the workplace as a result of tradition-based and research-based inquiry.
8. Compare the efficacy of randomized controlled trials, integrative reviews, or meta-analyses with practice-based evidence for continuous process improvement (PBE-CPI) to answer clinical research questions.
9. Specify institutions, units, teams, or individuals in the community that could be considered regional or national benchmark leaders in the provision of a specialized type of medical or nursing care.
10. Explore reasons for the disconnect that often exists between nurse researchers and educators studying evidence-based practice and nurses who seek to implement research into their practice.

INTRODUCTION

Nurses and other health care providers constantly strive to provide the best care for their patients. As new medications and health care innovations emerge, determining the best options can be challenging. This process has become more difficult in recent years as health care administrators, insurance companies, and other payers, accrediting agencies, and consumers demand the latest and greatest health care interventions. Nurses and physicians are expected to select health care interventions that are supported by research and other credible forms of evidence. They may also be expected to provide evidence to demonstrate that the care they deliver is not only clinically effective but also cost-effective, and satisfying, to patients. In light of these challenges, the term *evidence-based practice* has emerged as a descriptor of the preferred approach to health care delivery.

This chapter begins by defining the concept of evidence-based practice. Examples of when and where nurses are using evidence-based practice are provided, as are strategies for determining and applying these practices. In addition, the *who* of evidence-based practice is addressed regarding how nurses in various roles can support this approach to care. Finally, future implications are discussed.

WHAT IS EVIDENCE-BASED PRACTICE?

The term evidence-based practice is being used with increasing frequency among health care providers. Evidence-based practice has a variety of definitions and interpretations. The term evidence-based practice evolved in the mid-1990s when discussions of evidence-based medicine were expanded to apply to an interdisciplinary audience, which included nurses. David Sackett, one of the leaders of the movement, defined evidence-based medicine as "the conscientious and judicious use of current best evidence from clinical care research in the management of individual patients" (Sackett, Rosenberg, Gray, Haynes, & Richardson, 1996, p. 71). The Honor Society of Nursing, Sigma Theta Tau International (STTI) expanded this definition to address a broad nursing context with the following definition of evidence-based nursing practice: "An integration of the best evidence available, nursing expertise, and the values and preferences of the individuals, families and communities who are served" (STTI, 2005, p. 1).

Historically, various industries, in health care and beyond, have used the term *best practice* to describe the strategies or methods that work most efficiently or achieve the best results. This concept is often associated with the process of *benchmarking*, which involves identifying the most successful companies or institutions in a particular sector of an industry, examining their methods of doing business, using their approach as the goal or gold standard, and then replicating and refining their methods. Today, benchmarking data is one of the less scientific forms of evidence that is used, along with the results of formal research studies, to identify evidence-based nursing practices.

Consider This Today, most nurse experts agree that the best practices in nursing care are also evidence-based practices.

Although this process of identifying the best evidence-based practices has become more scientific, the ultimate goal remains to provide optimal patient care, with the goal of enhancing nursing practice and, in turn, improving patient or system outcomes.

Discussion Point

Are there any situations in which an evidence-based practice might not be considered the best practice?

WHY, WHEN, AND WHERE IS EVIDENCE-BASED PRACTICE USED?

Each week, new developments and innovations occur and are reported in health care—not only in research findings but also in the public media. Contemporary health care consumers are knowledgeable and demanding. They expect the most current, effective, and efficient interventions.

Why Is Evidence-Based Practice Important?

In their quest to provide the highest quality care for their patients, nurses are challenged to stay abreast of new developments in health care, even within the limits of their areas of specialization. Simultaneous with the growth of health care knowledge, health care costs have increased, and patient satisfaction has taken on greater importance. Administrators expect health care providers to satisfy their customers and to do it in the most clinically effective and cost-effective manner.

Control of health care costs was one of the early drivers of the evidence-based practice movement. As contracted and discounted reimbursement systems decreased revenue to hospitals and providers, it became increasingly apparent that some providers were capable of providing high-quality care in a more efficient and cost-effective manner than their peers. The practices of these industry leaders were quickly identified and emulated. Within the current litigious and cost-conscious health care environment, there remains a sense of urgency to select and implement the most effective and efficient interventions as quickly as possible.

Nurses are increasingly accepted as essential members, and often as leaders, of the interdisciplinary health care teams. To effectively participate and lead a health care team, nurses must have knowledge of the most effective and reliable evidence-based approaches to care, and as nurses increase their expertise in critiquing research, they are expected to apply the evidence of their findings to select optimal interventions for their patients.

The processes and tools of evidence-based practice can help nurses respond to these challenges. This approach to care is based on the latest research and other forms of evidence, as well as clinical expertise and patient preferences. All of these factors contribute to providing quality care that is clinically effective, cost-effective, and satisfying to health care consumers.

Discussion Point

What type of knowledge and education do nurses need to prepare them for leading evidence-based practice initiatives as described?

When and Where Is Evidence-Based Practice Used?

In recent years, the implementation of evidence-based practice has been identified as a priority across nearly every nursing specialty. Over the past decade, STTI, the International Honor Society for Nurses, has consistently received feedback from their membership surveys asking for support systems and resources to help nurses implement evidence-based practice. This feedback has been consistent across nursing specialties and across nursing roles and positions. Initiatives to help nurses understand and implement evidence-based practice have become a priority since that time. A review of recent literature yields case studies and recommendations for evidence-based practice implementation across several nursing specialties. These are shown in Table 2.1.

In addition to the universal application across nursing specialties, the concept of evidence-based practice is also valued across nursing roles and responsibilities. Stetler, Ritchie, Rycroft-Malone, and Charns (2014) discussed nurse leader behaviors that support evidence-based practice. Moseley (2012) discussed the role of evidence-based practice in clinical decision making for advanced practice nurses. Nursing faculty can implement a number of strategies to incorporate evidence-based practice into nursing curricula (Winters & Echeverri, 2012). Last but not least, staff nurses are frequently expected to participate in evidence-based practice initiatives (Brody, Barnes, Ruble, & Sakowski, 2012).

Evidence-Based Practice Around the World

A commitment to evidence-based practice is not limited to the United States. A few countries—in particular, Australia, Canada, and the United Kingdom—adopted this approach to care several years before it became popular in the United States. The Joanna Briggs Institute, which started at the University of Adelaide, Australia, in 1996, now has over 70 centers collaborating to provide evidence-based resources to health care providers around the world. The Registered Nurses Association of Ontario has been developing and distributing evidence-based nursing practice guidelines for more than a decade. Nursing Knowledge International (NKI), a subsidiary of STTI, also serves as an international clearinghouse and facilitator to promote international nursing communication, collaboration, and sharing of resources in support of evidence-based practice.

Consider This In the past decade, the concept of evidence-based practice has evolved and been embraced by nurses in nearly every clinical specialty, across a variety of roles and positions, and in locations around the globe.

How Do Nurses Determine Evidence-Based Practices?

Evidence-based practice begins with questions that arise in practice settings. Nurses must be empowered to ask critical questions in the spirit of looking for opportunities to improve nursing practice and patient outcomes. In any specialty or role, nurses can regard their work as a continuous series of questions and decisions.

TABLE 2.1 Evidence-Based Practice Across Nursing Specialties

Area of Specialization	Author and Year	Title or Theme	Type of Report
Administration	Brody et al. (2012)	Promoting EBP	Administrative strategies for engaging staff nurses in EBP
Critical care	Munaco, Dumas, and Edlund (2014)	Prevention of ventilator-associated events with EBP	Quality improvement project
Emergency	Popovich, Boyd, Dachenhaus, and Kusler (2012)	Emergency department improvement in patient flow using EBP	Protocol development to improve patient flow
Gerontology	Naylor et al. (2013)	Translating research into practice	Research study evaluating the translation of the Transitional Care Model into a large health plan
Medical–surgical	Magers (2013)	EBP utilization to reduce catheter-associated urinary tract infections in long-term acute care	Quality improvement project
Mental health	Alzayyat (2014)	EBP barriers in mental health nursing	Describes methods to overcome barriers to implementing EBP
Oncology	Choi et al. (2014)	EBP for cancer patient pain management	Describes implementation of EBP project
Pediatrics	Obrecht, Van Hulle Vincent, and Ryan (2014)	EBP change implementation for pediatric pain assessment scale	Describes EBP implementation of tool
Women's health	Wilson and Phelps (2013)	EBP in maternal/child inpatient hospital setting	Describes EBP dissemination and implementation

Note: EBP = evidence-based practice.

In a given day, a staff nurse may ask and answer questions such as "Should I give the analgesic only when the patient requests it, or should I encourage him to take it every 4 hours? Will aggressive ambulation expedite this patient's recovery, or will it consume too much energy? Will open family visitation help the patient feel supported, or will it interrupt her rest?"

A nurse manager or administrator might ask, "Who is the most qualified care provider for our sickest patient today? What is the optimal nurse-to-patient ratio for a specific unit? Do complication rates and sentinel events increase with less-educated staff? Do longer shifts result in greater staff fatigue and medication errors? Will higher-quality and more expensive mattresses decrease the incidence of pressure ulcers? What benefits promote nurse retention? How does the use of supplemental (or agency) staffing affect the morale of existing staff? Can this population be treated on an outpatient, rather than an inpatient, basis? What is the optimal length of time for a comprehensive home care assessment? How many patients can a nurse practitioner see in 8 hours?"

Likewise, a nurse educator may ask, "Is it more effective to teach a procedure in the simulation laboratory rather than on an actual patient? What are the most efficient methods of documenting continued competency? Do Web-based students perform as well on standardized tests as students in traditional classrooms?"

Each type of question can lead to important decisions that affect outcomes, such as patient recovery, organizational effectiveness, and nursing competency. The best answers and, consequently, the best decisions come from informed, evidence-based analysis of each situation. See Box 2.1 for a list of questions to assist the nurse in the process of evidence-based decision making for various nursing scenarios.

BOX 2.1 Key Questions to Ask When Considering Evidence-Based Practices

- Why have we always done "it" this way?
- Do we have evidence-based rationale? Or is this practice merely based on tradition?
- Is there a better (more effective, faster, safer, less expensive, more comfortable) method?
- What approach does the patient (or the target group) prefer?
- What do experts in this specialty recommend?
- What methods are used by leading, or benchmark, organizations?
- Do the findings of recent research suggest an alternative method?
- Is there a review of the research on this topic?
- Are there nationally recognized standards of care, practice guidelines, or protocols that apply?
- Are organizational barriers inhibiting the application of evidence-based practice in this situation?

FINDING EVIDENCE TO ANSWER NURSING QUESTIONS

Nurses rely on various sources to answer clinical questions such as those cited previously. A practicing staff nurse might consult a nurse with more experience, more education, or a higher level of authority to get help in answering such questions. Institutional standards or policy and procedure manuals are also a common reference source for nurses in practice. Nursing coworkers or other health care providers, such as physicians, pharmacists, or therapists, might also be consulted. Although all of these approaches are extremely common, they are more likely to yield clinical answers that are *tradition based* rather than *evidence based.*

If evidence-based practice is truly based on best evidence, nursing expertise, and the values and preferences of patients, then local expertise and tradition is not sufficient. However, the optimal source of best evidence is often a matter of controversy.

Discussion Point

In your preferred area of nursing specialization, what are some key questions and decisions that nurses address on a daily basis?

Discussion Point

What are the best sources of evidence for answering clinical questions?

Research is generally considered a more reliable source of evidence than traditions or the clinical expertise of individuals. However, many experts argue that some types of research are better, or stronger, forms of evidence than others. In medicine and pharmacology, the *randomized controlled trial* (RCT) has been considered the gold standard of clinical evidence. RCTs yield the strongest statistical evidence regarding the effectiveness of an intervention in comparison with another intervention or placebo. For many clinical questions in medicine and pharmacy, there may be multiple RCTs in the literature addressing a single question, such as the effectiveness of a particular drug. In such situations, an even stronger form of evidence is an *integrative review or meta-analysis* wherein the results of several similar research studies are combined or synthesized to provide the most comprehensive answer to the question.

In nursing literature, RCTs, meta-analyses, and integrative reviews are significantly less common than in medical or pharmaceutical literature. For many clinical questions in nursing, RCTs may not exist, or they may not even be appropriate. For example, if a nurse is considering how best to prepare a patient for endotracheal suctioning, it would be helpful to inform the patient what suctioning feels like. This type of question does not lend itself to an RCT, but rather to descriptive or qualitative research. In general, qualitative, descriptive, or quasi-experimental studies are much more common methods of inquiry in nursing research than RCTs or meta-analyses. Furthermore, the body of nursing research overall is newer and less developed than that of some other health disciplines. Thus, for many clinical nursing questions, research studies may not exist.

Recently, a research method has evolved that provides excellent support for evidence-based practice. Fittingly, this research method is referred to as *practice-based evidence for continuous process improvement* (PBE-CPI). PBE-CPI incorporates the variation from routine clinical practice to determine what works best, for which patients, under what circumstances, and at what cost. It uses the knowledge of frontline caregivers, who help to develop the research questions and define variables (Horn, DeJong, & Deutscher, 2012). This method can provide a more comprehensive picture than a randomized controlled study that only examines one intervention with a very limited population under strictly controlled, laboratory-like circumstances. Although research results are usually considered the optimal form of evidence, many other data sources have been used to support the identification of optimal interventions for nursing and other health care disciplines. Some of the additional sources are as follows:

- Benchmarking data
- Clinical expertise
- Cost-effectiveness analyses
- Infection-control data
- Medical record review data
- National standards of care
- Pathophysiologic data
- Quality improvement data
- Patient and family preferences

Another dilemma for the practicing nurse is the time, access, and expertise needed to search and analyze the research literature to answer clinical questions. Few practicing nurses have the luxury of leaving their patients to conduct a literature search. Many staff nurses practicing in clinical settings have less than a baccalaureate degree; therefore, they likely have not been exposed to a formal research course. Findings from research studies are typically very technical, difficult to understand, and even more difficult to translate into applications. Searching, finding, critiquing, and summarizing research findings for applications in practice are high-level skills that require substantial education and practice.

Discussion Point

If a practicing nurse has no formal education or experience related to research, what strategies should she or he use to find evidence that answers clinical questions and supports evidence-based practice?

SUPPORTING EVIDENCE-BASED PRACTICE

In light of the challenges of providing or implementing evidence-based practice, nurses must consider some alternative support mechanisms when searching for the best evidence to support their practice. Recommended mechanisms of support are summarized in Box 2.2.

Garner Administrative Support

The first strategy is to garner administrative support. The implementation of evidence-based practice should not be an individual, staff nurse–level pursuit. Administrative support is needed to access the resources, provide the support personnel, and sanction the necessary changes in policies, procedures, and practices. Recently, nursing administrators have had increased incentives to support evidence-based practice because this approach to care has become recognized as the standard expectation of organizations, such as the Joint Commission (formerly Joint Commission on Accreditation of Healthcare Organizations [JCAHO]), which accredits hospitals and other health care institutions. Evidence-based practice is also one of the expectations associated with the highly regarded Magnet Hospital Recognition program. Most nursing administrators who want their institutions to be recognized for providing high-quality care will understand the value of evidence-based practice and should therefore be willing to provide resources to support it.

BOX 2.2 Mechanisms to Promote Evidence-Based Practice

- Garner administrative support.
- Collaborate with a research mentor.
- Seek assistance from professional librarians.
- Search for sources that have already reviewed or summarized the research.
- Access resources from professional organizations.
- Benchmark with high-performing teams, units, or institutions.

BOX 2.3 Strategies for the New Nurse to Promote Evidence-Based Practice

- Keep abreast of the evidence—subscribe to professional journals and read widely.
- Use and encourage use of multiple sources of evidence.
- Find established sources of evidence in your specialty; do not reinvent the wheel.
- Implement and evaluate nationally sanctioned clinical practice guidelines.
- Question and challenge nursing traditions, and promote a spirit of risk taking.
- Dispel myths and traditions not supported by evidence.
- Collaborate with other nurses locally and globally.
- Interact with other disciplines to bring nursing evidence to the table.

Collaborate With a Research Mentor

One way nurse administrators can support the use of evidence-based practice is through the provision of nurse experts who can function as research mentors. Advanced practice nurses, nurse researchers, and nursing faculty are examples of nurses who may provide consultation and collaboration to support the process of searching, reviewing, and critiquing research literature and databases to answer clinical questions and identify best practices. Most staff nurses do not have the educational background, research expertise, or time to effectively review and critique extensive research literature in search of the evidence to support evidence-based practice. Research mentors can assist with these processes, whereas staff nurses can often provide the best insight on clinical needs and patient preferences. Box 2.3 includes a list of strategies for the new graduate nurse to promote evidence-based practice.

Seek Assistance From Professional Librarians

Another valuable type of support that is available in academic medical centers, and in some smaller institutions, is consultation from medical librarians. A skilled librarian can save nurses a tremendous amount of time by providing guidance in the most comprehensive and efficient approaches to search the health care literature to find research studies and other resources to support the implementation of evidence-based practice.

Search Already Reviewed or Summarized Research

A strategy nurses can use to expedite the search for evidence-based practice is to specifically seek references that have already been reviewed or summarized in the research literature. For example, some journals, such as *Evidence-Based Nursing* and *Worldviews on Evidence-Based Nursing*, specifically focus on providing summaries, critiques, and practice implications of existing nursing research studies. For example, recent issues of *Worldviews on Evidence-Based Nursing* included reviews and summaries on the following topics:

- Behavioral interventions
- Cognitive behavioral therapy
- Patient teaching
- Self-management of chronic metabolic diseases
- Support protocols for enteral nutrition

When conducting a literature search, use of keywords, such as "research review" or "meta-analysis," can assist the nurse in identifying research review articles that have been published on the topic of interest.

The *Cochrane Collaboration* is a large international organization composed of several interdisciplinary teams of research scholars that are continuously conducting reviews of research on a wide variety of clinical topics. The Cochrane Collaboration promotes the use of evidence-based practice around the world. The Cochrane reviews tend to focus heavily on evaluating the effectiveness of medical interventions, for example, comparing the effects of different medications for specific conditions. Therefore, many of the Cochrane review summaries are more useful for primary care providers, such as physicians and nurse practitioners, than for staff nurse clinicians. Some of the Cochrane projects of interest to nurses in direct care positions include their reviews of products designed to prevent pressure ulcers, nursing interventions for smoking cessation, interventions to help patients follow their medication regimens, and interventions to promote collaboration between nurses and physicians.

The Agency for Healthcare Research and Quality (AHRQ) is also a good resource for identifying research reviews and summaries that have been compiled by national panels of experts. One particularly helpful AHRQ resource is the *National Guideline Clearinghouse* (NGC), a link to which can be found on and is also available at www.guidelines.gov. The mission of the NGC is to "provide physicians and other healthcare providers … an accessible mechanism for obtaining objective, detailed information on clinical practice guidelines and to further their dissemination, implementation and use" (AHRQ, 2014, para. 2).

All of the practice guidelines available through this site are developed through systematic searches and reviews of research literature and scientific evidence by a professional organization, health care specialty association, or government agency. Nursing organizations that have contributed guidelines to the NGC include the American Association of Neuroscience Nurses; Association of Women's Health, Obstetric, and Neonatal Nursing; Emergency Nurses Association; the Oncology Nursing Society; and the Registered Nurses Association of Ontario. Each guideline includes an abstract summary and a list of recommended practices, strategies, or interventions for a specific clinical condition. The NGC contains more than 2,500 unique practice guidelines.

Access Resources From Professional Organizations

Professional nursing organizations can also provide a wealth of resources to support evidence-based practice. For example, the American Association of Critical Care Nurses has published several *Practice Alerts* that are relevant to nursing care in critical care units. These documents are based on extensive literature reviews conducted by national panels of nurse researchers and advanced practice nurses. They provide concise recommendations focused on areas where current common practices should change on the basis of the latest research. Some of the topics covered in the *Practice Alerts* include pain assessment in the critically ill adult, alarm management, and bathing of adult patients.

The Association of Women's Health, Obstetric, and Neonatal Nursing (AWHONN) also provides several resources to support evidence-based practice. The AWHONN Research-Based Practice Projects are designed to "translate research into nursing practice, ultimately advancing evidence-based clinical practice" (AWHONN, 2014, para. 1). Through this program, several nationwide, multiyear projects have been completed. Topics addressed through this mechanism have included management of women in second-stage labor, urinary continence for women, neonatal skin care, and cyclic pelvic pain and discomfort management.

AWHONN also sponsored an Evidence-Based Clinical Practice Guideline Program. Each of their guidelines includes clinical practice recommendations, referenced rationale statements, quality of evidence ratings for each statement, background information describing the scope of the clinical issue, and a quick care reference guide for clinicians. Neonatal Skin Care is an example of one of the guidelines produced through this program (AWHONN, 2014).

The Association of periOperative Registered Nurses (AORN), the Oncology Nursing Society (ONS), and STTI also provide Web-based resources to facilitate implementation of evidence-based practice. AORN has published *Guidelines for Perioperative Practice,* the ONS provides an *Evidence-Based Practice Resource Area,* and STTI publishes Web-based continuing education programs and several supportive publications, including *Worldviews on Evidence-Based Nursing.*

Discussion Point

What institutions, units, teams, or individuals can you identify in your region that would be considered regional or national benchmark leaders in the provision of a specialized type of medical or nursing care?

Benchmark With High-Performing Teams, Units, or Institutions

Finally, nurses can use benchmarking strategies to poll nurse experts from high-performing teams, units, or institutions to learn more about their practices for specific clinical problems or patient populations. Leaders of professional nursing organizations, such as STTI or the

National Association of Clinical Nurse Specialists, can help nurses locate and contact established nurse experts in various areas of specialization. Accrediting organizations, such as the Joint Commission, can assist in identifying institutions that are known as national leaders in providing specific types of care. The University of Iowa, Arizona State University, and McMaster University of Ontario are three North American institutions that have established reputations as leaders in evidence-based nursing practice.

Discussion Point

When the investigation reveals a need for an evidence-based change in practice, what strategies are useful for implementing change?

CHALLENGES AND OPPORTUNITIES: STRATEGIES FOR CHANGING PRACTICE

Nurses use several mechanisms for incorporating new research into current practice in the pursuit of promoting evidence-based practice. Perhaps the most common mechanism is through the development and refinement of research-based policies and procedures. Fortunately, the Joint Commission has mandated that health care institutions must implement formal processes for reviewing the latest research and ensuring that institutional policies and procedures are consistently revised in keeping with current research findings.

Protocols, algorithms, decision trees, standards of care, critical pathways, care maps, and institutional clinical practice guidelines are additional mechanisms used to incorporate new evidence into clinical practice. Each of these formats is used by health care teams to guide clinical decision making and clinical interventions. Although nurses often take the lead in developing or revising these devices, participation and buy-in from the interdisciplinary health care team are essential to achieve successful implementation and consistent changes in practice.

In addition to consensus from the interdisciplinary team, support from patients and their families is important. This element of the evidence-based practice process is frequently overlooked or not thoroughly considered. As previously mentioned, evidence-based nursing practice involves "an integration of the best evidence available, nursing expertise, and the values and preferences of the individuals, families and communities who are served" (STTI, 2005, p. 1).

If the review of evidence leads the health care team to recommend an intervention that is inconsistent with the patient's or family's values and preferences (such as a specific dietary modification or transfusion of blood products), the recommendation may lead to poor adherence or total disregard by the patient, not to mention a loss of the patient's trust and confidence in the health care team.

Discussion Point

Can you think of situations in which the latest research may be inconsistent with the values of an individual or group of patients?

Challenges to Implementing Evidence-Based Practice

Although evidence-based practice is being discussed and pursued by nurses around the world, several obstacles continue to inhibit the movement. Funk, Champagne, Wiese, and Tornquist (1991) originally studied this problem in 1991 and developed a survey instrument to quantify those barriers. Recently, Roe and Williams (2014) used this instrument as the first step in their project to promote implementation of evidence-based interventions for pressure ulcer prevention and wound care. In their study, they found that the biggest barrier for staff nurses was the overwhelming volume of research on these topics and the lack of time to read and synthesize that literature. Other researchers have also investigated the same type of questions with similar results (Research Study Fuels the Controversy 2.1).

Discussion Point

What obstacles would limit your involvement in the process of pursuing evidence-based practice?

Research Study Fuels the Controversy 2.1

Framework of Policy Recommendations for Implementation of Evidence-Based Practice: A Systematic Scoping Review

In 2013, these authors synthesized the results of 31 different research studies that were conducted in 17 different countries between 2001 and 2011. The focus of the review was to determine attitudes toward evidence-based practice as well as barriers and facilitators to implementation. Respondents for the studies included various health care providers.

Source: Ubbink, D. T., Guyatt, G. H., & Vermeulen, H. (2013). Framework of policy recommendations for implementation of evidence-based practice: A systematic scoping review. *BMJ Open, 3*(e001881), 1–12.

Study Findings

The majority of study respondents strongly believed that evidence-based practice was important and patient care was improved by the use of evidence-based practice. On the other hand, most health care providers did not feel their knowledge of evidence-based practice was sufficient. Some barriers to evidence-based practice included limited time to read and implement the evidence, lack of resources, and lack of evidence-based practice experience. Findings indicate the importance of educationally preparing nurses to implement evidence-based practice and providing the resources to facilitate the process.

Conclusions

Many nurses are experiencing success in promoting evidence-based practice. Organizations such as the AHRQ and the Cochrane Collaboration provide support to help clinicians overcome some of the barriers, such as the difficulties in obtaining and understanding research reports, and the lack of time to synthesize research findings into recommended practices. The many agencies that support teams of research experts to collect, critique, and summarize the research and other forms of evidence pave the way for frontline clinicians to find and adopt evidence-based practices.

Yet challenges continue. Too few nurses understand what evidence-based practice is all about. Organizational cultures may not support the nurse who seeks out and uses research to change long-standing practices rooted in tradition rather than science. In addition, a stronger connection needs to be established between researchers and academicians who study evidence-based nursing practice and staff nurses who must translate those findings into the art of nursing practice. Nursing cannot afford to value the art of nursing over the science. Both are critical to making sure that patients receive the highest quality of care possible.

For Additional Discussion

1. Can decision support tools such as algorithms, decision trees, clinical pathways, and standardized clinical guidelines ever replace clinical judgment?
2. Why does at least some level of disconnect exist between nurse researchers or faculty studying evidence-based practice and the nurses who seek to implement such research into their practice? Is the problem a lack of communication?
3. Do most nurses have access to evidence-based nursing research findings?
4. Are evidence-based practice findings consistent over time? Can you identify an evidence-based practice that was later found to be ineffective or inappropriate?
5. Should evidence-based practices be institution specific, or should they be more generalizable across different settings?

6. Is evidence-based nursing research grounded more in quantitative or qualitative research? Are both needed?
7. What can be done to increase the research knowledge base of practicing registered nurses (RNs), given that a significant proportion of those nurses have been educated at the associate-degree level?

References

Agency for Healthcare Research and Quality. (2014). *National guideline clearinghouse*. Retrieved November 13, 2014, from http://www.guideline.gov/about/index.aspx

Alzayyat, A. S. (2014). Barriers to evidence-based practice utilization in psychiatric/mental health nursing. *Issues in Mental Health Nursing, 35*, 134–143. doi:10.3109/01612840.2013.848385

Association of Women's Health, Obstetric and Neonatal Nursing. (2014). *Research-based practice projects*. Retrieved November 13, 2014, from http://www.awhonn.org/awhonn/content.do?name=03_JournalsPubsResearch%2F3G_ResearchBasedPracticeProjects.htm

Brody, A. A., Barnes, K., Ruble, C., & Sakowski, J. (2012). Evidence-based practice councils: Potential path to staff nurse empowerment and leadership growth. *The Journal of Nursing Administration, 42*(1), 28–33.

Choi, M., Kim, H. S., Chung, S. K., Ahn, M. J., Yoo, J. Y., Park, O. S.,... Geum, E. (2014). Evidence-based practice for pain management for cancer patients in an acute care setting. *International Journal of Nursing Practice, 20*, 60–69. doi:10.1111/ijn.121222

Funk, S. G., Champagne, M. T., Wiese, R. A., & Tornquist, E. M. (1991). Barriers to using research findings in practice: The clinician's perspective. *Applied Nursing Research, 4*(2), 90–95.

Horn, S. D., DeJong, G., & Deutscher, D. (2012). Practice-based evidence research in rehabilitation: An alternative to randomized controlled trials and traditional observational studies. *Archives of Physical Medicine and Rehabilitation, 93*(Suppl. 2), S127–S137.

Magers, T. L. (2013). Using evidence-based practice to reduce catheter-associated urinary tract infections. *The American Journal of Nursing, 113*(6), 34–42.

Moseley, M. J. (2012). The role of the advanced practice registered nurse in ensuring evidence-based practice. *Nursing Clinics of North America, 47*, 269-281. doi:10.1016/j.cnur.2012.02.004

Munaco, S. S., Dumas, B., & Edlund, B. J. (2014). Preventing ventilator-associated events: Complying with evidence-based practice. *Critical Care Nursing Quarterly, 37*(4), 384–392. doi:10.1097/CNQ.0000000000000039

Naylor, M. D., Bowles, K. H., McCauley, K. M., Maccoy, M. C., Maislin, G., Pauly, M. V., & Krakauer, R. (2013). High-value transitional care: Translation of research into practice. *Journal of Evaluation in Clinical Practice, 19*, 727–733. doi:10.1111/j.1365-2753.2011.01659.x

Obrecht, J., Van Hulle Vincent, C., & Ryan, C. (2014). Implementation of evidence-based practice for a pediatric pain assessment instrument. *Clinical Nurse Specialist CNS, 28*(2), 97–104. doi:10.1097/NUR.0000000000000032

Popovich, M., Boyd, C., Dachenhaus, T., & Kusler, D. (2012). Improving stable patient flow through the emergency department by utilizing evidence-based practice: One hospital's journey. *Journal of Emergency Nursing, 38*(5), 474–478. doi:10.1016/j.jen.2011.03.006

Roe, E., & Williams, D. L. (2014). Using evidence-based practice to prevent hospital-acquired pressure ulcers and promote wound healing. *American Journal of Nursing, 114*(8), 61–65.

Sackett, D. L., Rosenberg, W. M., Gray, J. A., Haynes, R. B., & Richardson, W. S. (1996). Evidence based medicine: What it is and what it isn't. *British Medical Journal, 312*(7023), 71–72.

Sigma Theta Tau International. (2005). *Evidence-based nursing position statement*. Retrieved November 13, 2014, from https://www.nursingsociety.org/about-stti/position-statements-and-resource-papers/evidence-based-nursing-position-statement

Stetler, C. B., Ritchie, J. A., Rycroft-Malone, J., & Charns, M. P. (2014). Leadership for evidence-based practice: Strategic and functional behaviors for institutionalizing EBP. *Worldviews on Evidence-Based Nursing, 11*(4), 219–226. doi:10.1111/wvn.12044

Wilson, B. L., & Phelps, C. (2013). Identifying and applying a targeted evidence-based practice change in the maternal/child health inpatient setting. *Nursing for Women's Health, 17*(6), 490–497. doi:10.1111/1751-486X.12077

Winters, C. A., & Echeverri, R. (2012). Teaching strategies to support evidence-based practice. *Critical Care Nurse, 32*(3), 49–54. doi:10.4037/ccn2012159

3

Developing Effective Leaders to Meet 21st-Century Health Care Challenges

Bernadette M. Melnyk, Kathy Malloch, and Lynn Gallagher-Ford

ADDITIONAL RESOURCES

Visit thePoint for additional helpful resources

- eBook
- Journal Articles
- WebLinks

CHAPTER OUTLINE

LEARNING OBJECTIVES

The learner will be able to:

1. Describe factors that are driving the need for innovative and transformational leaders in health care for the 21st century.
2. Identify nine health care leadership challenges of the 21st century.
3. Delineate three effective strategies to promote and sustain an evidence-based practice organizational culture.
4. Explain why effective leaders in the 21st century must engage in mentoring young leaders and succession planning today.

(continues on page 29)

5. Describe the characteristics required of leaders in order to effectively promote innovation and change.
6. Discuss the importance of teamwork, effective communication, and transdisciplinary/de-siloed work as they relate to health care outcomes.
7. List 13 essential characteristics of effective leaders.
8. Recognize the areas of change that have occurred as a result of the "electronic world."
9. Discuss the strengths and weaknesses of three leadership models: transactional, transformational, and complexity.
10. Distinguish the unique leadership components required in the complexity leadership model.

TODAY'S HEALTH CARE: IN CRITICAL CONDITION

The American health care system is in critical condition, with a tripling of costs over the past two decades, poor-quality services, wasteful spending, and a rise in medical errors (Hader, 2010). Half of the hospitals in the United States are functioning in deficit, and there are up to 200,000 unintended patient deaths every year (American Hospital Association, 2007). Furthermore, we are living in an era in which patients receive only approximately 55% of the care they should receive when they enter the health care system (Resar, 2006). The health care system is also facing the most severe shortage of health professionals, including physicians and nurses, it has ever encountered. The changing nature of morbidities in the United States (eg, a high prevalence of overweight/obesity, chronic diseases, and mental health disorders), the current condition of the health care system, and the severe shortage of health care professionals call for transformational and innovative leaders who will develop new models of transdisciplinary care and interprofessional education that will lead to the highest quality of evidence-based care and patient outcomes and, at the same time, decrease health care costs (ie, high-value health care) as well as limit the number of errors to attain high reliability (Melnyk, 2012).

This chapter presents nine critical leadership challenges for nurse leaders in the 21st century as well as 13 competencies needed to overcome these challenges. The chapter concludes with a discussion of leadership models for the 21st century and suggests that the complexity leadership model offers a new perspective for leadership and potential to support improved organizational performance.

TWENTY-FIRST-CENTURY LEADERSHIP CHALLENGES

The foregoing health care issues provide challenges or "character-builders" specific to nurse leaders in the 21st century. These challenges are listed in Box 3.1. Each individual nurse leader will have the opportunity to leverage the challenges of these times or be overwhelmed by them. Old models of autocratic, hierarchical leadership will not be adequate to handle the fast-paced, complex health care environment of the future. Leaders of today and in the future will need to be innovative, creative, flexible, engaging, courageous, relationship-based, and dynamic.

Leadership is not a "solo act"; it is imbedded in relationships, effective communication, shared ownership, and coaching and motivating others. Leadership must move from an autocratic, transactional model to innovative complexity leadership. Leaders who are steeped in traditional leadership styles and unwilling to grow and change their own practices will be particularly challenged by the dynamics of the health care environment that lies ahead. Leaders who are proactive and embrace

BOX 3.1 Nine 21st-Century Leadership Challenges

- Meeting expectations for increased productivity within budgetary constraints
- Advancing evidence-based practice
- Planning for succession and mentoring young nurse leaders
- Facilitating and enhancing teamwork and effective communication
- Embracing and supporting transdisciplinary health care
- Positioning nursing to influence decision making in organizational and health policy
- Promoting workplace wellness
- Striking a balance between technology and interpersonal relationships to deliver best care
- Creating cultures of innovation and change

new approaches, who are better suited for chaotic times, will be in the best position for dealing with the following challenges.

Meeting Expectations for Increased Productivity Within Rigorous Budgetary Constraints

Even in an era of major federal, state, and organizational budget reductions, leaders are expected to be highly productive with a scarcity of resources and financial constraints. In the theater of nursing, what exactly does "productive" encompass? Productivity includes both resource stewardship and delivery of the nursing "product" of safe, quality care. A major challenge for nurse leaders is to advocate for, attain, and maintain balance between these two key factors of nursing productivity. Nurse leaders need to use strategies where "caring management and financial constraints can coexist while promoting quality patient care" (Cara, Nyberg, & Brousseau, 2011).

Nurse leaders also need to understand and clearly articulate the inextricable connectedness of nurse engagement, productivity, and retention with caring and quality outcomes, which ultimately drive satisfaction and the financial well-being of the organization. Therefore, nurse leaders must be creative, innovative, entrepreneurial, and resourceful in garnering new resources and strategizing to maintain the core nursing value of caring to increase efficiency and to drive quality outcomes.

Advancing Evidence-Based Practice When Care in Many Health Care Institutions Remains Steeped and Mired in Tradition

Consider This A large number of medical errors occur because clinicians do not practice evidence-based health care.

The Institute of Medicine (IOM) named evidence-based practice (EBP) as a core competency for health care professionals (Greiner & Knebel, 2003). Shortly thereafter, the National Institutes of Health Roadmap initiative prioritized the acceleration of the transfer of knowledge from research into practice (Zerhouni, 2005; Research Study Fuels the Controversy 3.1). Furthermore, studies have supported that EBP enhances quality of care, improves patient outcomes, and decreases health care costs. Yet, in spite of all these, EBP is not the standard of practice in many health care organizations throughout the country (Harding, Porter, Horne-Thompson, Donley, & Taylor, 2014; Melnyk & Fineout-Overholt, 2015).

Findings from a survey of over 1,000 nurses randomly sampled from the American Nurses Association indicated that only one third of the nurses reported that their colleagues consistently implement EBP and only one third said they had EBP mentors. Further, the older the nurse, the less they were interested in gaining more

Research Study Fuels the Controversy 3.1

The Establishment of Evidence-Based Practice Competencies for Practicing Registered Nurses and Advanced Practice Nurses in Real-World Clinical Settings: Proficiencies to Improve Healthcare Quality, Reliability, Patient Outcomes, and Costs

In 2014, the first set of evidence-based practice (EBP) competencies for practicing nurses and advanced practice nurses was created. Consensus among a national panel of seven EBP experts was the first step in establishing the competencies followed by two rounds of a Delphi survey with 80 EBP mentors across the United States who validated them.

Source: Melnyk, B. M., Gallagher-Ford, L., Long, L. E., & Fineout-Overholt, E. (2014). The establishment of evidence-based practice competencies for practicing registered nurses and advanced practice nurses in real-world clinical settings: Proficiencies to improve healthcare quality, reliability, patient outcomes, and costs. *Worldviews on Evidence-Based Nursing, 11*(1), 5–15.

Study Findings

Two rounds of a Delphi survey with the 80 mentors resulted in a final set of 13 EBP competencies for practicing registered nurses and 11 additional competencies for advanced practice nurses. Leaders must create cultures and environments that support the implementation and sustainability of EBP. Integration of these competencies into health care system expectations, orientations, job descriptions, performance appraisals, and clinical ladder promotion process will enhance health care quality, safety, and consistency of health care interventions as well as reduce costs.

knowledge and skills in EBP (Melnyk, Fineout-Overholt, Gallagher-Ford, & Kaplan, 2012). Top barriers to EBP included time, organizational culture and politics, lack of EBP knowledge/education, lack of access to evidence/information, and leader/manager resistance.

Identification that leaders were a major barrier to EBP in this survey prompted yet another survey funded by Elsevier to further explore this finding. The survey with over 270 chief nurse executives across the United States revealed that although they believed in EBP, their own implementation of EBP was low. Further, although the chief nurses reported that their top priorities were health care quality and safety, EBP was rated as a low priority. These findings revealed a major disconnect in that many chief nurses do not see EBP as a direct pathway to quality and safety.

Therefore, leaders must have the knowledge and skills to create cultures of EBP that ignite a spirit of inquiry throughout the organization and cultivate an environment where EBP is the standard of care, not the exception. Unfortunately, although leaders report that they believe in the value of EBP, their own implementation of it is low (Sredl et al., 2011). It will be critical for nurse leaders to integrate evidence into their individual professional practices to deliver best leadership practice as well as to serve as EBP role models, which will influence their staff's EBP beliefs and implementation of evidence-based care. Recently developed tools, such as the new EBP competencies for practicing nurses and advanced practice nurses (Melnyk, Gallagher-Ford, Long, & Fineout-Overholt, 2014), will assist leaders in creating an infrastructure that supports EBP.

Discussion Point

As a new nurse leader, you are faced with an organization of nurses who in large part do not believe in or have the skills to deliver evidence-based care. What strategies would you embark upon early in your new role to begin to change that paradigm?

Planning for Leadership Succession and Mentoring Young Nurse Leaders

Continuity is a vital aspect of effective organizations; it is critical to strategic and operational goals. Disruption in an organization's continuity can have dire consequences. Disruption is particularly challenging in health care organizations because of the potential damage to confidence from the community and employees, the cost of unfinished business and negative impact on financing, and the harm to the organization's image and history (Bowen, 2014; Witt/Kieffer, 2004). Succession planning is the cure for this condition as the process is intended to create an internal leadership pipeline that identifies internal candidates to be promoted. These internal candidates require less time and effort to be oriented and are likely to be successful in their new position. This, in turn, allows organizations to accomplish at least two major goals during times of transition and turnover: (1) effective resource stewardship and (2) ongoing focus on accomplishing their strategic mission.

Succession planning also can be a very positive experience for the "up and coming" leaders in the organization. As individuals in the organization are given expanded opportunities, planned support, intentional mentorship, and effective and meaningful rewards and recognition, they develop their leadership portfolio and are less likely to be a "flight risk" (Blouin, McDonagh, Neistadt, & Helfand, 2006) to the organization.

Consider This Succession planning requires . . . planning! Have you thought about who will follow you and how you can influence their success?

One of the critical aspects of effective succession planning is mentoring. Studies have supported that nurses and physicians who have mentors tend to be more successful in and satisfied with their own careers (Beecroft, Santner, Lacy, Kunzman, & Dorey, 2006; Sambunjak, Straus, & Marusić, 2006). Mentoring can run the gamut from informal "in the moment" coaching to formal, planned meetings. "Giving talented future leaders the time, energy, advice, and experiences to gain new competencies and learn how to begin to prepare for future roles and responsibilities becomes the 'gift' a current leader can bestow upon a future leader" (Blouin et al., 2006, p. 328). Evidence has supported that mentoring programs decrease nursing turnover rates (Zucker et al., 2006). Both mentors and mentees benefit from the process of mentoring as professional and personal growth occurs.

Yet, despite all of its associated positive benefits, there has not been enough mentoring and empowering of young nurse leaders by more seasoned leaders in the nursing profession (Huston, 2010; Titzer & Shirey, 2013). As a result, the profession is highly vulnerable as large numbers of established nurse leaders will be retiring in the next decade and the resulting talent gap may cause nursing to lose much of the ground gained in health care in recent years. Intentional as well as informal mentoring of young leaders and strategic succession planning is an imperative for current nurse leaders in order to sustain the positive changes and significant outcomes cultivated during their tenures.

Facilitating and Enhancing Teamwork and Effective Communication

Communication has always been an important skill for all clinicians and teams with studies demonstrating the relationship between communication and patient safety. Effective communication among team members has been identified by the IOM as one of the markers of safe and highly reliable care (Kohn, Corrigan, & Donaldson, 2000).

Communication is not simply an exchange of information; it is a complex social process in which each party involved in the process brings history, assumptions, and expectations to the interaction (Lyndon, Zlatnik, & Wachter, 2011). "Effective (clinical) communication is clear, direct, explicit, and respectful" and "requires excellent listening skills, superb administrative support, and a collective commitment to move past traditional hierarchy and professional stereotyping" (p. 93). Communication, whether effective or ineffective, is jointly owned by all members of a team and each member is equally capable of engaging in good or bad communication tactics. Each member of the team enters the communication with different worldviews, values, fears, confidence level, and assumed place within the hierarchy. Effective communication requires conscious effort, shared commitment, and hard work.

Consider This Communication is a personal attribute and a learned skill. Do you have an understanding of your personal communication style? (How you communicate/how do you like to be communicated with?) There are many tools available that you can use to gain a better understanding of your style and how you interact with other individuals and teams and how you can modify your style to be more effective.

Leaders can significantly impact the success of teams and communication efforts in their organizations in a wide variety of ways. First, leaders must be effective communicators themselves and role model excellent communication skills in all settings. In addition, leaders are responsible to establish and uphold administrative structures to require and support effective teamwork and communication in their organizations. Finally, leaders must have the skills to effectively confront/manage conflicts that arise out of poor communications.

Embracing and Supporting Transdisciplinary Health Care

The complexity and multidimensional nature of health care and health problems require a different approach than the traditional, segregated, discipline-siloed approach to patient care that has often been the standard in health care organizations for decades. Transdisciplinary care has received a great deal of attention lately and is emerging as an essential requirement for health care. This approach includes true interprofessional decision making and trust among a variety of health care providers (Clark & Greenwald, 2013; Légaré, Ratté, Gravel, & Graham, 2008; Regan, Laschinger, & Wong, 2015). Transdisciplinary care assumes that merging the specialized knowledge from different health care disciplines together to act upon the same situation results in better and faster results for the recipient of that care (Vyt, 2008). Interprofessional collaboration, a key component of transdisciplinary care, has been demonstrated to improve patient care effectiveness for patients with chronic disease and a higher degree of work satisfaction in health care workers.

The challenge for leaders is to see the dynamics of health care through a contemporary lens, realize its complexities, and acknowledge that care must be evidence based and patient centered, both of which require a transdisciplinary, de-siloed approach. Leaders need to be well versed in tenets of this approach, able to model this approach in their leadership roles, and diligent in creating organizational settings and cultural milieus where this approach can thrive.

Positioning Nursing to Influence Decision Making in Organizational and Health Policy

Nurse leaders must not only be present in all health care and health policy venues but they must also be active contributors to key discussions and decision-making forums that influence the science and delivery of health care. They must also be proactive in assuring that nurses who are the best in representing certain topics are positioned at the organizational and health policy tables where those topics are being addressed. With an active presence at the "right tables," nurses are able to influence major decisions that positively influence health care quality, safety, and patient outcomes.

Discussion Point

Nurses are the largest sector of health care professionals, yet nurses rarely participate in health care policy decisions. Why does this dilemma persist? What can nurses (individually and as a united group) do to change this?

Promoting Workplace Wellness

Stress, burnout, and turnover continue to plague the nursing profession. This is particularly true for new graduates within the first year of employment (Cho, Laschinger, & Wong, 2006). In a recent study (Melnyk, Hrabe, & Szalacha, 2013), higher levels of workplace stress in new graduate nurses were associated with higher levels of depression and anxiety as well as lower levels of resiliency, job satisfaction, and healthy lifestyle beliefs. Furthermore, although nurses are typically great caregivers of others, their own health and wellness often suffer. In a recent Gallup (2012) survey, it was found that nurses have higher rates of smoking, obesity, hypertension, diabetes, and depression than physicians. Findings from another study by Spence Laschinger, Grau, Finegan, and Wilk (2011) found that, in addition to workload and bullying, psychological capital (ie, self-efficacy, optimism, hope, and resilience) was an important predictor of burnout in new nurses. Depression also has been found to be associated with prolonged absences from work (Franche et al., 2011).

Wellness includes physical, intellectual, mental, emotional, social, occupational, financial, environmental, and spiritual dimensions. Therefore, promoting workplace wellness in nurses is critical, whether they are new hires or long-term employees, not only to promote the health of nurses directly but also to enhance productivity and decrease absences and high turnover rates, which are very costly to the health care system. Workplace wellness requires a culture of respect and support, including definitive programs that address workplace abuse from patients as well as coworkers (Franche et al., 2011). Workplaces also must make healthy choices the easy choice to make.

Discussion Point

How healthy is your workplace, physically and emotionally?

What single action could you take to make your workplace healthier? When can you initiate that action? How healthy are you? What are you doing to promote *your* physical and emotional well-being? What single action could you take to make yourself healthier? When can you initiate that action?

Striking a Balance Between Technology and Interpersonal Relationships to Deliver Best Care

The impact of technology on health care in the past few decades has been startling, and this trend will surely continue into the future. The challenge for leaders as the next decades unfold will be in shifting from the current trend of technology driving our work to value-based health care quality and relationships as the drivers of our work, with technology supporting those drivers. Effective technology will need to be developed and designed with the "end users" (patients and providers) engaged, valued, and heard throughout the process.

Transformational and innovative leaders well versed in the concepts and language of technology development will be critical in forging the role and place of technology as an integrated component of health care in the future. They will need to understand and articulate the nonlinear and team-based nature of health care work, the innate complexity of the nature of life, and the essential requirement to deliver safe, timely, efficient, effective, equitable, patient-centered care through human interactions and relationships (Berwick, 2002).

Creating Cultures of Innovation and Change

An innovation is more than an idea—it is an idea that comes to fruition and sustains. Although leaders may say that innovation is important, they often do not model it themselves nor provide opportunities that foster innovation in others. For a change to be sustainable, it is not enough to simply create awareness about the change needed. To render a sustainable change, leaders must have the skills and capacity to manage the dynamics and processes associated with innovation as a lived experience (Porter-O'Grady & Malloch, 2010b).

To create a culture of innovation and change, leaders must acknowledge, embrace, and demonstrate engagement in innovation and change in their own leadership practices first. Only then are leaders able to help others to learn, embrace, and imbed the requirements of innovation and change into their individual practices.

Creating a culture of innovation and change is not a passive process; it requires active participation, role-modeling, and mentorship by the leaders involved. Leaders of organizations who do not model innovation are a barrier in creating and sustaining an innovative environment where positive change and outcomes continually occur (Melnyk & Davidson, 2009).

> **Consider This** Many people find change stressful. In addition, many people inherently resist change. Embracing change/innovation is a challenge for many traditional managers and leaders.

ESSENTIAL CHARACTERISTICS OF EFFECTIVE LEADERS

There are many characteristics that are essential for transformational and innovative leaders, of which 13 are detailed in Box 3.2. It is important to remember that titles do not produce effective leaders; leadership is derived from the combination of an individual's personal characteristics and how they mindfully act and interact with others. Informal leaders without titles who possess these characteristics are often far more respected than formal leaders with titles who do not possess these qualities.

Vision and the Ability to Inspire a Team Vision/Dream

> **Consider This** Nothing happens unless first a dream.
>
> —Carl Sandburg

There is nothing more important to achieving success than a potent dream/vision and an ability to inspire that vision in the team. The change efforts of many leaders fail because they focus too much on process and not enough on an exciting vision, although it does need to be recognized that vision without execution will also deter success. A motivational vision/dream will keep the energy of the leader and the team going when barriers, challenges, or fears are slowing or preventing outcomes from being achieved. Without an inspirational vision and a team who also buys into that vision, the likelihood of new initiatives being successfully attained is doubtful. In the health care environment of the future, characterized by constant change, switching directions, and continuous realignment of resources and priorities, the ability to set and achieve goals will be critical for a leader's success. Effective leaders in the 21st century will be those who can set a vision, guide others toward it, acknowledge progress along the way, and celebrate success relentlessly!

Passion for Patient Care and Making a Difference

> **Consider This** The main thing is to keep the main thing the main thing.
>
> —Stephen Covey

Historically, nurses have been perceived as *the* person on the health care team that "represents the patient" and "advocates for the patient." Placing the patient at the center of our work is not a stretch for nurses … it is

BOX 3.2 Thirteen Characteristics of Transformational and Innovative Leaders

- Vision and the ability to inspire a team vision/dream
- Passion for patient care and making a difference
- Transparency, honesty, integrity, and trust
- Effective communication skills
- The ability to lead/not micromanage
- Team, not "I," oriented
- Risk taking
- High level of execution
- Positive future orientation
- Innovative and entrepreneurial spirit
- Dedicated to coaching/mentoring
- Committed to motivating and empowering others to act/encouraging the heart
- Passion and persistence through the "character-building" experiences

part of nursing practice and it feels quite right to nurses. However, in the chaos and hustle-bustle of modern health care, it seems that this basic core value is lost at times. This simple idea must be reprioritized and be at the core of nursing, from the bedside to the leadership suite. It must remain an integral part of not only what defines us as clinicians but it must also be translated effectively to represent the value we bring to patients as well as to the health care delivery milieu.

When patient care is the focus of the leader's efforts, all of the trials and tribulations of the day take on a new perspective. As long as the first question to be answered is "what is the best thing to do for this patient?" a plan can be constructed to get there. With the patient as the focus, it is possible to connect staff with their passion for serving others and define a shared commitment to a set of beliefs about the way patients will be cared for, how families will be treated, how leadership will support that vision, and how staff will help each other. As health care becomes more complex, consumers become more educated, and expectations continue to escalate, having a clear and simple focus that drives the work being done will help nurse leaders to be effective and valued.

Transparency, Honesty, Integrity, and Trust

Consider This Few things help an individual more than to place responsibility upon him and to let him know that you trust him.

—Booker T. Washington

Transparency, honesty, and integrity are all critical elements for establishing trust. Over the past several decades and across many disciplines, much has been written about the importance of trust. It is considered by many to be the foundation or the basic building block for healthy relationships and effective functional teams. Leaders who are wise know that trust is critical to their success and they work every day to attain and to sustain it. Trust is a "two-way street" and to reap the full benefits of trust, a leader must develop relationships where he/she is trusted by team members *and* where team members are trusted by him/her as well. When words and actions match, when one is perceived as authentic, and when humility and reflection are common actions … trust will flourish. The benefits and rewards of relationships forged from trust are immeasurable, and it is in every nurse leaders' best interest to cultivate this attribute.

Discussion Point

As a nurse leader, you have a few nurse managers who hold things "tight to the vest" from their staff; they are not transparent. As a result, there is pervasive mistrust among the staff. How would you handle the situation?

Effective Communication Skills

Effective communication is critical to the safety of patients and the wellness of the workforce. By being effective communicators themselves and role modeling excellent communication skills at all times, leaders can significantly impact the success of teams and organizations. One of the earliest lessons presented in most nursing curriculums is to be attentive to verbal and nonverbal communication and to assess whether they are congruent in all interactions. This is a lesson that resonates whether one is taking care of a patient or presenting a strategic proposal at an executive board meeting. Words, tone, and nonverbal cues are all critically meaningful parts of communication. Effective leaders say what they mean, share as much information as they possibly can, and fully engage in their interpersonal interactions.

Within the scope of effective communication skills, the ability to listen cannot be emphasized enough. True listening to others is an incredibly powerful process. The effective listener not only obtains a tremendous amount of valuable information in the interaction but also begins, builds, or enhances their relationship with the other person.

However, it is not enough to simply have these skills and use them in the day-to-day operational context. Leaders must have the additional capacity and courage to use these skills effectively in the challenging times ahead in health care, to confront and manage the conflicts, dilemmas, and conundrums of the coming decades. Finally, in addition to being good communicators, leaders must fulfill their responsibility to establish and uphold administrative structures that assure effective teamwork and communication in their organizations.

The Ability to Lead/Not Micromanage

Consider This If you tell people where to go, but not how to get there, you'll be amazed at the results.

—General Patton

As a leader, it is critical to lead and sometimes to manage, but never micromanage. When you hire qualified people, you have to give them the freedom to carry out their jobs. Micromanagement is destructive at all levels and in every direction: vertical (manger/subordinate) as well as horizontal (peer/peer). When employees are micromanaged, they believe that their manager does not trust their work or judgment, which can often lead to employees' disengaging from their work and simply investing their time, but not their effort or creativity. The resulting dysfunctional work environment is characterized by employees feeling suffocated, which breeds contempt and distrust, both of which are extremely dangerous to teams, organizations, leaders, and, in the health care environment, patients! This cycle is a leader's nightmare.

Effective leaders understand and recognize the differences between managing and leading, and they choose to lead whenever possible. Managing people is a skill, whereas leading people is an art and it is an investment. It requires commitment, relationships, emotional intelligence, critical thinking, finesse, and time. The rewards and joys of effective leading compared to the dangers and drain of micromanaging make the effort to lead worthwhile every time.

> **Consider This** Informal leaders without a title can be more effective than leaders with a formal title.

Team, Not "I," Oriented

Teamwork is characterized by a set of interrelated activities accomplished by more than one person to achieve a common objective. Teamwork allows for engagement of many and the distribution of workload that enables each person to be more focused and efficient. Being on a team builds bonds among team members (being part of the team = being part of the solution), spawns creativity, and often generates a more robust outcome than could be achieved by a single individual. With all of this in mind, it would behoove any leaders to not squander the opportunity to work with and build effective teams.

Successful leaders understand the nature of teams and their role on a team. The effective leader, when working on a team, understands that the leader's goal is for the *team* to be successful. The effective leader knows that to be successful, each person must relinquish his or her own agenda for personal success and embrace the opportunity to share success with the team. Effective leaders understand that teams need different things from the leader at different stages of their development. A young team needs more direction and hand-holding, whereas a mature team needs more autonomy and freedom. The effective leader guides, motivates, listens to, critiques, and cheerleads the team, and in the end, earns the unique opportunity to celebrate successes as part of the team.

Risk Taking

> **Consider This** Progress always involves risk; you can't steal second base and keep your foot on first.
>
> —Frederick Wilcox

Many of the most successful people in life are the greatest risk takers. A definition of a risk taker is "a visionary change leader who can cope with the uncertainty that comes with change at the same time promoting innovation" (McGowan, 2007, p. 106). Risk taking is often related to "challenging the status quo." It requires a rigorous spirit of inquiry, relentless curiosity about the possibilities, and the courage to engage in both.

Risk taking is a complex undertaking that includes weighing risks against rewards and moving into a process/project with a clear vision of the benefits overshadowing the doubts. At the same time, successful risk takers proactively recognize the vulnerabilities of moving forward and develop "back up" plans to address unexpected problems.

Leaders of the future will necessarily have to be comfortable with taking risks because the health care environment in the coming decades is bound to be chaotic, unpredictable, messy, and frenetic. Every day in health care will be peppered with opportunities to be risk aversive or risk engaging, and those leaders who embrace and leverage risk effectively will be the success stories, looking at the others in their "rearview mirrors."

High Level of Execution

> **Consider This** We are judged by what we finish, not by what we start.
>
> —Unknown

Effective leaders understand that vision without execution will not lead to success, and so they begin their work with end point(s) in their mind and in their plan. They continuously think about outcomes, the bottom line, and/or the product to be delivered, but the critical difference of this attribute in great leaders is that they do this thinking/planning with finesse. They do not *only* focus on the outcome but also pay attention to the process and the people involved, but they never ever work without the end in mind.

Positive Future Orientation

Transformational leaders aim high, have a positive future orientation, and "live comfortably in the gap between reality and the organization's vision" (Balik & Gilbert, 2010, p. 14). They are never satisfied, and they are energized by dissatisfaction as opposed to being distressed by it. They convey a positive spirit in their organization as they look to the challenges ahead of them as opportunities, not obstacles (2010). Leaders in the chaotic health care environment of the future who address their work with this type of spirit and energy will be more likely to survive and thrive. The key to this attribute is that every individual gets to choose how they will face their day, and those leaders who choose a positive future orientation in their work will be more effective and more likely to *have* a positive future.

Innovative and Entrepreneurial Spirit

The current health care climate calls for leaders who are innovative and entrepreneurial. Resources are dwindling in most health care organizations, which require leaders to be more resourceful and creative in launching innovative and entrepreneurial initiatives that will lead to enhanced efficiency, revenue generation, and reduced costs. Leaders who create cultures of innovation and entrepreneurship will reap the benefits of an organization that thrives through uncertain times and budget constraints. According to Balik and Gilbert (2010), highly successful leaders in health care should "embrace a spirit of innovation, lead bold change, and find ways to lead from inside and outside health care—not only techniques, but changes in mind-set" and "learn to be prepared to lead an interdependent, agile organization with a non-hierarchical mentality that works as a team, with leaders defined by their actions, not by their title" (p. 256).

Dedication to Coaching/Mentoring

Coaching and mentoring young leaders is an imperative for nurse leaders in order to sustain the positive changes and significant outcomes cultivated during their tenure. The ability and desire to find and grow what is good in others is a hallmark of an effective leader. When you ask people ... "have you ever been mentored by someone?" they are immediately able to tell you who their mentor was and what that mentor did for them that was so life changing. Mentoring is a deep and powerful experience that enriches both the mentee and the mentor. Effective leaders understand the potential power to help others grow and engage in mentoring relationships in order to build effective young leaders and, ultimately, better organizations.

Discussion Point

What were the characteristics of individuals who have mentored you in your career? How did you know you were being mentored?

Is there someone in your work environment who you could/should be mentoring now? What can you do to begin that process?

Committed to Motivating and Empowering Others to Act/ Encouraging the Heart

The ability to truly motivate and empower others is a skill that effective leaders must possess. People are keenly aware of imposters when it comes to motivation and empowerment. The wise and effective leader knows that this aspect of leadership should only be fulfilled with pure and real intention or the results will be disastrous. Strategies and approaches to connecting with others to motivate them, grow them, and empower them, such as Kouzes and Posner's "encourage the heart," can serve leaders well in developing these attributes (Kouzes & Posner, 2007). These authors stress that leaders must make sure that people feel that what they do matters in their hearts. The practice of encouraging the heart is aligned with two commitments: (1) recognizing contributions by showing appreciation for individual excellence and (2) celebrating the values and victories by creating a spirit of community.

The sharing of stories can be an incredibly powerful tool for motivating and empowering others. Hearing about and relating to what others have lived, learned, or survived has served to help others for decades. Parents who have suffered the loss of a child who share their stories with other parents or with clinicians in training have demonstrated the power of storytelling. This type of exchange is emerging as a powerful tool for leaders to add to their toolkits (Melnyk & Fineout-Overholt, 2015).

Passion and Persistence Through the "Character-Building" Experiences

Consider This Many of life's failures are people who had not realized how close they were to success when they gave up.

—Thomas A. Edison

Passion is so critical, especially to avoid burnout and to keep you going when things get tough. Leaders need to know what their passion is and be able to access it and center on it when the environment intensifies. Persistence, described in the dictionary as an "enduring tenaciously," can be expressed quietly or loudly, but either way it is a key characteristic for effective health care leadership. Persistence is deeply connected to passion in that what you are passionate about you are likely to be persistent about. Nurse leaders must learn the power of passion and persistence and leverage both wisely to attain vision and goals.

Discussion Point

How many of these 13 essential characteristics have you mastered? Which of these characteristics do your coworkers, peers, direct reports, and supervisors attribute to you? What characteristics can you improve upon?

MODELS OF LEADERSHIP FOR THE 21ST CENTURY

Over the last 30 years, different types and styles of leadership have been used by nurse leaders. Both transactional and transformational models are commonplace in varying degrees in health care organizations. In spite of many successes with these models, nurse leaders continue to struggle with patient quality, financial limitations, time management, knowledge access, information sharing, and effective communication. Not surprisingly, leaders are continually searching for the holy grail of leadership, that ultimate, ideal model that effectively guides success in their respective organizations.

The work in today's health care organizations is increasingly complex and filled with digital tools and resources. Specifically, the digital world has changed when we work, where work takes place, and the media for information transfer. This digital revolution results in changes in clinical work processes, including relationships between and among employees, patients, and the community; and the speed at which information is processed, available, and shared. These changes challenge the best of traditional leadership models and render them ineffectual in many situations and settings. Understanding the dynamics of these changes is the first step in determining optimal leadership models that will be effective moving forward.

Scharmer and Käufer (2000) identified four areas of change as a result of the electronic world: media, time, space, and structure. *Media* is the first and refers to the form in which information is documented, shared, and transmitted. In the information age, the Internet has revolutionized how information is transmitted. Flash drives and discs are the norm for data storage. The digitization of information has dramatically reduced the size and format of information. Less physical space is required for papers and files. In many cases, the information is virtual, requiring only electronic storage space. It is now possible for information to be sent to nearly anyone, at anytime, anywhere in the world. The majority of documents can be digitized and thus provide for increased consistency and quality of information. For leaders, the written or typed modality is no longer the most reliable; digitized documentation of information is now the more effective and efficient media for information.

With the nearly open access to the Internet, *time* for work is now wide open as well. The open access to individuals at any time of the day or night increases the emphasis on speed and efficiency. Lag times are decreased allowing for almost instantaneous responses and actions. Given the emphasis on speed and efficiency, this new reality of time as an open concept requires leaders think differently about when work is done. Furthermore, the new reality blurs the work–personal time boundaries creating more challenges. Leaders are now required to shift the emphasis on specific times for work based on a traditional five-day, eight-hour day in which an individual is present in the workplace to different models. Now, the leader is required to recognize and value work products wherever they are done rather than time present in the workplace. In health care, different models for work time necessarily exist for those providing patient care. The blurring of boundaries for work time necessarily creates two significant challenges: (a) being physically present when there is value in presence and (b) in assuring separation of work and personal time for healthy work–life balance.

As time and media conceptualizations have evolved, the *space* required for work also has changed. While single offices are still commonplace, the actual time spent by individuals in offices is decreasing. The portability of media and ready access to the Internet allows for work to be completed in many locations rather than in the traditional office. It is now possible to perform work wherever the information is accessible. Conference calls and electronic communication have decreased the need for physical gatherings. Individuals gathering at common physical sites are less and less the norm. The trend is to increase flexible spaces for individual and group meetings while decreasing individual office spaces.

The final major change is organizational *structure*. Given the new realities of information and communication exchange, the underlying structure for how work is organized is now open and free flowing. These changes impact organizational structure in numerous ways. The traditional levels of authority diagrams, communication pathways, and span of control are now secondary guides for the organization rather than the primary expectations for communication and permissions. In the digital age, any employee or patient or community members can now communicate with anyone in the organization using electronic mail. Documents or pictures can be shared with anyone in the organization at any time without seeking multiple layers of permissions. For these reasons, it is no wonder that leaders are struggling to be effective and efficient. The rules and principles under which transactional and transformational leadership emerged originally are quite different in the digital age. In the next section, an overview of the strengths and weaknesses of transactional and transformational leadership models followed by the emerging complexity leadership model is presented. Table 3.1 presents a comparison of the three model characteristics. This information is designed to assist leaders in understanding leadership models from a historical perspective and also to determine the role of leaders and leadership for the future.

Transactional or *instrumental* leadership is the most common and well-known leadership style used in health care. In this model, the focus is on task orientation, leader direction, follower participation with the expectation of rewards, threats, or disciplinary action from the leader (Bass & Bass, 2008; see Table 3.1). Research specific to transactional leadership supports the belief that personality traits are consistently correlated with the emergence and effectiveness of leaders. In a transactional model, leaders expect followers to support their goals; a job for the follower is exchanged for support of the leader's vision. In a transactional model, leaders have traditionally relied on traits believed to support and facilitate the role of the leader. Examples of trait theories that focus on the behaviors of the leader include the following:

- Great man theory: Throughout history, great men such as Abraham Lincoln, John Kennedy, and Bill Gates emerged as leaders.
- Biological-genetic theories: Some individuals were born to lead, a natural leader.
- Traits of individuals specific to qualities: Intelligence, scholarship, gender, dependability, situation, age,

TABLE 3.1 Characteristics of Three Leadership Models

	Transactional	Transformational	Complexity
Focus	Planned work	Planned work	Emerging and transitional work
Locus of power	Individual leader-centric/ position; formal	Individual leader-centric/ position; formal	Team/group/relationship-centric network focus and informal
Work	Defined/prescribed; rule driven	Defined/prescribed; rule and principle driven	Emergent; principle driven
Communication direction	Top-down; authoritarian	Top-down; authoritarian	Multiple directions
Competencies	Plan, organize, direct, reward, punish	Plan, organize, direct, reward, punish, empower, collaborate	Facilitate, coach, collaborate
Organizational boundaries	Defined	Defined	Overlapping, informal

emotional competence, physique, fluency of speech, self-sufficiency, socioeconomic status, social activity, tact, popularity, and so on are common to leaders.

The limitations of transactional leadership include focus on a single individual as the source of knowledge and power; the role of the follower is to follow directions and support the vision of the leader. Creativity, self-actualization, and empowerment of followers are perceived as inappropriate in this model.

The second most common leadership model is *inspirational* or *transformational* and emphasizes the emotional and ideological appeals using exemplary behavior, confidence, symbolism, and intrinsic motivation (Bass & Bass, 2008). More recently, leaders have embraced the notion of transformational leadership, a style in which the leader forms relationships of mutual stimulation and elevation that converts followers into leaders (Bryman, Collinson, Grint, Jackson, & Uhl-Bien, 2011). In a transformational leadership model, the work of managing meaning, infusing ideological values, and co-creation of goals is recognized as processes of empowerment for both the leader and the follower. The exchange between the leader and the follower is elevated to include the value of personal growth for the follower.

Transformational leadership begins to engage followers to self-actualize and contribute to the organization and offers significant advantage over transactional leadership. The limitation of transformational leadership is the locus of power that still remains with the leader; the leader is expected to begin the empowerment processes to engage employees rather than employees being expected to lead from their position in the organization. Formal leaders, those designated with an official leadership position, are the norm while informal leadership is not recognized.

In spite of the advancements in the transformational leadership model, the ability for the organization to optimize the knowledge and competencies of all members of the organization in a fluid and timely manner is still limited. Continuing to rely on bureaucratic, top-down processes is counterproductive in the presence of the critical dynamics of the digital media, time, space, and structure advancements. Considerations for the changes resulting from the digital advancements are needed to support the uncertain, emergent, and highly interconnected nature of the environment as well as the organizational culture.

Congruency between the leadership model, namely, how work occurs, and the underlying assumptions, values, and artifacts of the organization are positively correlated and impact organizational efficiency and effectiveness (Casida & Pinto-Zipp, 2008). Thus, a new leadership model must necessarily integrate the organization culture and local environment. Advancing our current leadership models to address the identified challenges of overwhelming work volumes, fewer financial resources, and increases in complexity of providing patient care will provide an improved framework for leaders. The *complexity leadership model* offers a futuristic perspective for leadership and potential to support improved organizational performance.

Complexity leadership models are based on complexity leadership theory (CLT) and provide a new lens for leadership to increase effectiveness and efficiency (Uhl-Bien & Marion, 2008). This model recognizes health care organizations as networks of people, resources, knowledge, and other entities composed of overlapping, informal boundaries; leadership is both positional and informal, incorporating the full potential of human and social capital (Hanson & Ford, 2010, p. 6588).

The assumptions in a complexity leadership model are as follows:

- Positional and informal leaders fulfill diverse functions in the organization.
  - Positional leaders carry authority focused on managing organizational dynamics and enabling informal initiatives rather than directing or mandating behaviors.
  - Informal leaders emerge based on relationships.
- Control is difficult if not impossible; uncertainty is the norm.
- System boundaries cannot be defined as all interactions are human and interconnected.
- Leadership is the accountability of every individual in the organization specific to the assigned role.
- Power does not rest solely with an individual(s); power is distributed among the members of the organization and is located within relationships.
- High degrees of individual interactions are the norm.

Within the CLT model, three types of leadership functions are identified; *administrative, adaptive,* and *enabling.* Interestingly, CLT embraces some aspects of transactional and transformational leadership. The CLT model provides a more robust and congruent model for leadership. The *administrative* leadership component is somewhat similar to the transactional model. This work is about coordinating and planning organizational activities with less hierarchy and formality and thereby sustaining the framework of the organization. The goal is to minimize excessive control and bureaucracy and reinforce the adaptive work of others. The *adaptive* aspect of the model is about the emergence of optimal outcomes from interrelationships and interactions. Collaboration among individuals to produce collective best outcomes is the overall goal of the adaptive leadership role. Some similarities to the transformation model can be gleaned from the adaptive role. The *enabling* role is the new dimension and serves to foster and optimize adaptive work processes and mediate the tensions that occur between administrative and adaptive functions. Enabling leadership works to minimize bureaucratic controls, support the emergence of collective wisdom, and recognize the value of the multiple interactions of individuals as the way work occurs. This brief description of the CLT serves as the foundation for reframing the contemporary leadership model into a trimodal model to better meet the needs of today's challenges (Malloch, 2010).

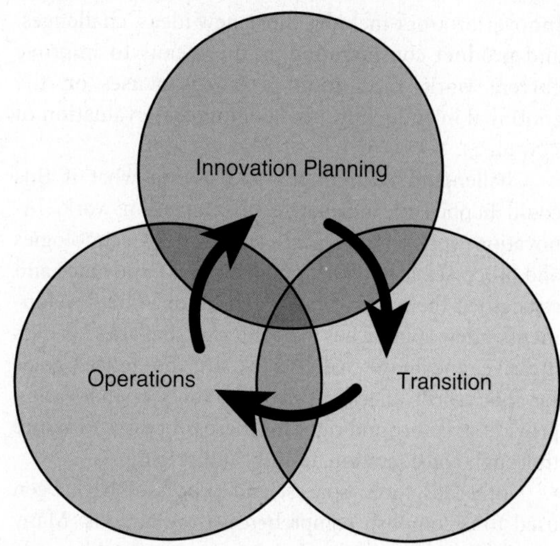

Figure 3.1 Trimodal Leadership.

The current work to meet the paradoxical nature of health care in which both stability and creativity are expected encompasses innovation and transition or transformation between operations and innovation. The organizational culture in a trimodal organization reinforces evidence-driven processes. It is also consistent with the work of innovation in which new ideas are encouraged, tested, validated, and implemented when evidence for improvement is available. The organizational culture also strongly supports the transition phase between innovation and operations. Oftentimes, new ideas are embraced and moved from innovation to operations without the necessary time to change to become embedded into the culture. Such changes are often discarded or at best modified. In the trimodal model, transition work is as important as operations and innovation work (Fig. 3.1).

The trimodal model reframes and identifies three vital work processes for leaders: operational stability, innovative leadership, and transformation from innovation to operations. These three categories are designed to manage the present, look to the future, and support the processes in between. A brief explanation of the three components excerpted from Porter-O'Grady and Malloch (2010a) follows.

Operations or the work of providing evidence-based patient care within a defined structure with supportive staff and resources comprises the majority of traditional health care work. This work is typically planned, funded, and evaluated within an operations model. Given the predictive nature of this work, it can be thought of as the technical work of an organization, provided by highly skilled professionals. Health care leaders balance and support multiple operational entities and initiatives, medical-surgical services, ambulatory services, pharmacy services, medical imaging, and others.

The new work, with greater variability and complexity, requires leaders to shift from an emphasis on operations to a model that values and integrates the work of change, innovation, and the transition between operations and innovation. It is unclear as to what the exact proportion of effort should be for each of these modes; however, it is clear that less time will be spent in operations, with increasing attention to innovation and transition to new levels of operational work.

Traditional operations change in several ways. The emphasis by operations on standardization shifts to one of accountability for work assignments and roles. There is a shift from an emphasis on rules to a focus on principles. Knowing that procedures will change, standardization and consistency must be continually challenged as new information and technologies are introduced. This approach recognizes the temporary nature of most work processes. The emphasis now shifts to the appropriateness of the work performed rather than the completion of checklists.

The second aspect of work in the trimodal model is innovation planning. In this model, innovation work is considered essential rather than optional.

Innovation work includes those new ideas, challenges, and product consideration as the means to improve current work. Innovation planning focuses on the continual introduction, challenging, and evaluation of new ideas.

Challenging assumptions and asking what if this could happen are normative in innovation work. Innovation work considers any and all new technologies and processes as potential opportunities to advance and strengthen the work of the organization. The development of new approaches to health care that are safer, less invasive, and more cost-effective are the desired goals for this aspect of leadership. The tools of innovation provide structure and rigor for these processes to assure thorough consideration, testing, and pricing.

Numerous tools, spaces, and processes have been used to accomplish comprehensive evaluations. Many organizations have created physical space for this work; however, the emphasis is more on thinking differently, researching available technologies and the needs of clients. This thinking work does not require a specific physical space, but rather a physical or virtual space that supports creative, safe, and respectful dialog. Necessarily, the structure for this work is loose to allow for creativity and openness.

The work of innovation planning is not only about looking at new ideas and products but also includes improving or eliminating current ineffective or poorly functioning processes. Furthermore, when organizations are faced with fewer resources, negative outcomes, or shortages of workers, the innovation planning team can begin to assist with creative dialogue to seek greater efficiencies without compromising on quality.

The third aspect of the trimodal model is the transition work that is needed to sustain change and transform work processes. The significance and complexity of facilitating and assuring an effective transition between innovation and operations is too often overlooked or underestimated. Once new ideas are identified and determined to be suitable for future work, sustainable pathways to modify roles, competencies, infrastructure, technology, funding, and the cultural norms must also evolve. Changing the culture requires much more than a single educational program; it requires persistence and focus. When innovations are introduced into a traditional culture without adequate transition support and modification of the existing work, the innovations are most likely to be considered fads and dismissed quickly. New ideas are considered burdens rather than opportunities to remain competitive and achieve the highest-quality outcomes. Participants are more likely to engage in new work at higher levels when they know the rationale for change, are able to test the knowledge in practice, and can support the ethical expectations for professional practice. Transition is about cultural transformation and requires time, reinforcement, and frequent course corrections to successfully embed new practices into the evolving culture at the point of service level.

Given that the needed leadership model necessarily emerges from the time, place, and circumstances in which the organization exists, the leader often relies on multiple leadership perspectives to achieve desired goals. For example, a transactional approach is appropriate when there are regulations to enforce; discussion about whether or not to comply is not appropriate or helpful unless the intent is to propose new regulation. Transformational behaviors—within a complexity leadership model—are appropriate when the focus is on individuals (Malloch, 2014). A complexity approach is most appropriate for the realities of today's health care world. For example, health care reform requirements, namely the emphasis on population health, coordination of care across the life span, and the delivery of value to health care users, are ideally supported by an open and networked approach that aligns the leadership behaviors and beliefs with the nature of this complex and uncertain work.

Understanding one's approach to decision making, conflict-utilization style, comfort with change, uncertainty, errors, and challenging assumptions are essential for the innovation leader. In addition, basic knowledge of innovation principles, collaboration at the highest and most uncommon levels to foster diversity, and comfort with coaching other to fully engage in the work of the organization are selected competencies that all member of the organization are likely to pursue. The following four principles provide guidance in assuring the alignment of work to be done with supportive leadership behaviors to achieve desired outcomes:

- Self-knowledge: Knowledge of personal ability to manage one's ego, to facilitate others to be fully engaged in the work, and courage to lead in all situations is necessary.
- Value: Value is created through full engagement of all individuals involved in the work of achieving improved health.
- Teamwork: Working in teams is a dynamic process and often requires specific direction from a leader rather than consensus building to achieve timely and value-based outcomes (Coutu, 2009; Frisch, 2008; Hansen, 2009).

- Evidence: When addressing challenges, consideration of available evidence and the need for innovation when evidence is lacking is important in determining what approach is needed for success—a traditional change process or an innovation strategy.

Conclusions

To be successful, leaders must possess important characteristics to overcome the major challenges that plague health care in the 21st century. Major challenges facing today's leaders include dwindling resources, organizations, and practices steeped in tradition, and intense pressures to achieve high-value, high-reliability organizations. Leaders must possess numerous essential characteristics, such as an ability to inspire a team vision, effective communication skills, integrity, and an ability to mentor and encourage their team to excel among others, in order to be effective. Although many leadership models exist, the complexity model combined with innovation leadership holds the most promise for best outcomes in dealing with 21st century leadership challenges.

For Additional Discussion

1. How do traditional attributes associated with the nursing profession (caring, advocacy, service, etc.) promote effective leadership in the 21st century? How might these traditional attributes hinder effective leadership in the 21st century?
2. How could traditional nursing attributes be proactively and thoughtfully leveraged to influence health care decisions in the 21st century?
3. Are health care leaders "walking the talk"/role-modeling EBP by integrating evidence into their daily management decision making? How can this leadership paradigm shift be enhanced?
4. How could formal leadership training for nurse managers and leaders impact hospitals in terms of saving money related to recruitment, nursing satisfaction, nurse wellness, and retention?
5. Compare and contrast the three leadership models identified in Table 3.1. How does each model facilitate patient safety? Also, how can each model be a barrier to patient safety?
6. Is there a model of leadership that better supports leadership at the point of service? Why? Why not?

References

American Hospital Association. (2007). *TrendWatch chartbook 2007: Trends affecting hospitals and health systems*. Retrieved from http://www.aha.org/aha/trendwatch/chartbook/2007/07chapter4.ppt#10

Balik, M. B., & Gilbert, J. A. (2010). *The heart of leadership: Inspiration and practical guidance for transforming your health care organization*. Chicago, IL: AHA Press.

Bass, B. M., & Bass, R. (2008). *Handbook of leadership: Theory, research, and management* (4th ed.). New York, NY: Free Press.

Beecroft, P. C., Santner, S., Lacy, M. L., Kunzman, L., & Dorey, F. (2006). New graduate nurses' perceptions of mentoring: Six-year program evaluation. *Journal of Advanced Nursing, 55*(6), 736–747.

Berwick, D. M. (2002). A user's manual for the IOM's "quality chasm" report. *Health Affairs, 21*(3), 80–90.

Blouin, A. S., McDonagh, K. J., Neistadt, A. M., & Helfand, B. (2006). Leading tomorrow's healthcare organizations: Strategies and tactics for effective succession planning. *The Journal of Nursing Administration, 36*(6), 325–330.

Bowen, D. J. (2014). The growing importance of succession planning. *Healthcare Executive, 29*(4),8.

Bryman, A., Collinson, D., Grint, K., Jackson, B., & Uhl-Bien, M. (Eds.). (2011). *The SAGE handbook of leadership*. London, England: Sage.

Cara, C. M., Nyberg, J. J., & Brousseau, S. (2011). Fostering the coexistence of caring philosophy and economics in today's health care system. *Nursing Administration Quarterly, 35*(1), 6–14.

Casida, J., & Pinto-Zipp, G. (2008). Leadership–organizational culture relationships in nursing units of acute care hospitals. *Nursing Economic$, 26*(1), 7–15.

Cho, J., Laschinger, H. K. S., & Wong, C. (2006). Workplace empowerment, work engagement and organizational commitment of new graduate nurses. *Nursing Leadership, 19*(3), 43–60.

Clark, R. C., & Greenwald, M. (2013). Nurse–physician leadership: Insights into interprofessional collaboration. *The Journal of Nursing Administration, 43*(12), 653–659.

Coutu, D. (2009). Why teams don't work. *Harvard Business Review, 87*(5), 99–103, 105.

Franche, R. L., Murray, E., Ibrahim, S., Smith, P., Carnide, N., Cote, P., . . . Koehoorn, M. (2011). Examining the impact of worker and workplace factors on prolonged work absences among Canadian nurses. *Journal of Occupational and Environmental Medicine, 53*(8), 919–927.

Frisch, B. (2008). When teams can't decide. *Harvard Business Review, 86*(10), 121–126.

Gallup. (2012). U.S. physicians set good health example. Retrieved from http://www.gallup.com/poll/157859/physicians-set-good-health-example.aspx

Greiner, A. C., & Knebel, E. (Eds.). (2003). *Health professions education: A bridge to quality.* Washington, DC: The National Academies Press.

Hader, R. (2010). The evidence that isn't... Interpreting research. *Nursing Management, 41*(9), 22–26. doi:10.1097/01.NUMA.0000387083.21113.09

Hansen, M. T. (2009). When internal collaboration is bad for your company. *Harvard Business Review, 87*(4), 83–88.

Hanson, W. R., & Ford, R. (2010). Complexity leadership in healthcare: Leader network awareness. *Procedia—Social and Behavioral Sciences, 2*(4), 6587–6596.

Harding, K. E., Porter, J., Horne-Thompson, A., Donley, E., & Taylor, N. F. (2014). Not enough time or a low priority? Barriers to evidence-based practice for allied health clinicians. *The Journal of Continuing Education in the Health Professions, 34*(4), 224–231.

Huston, C. J. (2010). *Professional issues in nursing: Challenges and opportunities* (2nd ed.). Philadelphia, PA: Lippincott Williams & Wilkins.

Kohn, L. T., Corrigan, J. M., & Donaldson, M. (Eds.). (2000). *To err is human: Building a safer health system.* Washington, DC: Institute of Medicine.

Kouzes, J. M., & Posner, B. Z. (2007). *The leadership challenge* (4th ed.). San Francisco, CA: Jossey-Bass.

Légaré, F., Ratté, S., Gravel, K., & Graham, I. D. (2008). Barriers and facilitators to implementing shared decision-making in clinical practice: Update of a systematic review of health professionals' perceptions. *Patient Education and Counseling, 73*(3), 526–535.

Lyndon, A., Zlatnik, M. G., & Wachter, R. M. (2011). Effective physician–nurse communication: A patient safety essential for labor and delivery. *American Journal of Obstetrics & Gynecology, 205*(2), 91–96.

Malloch, K. (2010). Innovation leadership: New perspectives for new work. *The Nursing Clinics of North America, 45*(1), 1–10.

Malloch, K. (2014). Beyond transformational leadership to greater engagement: Inspiring innovation in complex organizations. *Nurse Leader, 12*(2), 60–63.

McGowan, J. J. (2007). Swimming with the sharks: Perspectives on professional risk taking. *Journal of the Medical Library Association, 95*(1), 104–113.

Melnyk, B. M. (2012). Achieving a high reliability organization through implementation of the ARCC model for system-wide sustainability of evidence-based practice. *Nursing Administration Quarterly, 36*(2), 127–135.

Melnyk, B. M., & Davidson, S. (2009). Creating a culture of innovation in nursing education through shared vision, leadership, interdisciplinary partnerships and positive deviance. *Nursing Administration Quarterly, 33*(4), 1–8.

Melnyk, B. M., & Fineout-Overholt, E. (2015). *Evidence-based practice in nursing & healthcare: A guide to best practice* (3rd ed.). Philadelphia, PA: Wolters Kluwer.

Melnyk, B. M., Fineout-Overholt, E., Gallagher-Ford, L., & Kaplan, L. (2012). The state of evidence-based practice in US nurses: Critical implications for nurse leaders and educators. *The Journal of Nursing Administration, 42*(9), 410–417.

Melnyk, B. M., Gallagher-Ford, L., Long, L. E., & Fineout-Overholt, E. (2014). The establishment of evidence-based practice competencies for practicing registered nurses and advanced practice nurses in real-world clinical settings: Proficiencies to improve healthcare quality, reliability, patient outcomes, and costs. *Worldviews on Evidence-Based Nursing, 11*(1), 5–15.

Melnyk, B. M., Hrabe, D. P., & Szalacha, L. A. (2013). Relationships among work stress, job satisfaction, mental health, and healthy lifestyle behaviors in new graduate nurses attending the Nurse Athlete program: A call to action for nursing leaders. *Nursing Administration Quarterly, 37*(4), 278–285.

Porter-O'Grady, T., & Malloch, K. (2010a). *Innovation leadership: Creating the landscape of health care*. Sudbury, MA: Jones & Bartlett.

Porter-O'Grady, T., & Malloch, K. (2010b). Innovation: Driving the green culture in healthcare. *Nursing Administration Quarterly, 34*(4), E1–E5.

Regan, S., Laschinger, H. K., & Wong, C. A. (2015). The influence of empowerment, authentic leadership, and professional practice environments on nurses' perceived interprofessional collaboration. *Journal of Nursing Management*. doi:10.1111/jonm.12288

Resar, R. K. (2006). Making noncatastrophic health care processes reliable: Learning to walk before running in creating high reliability organizations. *Health Services Research, 41*(4, Pt. 2), 1677–1689.

Sambunjak, D., Straus, S. E., & Marusić, A. (2006). Mentoring in academic medicine: A systematic review. *The Journal of the American Medical Association, 296*(9), 1103–1115.

Scharmer, C. O., & Käufer, K. (2000). *Universities as the birthplace for the entrepreneuring human being*. Retrieved August 14, 2011, from http://www.ottoscharmer.com/docs/articles/2000_Uni21us.pdf

Spence Laschinger, H. K., Grau, A. L., Finegan, J., & Wilk, P. (2011). Predictors of new graduate nurses' well-being: Testing the job demands-resources model. *Health Care Management Review, 37*(2), 175–186.

Sredl, D., Melnyk, B. M., Hsueh, K. H., Jenkins, R., Ding, C. D., & Durham, J. (2011). Health care in crisis: Can nurse executives' beliefs about and implementation of evidence-based practice be key solutions in health care reform? *Teaching and Learning in Nursing, 6*, 73–79.

Titzer, J. L., & Shirey, M. R. (2013). Nurse manager succession planning: A concept analysis. *Nursing Forum, 48*(3), 155–164. doi:10.1111/nuf.12024.

Uhl-Bien, M., & Marion, R. (Eds.). (2008). *Complexity leadership, Part I: Conceptual foundations*. Charlotte, NC: Information Age.

Vyt, A. (2008). Interprofessional and transdisciplinary teamwork in healthcare. *Diabetes/Metabolism Research and Reviews, 24*(Suppl. 1), S106–S109.

Witt/Kieffer. (2004). *Putting succession planning in play: Identifying and developing the healthcare organization's successors*. Oak Brook, IL: Author.

Zerhouni, E. (2005). US biomedical research: Basic, translational, and clinical sciences. *JAMA, 294*(11), 1352–1358.

Zucker, B., Goss, C., Williams, D., Bloodworth, L., Lynn, M., Denker, A., & Gibbs, J. D. (2006). Nursing retention in the era of a nursing shortage: Norton Navigators. *Journal for Nurses in Staff Development, 22*(6), 302–306.

4

Advanced Practice Nursing
Where is the DNP Today?

Margaret J. Rowberg

ADDITIONAL RESOURCES

Visit thePoint the point for additional helpful resources

- eBook
- Journal Articles
- WebLinks

CHAPTER OUTLINE

LEARNING OBJECTIVES

The learner will be able to:

1. Provide an overview of doctoral degree program and graduate growth over the last 10 years.
2. Describe the driving and restraining forces for increasing the entry educational level for advanced practice nursing to that of a practice doctorate.
3. Describe the impetus for and controversies associated with the granting of the Doctor of Nursing Practice (DNP) degree.

According to the American Association of Colleges of Nursing (AACN) (2010), "The health system's increasing demand for front-line primary care, and the accelerating drive toward managed care, prevention, and cost-efficiency are driving a need for nurses with advanced practice skills in this country" (para. 16). There are four categories of nurses considered to be advanced practice registered nurses (APRNs) nurse practitioners (NPs), clinical nurse specialists (CNSs), certified nurse midwives (CNMs), and certified registered nurse anesthetists (CRNAs).

According to the most recent National Sample Survey of Registered Nurses, there were more than 254,000 APRNs in the United States in 2008 (U.S. Department of Health and Human Services, Health Resources and Services Administration (HRSA), 2010, p. 5–2). This number increased to more than 330,000 in 2014. Over 205,000 of the APRNs in the United States are NPs, according to the American Association of Nurse Practitioners (2014). The National Association of Clinical Nurse Specialists (NACNS) (2014) reports that there are more than 72,000 CNSs. Further, the American College of Nurse-Midwives (ACNM) (2014) stated that there were over 11,000 certified nurse-midwives (CNM), while the American Association of Nurse Anesthetists (AANA) (2015) confirm that there are more than 48,000 CRNAs in the U.S. Advanced practice registered nurses (APRNs) constitute nearly 10% of the RN workforce in this country (AACN, 2011).

APRNs have been making significant contributions to the health of the nation and around the world for almost 50 years, but they function in a health care system in the United States that is in need of change. In 1999, the Institute of Medicine (IOM) (1999) published its sentinel report *To Err Is Human: Building a Safer Health System* that stated that as many as 98,000 people die each year due to errors that occur while receiving health care. The IOM (2001) further reported, "research on quality of care reveals a health care system that frequently falls short in its ability to translate knowledge into practice, and to apply new technology safely and appropriately" (p. 3).

> **Discussion Point**
>
> How can nursing address the need for nurses who are educated with an emphasis on evidence-based practice?

Although the early IOM reports have been in existence for more than a decade, an unacceptable high number of errors continue to be reported. New safeguards have been put in place in most institutions, but nursing can and should be the key profession in leading the way to significant change to the health care system. According to the latest IOM (2011) report, "The Future of Nursing: Leading Change, Advancing Health,"

> *The nursing profession has the potential capacity to implement wide-reaching changes in the health care system...By virtue of their regular, close proximity to patients and their scientific understandings of care processes across the continuum of care, nurses have a considerable opportunity to act as full partners with other health care professionals and to lead in the improvement and redesign of the health care system and its practice environment.* (p. 23)

Unfortunately, however, although APRNs (or APNs) are skilled clinical practitioners, many do not have the knowledge and expertise needed to address the persistent professional issues that arise in the health care system. In response, the AACN initiated several task forces to assess these issues. In 2002, one expert group was asked "to examine the current status of clinical or practice doctoral programs, compare various models, and make recommendations regarding future development" (AACN, 2004, p. 1). The group was to determine whether a practice doctorate would be an appropriate degree for APRNs. Another task force was asked to assess how nursing could provide the kind of leadership needed in light of the issues in the health care system and the ever-increasing nursing shortage. Ultimately, the Board of the AACN proposed to its members that the Doctor of Nursing Practice (DNP) degree be developed.

Several nursing schools had existing practice doctorate programs, and many more were assessing whether to develop such a program. The AACN (2013b) thought it would be appropriate to develop a position about this degree because it believed that nursing had the "unparalleled opportunity and capability to address the critical issues that face the nation's current health care system" (p. 3). They also believed that nursing "has the answer to the predominant health care dilemmas of the future" (p. 3) and that "each of the prevailing health problems is suited to the nursing paradigm...Their amelioration is what nursing students are educated to do" (p. 4). Consequently, the AACN, upon task force recommendation, proposed furthering the development of a clinical practice doctoral degree.

Much has been written and published regarding the recommendations of the AACN task force. This chapter discusses the development of the DNP degree and offers some insight into the current trends, issues, and concerns surrounding this evolving role.

THE DOCTOR OF NURSING PRACTICE DEGREE

It is important to start the discussion of the DNP with the exact words from AACN to clarify why it recommended that this new degree be developed. In its classic position statement, the AACN (2004) stated:

> *Doctoral programs in nursing and other practice disciplines can be categorized into two distinct types: research-focused and practice-focused. The term practice, specifically nursing practice, as conceptualized in this document refers to any form of nursing intervention that influences health care outcomes for individuals or populations, including the direct care of individual patients, management of care for individuals and populations, administration of nursing and health care organizations, and the development and implementation of health policy. Preparation at the practice doctorate level includes advanced preparation in nursing, based on nursing science, and is at the highest level of nursing practice.*
>
> *What distinguishes this definition of practice from others is that it includes both direct care provided to patients by individual clinicians as well as direct care policies, programs, and protocols that are organized, monitored, and continuously improved upon by expert nurse clinicians.* (p. 3)

Consider This The definition of practice has been expanded to include policy and program development with ongoing continuous quality improvement strategies.

It is frustrating for APRNs to learn that despite the fact that the master's degree required many clinical hours and course credits, it often does not provide an education in areas such as leadership, health policy, practice management, information technology, process and outcomes evaluation, and similar topics that are vital to health care. Further, the IOM (2011) has recommended that nurses must "demonstrate new competencies in systems thinking, quality improvement, and care management and a basic understanding of health policy and research" (p. 31). APRNs are finding that they must take continuing education courses to help fill the gap. Schools of nursing have struggled to keep up with the increasing demand for this knowledge while maintaining a reasonable length to their master's degree programs. Consequently, the AACN responded to proactively move forward to develop the practice or clinical doctorate.

It is important to realize that doctoral programs are not new to nursing. "The first doctorate in nursing education was awarded by Columbia University in 1924. However, it wasn't until 1956 that there were graduate degrees specifically for nursing as a science, also from Columbia University" (NursingLink, 2015, para. 2). Not too soon after, other universities began awarding higher degrees in nursing, and the first PhDs in nursing research came from the University of Pittsburgh and New York University (NursingLink). When the first Doctor of Nursing Science (DNS/DNSc) programs were begun, schools stated that these degrees were "different" from a PhD, but it soon became clear that most of these programs were research-focused much like the PhD and not practice based.

Practice-based doctorates are also not new to nursing. The first program began at Case Western Reserve University (CWRU) in 1979 as a Doctor of Nursing (ND) degree. This degree was converted to the DNP. The school "has a long history of support and belief in the doctorate as the appropriate level of education for clinical nursing" practice (CWRU, 2013, para. 2).

There is some confusion, however, regarding the differences between a research doctorate (PhD or DNS/DNSc) and a practice doctorate (DNP or ND). The AACN (2006) provided an excellent explanation in its introduction to the *DNP Essentials* document:

> *Doctoral programs in nursing fall into two principal types: research-focused and practice-focused. Most research-focused programs grant the Doctor of Philosophy degree (PhD), while a small percentage offers the Doctor of Nursing Science degree (DNS, DSN, or DNSc). Designed to prepare nurse scientists and scholars, these programs focus heavily on scientific content and research methodology; and all require an original research project and the completion and defense of a dissertation or linked research papers. Practice-focused doctoral programs are designed to prepare experts in specialized advanced nursing practice. They focus heavily on practice that is innovative and evidence-based, reflecting the application of credible*

research findings. The two types of doctoral programs differ in their goals and the competencies of their graduates. They represent complementary, alternative approaches to the highest level of educational preparation in nursing. (p. 3)

One of the major issues that supported the move to the practice doctorate was the need for many APRN programs to increase the "number of didactic and clinical clock hours far beyond the requirements of master's education in virtually any other field. Many NP master's programs now exceed 60 credits and cannot be completed in less than three years" (AACN, 2004, p. 7). As a result, in its position statement on the practice doctorate, AACN (2004) suggested that:

In response to changes in health care delivery and emerging health care needs, additional knowledge or content areas have been identified by practicing nurses. In addition, the knowledge required to provide leadership in the discipline of nursing is so complex and rapidly changing, that additional or doctoral level education is needed. (p. 7)

Based on the work of the task force, the AACN (2004) endorsed the Position Statement on the Practice Doctorate in Nursing recommending that all advanced practice nursing education change from graduating APRNs with master's degrees to doctoral degrees by 2015. AACN (2006) then continued its work in this area and approved a document titled "*The Essentials of Doctoral Education for Advanced Practice Nursing*." These *Essentials* are similar in focus to the *Essentials of Baccalaureate Education for Professional Nursing Practice* (AACN, 2008). This *DNP Essentials* document provided schools of nursing with the key content areas that should be included in the DNP curriculum. It was not intended to be prescriptive of actual courses but to provide guidelines and standards around which faculty can develop the courses that they feel are appropriate to their DNP degree. These essentials are shown in Box 4.1, as well as on the AACN Web site.

In the years since these documents have been published, many changes have occurred. It is interesting to note that schools adopted the recommendations with less resistance than previously seen in nursing. Two hundred forty-three DNP programs are currently enrolling students at schools of nursing nationwide, and an additional 59 DNP programs are in the planning stages (AACN, 2014a). NP programs are the ones moving most quickly to the DNP. The American Nurses Association (ANA) issued its first position statement on the DNP in 2010 but "supports both master's and doctoral level of preparation as entry into APRN practice through a period of transition" (ANA, 2010, p. 9).

Though the change to the DNP by schools of nursing has occurred with little controversy, some nursing leaders continue to debate its necessity (Cronenwett et al., 2011; Dreher, 2011; Fontaine & Langston, 2011; Gilliss & Hill, 2011; Malone, 2011). Nursing historically has been unwilling to accept innovation in a timely manner. It has been more than 50 years and yet nursing continues its discussion on the appropriate degree for entry into practice. The current argument has become whether to adopt the DNP as entry into practice for APRNs but the acceptance of the DNP has occurred in a fairly short time period and may be reflective of a

BOX 4.1 The Essentials of Doctoral Education for Advanced Practice Nursing

1. Scientific underpinnings for practice
2. Organizational and systems leadership for quality improvement and systems thinking
3. Clinical scholarship and analytical methods for evidence-based practice
4. Information systems/technology and patient care technology for the improvement and transformation of health care
5. Health care policy for advocacy in health care
6. Interprofessional collaboration for improving patient and population health outcomes
7. Clinical prevention and population health for improving the nation's health
8. Advanced nursing practice

Source: American Association of Colleges of Nursing (AACN) (2006). *The essentials for doctoral education for advanced practice nursing.* Retrieved from: http://www.aacn.nche.edu/DNP/pdf/Essentials.pdf

better understanding by nursing leaders that, due to the persistent health care system issues, nursing must finally be one of the leaders in change.

WHAT DO THE APRN ORGANIZATIONS THINK?

Some of the APRN organizations were quick to respond to the recommendation to adopt the DNP degree as the entry into practice for APRNs by 2015. The National Organization of Nurse Practitioner Faculties (NONPF) began work on the practice doctorate in 2001. In April 2011 and amended in 2012, it released its final document on the core competencies for NP education and practice at the doctoral level. In the end, the NONPF decided that it could not support the 2015 deadline for NP programs to prepare graduates at the doctoral level (NONPF, 2012) but acknowledged that the DNP is a worthwhile goal for NP programs to attain and recommended that programs transition at a pace that would continue to ensure quality.

Consider This All advanced practice nursing organizations have established their own guidelines for changing advanced practice entry to doctoral education.

The other three advanced practice specialties (CNS, CNM, and CRNA) have taken a more conservative approach to the DNP recommendation. Their representative associations have published position statements that offer different views on the topic.

The NACNS (2009) decided to remain neutral about the recommendation and has requested ongoing dialogue to tackle lingering concerns. The association did state that the "NACNS supports CNS education at the master's or the doctoral level, including programs that offer the practice doctorate, providing that established, validated CNS competencies and education program standards are met. NACNS does not support eliminating MSN programs and moving to practice doctorate programs as the exclusive point-of-entry into CNS practice" (para. 2).

The CNM stated that though they see the DNP as an option, it "will not be a requirement for entry to practice for CNMs or CMs (certified midwives)" (American College of Nurse Midwives [ACNM], 2009, para. 1). The ACNM believes that midwives, for decades, "regardless of terminal degree, are safe, cost-effective providers of maternity and women's health care" (ACNM, 2012, para. 3).

In an effort to thoroughly examine the issues and arrive at a logical decision, the AANA (2007) commissioned a task force that did an extensive study of the issue and published support for mandating the DNP but decided that the timeline should be extended to 2025 based on the outcomes of the study (para. 4).

ISSUES AND CONCERNS—WHERE ARE WE NOW?

Much of the initial concern over the DNP was resolved with AACN's clarification of the role and its ultimate release of the *DNP Essentials* document. However, some issues persist and others have evolved. These concerns include the timing of the recommendation; questions over the DNP not including adequate theory; the effect of the DNP on nursing education; concern that DNP graduates who become faculty members may not be able to attain tenure; and apprehension about DNP programs having the same degree of rigor as other doctoral programs. It is unclear why nurses feel compelled to continue to argue over a practice doctorate when the IOM is demanding that nursing develop a degree that focuses on practice and the clinical setting.

Discussion Point

Do the concerns raised seem logical and reasonable? Are there other significant concerns that should also be considered?

Timing

Cronenwett et al. (2011) argued that the timing may have been right when AACN originally introduced the DNP but due to changes in the economy, it is no longer appropriate to introduce new programs. They further counter with the comment "the evolution of the DNP... is a reflection of societal changes, increasing health care demands and ongoing emphasis on quality" (p. 115).

Now is an appropriate time as nursing programs are looking at ways to strengthen its education at all levels in an effort to ensure inclusion of the IOM competencies into curriculum. Drayton-Brooks, Barksdale, and Werner (2011) feel the move to the "DNP is a glowing example of the profession's responsiveness to the need for changing education requisites, practice improvement and knowledge transition in the health care delivery system" (p. 115).

This author believes that having only a research-focused doctoral degree in nursing limits the dissemination of the important outcomes nursing has achieved. The main focus of PhD programs is the development of research, which does not always include implementation of that research. DNP graduates have the coursework and clinical practice preparation to utilize the work of the PhD or DNS nurse through implementation of the research to effect change and improve care.

Cronenwett et al. (2011) also recommended that APRN education remain at the master's level and the DNP be awarded only as a post-master's degree. Much commentary occurred because of these recommendations. Malone (2011) agreed, "We (the National League for Nursing) have long held that to exclude nurses from a variety of entry points ... is short-sighted" (p. 117). This author would argue that the data are clear that schools cannot continue to educate APRNs at the master's level and be able to keep the program to a reasonable length. As previously stated, the health care system desperately needs nurses with the knowledge of policy, practice management, informatics, and the other topics that cannot be included in the current master's curriculum.

Gilliss and Hill (2011) also agreed with Cronenwett and colleagues and "look forward to the authors' future thinking" (p. 120). Fontaine and Langston (2011) presented a doomsday response when they remarked that "the 2015 date has served to confuse the profession and the public, create anxiety in faculty and current master's students and leads to yet another division of the nursing profession" (p. 121). Drayton-Brooks et al. (2011) suggest, "The recent focus in their (Cronenwett et al., 2011) analysis on 2015 and the potential consequences of a 'mandated transition' suggests an intention to generate fear rather than offer a consideration of how both practice and research-focused degrees can co-exist with a common aim to transform health care" (p. 116).

The public does get confused about nursing and its role because there is no clear designation as to which individuals in the clinical setting are registered nurses. One could agree that faculty may indeed be anxious but their greatest concern is the need to squeeze the required content into a master's degree. This discussion then appears to perpetuate the never-ending turmoil within the nursing profession and prevents its leaders from focusing on the more important issues in the health care system.

Instead of embracing change as supported by the IOM, these nursing leaders are insisting on continuing along the same path in which nursing has been trapped for decades. As Benner, Sutphen, Leonard, and Day (2010) discuss in the Carnegie report, *Educating Nurses: A Call for Radical Transformation*, the major goal in education should be to "focus on changes in teaching and learning that will unburden overloaded curricula" (p. 8). To accomplish this, they recommend "approaches to teaching and student learning that will best prepare both today's and tomorrow's nurses" (p. 8). Though these authors are speaking mainly about baccalaureate education, these same words can and should be applied to master's education of the APRN and provide the logic for the need to continue the move to the DNP.

Though Cronenwett et al. (2011) present their argument for the DNP as only a post-master's degree, they are expressing the usual nursing clash over innovative ideas. As Dreher (2011) suggests, the argument against the DNP is the same resistance that nursing leaders have presented over the BSN as entry into practice and the master's degree as the level needed for APRN certification (p. 126). In this author's opinion, nursing cannot afford, in light of the IOM recommendations, to drag its feet in implementing this change.

Dreher (2011) suggests that though Cronenwett et al. (2011) support the PhD, they "disdain the need to establish practice doctorates to place the profession in equal status among other practice doctorates, eg, pharmacy, medicine, dentistry, clinical psychology, podiatry, optometry, physical therapy" (p. 126).

Potempa (2011) adds to the discussion in her assertion,

> *Compelling arguments can be made that students and the profession are better served by programs that move baccalaureate graduates seamlessly into DNP programs without a break in their studies. Using this model, students may indeed progress more quickly to the terminal degree and incur fewer educational expenses than students who complete a master's program and then return to school years later to complete a doctorate.* (p. 124)

Though the discussions continue, the evidence is clear that schools of nursing are adopting the DNP at record speed and nurses are flocking to these programs to obtain this degree. As evidence, the AACN (2014b) Annual Report states in 2013 "5,145 are enrolled in research-focused doctoral programs, and 14,688 are enrolled in practice-focused doctoral programs in nursing" (p. 3), a change of only 35 research-focused students from 2012 while an increase of over 3,000 students enrolled in practice-focused programs (AACN, 2013a).

Effect of the DNP on Nursing Education

Important questions have been raised over the effect of the DNP on nursing education. One such concern is how schools that do not offer doctorates will approach the DNP recommendation. An example of this issue occurred in the state of California where there is a two-tiered classification of higher education—the University of California (UC) system and the California State University (CSU) system. The CSU system by design was not meant to award doctoral degrees because this role was designated for the UC system.

There has been extensive discussion about the DNP at the Chancellor's level for both systems. The doctoral barrier was broken when a bill was passed that allowed a school within the CSU system to award educational doctorates (Goulette, 2008, p. 8). This law provided the impetus for allowing the DNP in the CSU. In 2010, Assembly Bill 867 (Nava & Arambula, 2010) CSU: Doctor of Nursing Practice Degree passed the California legislature and was signed into law. This bill allowed the CSU to offer three pilot DNP programs in the state. In fall 2012, two post-master's DNP programs were launched. These programs were developed as a joint effort between CSU Fullerton, CSU Long Beach, and CSU Los Angeles in southern California. The second is located in northern California as a joint effort between CSU Fresno and San Jose State University. The first classes graduated 59 graduates in May 2014 (CSU, 2014).

Another concern expressed about the effect of the DNP on nursing education relates to the actual content of each DNP program. During the many early discussions (Fulton & Lyon, 2005; Meleis & Dracup, 2005; Milton, 2005), comments were made that there were great differences in program content among DNP programs. Grey (2013) suggests that programs vary in content from advanced clinical practice to "administration, policy, and leadership" (p. 463). She further states that while "the original intent of the professional DNP was to educate APNs for population-based care," the components of "leadership, policy, education and management...comprise most of the content in post-master's DNP programs" (p. 463). Finally, she states, "there must be consensus about what the degree means and what capabilities can be expressed by those who hire DNP graduates" (p. 463). One could also argue that there is considerable variance in content in PhD programs, but it should be expected that content in either degree will vary depending on its focus.

The literature has been questioning the DNP since the beginning. In their early comments on the DNP, Meleis and Dracup (2005) began some of the discussion when they stated "all doctoral education must be designed to help define, generate, develop, translate and test the substantive base of knowledge in nursing" (para. 12). This statement implies that practice doctorates will not contribute to this knowledge base. Edwardson (2010) agrees, arguing,

> *The scholarship (of the DNP) focuses on integration, application, and teaching of knowledge. The scholarship of the DNP graduate may add to the store of generalizable knowledge, but in most cases will be more local and practical in nature than that developed by the PhD-prepared nurse. They will be able to exploit the evidence base to strengthen evidence-based practice.* (p. 138)

Melnyk (2013) states it best when she discusses the issues between PhD and DNP education. She feels the confusion occurs because some DNP programs are requiring the same rigorous research they require for PhD candidates and that PhD faculty are designing and teaching DNP content. These PhD-prepared faculty, therefore, do not understand the difference between evidence-based practice and translational research. Instead of having DNP students conduct rigorous research, which was not the original intent of the DNP, faculty should be helping DNP students understand how to use the evidence "that was generated through research to improve practice" (para. 9).

The *DNP Essentials* document describes the requirements of the DNP student final project, which may focus on "manuscripts submitted for publication, systematic review, research utilization project, practice topic dissemination, substantive involvement in a larger endeavor, or other practice project" (AACN, 2006, p. 20). Melnyk (2013) feels that the *Essentials* "clearly indicates that a DNP project should be a practice application demonstrating a synthesis of a student's work, creating a basis for future scholarship" (para. 9). A review of some outstanding DNP projects found that they met and exceeded these criteria. These projects have been defining, translating, and testing the research. An excellent example is A. Matos-Pagan (personal communication) who developed a coalition of nurses who were trained to respond to disasters on the island of Puerto Rico. Her work has continued and is now expanding to other islands in the Caribbean. Examples of other DNP student projects can be found at a Web site dedicated to the DNP (Doctors of Nursing Practice, 2015).

Consider This Student DNP projects are utilizing research and translating them into positive outcomes in practice.

There has also been concern that the practice doctorate or DNP will detract from nurses applying to PhD programs. Quite to the contrary, the DNP ensures that the PhD will remain focused on research. Because there were no other options, nurses pursued a PhD degree but having both degrees now offers nurses the choice of selecting a program that will best meet their needs. Box 4.2 provides a table of the key differences between the DNP and PhD. Based on conversations with several directors of DNP programs, nurses, particularly APRNs, had not considered pursuing a doctorate because their

BOX 4.2 Key Differences Between DNP and PhD/DNS Programs

	DNP	PhD/DNS
Program of study	*Objectives:* Prepare nurse leaders at the highest level of nursing practice to improve patient outcomes and translate research into practice *Competencies:* See AACN's *Essentials of Doctoral Education for Advanced Nursing Practice* (2006)	*Objectives:* Prepare nurses at the highest level of nursing science to conduct research to advance the science of nursing *Content:* See *The Research-Focused Doctoral Program in Nursing: Pathways to Excellence* (2010)
Students	Commitment to practice career Oriented toward improving outcomes of patient care and population health	Commitment to research career Oriented toward developing new nursing knowledge and scientific inquiry
Program faculty	Practice or research doctorate in nursing, and expertise in area of teaching Leadership experience in area of role and population practice High level of expertise in practice congruent with focus of academic program	Research doctorate in nursing or related field Leadership experience in area of sustained research funding High level of expertise in research congruent with focus of academic program
Resources	Mentors and/or preceptors in leadership positions across practice settings Access to diverse practice settings with appropriate resources for areas of practice Access to financial aid Access to information and patient-care technology resources congruent with areas of study	Mentors and/or preceptors in research settings Access to research settings with appropriate resources Access to dissertation support dollars and financial aid Access to information and research technology resources congruent with program of research
Program assessment and evaluation	*Program Outcome:* Health care improvements and contributions via practice, policy change, and practice scholarship Receives accreditation by nursing accreditor	*Program Outcome:* Contributes to health care improvements via the development of new knowledge and scholarly products that provide the foundation for the advancement of nursing science Oversight by the institution's authorized bodies (ie, graduate school) and regional accreditors

Reprinted with permission from William O'Connor, Director of Publications, American Association of Colleges of Nursing, April 14, 2015 via electronic mail.

only option was research-based PhD degrees. The rapid growth of DNP programs nationwide reflects that nurses would indeed like to obtain doctoral degrees but want them to be relevant to their clinical practice.

Consider This Many nurses never pursued doctoral degrees because the PhD degree was their only option.

It has been expressed that the DNP will not increase the number of nursing faculty because there are no teaching courses included in the curriculum (Malone, 2011). The AACN (2004), in fact, stated that the DNP graduates, as well as PhD graduates, would need additional education if their intent is to teach at the collegiate level (p. 13). Consequently, all persons who wish to be educators need to understand that neither of these nursing doctorates will prepare them to teach at the collegiate level, and they must pursue additional coursework that focuses on teaching. The unfortunate outcome for California since the passing of Assembly Bill 867 (Nava & Arambula, 2010) is that the DNP programs must "focus on the preparation of clinical faculty to teach in postsecondary nursing education programs" (para. 2). Consequently, these programs must include coursework on curriculum development and a teaching practicum. Though a good addition, it detracts from the original intent of the DNP by the AACN.

Concern That DNP Graduates Who Become Faculty Cannot Attain Tenure

Another common concern that arises about DNP graduates is that they may not be able to obtain tenure and equal status with PhDs in academia. The AACN (2012) states on its Web site,

> *Though primarily an institutional decision, AACN is confident that a DNP faculty member will compete favorably with other practice doctorates in tenure and promotion decisions, as is the case in law, education, audiology, physical therapy, pharmacy, criminal justice, public policy and administration, public health, and other disciplines.* (para. 11)

It goes on to say that

> *AACN data from 2011 show that doctoral students who also teach are just as likely to have a DNP as a PhD. This indicates that graduates of both types of doctoral programs are finding teaching positions.* (para. 11)

A small survey of DNP directors by this author found though that there would, in fact, be some challenges for DNP-educated faculty to obtain tenure. One DNP director commented that no faculty at her institution, including herself, would receive tenure if he or she is not involved in extensive research (K. White, personal communication). O'Dell (2010), co-founder of Doctors of Nursing Practice, LLC, did state,

> *Many colleges of nursing are not offering tenure to DNP-prepared graduates. Some say that tenure should be reserved for researchers that generate new nursing knowledge, and that a DNP does not have the education or even the expectation to produce original scholarly work.* (para. 3)

He went on to say that the lack of being offered tenure is creating issues on some campuses but also felt that some universities "are entrenched in very old traditions" (para. 5) and obtaining tenure for DNPs may take some time. Meleis (2011) exhibits this narrow view when she states "Advancing knowledge, building disciplines, and mentoring others to continue in the same traditions require solid education in nursing science" (p. 281). Zychowicz (2011) counters with

> *scholarship, service and teaching are cornerstones of most, if not all, promotion and tenure criteria... Boyer's work challenges us to consider non-research aspects of scholarship. Boyer identifies four areas of scholarship: discovery, application, integration, and teaching. Applying Boyer's definition of scholarship, it is clear how DNP-prepared faculty members contribute to scholarship of nursing through non-research work.* (p. 281)

Bellini, McCauley, and Cusson (2012) make the point that there is "widespread lack of appreciation and acceptance of clinical scholarship as a worthy endeavor by many traditional nursing faculties" (p. 550). They further believe that the "thoughtful evaluation and redesign of many traditional frames of reference pertaining to exactly what does and does not qualify as nursing scholarship" (p. 550) must occur and is "an essential paradigm shift for nursing…if we are to further the influence of the discipline" (p. 550).

Nicholes and Dyer (2012) conducted an Internet-based survey inviting 200 randomly chosen faculty of schools of nursing around the United States. There was a 33.8% response rate of 65 participants (p. 14). These participants included PhD, DNP faculty, and deans. "In 61.3% (n = 38) of the institutions, DNP faculty were eligible for tenure" (p. 15).

Three themes emerged as benefits for allowing DNPs to achieve tenure (Nicholes & Dyer, 2012). "The most common benefit cited…was related to the recruitment and retention of quality faculty" (p. 15). Allowing the DNP to achieve tenure aids in this goal. The other two benefits were the clinical component that DNPs bring and that DNPs were capable of achieving the rigorous standards of scholarship.

Concerns that surfaced in the Nicholes and Dyer (2012) study were the beliefs that "DNP faculties lack the preparation for contributing to the body of scholarly research" (p. 17). "Allowing DNP faculty eligibility for tenure will diminish the progress nursing has made in academia" and "concern regarding success of DNP faculty in producing traditional research and the notion that a practice degree is not viewed as an academic equivalent to PhD" (p. 17). The final evaluation though was that "DNP faculty be held to the same standards as the PhD faculty" (p. 17). The other "view was that the requirements are the same as any other terminal degree in regard to teaching and service, but the research component may differ. The differences were through clinical practice and the use of evidence-based research" (p. 17).

Similar concerns were raised in research undertaken by Udlis and Mancuso (2015), although they suggested that the role ambiguity in research, academe, and academic leadership tends to obscure the distinctness and

Research Study Fuels the Controversy 4.1

A quantitative, descriptive, cross-sectional design study was conducted in spring of 2013. Questionnaires were used at two large Midwestern conferences, where one consisted of mostly PhD-prepared, academic and research nurses while the other was attended by mostly master's-prepared advance practice nurses. The survey consisted of 21 items, which questioned the clarity of the role of the DNP-prepared nurse, using a 4-point scale. The researchers also collected demographic information of each respondent.

There were 340 participants, mostly White women, who held at least an MSN degree. Slightly more than half of the respondents worked in an academic setting and two thirds of them identified themselves as faculty. Sixty-eight percent of the participants said they were APRNs.

Source: Udlis, K. A., & Mancuso, J.M. (2015, February). Perceptions of the role of the doctor of nursing practice-prepared nurse: Clarity or confusion. *Journal of Professional Nursing,* 1-10. doi:10.1016/j.profnurs.2015.01.004.

Study Findings

Seventy-three percent of respondents were clear that both the PhD and the DNP are terminal degrees with the majority (85%) agreeing that DNPs "will be able to articulate nursing's contribution to health care" (p. 6). About half had concerns about DNPs helping to "unify and strengthen the profession" (p. 6).

A large majority (81%) felt that DNPs were prepared to be successful in "complex leadership roles that influence change in health care delivery systems, policy, and interprofessional collaboration" (p. 6). At the same time, slightly less than half of the respondents felt that DNPs would be able to hold leadership positions in the academic setting.

Only slightly more than half (55%) felt that DNPs would help improve the faulty shortage and less than half (46%) felt they were prepared to teach. Interestingly, though, 63% believed that tenure requirements should be the same for both degrees. It was also believed that the DNP faculty would replace master's prepared faculty. There was also great support (88%) that DNPs would "bridge the gap between science and practice and substantially contribute to nursing scholarship" (p. 6). More than half of the respondents (57%) felt that the "DNP degree prepares individuals to develop knowledge generating research" (p. 6).

There was much agreement that the DNP degree was similar to physicians, dentists, and pharmacists and that they will improve health care outcomes. There was also agreement that the DNP will help increase salaries and professional respect but few (19.5%) felt that "employers would prefer DNP graduates over MSN graduates in the clinical setting" (p. 7).

The researchers then divided the respondents by degree and analyzed the results again. In the understanding category, it was found that 80% of DNPs felt that was substantial overlap in the expectations for DNPs and PhDs as compared to only 24% of PhD-prepared nurses, 53% of MSN nurses, and 33% of PSN participants (p. 7). Further, almost all (97%) of DNPs versus only 51% of PhDs felt the DNP is a terminal degree. There was also disparity that DNPs will "strengthen

(*continued*)

Research Study Fuels the Controversy 4.1 (continued)

and unify the profession," and 80% DNPs agree compared to 34% for PhDs and 45.5% for MSNs (p. 7).

For leadership, the greatest concern was over the ability of DNP nurses to assume academic leadership roles. Eighty-four percent of DNPs versus only 19% of PhD participants felt DNPs were prepared for these positions.

There were great disparities related to the faculty role for DNPs. The majority (84%) of DNPs believed they could help relieve the faculty shortage while only 50% of PhDs, 54% of MSNs, and 38.5% of BSN nurses agreed (p. 7). PhDs did not feel that DNP graduates are prepared for "the rigors of the faculty role" (p. 7) with only a 19% responding in the positive. At the same time, 76% of DNPs felt they could meet the requirements. There was further disagreement about whether the requirements for tenure should be the same for both degrees. Only 35% of PhDs compared to 84% of DNPs felt the requirements should be the same. The majority of all nurses in the study believed that DNPs would contribute to nursing scholarship.

When the participants were asked whether employers would prefer DNP graduates over MSNs, only 13% of MSNs agreed. Even DNPs did not fully agree at only 30% and PhDs at 23%. Interestingly, the BSN nurses were more accepting of this premise at 46% (p. 7). Slightly less than half (49%) of MSNs agreed with the idea that DNP is an "entry-level advanced practice degree parallel to physicians, dentists and pharmacists" (p. 7). Finally, the overall majority of all nurses, no matter their degree, believed that DNPs would improve health outcomes.

The authors concluded that "role ambiguity was prevalent among the sample of nurses surveyed...There are multiple levels of confusion concerning research, academia, and academic leadership, and scholarship, which tend to obscure the distinctness and individuality of the DNP degree, thus impacting role identity. The roles of the DNP-prepared nurse are forming and evolving" (pp. 8-9). "To further reduce role stress, strain, and ambiguity and successfully function...the distinctive and necessary contributions of the DNP-prepared nurse must be embraced, valued, and operationalized" (p. 9). The authors believe the degree will continue to be challenged if these contributions are not accepted.

individuality of the DNP degree, thus impacting role identity (Research Study Fuels the Controversy 4.1).

This author did not find any barriers to achieve tenure in a college composed of the sciences including chemistry, physics, and biology as well as mathematics. It was found through a Web search that for most nursing faculty career opportunities the applicant needed to have a master's in nursing and an undefined doctorate in nursing or related field with some universities actively seeking applicants who have the DNP (HigherEdJobs, 2015a,b,c).

Consider This Resistance to hiring nursing faculty with DNP degrees for tenure track positions in universities may be decreasing.

Do DNP Programs Have the Same Amount of Rigor as Other Doctoral Programs?

One must question whether there should be a concern about rigor as part of the discussion on the DNP. Bellini and Cusson (as cited in Dreher & Smith Glasgow, 2011) suggest that maybe the word "rigor" should not be used and propose that the word "scholarship" be used instead. "As rigor tends to be synonymous with traditional research methodology, scholarship is a broader concept that may actually lend some clarity to our current dilemma" (p. 131). They further propose,

> *While the level of rigor of DNP programs as perceived by some might not necessitate a level consistent with what is expected in a PhD program, the outcomes may offer significant benefits in terms of valuable learning experiences consistent with clinical scholarship and development of leadership abilities, thereby establishing the DNP as a truly learned individual, respected in the academic setting and valuable in the practice setting.* (p. 130)

There are distinct differences between research-based and practice-based degrees but both are completed in universities, which must meet the standards of the professional accrediting bodies. The notion that DNPs would not be able to achieve the rigor of such scholarly institutions is not supported by any data. Edwardson (2010) discusses the concern over rigor between the

DNP and PhD but emphasizes that these degrees have different purposes and thus should not include the same content. She states, "The PhD degree has as its express purpose the preparation of scholars to articulate and generate knowledge for the discipline" (p. 137). She further suggests:

> *The purpose of the DNP, on the other hand, is to prepare practitioners to take the knowledge created by researchers and theoretical scholars and use it in the delivery of services and advancement of policies that support high-quality health care. This is not to say that the DNP-prepared nurse does not engage in scholarship. Rather, the scholarship focuses on integration, application, and teaching of knowledge. The scholarship of the DNP graduate may add to the store of generalizable knowledge, but in most cases will be more local and practical in nature than that developed by the PhD-prepared nurse. They will be able to exploit the evidence base to strengthen evidence-based practice.* (p. 138)

Consider This DNP graduates base their practice on the latest evidence as defined in the third item of the DNP Essentials document.

In addition, the Commission on Collegiate Nursing Education (CCNE), the independent accrediting agency for the AACN, released a press report stating, "In a move consistent with other health professions... [CCNE] has decided that only practice doctoral degrees with the DNP title will be eligible for CCNE accreditation" (AACN, 2005, para. 1). This support by the CCNE reinforces that these programs do indeed meet the rigor of any doctoral degree.

Finally, with the development of the *DNP Essentials*, the AACN (2006) laid the groundwork for a strong and rigorous curricular model. The suggestion that the PhD is the only worthwhile doctoral program and that the DNP could not be as rigorous or as valuable to the profession is disrespectful to the many outstanding institutions that have initiated DNP programs. Edwardson (2010) supports this belief when she states that "this is a real concern only if schools of nursing fail to insist on comparable rigor in the two programs" (p. 138) and suggests that "DNP preparation will deliberately prepare clinicians who base their practices in quality evidence and fill an important gap in practice such as being the principal providers of primary care" (p. 138).

Concern That the DNP Curriculum Does Not Include Theory

When the discussion on the DNP first began, Whall (2005) and Milton (2005) questioned the lack of theory in DNP programs. Algase (2010) in her recent editorial supports this premise. She goes so far as to suggest that theory must be part of DNP education; otherwise DNPs will be "less equipped than those with research-focused doctorates" (p. 93). While these authors imply that DNP graduates have lesser knowledge, they miss the point that theories are often integrated throughout a curriculum depending on the particular course and topic. The fact that these theories may not be nursing theories may be an issue for some, but nursing in the 21st century does not practice in a vacuum. The profession must consider that nurses are working as part of an interdisciplinary team and need to understand many types of theories. The inability to understand nonnursing theories has been one of the major barriers for nurses effecting significant change. In addition, because the BSN curriculum includes courses that discuss a number of theories, professional nurses have the needed theoretical background.

Business, leadership, and organizational theories, not just nursing theories, are crucial for nurse leaders working to transform the health care system, making acquisition of this knowledge vital for the DNP. Leaders require knowledge of all conceptual theories if they are to be successful in their attempts at change.

Consider This The nursing profession must understand theories from all disciplines if it is to effect change in the health care system.

RECENT DEVELOPMENTS

A document released by the American Academy of Family Physicians (AAFP, 2012) states that "the 2010 survey found 26 percent of patients identified nurse practitioners as medical doctors and another 5 percent were unsure" (para. 3). It goes on to say, "Moreover, more than one third of respondents (35%) thought a doctor of nursing practice (DNP) was a medical doctor...In short, more than half of respondents could not identify a DNP as a member of the *nursing*, not medical, profession" (para. 3). Earlier in the document, the statement is made that there is "profound confusion about whether a physician or other health professional is providing their care" (para. 2). The data that the AAFP presents does not support that the general public has concerns over who is providing the care. In fact, their data actually support the need for DNPs because only a minority of the survey respondents had issues with advanced practice nurses. The key concern is whether patients are receiving quality care from whatever provider they see.

Another document was published in 2009 by the American College of Physicians (ACP, 2009) and has not been updated. In this document the ACP takes the position that physicians are the "most appropriate health care professionals for many patients" (p. 1). It further suggests that the reason nursing decided to move to the DNP was "to improve the quality of NP education" (p. 5). There has never been a question about the quality of NP education. One of the main reasons programs are moving to the doctoral level is to finally award a degree that reflects the number of units taken by students. As stated in the AACN (2004) position statement on the practice doctorate in nursing,

> *The growing complexity of health care, burgeoning growth in scientific knowledge, and increasing sophistication of technology have necessitated master's degree programs that prepare APNs to expand the number of didactic and clinical clock hours far beyond the requirements of master's education in virtually any other field.* (para. 22)

It furthers states that,

> *In response to changes in health care delivery and emerging health care needs, additional knowledge or content areas have been identified by practicing nurses. In addition, the knowledge required to provide leadership in the discipline of nursing is so complex and rapidly changing that additional or doctoral level education is needed.* (para. 23)

The ACP (2009) also states that the education of physicians and NPs are not equivalent and feels that NPs cannot function in the same capacity as physicians because physicians have so much more education than NPs. The document states:

> *Training of physicians involves 4 years of premedical college education, 4 years of medical school that includes 2 years of clinical rotations, 3 years or more of clinical residency training with up to 80-hour workweeks, additional fellowship subspecialty training, and continuing medical education.* (p. 9)

This statement notes that NPs do not spend an equivalent amount of time in their education and suggests they cannot function at the expected level needed for their chosen area of practice. NPs do, however, spend 4 years in the baccalaureate nursing education, and 2 to 3 additional years obtaining a master's degree or now 3 to 4 years obtaining a DNP while typically working as a registered nurse and gaining needed clinical experience. The question must be asked whether NPs need additional years of education and advanced clinical training to perform the role. Since NPs have been providing quality care for 50 years, it is clear that nursing is providing the needed level of education for these health care providers and is responsive when required as is seen in the move to the DNP.

Most NP programs require at least 1 year of clinical experience as a registered nurse before applying to the NP program and must have received a bachelor's degree in nursing. In this author's experience as a former NP program coordinator, most NP students have 5 to 20 years of experience as a nurse. In the end, it is not unusual for an NP to have 7 to 9 or more years of collegiate education and many more years practicing as a registered nurse before taking on the APRN role.

At the same time, there has never been the suggestion that NPs and physicians practice the same but it also does not mean that one practices better or more safely than the other. Physicians practice from a medical model while nursing practices from the nursing model. The main difference between these models is that nurses emphasize health promotion and disease prevention: a key component of NP practice and one that many patients value. It is interesting to note that in recent years medical schools are now talking about the importance of health promotion and disease prevention, partially in response to the quality and safety movement.

The ACP (2009) document does encourage collaboration. As stated in the IOM report, *Health Professions Education: A Bridge to Quality (2003)*, health care professionals "work in interdisciplinary teams - cooperate, collaborate, communicate and integrate care in teams to ensure that care is continuous and reliable" (IOM, 2003 p. 45), NPs have always advocated that all health care providers, including physicians, NPs, physical therapists, pharmacists, and respiratory therapists, among others, work together to provide the highest quality of care but it does not mean that the physician is or should be the lead/main provider.

It is unfortunate that physician organizations continue to believe that the health care system is a pyramid and that they are at the pinnacle with the right to direct all other health care professionals. Physicians have no legal right to attempt to regulate APRNs or to state that NPs must function under the direct supervision of a physician. Boards of nursing are the legal bodies that regulate nursing and monitor its practice. State Nurse Practice Acts clarify the role and function of a nurse. One can only imagine the backlash if nursing tried to tell physicians how to practice. Unfortunately, the medical community seems determined to continue its long history of trying to defend what it believes is its turf.

Consider This The medical community has no legal right to attempt to regulate APRNs or to state that they must function under the direct supervision of a physician.

The goal instead should be to work in collaboration and as a team, given that all health care professionals make significant contributions to the health of the patient. One would think that the medical profession would focus on the more important issue of providing safe and high-quality care instead of wasting time and energy trying to regulate other providers who have extensive documentation of their worth. Any concern over the quality of care provided by APRNs has been eliminated in multiple studies. The most recent one by Newhouse et al. (2011) reviewed the literature from 1990 to 2008 on care provided by APRNs in comparison with physician care.

The results indicate that APRNs provide effective and high-quality patient care, have an important role in improving quality of patient care in the United States, and could help to address the concerns about whether care provided by APRNs can safely augment the physician supply to support reform efforts aimed at expanding access to care (p. 1).

Another recent development was the AMA resolution (Sorrel, 2008), which called for limitations on the use of the term "doctor" and suggested that it be restricted to physicians, dentists, and podiatrists. After much discussion, however, the terminology was changed to say that all professionals must clearly identify their qualifications and credentials to patients. A floor amendment was approved that AMA will support legislation to "make it a felony for non-physician health care professionals to misrepresent themselves as physicians" (Sorrel, 2008, p. 25).

Why some physicians believed it was necessary to make such an amendment is unclear, given that it has always been illegal to misrepresent oneself as a licensed health care professional. Unfortunately, the ACP (2009) also felt compelled to discuss this issue in its monograph and suggests that the use of the term "doctor" by NPs could lead to confusion by the public. Patients are highly informed today and are more than capable of distinguishing among the many health care providers. It is unclear why physicians have such great concern about NPs who have doctorates when so many health care providers today also have doctoral degrees. Most NPs clearly emphasize to their patients that they are NPs and not physicians.

Nursing must continue to be vigilant about these attempts to encroach on its right to practice. The IOM (2011) is recommending that all levels of nursing be allowed and encouraged to perform to the full scope of their practice. Nurses must be strong advocates for the profession by joining and being actively involved in professional associations that focus on monitoring practice issues and voting for legislators who will support the role. Legislators must be kept informed of nursing practice and its meaning and provide documentation of its outstanding patient outcomes. Nursing must define nursing before others take away our freedom to practice.

Consider This Nursing must continue to be vigilant about these attempts to encroach on its right to practice.

Conclusions

The controversy over the clinical practice doctorate will probably continue for many years, but advanced practice registered nursing must continue to evaluate what level of education is needed to provide the quality of care for patients in today's health care system. Of equal importance is that individual APRNs must learn from the lessons of the past and develop the skills needed to survive as a vital constituent of the health care system in the 21st century. There is little doubt that advanced practice nursing makes valuable contributions to the health care system. The movement to the DNP is a crucial part of that process.

For Additional Discussion

1. Can the public appropriately distinguish among the many doctoral degrees offered by universities?
2. Will offering the DNP decrease the number of PhD candidates?
3. Is it necessary for DNP graduates to have coursework in nursing theory?
4. Should the medical profession be allowed to dictate the scope of practice for DNPs or other nurses?

References

Algase, D. (2010). Essentials of scholarship for the DNP: Are we clear yet? [Editorial]. *Research and Theory for Nursing Practice, 24*(2), 91–93.

American Academy of Family Physicians. (2012). *Patient perceptions regarding health care providers.* Retrieved from http://www.aafp.org/dam/AAFP/documents/about_us/initiatives/PatientPerceptions.pdf

American Association of Colleges of Nursing. (2004). *AACN Position statement on the practice doctorate in nursing.* Retrieved from http://www.aacn.nche.edu/publications/position/DNPpositionstatement.pdf

American Association of Colleges of Nursing. (2005). *Commission on Collegiate Nursing Education moves to consider for accreditation only practice doctorates with the DNP degree title.* Retrieved from http://www.aacn.nche.edu/news/articles/2005/commission-on-collegiate-nursing-education-moves-to-consider-for-accreditation-only-practice-doctorates-with-the-dnp-degree-title

American Association of Colleges of Nursing. (2006). *The essentials of doctoral education for advanced nursing practice.* Retrieved from http://www.aacn.nche.edu/DNP/pdf/Essentials.pdf

American Association of Colleges of Nursing. (2008). *The essentials of baccalaureate education for professional nursing practice.* Retrieved from http://www.aacn.nche.edu/education/pdf/BaccEssentials08.pdf

American Association of Colleges of Nursing (AACN). (2010). Your nursing career: A look at the facts. Retrieved from ww.aacn.nche.edu/students/your-nursing-career/facts

American Association of Colleges of Nursing. (2011). *Nursing fact sheet.* Retrieved from http://www.aacn.nche.edu/media-relations/fact-sheets/nursing-fact-sheet

American Association of Colleges of Nursing. (2012). *Frequently asked questions.* Retrieved from http://www.aacn.nche.edu/dnp/about/frequently-asked-questions

American Association of Colleges of Nursing. (2013a). 2013 Annual Report: Moving the conversation forward. Advancing nursing education. Retrieved from http://www.aacn.nche.edu/aacn-publications/annual-reports/AnnualReport13.pdf

American Association of Colleges of Nursing (AACN). (2013b). *Competencies and curricular expectations for clinical nurse leader education and practice.* Retireved from http://www.aacn.nche.edu/cnl/CNL-Competencies-October-2013.pdf

American Association of Colleges of Nursing. (2014a). *DNP fact sheet.* Retrieved from http://www.aacn.nche.edu/media-relations/fact-sheets/dnp

American Association of Colleges of Nursing. (2014b). Annual report 2014: Building a framework for the future. Advancing higher education in nursing. Retireved from http://www.aacn.nche.edu/aacn-publications/annual-reports/AnnualReport14.pdf

American Association of Nurse Anesthetists. (2007). *AANA Position on doctoral preparation of nurse anesthetists.* Retrieved from http://www.aana.com/ceandeducation/educationalresources/Documents/AANA_Position_DTF_June_2007.pdf

American Association of Nurse Anesthetists. (2015). *Who we are.* Retrieved from http://www.aana.com/aboutus/Pages/Who-We-Are.aspx

American Association of Nurse Practitioners. (2014). *NP fact sheet.* Retrieved from http://www.aanp.org/all-about-nps/np-fact-sheet

American College of Nurse-Midwives. (2009). *Mandatory degree requirements for entry into midwifery practice.* Retrieved from http://www.midwife.org/

ACNM/files/ACNMLibraryData/UPLOADFILENAME/000000000076/Mandatory%20Degree%20Requirements%20Position%20Statement%20June%202012.pdf

American College of Nurse-Midwives. (2012). *Midwifery education and the Doctor of Nursing Practice (DNP).* Retrieved from http://www.midwife.org/ACNM/files/ACNMLibraryData/UPLOADFILENAME/000000000079/Midwifery%20Ed%20and%20DNP%20Position%20Statement%20June%202012.pdf

American College of Nurse-Midwives. (2014). *Essentialfacts about midwives.* Retrieved from http://www.midwife.org/Essential-Facts-about-Midwives

American College of Physicians. (2009). *Nurse practitioners in primary care* [Policy Monograph]. Philadelphia, PA: American College of Physicians.

American Nurses Association. (2010). *Position statement.* Retrieved from http://www.doctorsofnursingpractice.org/wp-content/uploads/2014/08/ANA_Position_Statement_on_DNP_as_a_Terminal_Degree_6_14_2010.pdf

Bellini, S., McCauley, P., & Cusson, R. M. (2012). The doctor of nursing practice graduate as faculty member. *Nursing Clinics of North America, 47*(4), 547–556. doi:10.1016/j.cnur.2012.07.004

Bellini, S., & Cusson, R. M. (2011). The role of the practitioner. In H. M. Dreher & M. E. Smith Glasgow (Eds.), *Role development for advanced nursing practice* (pp. 123–135). New York, NY: Springer.

Benner, P., Sutphen, M., Leonard, V., & Day, L. (2010) *Educating nurses: A call for radical transformation.* San Francisco, NC: Jossey-Bass/The Carnegie Foundation for the Advancement of Teaching.

California State University. (2014). *CSU Doctor of nursing practice degree programs.* Retrieved from http://www.calstate.edu/dnp/

Case Western Reserve University. (2013). *History of the DNP at FPB.* Retrieved from http://fpb.case.edu/DNP/history.shtm

Cronenwett, L., Dracup, K., Grey, M., McCauley, L., Meleis, A., & Salmon, M. (2011). The doctor of nursing practice: A national workforce perspective. *Nursing Outlook, 59*, 9–17. doi:10.1016/j.outlook.2010.11.003

Doctors of Nursing Practice. (2015). DNP scholarly projects. Retrieved from http://www.doctorsofnursingpractice.org/resources/dnp-scholarly-projects/

Drayton-Brooks, S. M., Barksdale, D. J., & Werner, K. E. (2011). An alternative view of the doctor of nursing practice. *Nursing Outlook, 59*, 115–116. doi:10.1016/j.outlook.2010.11.003

Dreher, M. (2011). The doctor of nursing practice: A national workforce perspective—A response. *Nursing Outlook, 59*, 126–127. doi:10.1016/j.outlook.2011.03.013

Edwardson, S. (2010). *Doctor of philosophy and doctor of nursing practice as complementary degrees. Journal of Professional Nursing, 26*(3), 137-140. doi: 10.1016/j.profnurs.2009.08.004.

Fontaine, D., & Langston, N. (2011). The master's is not broken: Commentary on "The doctor of nursing practice: a workforce perspective." *Nursing Outlook, 59*, 121–122. doi:10.1016/j.outlook.2011.03.003

Fulton, J., & Lyon, B. (2005). The need for some sense making: Doctor of nursing practice. *The Online Journal of Issues in Nursing, 10*(3). Retrieved from http://eds.b.ebscohost.com/eds/detail/detail?sid=236fcebb-25c7-4772-a723-43df25024239%40sessionmgr114&vid=3&hid=119&bdata=JnNpdGU9ZWRzLWxpdmU%3d#AN=2009086366&db=rzh

Gilliss, C., & Hill, M. (2011). Commentary: The doctor of nursing practice—A national workforce perspective. *Nursing Outlook, 59*, 119–120. doi:10.1016/j.outlook.2011.03.014

Goulette, C. (2008). *A look at current state legislation and government-related issues.* Retrieved from Advance Healthcare Network—For Nurses website: http://nursing.advanceweb.com/Article/From-the-Hill-4.aspx

Grey, M. (2013). The doctor of nursing practice: Defining the next steps. *Journal of Nursing Education*, 52(8), 462–465.

HigherEdJobs. (2015a). *Assistant professor of nursing.* Retrieved from https://www.higheredjobs.com/faculty/details.cfm?JobCode=176059502&Title=Assistant%20Professor%20of%20Nursing

HigherEdJobs. (2015b). *Faculty, College of nursing & health professions—FNP.* Retrieved from https://www.higheredjobs.com/faculty/details.cfm?JobCode=176050992&Title=Faculty%20%2D%20College%20of%20Nursing%20%26%20Health%20Care%20Professions%20%2D%20FNP

HigherEdJobs. (2015c). *Full-time faculty—Undergraduate nursing.* Retrieved from https://www.higheredjobs.com/faculty/details.cfm?JobCode=176065422&Title=Full%2Dtime%20Faculty%20%2D%20Undergraduate%20Nursing

Institute of Medicine of the National Academies. (1999). *To err is human: Building a safer health system.* Washington, DC: National Academies Press.

Institute of Medicine of the National Academies. (2001). *Crossing the quality chasm.* Washington, DC: National Academies Press.

Institute of Medicine of the National Academies. (2003). *Health professions education: A bridge to quality.* Washington, DC: National Academies Press. Retrieved from http://books.nap.edu/openbook.php?record_id=10681&page=45

Institute of Medicine of the National Academies. (2011). *The future of nursing: Leading change, advancing health.* Washington, DC: National Academies Press.

Malone, B. (2011). Commentary on "The doctor of nursing practice: A national workforce perspective." *Nursing Outlook, 59*, 117–118. doi:10.1016/j.outlook.2011.03.002

Meleis, A. I. (2011). DNPS as tenured faculty. *The Journal for Nurse Practitioners, 7*(4), 280–281.

Meleis, A. I., & Dracup, K. (2005, September 30). The case against the DNP: History, timing, substance, and marginalization. *The Online Journal of Issues in Nursing, 10*(3). Retrieved from http://www.nursingworld.org/MainMenuCategories/ANAMarketplace/ANAPeriodicals/OJIN/TableofContents/Volume102005/No3Sept05/tpc28_216026.aspx

Melnyk, B. M. (2013). Distinguishing the preparation and roles of Doctor of Philosophy and Doctor of Nursing Practice graduates: National implications for academic curricula and health care systems. *Journal of Nursing Education, 52*(8), 442–448. doi:10.3928/0148434-20130719-01

Milton, C. L. (2005). Scholarship in nursing: Ethics of a practice doctorate. *Nursing Science Quarterly, 18*(2), 113–116.

National Association of Clinical Nurse Specialists. (2009). *Position statement on the nursing practice doctorate.* Retrieved from http://www.nacns.org/docs/DNP-Statement1507.pdf

National Association of Clinical Nurse Spcialists. (2014). *Who are clinical nurse specialists?* Retrieved from http://www.nacns.org/docs/pr-CNSWeekTop10.pdf

National Organization of Nurse Practitioner Faculties. (2012). *Nurse practitioner core competencies.* Retrieved from http://c.ymcdn.com/sites/www.nonpf.org/resource/resmgr/competencies/npcorecompetenciesfinal2012.pdf

Nava and Arambula. (2010). AB 867. Retrieved from http://www.leginfo.ca.gov/pub/09-10/bill/asm/ab_0851-0900/ab_867_bill_20100928_chaptered.html

Newhouse, R., Stanik-Hutt, J., White, K., Johantgen, M., Bass, E., Zangaro, G., . . .Weiner, J. (2011). Advance practice nurse outcomes 1990–2008: A systematic review. *Nursing Economic$, 29*(5), 1–22. Retrieved from https://www.nursingeconomics.net/ce/2013/article3001021.pdf

Nicholes, R. H., & Dyer, J. (2012). Is eligibility for tenure possible for the doctor of nursing practice-prepared faculty? *Journal of Professional Nursing, 28*(1), 13–17.

NursingLink. (2015). *PhD in nursing explained.* Retrieved from http://nursinglink.monster.com/education/articles/189-phd-in-nursing-explained

O'Dell, D. (2010, June 26). *DNP discussions: Tenure for DNP graduates* [Web log comment]. Retrieved from http://community.advanceweb.com/blogs/np_7/archive/2010/06/26/tenure-for-dnp-graduates.aspx

Potempa, K. (2011). The DNP serves the public good. *Nursing Outlook, 59*, 123–125. doi:10.1016/j.outlook.2011.03.001

Sorrel, A. L. (2008). *AMA Meeting: Physicians demand greater oversight of doctors of nursing.* Retrieved from http://www.ama-assn.org/amednews/2008/07/07/prsd0707.htm

Udlis, K. A., & Mancuso, J.M. (2015). Perceptions of the role of the doctor of nursing practice-prepared nurse: Clarity or confusion. *Journal of Professional Nursing,* 0(0), 1–10. doi:10.1016/j.profnurs.2015.01.004

U.S. Department of Health and Human Services, Health Resources and Services Administration. (2010). *The registered nurse population. Findings from the 2008 National Sample Survey of Registered Nurses.* Retrieved from http://bhpr.hrsa.gov/healthworkforce/rnsurveys/rnsurveyfinal.pdf

Whall, A. (2005). "Lest we forget": An issue concerning the Doctorate in Nursing Practice (DNP). *Nursing Outlook, 53*(1), 1.

Zychowicz, M.E. (2011). DNPS as tenured faculty. *The Journal for Nurse Practitioners, 7*(4), 280-281.

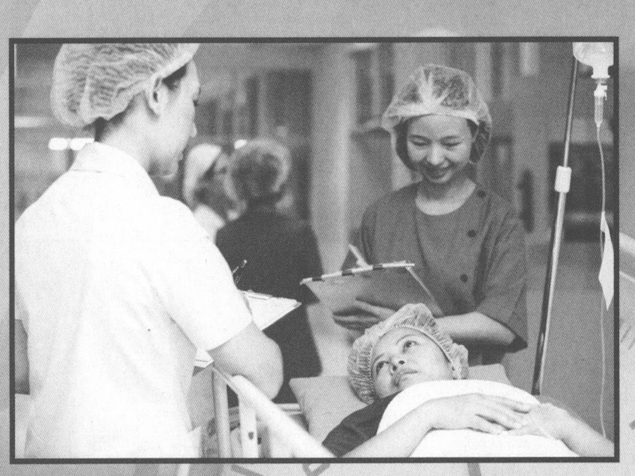

2

Workforce Issues

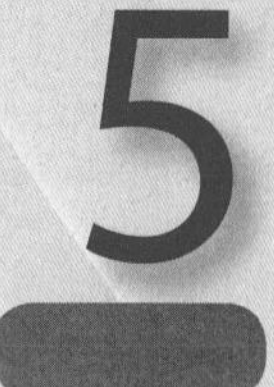

Is There a Nursing Shortage?

Carol J. Huston

ADDITIONAL RESOURCES

Visit thePoint for additional helpful resources

- eBook
- Journal Articles
- WebLinks

CHAPTER OUTLINE

LEARNING OBJECTIVES

The learner will be able to:

1. Explore factors affecting the current supply of registered nurses (RNs) in the United States as well as the current and projected demand through 2020.
2. Compare regional differences in the supply and demand for RNs in the United States.
3. Discuss consequences of the current shortage on quality of health care, current working conditions for RNs, and RN retention rates.
4. Identify the relationship between the current nursing shortage and the state of the national economy.
5. Analyze the impact of salary as an incentive for resolving nursing shortages.
6. Address the educational challenges inherent in solving the nursing shortage given unfilled faculty positions, resignations, projected retirements, low faculty pay schedules, and the shortage of students being prepared for the faculty role.
7. Identify specific strategies being used to recruit and retain older nurses in the workforce.
8. Differentiate between and provide examples of both short- and long-term solutions to nursing shortages.
9. Outline strategies directed at both supply and demand factors that have been proposed in an effort to reduce the current nursing shortage and analyze the efficacy of each.
10. Reflect upon his or her personal commitment to a career in professional nursing.

INTRODUCTION

As government and private insurer reimbursement declined in the 1990s and managed care costs soared, many health care organizations, and hospitals in particular, began downsizing to achieve cost containment by eliminating registered nursing jobs or by replacing registered nurses (RNs) with unlicensed assistive personnel. Even hospitals that did not downsize during this period often did little to recruit qualified RNs.

This downsizing and shortsightedness regarding recruitment and retention contributed to the beginning of an acute shortage of RNs in many health care settings by the late 1990s. The health care quality and safety movement also exacerbated this shortage in the late 1990s as research emerged to demonstrate the relationship between nurse staffing and patient outcomes and the public became aware of how important an adequately sized workforce was to patient safety. Unlike earlier nursing shortages, which typically lasted only a few years, this shortage was longer and more severe than earlier nursing shortages. Indeed, as of 2010, the overwhelming majority of states in the United States were reporting nursing shortages, ranging from a shortage of 200 nurses in Alabama to a shortage of 47,600 nurses in California (Trust for America's Health, 2015).

When the economy soured, however, early in the second decade of this century, new graduate nurses began struggling to find jobs and vacancy rates fell at most hospitals across the country. This occurred, at least in part, because a large number of part-time nurses sought full-time employment and the economy delayed some nurses from cutting back on their work hours or seeking retirement. Thus, the economic crisis obscured whether a nursing shortage continued to exist.

Consider This The recent economic crisis has obscured whether a nursing shortage exists.

Wood (2012) notes, however, that while economists say the recession is over and that consumer confidence is improving, nurses are still hanging on to their jobs. She notes, however, that retirements will come and the next shortage could be even worse than the one encountered just a few years ago. Staiger agrees, arguing that when the economy improves, and the mostly married, female workforce quits, reduces working hours to part-time or reaches retirement age, a shortage of nurses is expected again (Ostrow, 2012).

The American Association of Colleges of Nursing (AACN, 2014a) concurs arguing that given the fluctuations in the economy, it is difficult to "accurately project how long the nation will take to recover and exactly when old workforce patterns may re-emerge. In the short term, the changing characteristics of employment options for new nurses are causing frustration to many new graduates who expected a different occupational outlook from what currently exists in many places" (para. 10). Indeed, Schepp (2013) noted that more than a third (36%) of newly licensed RNs who graduated in 2011 weren't working as RNs 4 months after graduation, according to a survey by the National Student Nurses Association.

To more accurately assess the depth or significance of any current nursing shortage then, data must be examined regarding both the demand for RNs and the supply. Assessing the demand for RNs is, in many ways, more complicated than assessing the supply. However, from an economic perspective, the most recent nursing shortage was driven more by the supply side of the supply/demand equation than the demand side. Supply shortages are more difficult to solve than demand-induced shortages because they require longer-term solutions.

Consider This Supply shortages are more difficult to solve than demand-induced shortages because they require longer-term solutions

This chapter will explore whether a current nursing shortage exists by examining the present and projected demand for RNs, as well as the supply. In addition, the potential consequences of an unaddressed shortage will be examined, together with strategies needed to keep the shortage from reappearing.

THE DEMAND FOR NURSES

Demand is defined by the *Merriam Webster's Online Dictionary* (2014a) as the quantity of a commodity or service wanted at a specified price and time. In the case of nursing, demand would be the amount of a good or service (in this case, an RN) that consumers (in this case, an employer) would be willing to acquire at a given price. A shortage occurs when employers want more employees at the current market wages than they can get. Demand then is derived from the health status of a population and the use of health services.

The demand for professional nurses in both the short- and long-term future continues to increase. In fact, employment of RNs is expected to grow much faster than average for all occupations through 2022. Indeed, the U.S. Bureau of Labor projections reported that the RN workforce is expected to grow from 2.71 million in 2012 to 3.24 million in 2022, an increase of 526,800 or 19%. The Bureau also projects the need for 525,000 replacement nurses in the workforce bringing the total number of job openings for nurses due to growth and replacements to 1.05 million by 2022 (AACN, 2014b). Similarly, AACN (2014b) notes that according to the 2012 "United States Registered Nurse Workforce Report Card and Shortage Forecast," a shortage of RNs is projected to spread across the country between 2009 and 2030, with the shortage being felt most intensely in the Southern and Western United States.

Causes of Increased Demand

There are multiple factors driving this demand, including a growing population, medical advances that increase the need for adequately educated nurses, and the increased acuity of hospitalized patients. Other factors driving demand are the technological advances in patient care and an increasing emphasis on health care prevention.

In addition, a growing elderly population with extended longevity and more chronic health conditions requires more nursing care. As life expectancy in the United States increases, more nurses will be needed to assist the individuals who are surviving serious illnesses and living longer with chronic diseases. The AACN (2014a) concurs, suggesting that as baby boomers enter their retirement years, their demand for care is escalating and health care reform will soon provide subsidies for more than 30 million citizens to more fully use the health care system. As a result, the demand for health care is expected to steadily increase in the next few decades and the numbers of nurses to care for these patients will lag behind.

THE SUPPLY OF NURSES

Supply refers to the quantity of goods or services that are ready for use or purchase (*Merriam Webster's Online Dictionary*, 2014b). Currently, hospitals employ about 61% of working nurses. Seven percent of RNs hold jobs in physician offices, 6% in home health care services, 7% in nursing care facilities, and 6% in government (Bureau of Health Statistics, 2014–2015).

To evaluate the supply of RNs in the United States, it is necessary to look at both RNs who are currently working and those who are eligible to work, but do not. In addition, the current and potential student pool must be part of the supply discussion.

The United States currently has about 3 million RNs filling about 2.7 million jobs (Bureau of Health Statistics, 2014–2015). Despite declining vacancy rates, particularly at hospitals, this does not appear to be enough to meet either short- or long-term needs in hospitals or other health care settings. "In June 2011, *Wanted Analytics* reported that employers and staffing agencies posted more than 121,000 new job ads for RNs in May, up 46% from May 2010. About 10% of that growth, or 12,700, were ads placed for positions at general and surgical hospitals, where annual turnover rates for RNs average 14%" (AACN, 2014b, para. 4).

The bottom line is that the supply of RNs is expected to grow minimally in the coming decade, but large numbers of nurses are expected to retire. It must be noted, however, that despite evidence suggesting a significant current and projected nursing shortage, new nurse graduates in many parts of the country report having difficulty finding jobs, particularly in hospital settings. In addition, Magnet hospitals prefer to hire baccalaureate graduates, making it more difficult for nurses educated in diploma or associate degree programs to find jobs. The 2010 IOM report, *The Future of Nursing*, recommends a rapid escalation of baccalaureate degree completion for RNs, and this too will further job-hunting challenges for newly graduated associate degree and diploma-educated nurses in the coming decade.

The current restricted job market for new graduate nurses, however, most likely reflects the current low vacancy rate in hospitals related to economy-induced delayed retirements and hiring freezes. The reality is that hospitals are hiring nurses, but they are attempting to hire experienced nurses whenever possible.

Discussion Point

Why are nursing school applications surging to record highs at a time when new graduate nurses are reporting difficulty finding jobs?

Enrollment in Nursing Schools

The number of students enrolled or projected to enroll in nursing programs is also an important factor in

TABLE 5.1 Number of Candidates Taking the National Council Licensure Examination for Registered Nurses (NCLEX-RN): First-Time, US-Educated Candidates Only

Program	2008	2009	2010	2011	2012	2013
Diploma	3,666	3,677	3,753	3,476	3,173	2,840
Baccalaureate	49,739	52,241	55,414	58,246	62,535	65,406
Associate	75,545	78,665	81,618	82,764	84,517	86,772
Total	129,121	134,708	140,889	144,583	150,266	155,098

Source: National Council State Boards of Nursing. (2014). *NCLEX pass rates.* Retrieved November 30, 2014, from https://www.ncsbn.org/1237.htm

determining RN supply. Unfortunately, some schools of nursing have closed nursing programs due to funding cuts or to reduce program size. Still others have been forced to turn away potential students because of a lack of faculty. Despite this, enrollment in nursing schools has steadily increased every year for almost a decade (Table 5.1). Unfortunately, however, these increases are not adequate to replace those nurses who will be lost to retirement in the coming decade.

AACN (2014b) suggests that the 2.6% increase in entry-level baccalaureate programs in nursing in 2013 is not sufficient to meet the projected demand for nursing services. Unfortunately, enrollment increases are not possible without a significant boost in federal and state funding to prepare new faculty, enhance teaching resources, and upgrade nursing school infrastructure. More money is needed in the form of nursing scholarships and loans to encourage young people to enter nursing. In addition, individual nurses and professional organizations must support legislation to improve financial access to nursing education. The Tri-Council for Nursing (comprising the AACN, the American Nurses Association, the American Organization of Nurse Executives, and the National League for Nursing) has urged nurses to advocate for increased nursing education funding under Title VIII of the Public Health Service Act, as well as other publicly funded initiatives, so that there will be the necessary capacity and resources to educate future nurses.

There have been increases in federal money for nursing education over the last decade. The passage of legislation such as the 2002 Nurse Reinvestment Act encouraged more students to choose nursing as a career and helped students financially to complete their education. It also encouraged graduate students to complete their studies and assume teaching positions in nursing schools. In addition, many states introduced or passed legislation designed to improve working conditions and attract more nurses.

In addition, some hospitals have joined forces with local schools of nursing to offer scholarships in exchange for a student's willingness to work in that institution after graduation. Hospitals are also lending master's and doctorally prepared nurses such as nurse practitioners, clinical nurse specialists, and clinical nurse leaders to supplement faculty positions.

Private foundations have also stepped up to offer funding for nursing education. For example, in 2008, the Robert Wood Johnson Foundation (RWJF) joined with the AACN to create the RWJF New Careers in Nursing (RWJF, 2013). Through grants to schools of nursing, the program funds more than 1,500 scholarships of US$10,000 each annually to schools that offer accelerated baccalaureate and master's nursing programs. Similarly, foundations set up by nursing organizations such as the Association of Perioperative Registered Nurses, the National Student Nurses' Association, and the American Nurses Association provide scholarships and financial assistance to students and RNs pursuing degrees in nursing.

Ironically, recruitment efforts into the nursing profession in the last decade have been very successful, and the problem is no longer a lack of nursing school applicants. Indeed, enrollment in nursing programs of education has increased steadily since 2001. The problem is that there are inadequate resources to provide nursing education to those interested in pursuing nursing as a career, including an insufficient number of clinical sites, classroom space, nursing faculty, and clinical preceptors. As a result, qualified applicants are turned away, despite the current shortage of nurses. Indeed, the AACN (2014b) reported that 79,659 qualified applicants were turned away from baccalaureate and graduate nursing programs alone in 2012. Almost two thirds of the nursing schools responding to the survey pointed to faculty shortages as a reason for not accepting all qualified applicants into their programs (AACN, 2014b).

Educational costs are also a deterrent to increasing nursing school enrollment. Nursing is often called an "expensive major" given relatively low faculty-to-student ratios in clinical courses and the need for financially strapped states to subsidize the cost of education at state universities.

Discussion Point

Should the increased cost of nursing education be passed on to students? Would students enrolled in public universities be willing to pay more for their education than students in other majors?

The greatest challenge, however, to increasing nursing school enrollment, is an inadequate number of nursing faculty to teach students interested in pursuing nursing as a career. According to a Special Survey on Vacant Faculty Positions released by AACN in October 2013, a total of 1,358 faculty vacancies were identified in a survey of 680 nursing schools with baccalaureate and/or graduate programs across the country, creating a national nurse faculty vacancy rate of 8.3% (AACN, 2014c). Besides the vacancies, schools cited the need to create an additional 98 faculty positions to accommodate student demand. Most of the vacancies (86.9%) were faculty positions requiring or preferring a doctoral degree. The top reasons cited by schools having difficulty finding faculty were a limited number of doctorally prepared faculty (31%), and noncompetitive salaries compared with positions in the practice arena (28.4%; AACN, 2014c).

Research conducted by the National League for Nursing (NLN) and the Carnegie Foundation Preparation for the Professions Program found an aging, overworked faculty earning far less than nurses entering clinical practice (NLN, 2015). In fact, this study reported that nurse faculty earned only 76% of the salary that faculty in other academic disciplines earned and that they earned far less than their RN counterparts in clinical practice. This lack of competitive pay for nurse educators is a significant obstacle to recruiting new nursing faculty.

> *At the professor rank, nurse educators suffered the largest deficit with salaries averaging 45% lower than those of their non-nurse colleagues. Associate and assistant nursing professors were also at a disadvantage, earning 19% and 15% less than similarly ranked faculty in other fields. Those employed as nursing instructors experienced the only advantage, with salaries averaging 8% higher than those of non-nurses.* (NLN, 2015, para. 2)

Increasing the number of nursing students in the pipeline as a strategy for addressing the current nursing shortage clearly depends on having enough qualified faculty to teach them. Clearly, the same energy that was directed at recruiting young people for nursing must now be directed at recruiting nursing faculty.

In response, programs have been created both to encourage nurses to consider careers in nursing education and to support them in that role. For example, the Division of Labor Workforce Investment Act has created a Faculty Loan Repayment Program, for nurses willing to serve in faculty roles after graduation. Furthermore, the NINR, the Agency for Health Care Research and Quality Department of Veterans Affairs, and other private foundations have funds available to enhance nursing education and faculty development.

In addition, AACN and the Johnson & Johnson Campaign for Nursing's Future announced the creation of a Minority Nurse Faculty Scholars program in 2008 (AACN, 2014c). This program seeks to address the nursing faculty shortage and diversity of the faculty population by providing financial support to graduate nursing students from minority backgrounds who agree to teach in a school of nursing after graduation. In late 2012, the Jonas Nurse Leaders Scholar Program expanded nationally and now provides funding and support to 198 doctoral nursing students in 87 schools across the United States, making it one of the largest programs addressing the nation's dire shortage of doctorally prepared nursing faculty (AACN, 2014c).

To support the retention of new nursing faculty, the Elsevier Foundation awarded a grant to the Sigma Theta Tau International (STTI) Foundation for Nursing in 2009 to create a Nurse Faculty Mentored Leadership Development Program. Early career nurse educators with an advanced degree were selected to receive 18 months of leadership training designed to help them overcome the challenges of transitioning from nursing practice to faculty (Elsevier Foundation, 2014). "The program reflects the Elsevier Foundation's effort to alleviate the nurse faculty crisis by providing knowledge, skill development

BOX 5.1 Long-Term Strategies for Addressing the Nursing Faculty Shortage

1. Recruitment
   - Provide a positive image for a career in nursing education.
   - Provide incentives for part-time and adjunct faculty to return to school to earn doctoral degrees.
   - Provide fellowships or tuition forgiveness in exchange for teaching service.
   - Develop mentoring/support programs for new academics.
2. Retention
   - Provide salaries and benefits for nursing faculty similar to that in nonacademic settings.
   - Establish positive work environments and reasonable teaching assignments.
   - Recognize and reward teaching excellence.
   - Create academic environments that foster innovation.
   - Fund faculty development and mentorship programs.
3. Collaboration
   - Partner with health care stakeholders to create support for higher education in nursing.

opportunities and support to retain new nurse educators who have transitioned into the role" (Elsevier Foundation, 2014). Other long-term strategies for addressing the nursing faculty shortage are shown in Box 5.1.

Consider This Unfilled faculty positions, resignations, and projected retirements continue to pose a threat to the nursing education workforce.

Part-Time and Unemployed Nurses: An Untapped Pool?

Some experts have suggested that too much emphasis has been placed on recruiting young people to solve the nursing shortage and that supply could more easily be increased by bringing unemployed or part-time nurses back to nursing full-time. The reality, however, is that the percentage of RNs who are not employed in nursing has dropped significantly since 1977, from more than one in four RNs to one in six (Buerhaus, Staiger, & Auerbach, 2009b). In addition, the number of RNs working full time increased from 68% in 1977 to just greater than 70% in 2004, and the number of hours during a given week worked by both full- and part-time RNs combined increased by approximately 6.5% between 1983 and 2006 (Buerhaus et al., 2009b). Thus, the pool of part-time and unemployed nurses has already been tapped.

In addition, the literature on reentry of RNs into the workplace is often pessimistic, suggesting that such programs take a great deal of effort for the results they provide. Yet, Buerhaus et al. (2009b) suggest that the current shortage has been lessened, at least in part, by the reentry of older RNs into employment. This was especially true earlier in the past decade when the US economy first began to stall. In fact, the "employment growth of older RNs (over the age of 50) has increased every year since 2000 for an astounding net gain of more than 257,000 full time equivalent (FTE) RNs" (Buerhaus et al., 2009b, p. 119). In contrast, the total net employment growth of RNs aged 21 to 34 was only roughly 36,000, which was effectively negated by a similar net decrease in employment (roughly 40,000 FTE RNs) by RNs aged 35 to 59. Buerhaus et al. warned, however, that the increased demand by boomers and the aging workforce will make the reentry of older RNs only a brief reprieve in a shortage that is far from over.

Using Foreign-Born Nurses to Relieve the Shortage

The shortage has also been alleviated at least in part by the importation of RNs from foreign markets. Buerhaus, Staiger, and Auerbach (2009a) suggested that the number of foreign-born RNs in the US workforce between 1994 and 2001 averaged 6.0% each year. By 2002, it doubled to 12.5%. After a temporary decline in 2005, likely related to the expiration of work visas, the employment of foreign-born nurses surged forward again in 2006, outstripping the growth in employment among nurses born in the United States: "Overall, the rapid growth in employment of foreign-born RNs accounts for more than one third (37%) of the total growth of total RN employment in the United States since 2002" (Buerhaus et al., 2009a, p. 118).

Widespread, transnational nursing migration is likely to continue for some time, given the success hospitals have had with foreign recruitment and the time required to strengthen the domestic nurse supply pipeline. Such practice, however, could potentially have negative implications in terms of the domestic job market and health care quality. In addition, using foreign-born labor has complex international implications, creating a drain on some countries' health care systems while shoring up the economies of countries that purposefully export their workers. Because the importation of nurses has such complex ramifications, a separate chapter is devoted to its discussion (see Chapter 6).

ROOTS OF THE SHORTAGE

Many factors contribute to the current nursing shortage in acute care settings, including an aging workforce, high turnover due to worker dissatisfaction, inadequate long-term pay incentives, and an increasing recognition by nurses that they can make more money and act more autonomously as free agents than as full-time employees of a health care organization. These factors and others (Box 5.2) will be discussed in this section.

Nursing as a "Graying" Population

Nursing is a graying population—even more so than the population at large. This means that the nursing workforce is retiring at a rate faster than it can be replaced. According to a 2013 survey conducted by the National Council of State Boards of Nursing and The Forum of State Nursing Workforce Centers, 55% of the RN workforce is age 50 or older (AACN, 2014b). In addition, the Health Resources and Services Administration projects that more than 1 million RNs will reach retirement age within the next 10 to 15 years (AACN, 2014b).

Given the demographics of the nursing workforce, an aging pattern is expected to continue over the next decade. Indeed, the average age of the working nurse has been increasing for some time, reflecting a two- to three-decade-long trend toward older students entering nursing education programs, as well as a general decline in interest in nursing as a career among younger people.

Indeed, retirement projections for the profession continue to be grim. Ostrow (2012) suggests that the nursing shortage will explode once again by 2020 when a glut of retirees will leave a new gap to fill. Although many nurses have temporarily delayed retirement due to the recession, a wave of retiring nurses is coming and this will result in an "intellectual drain of institutional and professional nursing knowledge" (Wood, 2011, para. 15). The loss of so many experienced nurses and institutional memory at the same time would almost certainly have an impact on the stability as well as quality of care. Wood (2012) agrees, noting that younger nurses need the knowledge and mentoring that older, more experienced nurses can provide and that the health care system will lose critical clinical and institutional knowledge that creates a safety net for patients and novice nurses in the complexity of today's health care.

Discussion Point

What factors have led to the "graying" of the nursing workforce? Does there appear to be any short-term resolution of these factors?

BOX 5.2 Causes of the Current Nursing Shortage

- Increasing elderly population (more individuals who are chronically ill)
- Increased acuity in acute care settings, requiring higher-level nursing skills
- Downsizing and restructuring of the late 1990s, which eliminated many RN positions
- A relatively healthy economy in the late 1990s and early 2000s, which encouraged some nurses to change from full-time employment to part-time or to quit
- Aging RN workforce
- Workplace dissatisfaction
- Women choosing fields other than nursing for a career
- Aging faculty for RN programs
- Inadequate nursing programs to accommodate interested applicants
- Low ceiling on wages for RNs without advanced degrees
- Future educator pool for RNs more limited than demand

Discussion Point

Why is there so little discussion about the "expertise gap" that will occur as a result of impending nursing retirements?

The Nursing Faculty Are Grayer Yet

To further confound the nursing shortage and efforts to address it, the average age of nursing faculty members continues to increase, narrowing the number of productive years nurse educators can teach. AACN (2014c) notes in their *2012–2013 Salaries of Instructional and Administrative Nursing Faculty in Baccalaureate and Graduate Programs in Nursing*, that the average ages of doctorally prepared nurse faculty holding the ranks of professor, associate professor, and assistant professor were 61.3, 57.7, and 51.5 years, respectively. For master's degree-prepared nurse faculty, the average ages for professors, associate professors, and assistant professors were 57.2, 56.8, and 51.2 years, respectively. AACN concludes that a wave of faculty retirements is expected across the United States over the next decade.

One must question where the faculty will come from to teach the new nurses needed to solve the current shortage. In addition, given the lag time required to educate master's- or doctorally prepared faculty, the faculty shortage may end up being the greatest obstacle to solving the current nursing shortage.

Consider This Even if enough students can be recruited to become nurses, there will likely not be enough faculty to teach them.

Cusson (2014) suggests a two-prong approach to the nurse faculty shortage. She suggests a short-term approach of creating incentives for part-time and clinical adjunct faculty to return to school for advanced degrees and providing built-in periodic raises and use of a full-time clinical coordinator to support these faculty, so they can be more closely connected to the school's curriculum and mission. The long-term approach is to recruit graduate students to join the ranks of their professors as well as providing scholarship support for students interested in a teaching career.

Fortunately, many foundations and funders have stepped forward to do just this. In June 2011, the AACN and the Jonas Center for Nursing Excellence entered into a collaboration to increase the number of doctorally prepared faculty available to teach in nursing schools nationwide. This initiative supports 150 new doctoral students across all 50 states, providing financial assistance, leadership development, and mentoring support to expand the pipeline of future nurse faculty into research-focused (PhD, DNS) and practice-focused (DNP) doctoral nursing programs (AACN, 2014c).

The Free Agent Nurse

An increase in the number of free agent nurses is another aspect that must be examined in assessing supply and demand factors of the current nursing shortage. Full-time employment of nurses is decreasing. Instead, nurses are increasingly assuming the role of *free agent*, a term more common to Generation X than their older counterparts, and this contributes to a shortage in acute-care agencies. A free agent nurse is often an independent contractor who sells his or her services to an employer, with the condition that he or she maintains control over the number of hours they are willing to work and working conditions.

Per-diem and *traveling nurses* are two types of free agents. The relationship between the free agent and his or her employing organization is based on a free and open exchange, more of a partnership than an unequal dependency relationship. Typically, the free agent nurse makes a higher hourly wage than other full-time or part-time employees in a health care organization in exchange for not receiving health care and retirement benefits. Such nurses also have greater control over if and when they want to work.

Historically, health care organizations have sought to employ full-time workers (employees) so that they could better control the availability of needed human resources. However, the free agent model of nursing is gaining momentum in health care organizations as they recognize that they need to supplement their full-time employee pool with these skilled workers and that significant benefit costs can be saved from using free agent or temporary workers.

Critics of the increased use of free agent nurses, particularly traveling nurses, suggest that this practice may negatively affect the quality of care related to inconsistency of caretakers and a reduced ability to determine the competencies of the specific free agent nurse. More research is needed, however, on the effect of the free agent nurse on the current nursing shortage.

Workplace Dissatisfaction

Perhaps one of the most significant yet least addressed factors leading to the current RN shortage is workplace dissatisfaction, resulting in high turnover levels and nurses leaving the profession. Long shifts, low autonomy, mandatory overtime, and being forced to work during weekends, nights, and holidays prompt many nurses to look for other jobs.

A recent RWJF study found that an estimated 17.5% of newly licensed RNs leave their first nursing job within the first year and one in three (33.5%) leave within 2 years (New York University, 2014). Twibell et al. (2012) suggest this turnover for new nurses is primarily related to heavy workloads and an inability to ensure patient safety. In addition, new nurses express disillusionment about scheduling, lack of autonomous practice, and the lack of intrinsic and extrinsic workplace rewards. Lastly, new nurses report dissatisfying relationships with peers, managers, and interprofessional colleagues and insufficient time with patients (Twibell et al., 2012).

Consider This Nursing shortages cannot be resolved until we address the underlying issues of worker dissatisfaction that caused them in the first place.

Is Pay an Issue?

Salaries also provide mixed incentives for young people to become nurses and for nurse retention. The economy at the end of the 20th century was fairly strong, with low unemployment and rising consumer confidence. This resulted in some RNs, who were often the second breadwinner in the family unit, reducing their work hours or leaving the workplace entirely. Many of these same RNs, however, returned to work in the past decade as a result of declining stock market values, a rising recession, and lower levels of consumer confidence.

Wages for RNs have, however, increased with rising demand and progression of the shortage. The median annual wage of RNs as of 2012 was $64,470 (Bureau of Health Statistics, 2014). RNs employed by the government had the highest median wages at $68,540 and nurses working in physician offices had the lowest at $58,420. Experienced nurses (more than 20 years), on average, earn significantly more than those with less than 1-year experience ($67,000 median salary as compared to $51,000; PayScale, 2014a).

Discussion Point

Historically, nursing has been considered an altruistic profession. How critical do you think pay is as a motivator for people who want to become nurses today?

Average base salaries for nurse practitioners in 2014 ranged from US$69,992 to US$102,382 with bonuses and profit sharing adding up to US$20,000 additional wages annually (PayScale, 2014b). Similarly, according to the American Academy of Nurse Practitioners, the average salary of a nurse practitioner, across settings and specialties, was $94,050 (AACN, 2014b).

In contrast to the findings for staff nurses, salary is clearly a deterrent for nursing faculty, although Cusson (2014) suggests that flexible hours, the ability to work from home, generous benefit packages (particularly at state institutions), and academic calendars provide opportunities for a better lifestyle than do many clinical positions. PayScale (2014c) reported that the median salary in 2014 for a nurse educator was $67,025 (PayScale, 2014c). In contrast, AACN (2014c) reported that master's prepared faculty earned an annual average salary of $80,690 in 2013.

One reason that nursing faculty salaries are so poor comparatively is that nursing education has never had the same federal funding support as medical education. In addition, securing advanced academic degrees is costly. Indeed, many graduate students who may have become educators in the past are now opting instead for better-paying positions in clinical and private practice. Clearly, increasing faculty salaries and providing tuition support for graduate students considering a career as a nursing faculty will be an essential part of addressing the increasing faculty shortage.

Discussion Point

What incentives should be offered to nurses who earn a master's or doctoral degree to become nursing faculty members rather than advanced practice nurses engaged in clinical practice?

Retention: An Undervalued Strategy

Some organizational turnover is normal and, in fact, desirable since it infuses the organization with fresh ideas. It also reduces the probability of *groupthink*, in which everyone shares similar thought processes, values, and goals (Marquis & Huston, 2015). However, excessive or unnecessary turnover reduces the ability of the organization to produce its end product. Thus, retention becomes a critical goal when workforce shortages exist and the achievement of desired outcomes is critical to organizational success.

Unfortunately, many highly trained, employable nurses are *voluntarily* leaving the profession because they are dissatisfied with their work or the environment in which they work. Annual turnover in acute care hospitals is currently approximately 16.5%, up from 14.7% in 2012 (Nursing Solutions Inc, 2014). Similarly, the turnover rate for bedside RNs also increased during this same time period to 14.2%, up from 13.1% in 2012. RNs working in surgical services recorded the lowest turnover rate at 10.7%. Nurses working in Med/Surg experienced a higher turnover rate than any other nursing specialty at 24% (Nursing Solutions Inc, 2014).

High levels of turnover are disruptive to organizational functioning and threaten the quality of patient care. High turnover rates are also generally expensive. According to Nursing Solutions Inc (2014), the average cost of turnover for a bedside RN ranges from $44,380 to $63,400 resulting in the average hospital losing $4.21M to $6.02M. Each percent change in RN turnover will cost the average hospital an additional $359,650.

Not all health care organizations, however, have high turnover rates. Organizations perceived to be employers of choice, such as magnet hospitals, retain their employees and are more capable of replacing losses than less-sought-after employers. Therefore, having a healthy work environment provides an advantage in the competition for scarce nursing resources. Clearly, organizations that pay attention to the employee market and understand what people are looking for in the work environment have a better chance to recruit and retain top talent.

Many strategies have been suggested for promoting the retention of workers. A literature review by Lartey, Cummings, and Profetto-McGrath (2014) suggested that no single intervention can be shown to promote RN retention; instead, team work and individually targeted strategies including mentoring, leadership interest, and in-depth orientation increased job satisfaction and produced higher retention results (Research Study Fuels the Controversy 5.1).

Consider This Retention of precious nurse resources must be a very real part of the solution to the nursing shortage; health care institutions must make a commitment to improving working conditions for nurses.

Research Study Fuels the Controversy 5.1

Interventions to Promote RN Retention

This systematic review of the literature synthesized evidence-based interventions that promote the retention of experienced RNs in health care settings. Six electronic databases—CINAHL, PsychInfo, EMBASE, Medline, Cochrane library, SCOPUS—were searched for this study. The titles and abstracts of the articles were reviewed and assessed for articles describing interventions that measured retention among RNs in a health care setting.

Source: Lartey, S., Cummings, G., & Profetto-McGrath, J. (2014). Interventions that promote retention of experienced registered nurses in health care settings: a systematic review. *Journal of Nursing Management, 22*(8), 1027–1041. doi:10.1111/jonm.12105

Study Findings

While many studies in the literature have focused on the retention of new graduate nurses and strategies that increase job satisfaction, little research has been published on interventions that increase the retention of experienced nurses. This review, in line with findings from another review, found little evidence of the effectiveness of any specific intervention targeting the retention of this group. Given that retention is influenced by many factors such as flexible scheduling, money, health benefits, mentorship opportunities, organizational focus on retention, management practices and recognition, work environment, and retirement plans, the results of this review do not point to one particular intervention that could be implemented to influence experienced nurse retention. The researchers concluded that health care settings need a combination of these interventions to increase the retention of their experienced nursing staff.

CONSEQUENCES OF NURSING SHORTAGES

What are the consequences of a nursing shortage? To answer this question, it is critical first to recognize that patient outcomes are sensitive to nursing interventions and that, as a result, nurse staffing (total hours of care, as well as staffing mix) affects patient outcomes. This supposition is certainly supported by a review of the literature, which increasingly suggests that RN staffing affects patient outcomes such as inpatient mortality and other measures of quality of hospital care. Indeed, numerous studies have been conducted to describe the relationship between nurse staffing levels and clinical outcomes of patients at both the hospital and unit levels. These studies are summarized in Chapter 9.

ADDITIONAL STRATEGIES FOR SOLVING A NURSING SHORTAGE

Just as the issues that caused nursing shortages are complex, so too must be the solutions. Only some of the solutions that have been presented to address the current nursing shortage are included here, including redesigning the workplace, increasing the number of nursing students in the pipeline, importing foreign nurses, improving nursing's image, and increasing the faculty pool. In addition, Box 5.3 includes a list of 11 strategies created by the Honor Society of Nursing, STTI (1999–2014) for reducing the current shortage.

Redesigning the Workplace for an Older Workforce

The age of the current nursing workforce is an important factor in the current nursing shortage because nursing can be both physically and mentally taxing, even to the young. Some experts have suggested that more attention should be given to retaining older workers or bringing retired nurses back into the workforce since these employees are generally more productive, more reliable, and highly experienced. Some adaptations of the working environment may be needed, however, to meet the needs and limitations of an aging workforce such as flexible work shift options and job sharing.

In addition, RNs must be made to feel valued, and physician–nurse relationships reflecting collegiality and collaboration should be fostered. In addition, environments of shared governance should be created in which nurses actively participate in all decision making related to patient care. Staff nurses should feel empowered, and autonomy should be encouraged. Additional strategies for retaining older workers are shown in Box 5.4.

BOX 5.3 Strategies for Addressing Nursing Shortages

- Demonstrate to health care leaders that nurses are the critical difference in the US health care system.
- Reposition nursing as a highly versatile profession in which young people can learn science and technology, customer service, critical thinking, and decision-making skills.
- Construct practice environments that are interdisciplinary and build on relationships among nurses, physicians, other health care professionals, patients, and communities.
- Create patient care models that encourage professional nurse autonomy and clinical decision making.
- Develop additional evaluation systems that measure the relationship of timely nursing interventions to patient outcomes.
- Establish additional standards and mechanisms for recognition of professional practice environments.
- Develop career enhancement incentives for nurses to pursue professional practice.
- Evaluate the effects of the nursing shortage on the preparation of the next generation of nurse educators, nurse administrators, and nurse researchers and take strategic action.
- Implement and sustain a marketing effort that addresses the image of nursing and the recruitment of qualified students into nursing as a career.
- Promote higher education to nurses of all educational levels.
- Develop and implement strategies to promote the retention of RNs and nurse educators in the workforce.

Source: Honor Society of Nursing, Sigma Theta Tau International. (1999–2014). *Facts on the nursing shortage in North America.* Retrieved November 30, 2014, from http://www.nursingsociety.org/Media/Pages/shortage.aspx. Reprinted with permission.

BOX 5.4 Strategies for Retaining Older Workers

- Flexible shift options with more options for shorter shifts
- Job-sharing
- Work redesign to limit physical energy expenditure
- Use lift teams, special beds, and equipment to reduce work-related injuries and strain
- Benefit packages that recognize the needs of mature workers
- Recognize and use experienced workers as mentors and preceptors

Changing Nursing's Image

Price and McGillis Hall (2014) note that stereotypical imaging and messaging of the nursing profession have been shown to shape nurses' expectations and perceptions of nursing as a career, which has implications for both recruitment and retention. Students interested in nursing may be dissuaded from choosing it as a career based on negative, stereotypical images, especially those that position the profession as inferior to medicine. Thus, strategies for future recruitment and socialization within the nursing and the health professions need to include contemporary and realistic imaging of both health professional roles and practice settings (Price & McGillis Hall, 2014). This will not be an easy task, given the historical roots of nursing stereotypes and the profession's long history of being unable to effectively change public perceptions regarding professional nursing roles and behaviors (see Chapter 24).

Conclusions

Many factors led to a significant professional nursing shortage in the early 21st century. Predictions are that this shortage will recur by 2020 as the economy continues to improve, demand increases, and an aging workforce retires. Health care providers, the public, and legislators are beginning to recognize that both the problem and the potential consequences could be severe. One would be hard-pressed to find a congressperson or senator who would not identify health care workforce shortages as one of the most serious issues affecting health care today.

Yet, efforts to proactively address the coming shortage have, to date, been few and far between. Short-term solutions to the shortage have been attempted, including importing foreign nurses and increasing federal money for nursing education. The passage of current legislation has encouraged more students to choose nursing as a career and has helped students financially to complete their education. It has also encouraged graduate students to complete their studies and assume teaching positions in nursing schools. Long-term planning and aggressive intervention, however, will be needed for some time at the national and regional levels to ensure that an adequate, highly qualified nursing workforce will be available in the future to meet health care needs in the United States.

More must be done to address the predicted future nursing shortage, and it is increasingly obvious that multiple solutions to the shortage will be needed. These solutions will require the best thinking of experts and will likely reshape fundamental core underpinnings that have been a part of the nursing work world for decades, if not centuries.

For Additional Discussion

1. In what ways do other professions do a better job of attracting younger workers—both men and women?
2. Are salaries a significant driver in the current nursing shortage? At what level would salaries not be a factor?
3. How would increasing the educational level for entry into practice affect the current nursing shortage?
4. Will the demand for RNs in the future be affected by growing technological developments?

(continued)

5. Why has the nursing workforce historically suffered some degree of a shortage every 10 to 15 years?
6. If magnet hospital criteria (increased number of BSN educated nurses on staff) become the baseline for organizational structure and performance, would nursing shortages exist?
7. Why are starting salaries for nurses with master's and doctoral degrees in academia so low?
8. Why do many health care organizations choose to expend more money on recruitment than on retention strategies? Which is more effective in the short term and in the long term?
9. Is implementation of mandatory minimum staffing ratios in acute care hospitals likely to reduce the nursing shortage in California?

References

American Association of Colleges of Nursing. (2014a). *Joint statement from the Tri-Council for Nursing on recent registered nurse supply and demand projections.* Retrieved November 29, 2014, from http://www.aacn.nche.edu/Media/NewsReleases/2010/tricouncil.html

American Association of Colleges of Nursing. (2014b). *Fact sheets: Nursing shortage.* Retrieved from http://www.aacn.nche.edu/Media/FactSheets/NursingShortage.htm

American Association of Colleges of Nursing. (2014c). *Fact sheet: Nursing faculty shortage.* Retrieved November 30, 2014, from http://www.aacn.nche.edu/media-relations/fact-sheets/nursing-faculty-shortage

Buerhaus, P. I., Staiger, D. O., & Auerbach, D. I. (2009a). *The future of the nursing workforce in the United States: Data, trends, and implications.* Boston, MA: Jones & Bartlett Learning.

Buerhaus, P., Staiger, D., & Auerbach, D. (2009b). The recent surge in nurse employment: Causes and implications. *Health Affairs, 28*(4), w657–w668.

Bureau of Health Statistics, U.S. Department of Labor. (2014). *Registered nurses.* Retrieved November 30, 2014, from http://www.bls.gov/ooh/Healthcare/Registered-nurses.htm

Bureau of Health Statistics, U.S. Department of Labor. (2014–2015). *Occupational outlook handbook—Registered nurses* (2014–2015 ed.). Retrieved November 30, 2014, from http://www.bls.gov/ooh/healthcare/registered-nurses.htm#tab-3

Cusson, R. (2014, March 20). How colleges can deal with the shortage of nursing professors. *UConn Today.* Retrieved November 30, 2014, from http://today.uconn.edu/blog/2014/03/how-colleges-can-deal-with-the-shortage-of-nursing-professors/

Demand. (2014a). In *Merriam Webster's online dictionary.* Retrieved November 30, 2014, from http://www.merriam-webster.com/dictionary/demand

Elsevier Foundation. (2014). *Preparing nurse educators to confront the nursing shortage.* Retrieved November 29, 2014, from http://www.elsevierfoundation.org/stories/preparing-nurse-educators-to-confront-the-nursing-shortage/

Honor Society of Nursing, Sigma Theta Tau International. (1999–2014). *Facts on the nursing shortage in North America.* Retrieved November 30, 2014, from http://www.nursingsociety.org/Media/Pages/shortage.aspx

Lartey, S., Cummings, G., & Profetto-McGrath, J. (2014). Interventions that promote retention of experienced registered nurses in health care settings: A systematic review. *Journal of Nursing Management, 22*(8), 1027–1041. doi:10.1111/jonm.12105

Marquis, B., & Huston, C. (2015). *Leadership roles and management functions in nursing* (8th ed.). Philadelphia, PA: Lippincott Williams, & Wilkins.

National League for Nursing. (2015). *NLN nurse educator shortage fact sheet.* Retrieved from http://www.nln.org/docs/default-source/advocacy-public-policy/nurse-faculty-shortage-fact-sheet-pdf.pdf?sfvrsn=0

New York University. *Nearly one in five new nurses leave first job within a year, according to survey of newly-licensed registered nurses* (2014, September 8). Retrieved November 30, 2014, from http://www.nyu.edu/about/news-publications/news/2014/09/08/nearly-one-in-five-new-nurses-leave-first-job-within-a-year-according-to-survey-of-newly-licensed-registered-nurses.html

Nursing Solutions Inc. (2014). *2014 National healthcare and RN retention report.* Retrieved November 30, 2014, from http://www.nsinursingsolutions.com/

Files/assets/library/retention-institute/National-HealthcareRNRetentionReport2014.pdf

Ostrow, N. (2012, March 21). Nursing shortage is over in U.S. until retirement glut hits. *Bloomberg News.* Retrieved November 30, 2014, from http://www.bloomberg.com/news/2012-03-21/nursing-shortage-in-u-s-is-over-temporarily-researchers-find.html

PayScale. (2014a). *Registered nurse (RN) salary.* Retrieved November 30, 2014, from http://www.payscale.com/research/US/Job=Registered_Nurse_(RN)/Hourly_Rate

PayScale. (2014b). *Nurse practitioner (NP) salary (United States).* Retrieved November 29, 2014, from http://www.payscale.com/research/US/Job=Nurse_Practitioner_(NP)/Salary

PayScale. (2014c). *Nurse educator salary (United States).* Retrieved November 30, 2014, from http://www.payscale.com/research/US/Job=Nurse_Educator/Salary

Price, S. L., & McGillis Hall, L. (2014). The history of nurse imagery and the implications for recruitment: A discussion paper. *Journal of Advanced Nursing, 70*(7), 1502–1509. doi:10.1111/jan.12289

Robert Wood Johnson Foundation. (2013). *About NCIN.* Retrieved November 29, 2014, from http://www.newcareersinnursing.org/about-ncin

Schepp, D. (2013, March 5). Is there a nursing shortage? *AOL Jobs.* Retrieved November 29, 2014, from http://jobs.aol.com/articles/2013/03/05/is-there-a-nursing-shortage-infographic/

Supply. (2014b). In *Merriam Webster's online dictionary.* Retrieved November 30, 2014, from http://www.merriam-webster.com/dictionary/supply

Trust for America's Health. (2015). *State data: Nursing shortage estimates (2010).* Retrieved August 29, 2015, from http://healthyamericans.org/states/states.php?measure=nursingshortage

Twibell, R., St. Pierre, J., Johnson, D., Barton, D., Davis, C., Kidd, M., & Rook, G. (2012, June). Tripping over the welcome mat: Why new nurses don't stay and what the evidence says we can do about it. *American Nurse Today, 7*(6). Retrieved November 30, 2014, from http://www.americannursetoday.com/tripping-over-the-welcome-mat-why-new-nurses-dont-stay-and-what-the-evidence-says-we-can-do-about-it/

Wood, D. (2011, June 10). Nurses continue to delay retirement. *Nursezone.com.* Retrieved June 14, 2011, from http://www.nursezone.com/Nursing-News-Events/more-news/Nurses-Continue-to-Delay-Retirement_37086.aspx

Wood, D. (2012). Retirees and new graduate nurses: The wild cards impacting the nursing shortage. *Nursezone.com.* Retrieved November 30, 2014, from http://www.nursezone.com/Nursing-News-Events/more-news/Retirees-and-New-Graduate-Nurses-The-Wild-Cards-Impacting-the-Nursing-Shortage_36300.aspx

Importing Foreign Nurses

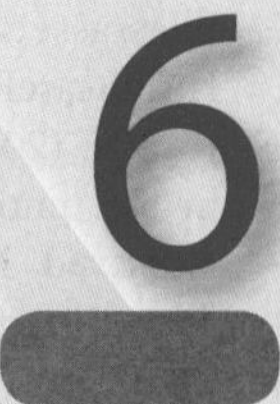

Carol J. Huston

ADDITIONAL RESOURCES

Visit thePoint for additional helpful resources

- eBook
- Journal Articles
- WebLinks

CHAPTER OUTLINE

LEARNING OBJECTIVES

The learner will be able to:

1. Examine how the scope of global nurse migration has changed over the last decade.
2. Analyze "push" and "pull" factors that encourage nurses to migrate internationally.
3. Identify primary donor and recipient countries of migrating nurses.
4. Explore potential negative effects of international migration, including "brain drain" from donor countries.
5. Apply the ethical principles of autonomy, utility, and justice in arguing for or against global nurse recruitment and migration.
6. Explore the ethical dimensions of nurse migration.
7. Outline common key components of position statements on nurse migration adopted by professional associations such as the International Council of Nurses, the International Centre on Nurse Migration, AcademyHealth, and the World Health Organization.
8. Explore national and international efforts to develop best practices or regulatory oversight of international nurse recruitment and migration.
9. Differentiate between the types of work visas foreign nurses use to gain entry for employment in the United States.

(continues on page 79)

10. Outline the certification process required by the Commission on Graduates of Foreign Nursing Schools for migratory nurses to be able to take the NCLEX examination and obtain visas for work in the United States.
11. Discuss the need for ongoing cultural, professional, and psychological support for foreign nurses after their arrival in their importer country to assist them in successful socialization.
12. Reflect on personal beliefs and values regarding the use of widespread international recruitment and nurse migration to address nursing shortages.

INTRODUCTION

Many countries have experienced cyclical shortages of nurses, but typically they were caused by increasing demand outstripping a static or slowly growing supply of nurses. The current situation is different. Demand continues to grow while supply decreases as a result of an aging workforce, projected increases in nursing retirements in the coming decade, and an inadequate number of new graduates from nursing education programs. Indeed, many of the developed countries in the world are reporting nursing shortages. In 2013, the International Council of Nurses Workforce Forum noted that most industrialized countries are or will be imminently facing a nursing shortage due to the increased demands for health care (Hongyan, Wenbo, & Junxin, 2014).

One increasingly common means of alleviating these shortages has been to recruit foreign nurses. International recruitment and *nurse migration*—moving from one country to another in search of employment—has been viewed as a relatively inexpensive, "quick-fix" solution to health care worker shortages. The current situation, however, is different from the past, when nurse migration was mostly based on individual motivation and typically followed previous colonial ties. Now there is active planning of large-scale international nurse recruitment, often from developing countries that can least afford to lose their most highly educated health care workers.

This has significant local and regional implications. For example, Aiken, Buchan, Sochalski, Nichols, and Powell (2013) note that nurse migration from developing countries is occurring at the same time that international resources are finally available to address HIV/AIDS and improve immunization coverage around the world. However, this effort has been undermined by the severe shortage of health personnel in countries like Botswana.

A recruiting onslaught affects the ability of developing countries to develop sustainable health care systems and provide appropriate care to their citizens. Indeed, few donor nations are prepared to manage the loss of their nurse workforce to such widespread migration. In addition, developing countries often recruit from each other, even within the same geographical region. Table 6.1 summarizes the current dynamic nature of nurse migration in select countries around the world.

GLOBAL MIGRATION OF NURSES: "PUSH" AND "PULL" FACTORS

To understand what is driving the global migration of nurses, it is first necessary to examine what are known as the "push" and "pull" factors of nursing migration. *Push factors* are those factors that push or drive nurses to want to leave their countries to go to another. Low pay, inadequate opportunities for career advancement or continuing education, sociopolitical instability, and unsafe workplaces are examples of push factors. Other factors that act as push factors in some countries include the risk of human immunodeficiency virus and acquired immunodeficiency disease to health system workers, concerns about personal security in areas of conflict, and economic instability.

Consider This Nurses migrate for many reasons and the push/pull factors to migrate are in constant imbalance.

Pull factors are those factors that draw the nurse toward a different country. Pull factors typically include higher pay, more-developed career structures, opportunities for further education and professional development, and, in some cases, safety from the threat of violence (more prevalent in less-developed countries). Other pull factors, such as the opportunity to travel or to participate in foreign aid work, also influence some nurses. A summary of push and pull factors for nurse migration is given in Table 6.2.

TABLE 6.1 Effect of Push–Pull Migration on Select Countries

Africa	Hongyan et al. (2014) note that Sub-Saharan Africa suffers from 25% of the world's disease burden, yet they only have 1.3% of the trained health workforce. Thus, the nursing shortage is more severe and felt more strongly in the source countries. The migration drains the source countries of desperately needed skilled personnel. A 2014 study by Silvestri et al. (2014) suggests that a significant proportion of nursing students in Africa intend to work abroad or in cities after training. Similarly, George and Reardon (2013) found that more than a third (37%) of the medical and nursing student respondents in South Africa intended to work or specialize abroad and the majority intended to leave South Africa within 5 years of completing their medical or nursing. Poor working conditions within the health sector, such as long work hours, high patient loads, inadequate resources, and occupational hazards, influenced these students' decisions to consider migration.
Australia	Australia has long imported foreign nurses to supplement its health care workforce and numbers are only increasing. In fact, the permanent migration of foreign registered nurses to Australia has increased sixfold since the year 2000 (Finnish Medical Society, 2013). Australia is identified though as both a primary donor and a recipient country for migrant nurses and primarily recruits from the United Kingdom and New Zealand. Hongyan et al. (2014) suggest that Australia gains an indirect economic benefit from migrating nurses. In Australia, foreign-educated nurses are required to complete a 1- or 2-year pre-registration nurse course as well as language classes prior to employment. Individual nurses pay up to $20,000 per year for these courses. In addition, these nurses pay for their basic living costs. Thus, training migrant nurses is a profitable industry and contributes to their national economy.
Canada	Canada is both a source and a destination country for international nurse migration, with an estimated net loss of nurses. The United States is a major beneficiary of Canadian nurse emigration, resulting from the reduction of full-time jobs for nurses in Canada due to health system reforms. FWCanada Inc. (2014) notes there are two Canadian immigration programs foreign RNs can qualify for without the need of a job offer from a Canadian employer. The Quebec Skilled Worker program has long allowed foreign nurses to qualify for permanent residence. In August 2013, the Quebec government made changes to the program to allow nurses to earn even more points under this program. As a result, the permanent migration of foreign nurses to Canada has increased threefold since the year 2000 (Finnish Medical Society, 2013). The other program is the Nova Scotia Provincial Nominee Program known as the Regional Labor Market Demand Stream. This program has designated 26 occupations that are in high demand in the province and has imposed relatively low barriers to apply.
China	Many Chinese nurses intend to migrate due to limited job opportunities, low salary, and low job satisfaction. Commercial recruiters have expressed a strong interest in recruiting Chinese nurses, but there are limited examples of successful ventures. It is likely that China will become an important source of nurses for developed nations in the coming years.
India	Despite an extremely low nurse-to-population ratio in India, large-scale nurse migration to other countries is increasing. Low wages, heavy workloads, poor working conditions, and a lack of respect are push factors for many Indian nurses to migrate.
Ireland	As late as 25 years ago, Ireland had an abundant pool of nurses. Ireland now though actively recruits nurses from overseas. Thus, Ireland has moved from being a traditional exporter of nurses to an importer.
Lebanon	Lebanon is a source/donor country to the Persian Gulf, North America, and Europe. The primary push factors are poor working conditions and a lack of autonomy in decision making.
New Zealand	New Zealand has been both a source and destination country since the beginning of the 21st century. The movement of New Zealand RNs to Australia is expedited by the Trans-Tasman Agreement, whereas the entry of foreign RNs to New Zealand is facilitated by nursing being an identified priority occupation. As of March 2015, immigration requirements in New Zealand were tightened so that registered nurses seeking "essential skill" visas under the critical care and emergency, medical, or perioperative categories would have to have 5 years relevant experience rather than 3 years (NZ Tightens Migration Criteria, 2014).

(*continued*)

TABLE 6.1 Effect of Push–Pull Migration on Select Countries (*continued*)

Philippines	The Philippines is a source country for nurse migration. National opinion has generally focused on the improved quality of life for individual migrants and their families and on the benefits of remittances to the nation; however, a shortage of highly skilled nurses and the massive retraining of physicians to become nurses elsewhere has created severe problems for the Filipino health system, including the closure of some hospitals.
Saudi Arabia	Saudi Arabia now gets most of its nurses from the Philippines—the same place where most countries, including the United States, are doing the majority of their recruiting.
South Korea	A recent study of South Korean nursing students found that 69.8% of respondents intended to migrate abroad, if possible, or absolutely in the future (Lee & Moon, 2013). The two most common reasons for their intended migration were economic (salary) (29.7%) and professional development (28.2%). Working conditions, however, was the most prevalent reason for the decision regarding the destination and place to work.
United Kingdom	Both a donor and recipient county, nurse migration is common in the UK. A significant uptick in Bulgarian and Romanian nurse migration to the UK occurred in 2014 as a result of changes in immigration restrictions. Bulgaria and Romania were no longer subject to transitional employment restrictions as of January 1, 2014 (Office for National Statistics, 2014).
United States	Nurse immigration to the United States has tripled since 1994. Foreign-educated nurses are located primarily in urban areas, most likely to be employed by hospitals, and somewhat more likely to have a baccalaureate degree than native-born nurses.

It is important to remember that developed countries, such as Australia, the United Kingdom, the United States, Norway, Australia, Ireland, and Saudi Arabia, are the primary destinations of most migrant nurses, and developing nations are primarily the donors. Some developed countries, such as the United Kingdom and Australia, are both a source and recipient for the migrating nurses (Hongyan et al., 2014). Destination countries are able to recruit nurses as a result of a large number of pull factors. Many internationally recruited nurses suggest they would have preferred to remain in their home country with family and friends and in a familiar culture and environment, but push and pull factors overwhelmingly influenced their decision to migrate.

Consider This Developed countries are often the recipients of migrant nurses and developing countries are often the donors. In essence then, developing countries are supporting the health care infrastructure of more developed countries, often at the expense of their own country.

TABLE 6.2 Push and Pull Factors for Nurse Migration

Push Factors	Pull Factors
Low pay	High pay
Inadequate opportunities for career advancement or continuing education	More developed career structures or opportunities for further education and professional development
Sociopolitical instability	Increased quality of life
Unsafe workplaces	Safety from the threat of violence
Practice restrictions	Family members in destination country
High workloads	Adventure/love of travel
Poor living conditions (housing, food, water)	Humanitarian motives
Remittance income	Recognition and status
Economic instability	Political stability

EFFECTS OF GLOBAL MIGRATION ON DEVELOPING COUNTRIES

A review of the literature suggests that different countries have experienced different effects as a result of the push–pull of international nurse migration. In some cases, aggressive recruitment, by which large numbers of recruits are sought, may significantly deplete a single health facility or contract an important number of newly graduated nurses from a single educational institute. This has significant local and regional implications since not only is critical intellectual capital taken away from the developing country but that country's health outcomes are likely to worsen.

The Philippines has long been the number one exporter of nurses worldwide. China, with the second largest nursing workforce in the world (2.2 million nurses), is another country actively seeking to export nurses. Yet, a shortage of nurses has haunted China for years and the situation is showing no sign of improvement (Qun & Xiaojing, 2014). A shortfall of 180,000 nurses was reported in south China's Guangdong Province in 2014. Similarly, Hebei Province reports having only 1.52 nurses for every 1,000 people, failing to reach the World Health Organization standard, which requires 2 nurses for every 1,000. By the end of 2013, in the whole country, there were only 1.85 for every 1,000 people (Qun & Xiaojing, 2014).

India is also gaining ground as one of the world's leading nurse exporters, despite having an extremely low nurse-to-population ratio, with the major destinations being the Gulf countries and the Organization for Economic Cooperation and Development (Kodoth & Jacob, 2013). Poor pay as well as poor working and living conditions are significant push factors.

Nonetheless, recent reports from South Africa, Ghana, China, the Caribbean, and even the Philippines highlight that such a significant outflow of nurses has had negative effects, including reductions in the level and quality of services and the loss of specialist skills. Similarly, African countries, particularly those in sub-Saharan Africa, have lost a substantial proportion of their skilled workforce through migration. In fact, a recent study suggested that more than a third (37%) of the medical and nursing student respondents intended to work or specialize abroad and the majority intended to leave South Africa within 5 years of completing their medical or nursing studies (George & Reardon, 2013). Poor working conditions within the health sector, such as long work hours, high patient loads, inadequate resources, and occupational hazards, influenced these students' decisions to consider migration.

This was the case in research conducted by Likupe (2013) where nurses from sub-Saharan Africa identified poor remuneration, lack of professional development in the home countries, poor health care and systems, language and education similarities, and easy availability of jobs and visas as their push factors to leave Africa. These nurses stressed that they would like to stay in their own countries and help develop health care there, but reasons for moving were often strong and apparently not within their control. Research by George, Atujuna, and Gow (2013) supported that assertion that the migration of health workers from South Africa was not occurring as a result of lower salaries alone. Instead, the consideration to move was determined by other factors including age, levels of stress experienced, and the extent to which health workers were satisfied at their current place of work.

The movement of health workers both within and outside of South Africa has been recognized as a major problem for the health sector, increasing the strain on the already burdened public health sector, increasing the workload for those who stay, and leading to a shortage of skills and subsequent loss of capacity for health systems to deliver adequate health care (George et al., 2013).

Consider This The positive global economic/social/professional development associated with international migration must be weighed against the substantial brain and skills drain experienced by donor countries.

Remittance Income

Some national governments and government agencies have, however, actually encouraged the outflow of nurses from their country, including Fiji, Jamaica, India, Mauritius, South Africa, and the Philippines. For many years, the Philippine government actively endorsed and facilitated initiatives aimed at educating, recruiting, training, and placing nurses around the world. This was likely the result of a financial imperative, to encourage the generation of *remittance income*.

The International Centre on Nurse Migration (ICNM) (2014, para. 2) agrees, noting that "nurses' remittances represent an important course of added income and stability for individuals, families, and communities around the world. These funds lessen the burden on health systems by improving access to food, housing, and education—all three significant social determinants of health." In fact, the ICNM (2014) notes that migrants sent more than $414 billion back home in 2013.

Indeed, labor is the most profitable export of Philippines, with somewhere between 4 and 5 million citizens working around the globe and generating remittance income annually (Philippines Economy, 2014). Similarly, remittances from migrants are recognized as an important source of resilience for households in African countries, especially in light of the fact that the monetary value of remittances to Africa now exceeds that of aid (United Nations University, 2012).

Consider This Migrating nurses often send remittances back home to support their families and bolster the economy; in addition, some workers later return home with enhanced skills and experience.

In addition, some donor countries overproduce nurses with the intent of export. For example, the mass export of nurses from the Philippines is a response to a labor market oversupply. According to Reuben Seguritan, general counsel of the Philippine Nurses Association of America, the Philippines is the world's largest supplier of foreign-trained nurses with 429 nursing schools and 80,000 nursing students (Rodis, 2013). Indeed, 20% of all the registered nurses in California are Filipinos, a considerably large percentage since Filipinos number only 2.3 million (officially 1.2 million) out of a state population of 38 million (Rodis, 2013).

Yet, the deployment of nurses from the Philippines also poses threats to its own health care infrastructure. Masselink and Lee (2013, p. 90) note, however, that resultant impacts on the Filipino health care infrastructure appear to be less important philosophically than perceived potential benefits, noting that "Philippine government officials cast nurses as global rather than domestic providers of health care, implicating them in development more as sources of remittance income than for their potential contributions to the country's health care system." Masselink and Lee suggest that this orientation is motivated not simply by the desire for remittance revenues, but also as a way to cope with overproduction and lack of domestic opportunities for nurses in the Philippines.

Brain Drain

It is *brain drain* that is one of the most critical negative consequences of widespread nursing migration from developing countries. Brain drain refers to the loss of skilled personnel and the loss of investment in education that is experienced when those human resources migrate elsewhere. Thus, brain drain typically occurs when the skilled professionals from less-developed countries migrate to more-developed countries, resulting in these developing countries losing their most highly skilled and educated workforce. In addition, resource-limited nations have overwhelmingly become donor countries. This is especially true for countries like South Africa, Ghana, India, and Pakistan where nurses are central to the health care systems and indeed are the most visible health care providers in those systems (Delucas, 2014). The consequences of this large scale and nonstrategic migration are far reaching including a breakdown of national health care infrastructures and the inability of many donor countries to meet the health care needs of their own citizens.

Complaints of brain drain are heard from donor countries such as India, the Philippines, South Africa, and Zimbabwe. These nations argue that their human health care resources are being extracted at a time when they are needed most. This is the case even in many of the countries that have historically encouraged the exportation of their nurses. This suggests that the individual's right to choose cannot be easily negated simply because the donor country does not want to lose its highly educated human resources. Clearly, many nursing organizations and nursing leaders have begun to recognize the negative effects of international migration on "supplier" countries, but efforts to address the problem have been inadequate.

Finally, one must consider whether recruiting foreign nurses to solve acute staffing shortages is simply a poorly thought-out quick fix to a much greater problem and whether, in doing so, not only are donor nations harmed but also the issues that led to the shortage in the first place are never addressed. Certainly, one must at least question whether wholesale foreign nurse recruitment would even be necessary if importer nations made a more concerted effort to improve the working conditions, salaries, empowerment, and recognition of the home-born nurses they already employ.

Consider This Importing foreign nurses to solve the nursing shortage only puts a Band-Aid on the problem. The factors that led to the nursing shortage in the first place still need to be resolved.

This was clearly the case in research conducted by Zander, Blümel, and Busse (2013). Relevant push factors for migrating from Germany were identified for 1,508 German hospital nurses. Results suggested that the way

Research Study Fuels the Controversy 6.1

Reducing Pull Factors as a Retention Strategy

This study examined the motives of German hospital nurses to migrate, comparing working conditions in Germany to five destination and three source countries. In addition, the researchers examined whether working conditions in destination countries were better than in source countries. The impact of these push factors on the stated "intention-to-leave" of 1,508 hospital nurses in Germany was assessed using multivariate data analysis. Descriptive statistics were used to illustrate comparisons across all countries using a total sample of 27,451 nurses from 328 hospitals.

Source: Zander, B., Blümel, M., & Busse, R. (2013). Nurse migration in Europe—Can expectations really be met? Combining qualitative and quantitative data from Germany and eight of its destination and source countries. *International Journal of Nursing Studies, 50*(2), 210–218. doi:10.1016/j.ijnurstu.2012.11.017

Study Findings

All push factors showed a positive association with the risk for nurses to leave their current jobs, with "poor working environment" having the most pronounced relationship. On average, 4 out of 5 destination countries received better ratings than Germany (with 5/5 for "sufficient nursing staff," "recognition," "decision-making power," and "collaboration between nurses and physicians" but only 1/5 for "advanced training prospects"), while 2 out of 3 source countries received worse ratings than Germany. Results suggested that the way to retain and attract nurses on the short term is to invest in better working environments. German nurses would indeed find more satisfying conditions abroad in most cases—findings that encourage a revision of work-related aspects in German hospitals.

to retain and attract nurses on the short term was to invest in better working environments at home (Research Study Fuels the Controversy 6.1).

Discussion Point

If the money that is being spent on recruitment and immigration of foreign nurses was instead spent on resolving the domestic nursing issues that led to a shortage in the first place, would international nurse recruitment even be necessary?

GLOBAL NURSE RECRUITMENT AND MIGRATION AS AN ETHICAL ISSUE

Controversy regarding the ethics of international recruitment of nurses is not new. Whenever resources are limited, ethical issues regarding their allocation are likely to arise. In the case of global nurse recruitment and migration, the ethical principles of autonomy, utility, and justice seem most relevant. Certainly, there must be some sort of a balance between the right of individual nurses to choose to migrate (autonomy), particularly when push factors are overwhelming, and the more utilitarian concern for the donor nations' health as a result of losing scarce nursing resources.

International law clearly guarantees an individual the right to freedom of movement and residence (as established in the Universal Declaration of Human Rights; United Nations General Assembly, 1948) and the International Covenant on Civil and Political Rights (Office of the United Nations High Commissioner for Human Rights, 1976). The individual's right to migrate is central to self-determination.

Discussion Point

Should the right for the individual nurse to migrate (autonomy and self-determination) override what might be best for the donor nation (utilitarianism)?

Justice, or fairness, however, is another ethical principle that seems appropriate to this discussion because it examines how social and material goods are distributed to or withheld from members of a group or society, particularly in relation to fairness. Both recipient and donor countries have strong moral obligations to work toward fairer distributions of health care services as the fate of other communities cannot be ignored. Donkor and Andrews (2011) agree, arguing that nursing migration from developing countries has resulted in unbearable caseloads, decreased job satisfaction, and emotional fatigue on the part of the remaining nurses. As such, they argue that it is a global concern requiring all stakeholders to move beyond traditional stereotypes and to instead be flexible and forward looking.

Consider This The majority of countries importing foreign nurses are primarily White, and donor nations typically export nurses of color. The issue of race and the global economics of nursing should be examined in terms of effect on both supplier and donor countries.

Wild (2012) concurs, suggesting that there are many issues related to migration that have profound ethical relevance. For example,

> *Who deserves what in terms of health (care), and which role does citizenship or nationality play? How far should the responsibility of the receiving country go in terms of the health of migrants and why? Can restrictions to health care as a political instrument of deterrence be morally justified? Should there be a difference regarding health care between subgroups of migrants, for example, between forced and economic migrants, between legal and undocumented migrants, or between children and adults?* (p. 12)

The ethical significance of these questions becomes especially salient in times of rising pressure on political parties to protect nation's citizens' resources.

Wild (2012) goes on to suggest that

> *there are bioethical justice theories for societies and, increasingly, theories on global health ethics that consider affluent countries' obligations toward developing countries. But there seems to be a blind spot when it comes to the specific question of what happens if people move into the boundaries, that is, into the sphere of responsibility of a country. There is no wider debate in bioethics on moral responsibilities that explicitly addresses the different groups of migrants, whether differential treatment for citizens can ever be morally justified, and how these moral evaluations should find their way into public and institutional policies.* (p. 12)

In addition, migration numbers have increasingly become feminized. "The immigration of highly skilled women is higher when the source country is poorer. This impacts negatively on three key education and health indicators in source countries: infant mortality rate, under-five mortality, and secondary school enrollment rate by gender" (Finnish Medical Society, 2013, p. 6).

The following question then must be asked: Does global recruitment violate the principle of justice, particularly if such migration does not solve the underlying shortage and when such retention is done at the expense of the donor country? Clearly, donor countries have an ethical obligation to do what they can to provide their nurses with a safe, satisfying, and economically rewarding work environment. Importer countries have an ethical obligation to do what is necessary to be more self-reliant in meeting their professional workforce needs and to avoid recruiting nurses from those countries that can least afford to experience brain drain. Finally, professional health care associations must lead the way in addressing how best to respond to these ethical concerns.

PROFESSIONAL ORGANIZATIONS RESPOND

Given the current extent of nurse migration and the multiplicity of ethical dilemmas associated with it, many professional organizations, representing nurses from around the world, have weighed in on the issue. Some have provided formal position statements to guide both donor and importer countries. Others have attempted to provide guidance to the individual nurse considering global migration.

The International Council of Nurses

One international agency, the International Council of Nurses (ICN), has issued several position statements arguing for ethics and good employment practices in international recruitment (Box 6.1). The ICN, a federation of more than 130 national nurses' associations, represents more than 16 million nurses worldwide (ICN, 2013). The *ICN Position Statement: Nurse Retention and Migration* authored in 1999 and revised in 2007 confirms the right of nurses to migrate, as well as the potential beneficial outcomes of multicultural practice and learning opportunities supported by migration, but acknowledges potential adverse effects on the quality of health care in donor countries (ICN, 2007a).

The ICN (2007a) position statement also condemns the practice of recruiting nurses to countries where authorities have failed to implement sound human

BOX 6.1 ICN Position Statement on Nurse Retention, Transfer, and Migration (1999)

ICN and its member associations firmly believe that quality health care is directly dependent on an adequate supply of qualified nursing personnel.

ICN recognizes the right of individual nurses to migrate, while acknowledging the possible adverse effect that international migration may have on health care quality.

ICN condemns the practice of recruiting nurses to countries where authorities have failed to address human resource planning and problems that cause nurses to leave the profession and discourage them from returning to nursing.

In support of the above, ICN does the following:

- Disseminates information on nursing personnel needs and resources and on the development of fulfilling nursing career structures
- Provides training opportunities in negotiation and socioeconomic welfare–related issues
- Disseminates data on nursing employment worldwide
- Takes action to help reduce the serious effects of any shortage, maldistribution, and misutilization of nursing personnel
- Advocates adherence nationally to international labor standards
- Condemns the recruitment of nurses as a strike-breaking mechanism
- Advocates for open and transparent migration systems (recognizing that some appropriate screening is necessary to ensure public safety)
- Supports a transcultural approach to nursing practice
- Promotes the introduction of transferable benefits, for example, pension

National nurses' associations are urged to do the following:

- Encourage relevant authorities to ensure sound human resources planning for nursing
- Participate in the development of sound national policies on immigration and emigration of nurses
- Promote the revision of nursing curriculum for basic and postbasic education in nursing and administration to emphasize effective nursing leadership
- Disseminate information on the working conditions of nurses
- Discourage nurses from working in other countries where salaries and conditions are not acceptable to nurses and professional associations in those countries
- Ensure that foreign nurses have conditions of employment equal to those of local nurses in posts requiring the same level of competency and involving the same duties and responsibilities
- Ensure that there are no distinctions made among foreign nurses from different countries
- Monitor the activities of recruiting agencies
- Provide an advisory service to help nurses interpret contracts and assist foreign nurses with personal and work-related problems, such as institutional racism, violence, and sexual harassment
- Provide orientation for foreign nurses on the local cultural, social, and political values and on the health system and national language
- Alert nurses to the fact that some diplomas, qualifications, or degrees earned in one country may not be recognized in another
- Assist nurses with their problems related to international migration and repatriation

Source: International Council of Nursing. (2007a). *Position statement: Nurse retention and migration*. Retrieved January 19, 2015, from http://www.icn.ch/images/stories/documents/publications/position_statements/C06_Nurse_Retention_Migration.pdf

resource planning and to seriously address problems that cause nurses to leave the profession and discourage them from returning to nursing. The position statement also denounces unethical recruitment practices that exploit nurses or mislead them into accepting job responsibilities and working conditions that are incompatible with their qualifications, skills, and experience. The ICN and its member national nurses' associations call for a regulated recruitment process based on ethical principles that guide informed decision making and reinforce sound employment policies on the part of governments, employers, and nurses, thereby supporting fair and cost-effective recruitment and retention practices.

In addition, the ICN adopted a second position paper on ethical nurse recruitment in 2001 that was also revised and reaffirmed in 2007 (ICN, 2007b).

BOX 6.2 ICN Principles of Ethical Nurse Recruitment

Effective planning and development strategies must be introduced, regularly reviewed, and maintained to ensure a balance between supply and demand of nurse human resources.

1. Nursing legislation must authorize regulatory bodies to determine nurses' standards of education, competencies, and standards of practice and to ensure that only individuals meeting these standards are allowed to practice as a nurse.
2. Because the provision of quality care relies on the availability of nurses to meet staffing demand, nurses in a recruiting region/country and seeking employment should be made aware of job opportunities.
3. Nurses should have the right to migrate if they comply with the recruiting country's immigration/work policies (e.g., work permit) and meet obligations in their home country (e.g., bonding responsibilities, tax payment).
4. Nurses have the right to expect fair treatment (e.g., working conditions, promotion, and continuing education).
5. Nurses and employers are to be protected from false information, withholding of relevant information, misleading claims, and exploitation (e.g., accurate job descriptions, benefits/allocations/bonuses specified in writing, authentic educational records).
6. There should be no discrimination between occupations/professions with the same level of responsibility, educational qualification, work experience, skill requirement, and hardship (e.g., pay, grading).
7. When nurses' or employers' contracted or acquired rights or benefits are threatened or violated, suitable machinery must be in place to hear grievances in a timely manner and at reasonable cost.
8. Nurses must be protected from occupational injury and health hazards, including violence (e.g., sexual harassment) and made aware of existing workplace hazards.
9. The provision of quality care in the highly complex and often stressful health care environment depends on a supportive formal and informal supervisory infrastructure.
10. Employment contracts must specify a trial period when the signing parties are free to express dissatisfaction and cancel the contract with no penalty. In the case of international migration, the responsibility for covering the cost of repatriation needs to be clearly stated.
11. Nurses have the right to affiliate to and be represented by a professional association and/or union to safeguard their rights as health professionals and workers.
12. Recruitment agencies (public and private) should be regulated, and effective monitoring mechanisms, such as cost-effectiveness, volume, success rate over time, retention rates, equalities criteria, and client satisfaction, should be introduced.

Source: Adapted from International Council of Nurses. (2007b). *Position statement: Ethical nurse recruitment.* Retrieved January 19, 2015, from http://www.icn.ch/images/stories/documents/publications/position_statements/C03_Ethical_Nurse_Recruitment.pdf

This document identifies principles (Box 6.2) necessary to create a foundation for ethical recruitment, whether international or intranational contexts are being considered. The ICN suggests that all health sector stakeholders—patients, governments, employers, and nurses—will benefit if this ethical recruitment framework is systematically applied.

The International Centre on Nurse Migration

Another organization, the International Centre on Nurse Migration (ICNM), established in 2005, represents a collaborative project launched by the ICN and the Commission on Graduates of Foreign Nursing Schools (CGFNS). The ICNM serves as a global resource for the development, promotion, and dissemination of research, policy, and information on global nurse migration (ICNM, 2014). The ICNM Web site includes commissioned papers on nurse migration, publication links, fact sheets, and e-newsletters.

The AcademyHealth Project: Achieving Consensus on Ethical Standards of Practice for International Nurse Recruitment

AcademyHealth, a professional society of individuals and affiliated organizations throughout the United States and abroad, has also taken an active role in working to assure the ethical recruitment of international nurses (AcademyHealth, 2008–2012). Funded through a grant from the John D. and Catherine T. MacArthur Foundation in collaboration with the O'Neill Institute for National and Global Health Law at Georgetown University, AcademyHealth convened a task force of recruiters, hospitals, and foreign-educated nurses to develop draft standards of practice about global nurse recruitment, as well as recommendations on how to institutionalize these standards. This collaboration led to the release of a *Voluntary Code of Ethical Conduct for the Recruitment of Foreign Educated Nurses to the United States*. The code was designed to increase transparency and accountability throughout the process of international recruitment and ensure adequate orientation for foreign-educated nurses. It also provided guidance on ways to ensure recruitment is not harmful to source countries. This document was endorsed by the National Council of State Boards of Nursing (NCSBN).

The World Health Organization

Another international organization involved in establishing guidelines for nurse migration is the World Health Organization (WHO). In an effort to balance the right of workers to migrate with a need to assure that global health care needs are met, the WHO launched the *Health Worker Migration Policy Initiative* in 2007 (WHO, 2015). The initiative brought together professional organizations and other groups to create a code, which emphasized the positive benefits of health worker migration and minimized its negative impacts, and that spread the benefits of health worker migration more equitably among developed and developing nations.

The code, as called for by a resolution of the World Health Assembly in 2004, promoted ethical recruitment, protects migrant health workers' rights, and encourages governments in both developed and developing nations to actively address the push and pull factors that promote nurse migration (WHO, 2015). The Code of Practice was the first of its kind on a global scale for migration. In 2011, the Sixty-Third World Health Assembly unanimously passed a resolution to adopt the Code of Practice, acknowledging the global dimension and complexities of the health workforce crisis and the interconnected nature of both the problems and the solutions (WHO, 2015). In addition, the 2004 WHO Resolution 57.19 urged member states to mitigate the adverse effects of health care worker migration by forming country and regional agreements such as the South Africa/United Kingdom Memorandum of Understanding, the Pacific Code, and the Caribbean Community agreement.

THE MISTREATMENT OF FOREIGN NURSES

Despite the costs and investment of time and energy that goes into recruiting foreign nurses, some health care organizations treat imported nurses poorly once they arrive. Some migrant nurses receive substandard jobs or wages or are subjected to illegal practices by their employers.

In addition, some recruiting firms charge foreign nurses an upfront fee, a practice that has been found illegal in connection with the recruitment of temporary farm workers in the United States and that is prohibited in the U.K. Code of Practice for the International Recruitment of Health Care Professionals. In addition, many recruiters charge migrant nurses a "buyout" or breach fee for resigning before the end of their employment contract. This is because placement agencies often charge health care organizations a significant fee, depending on the state and the nurse's experience, to bring in a foreign nurse. It should be noted, however, that recent research by Spetz, Gates, and Jones (2014) actually found that internationally educated nurses reported higher annual earnings than their US-educated counterparts. The researchers suggested this is because foreign nurses are more likely to work full time and hold multiple positions. Salary differences, however, were generally insignificant when setting and job title were controlled.

Consider This Recruiting internationally may be a quick-fix solution, but it is far from clear that it is always a cost-effective solution.

There are also reports that overzealous recruiters have made false promises to foreign nurses regarding job opportunities and wages and virtually forced the newly migrated RNs to work long hours in substandard working conditions. Part of the reason for this is that private for-profit agencies have increasingly become involved in the search for nursing personnel, and there is generally no designated body that regulates or monitors the content of contracts offered. Internationally recruited nurses may be particularly at risk of exploitation or abuse due to the difficulty of verifying the terms of employment as a result of distance, language barriers, cost, and naiveté. These questionable hiring or employment practices are shown in Box 6.3.

Consider This Due to the lack of regulatory oversight of global nurse migration contracting, foreign nurses are at increased risk for employment under false pretenses and may be misled as to the conditions of work, remuneration, and benefits.

BOX 6.3 Questionable Practices Reported by International Nurses

- Changing contracts from the time a nurse departs his/her home country and on arrival in sponsor country without consent
- Paying lower wages than the prevailing rate or less than the hours worked
- Charging high breach fees
- Inadequate orientation to clinical agencies
- Imposing excessive work demands or mandatory overtime
- Retaining green cards, delays in processing social security numbers and RN permits
- Threats that nurses will be reported to immigration authorities
- Providing substandard housing

Discussion Point

Should there be greater regulatory oversight of foreign nurse recruitment? If so, who should be charged with this responsibility?

ASSIMILATING THE FOREIGN NURSE THROUGH SOCIALIZATION

The ethical obligation to the foreign nurse does not end with his or her arrival in a new country. The move from one cultural context to another can be very stressful. Many migrant nurses are afraid to express dissatisfaction or to ask for help for fear they will no longer have a job or because they fear being sent home. In addition, many of the families left behind in donor countries count on the migrant RN sending money home to improve their living standard. All of these factors place migrated nurses at increased risk for abuse and failure to assimilate. As a result, sponsoring countries must do whatever they can to see that migrant nurses are assimilated into new work environments.

Xu (2010) contends that there are typically four broad categories of transitional challenges faced by international nurses who migrate (Box 6.4). The first is language and communication challenges. Not only do most foreign nurse migrants have an inadequacy of language preparation but they are also unfamiliar with accent, slang, and other language nuances. As a result, they find it difficult to relate to patients, families, and other health care team members, to speak up for themselves, and to advocate for their patients.

The second challenge identified by Xu is the variance in nursing practice across different countries. These include role and expectations of the nurse, scope of practice, legal environment, accountability, professional autonomy, health care technology, and relationships between nurses and physicians.

The third challenge is marginalization, discrimination, and racism. Many migrant nurses experience unfair treatment (such as higher patient loads than others or being passed over for promotions) and racism, which results in stereotyping and rejection by patients and peers. In addition, the risk of being bullied is higher in this population.

BOX 6.4 Broad Categories of Transitional Challenges Facing International Nurse Migrants

1. Language and communication
2. Differences in nursing practice
3. Marginalization, discrimination, and racism
4. Cultural displacement and adjustment

Source: Xu, Y. (2010). Transitioning international nurses: An outlined evidence-based program for acute care settings. *Policy Politics & Nursing Practice, 11*(3), 202–213.

Finally, the fourth challenge is cultural displacement and adjustment. Cultural uprooting can lead to perceptions of not belonging. In addition, Xu suggests that cultural adjustment often results in communication barriers as well as interpersonal conflicts based on differences in culture-based values, norms, and expectation.

Hongyan et al. (2014) agree, suggesting that it is often difficult for foreign RNs to form working relationships with the host nurses in a health care organization due to feelings of isolation, loneliness, and depression. Long-term geographical separation from their family leads many of these nurses to have feelings of insecurity regarding their marriages and sadness over the lost emotional connection with their children. When immigrant nurses are able to establish a good relationship with their colleagues, the nurses are more motivated to stay in their work and the safety and quality of care is increased.

Xu (2010) suggests that "given the documented transitional challenges facing international nurses and the initial evidence of associated real and potential risks to patient safety and quality of care, transition of international nurses should be regarded as a regulatory requirement" (p. 210). Xu also suggests that such transition programs will likely be required by regulatory agencies in the foreseeable future in the United States as well as the United Kingdom and Australia and that these programs must be qualitatively different from those designed for domestic nurse hires to address the unique transitional needs of foreign migrant nurses.

THE INTERNATIONAL COMMUNITY ADDRESSES THE PROBLEM

The nursing shortage and resulting global migration issues have led several national governments to intervene, and, as a result, some countries have made progress in tackling the ethical issues associated with global recruitment and migration of nurses.

Some Governments Respond

Within the last few years, many countries, including the United States, have published national nursing strategies for dealing with staff shortages. Norway has issued a policy statement on the ethics of international recruitment. The Netherlands, Ireland, and the Scandinavian countries also have good-practice guidelines on international recruitment or are looking at developing guidelines. The United Kingdom, while allowing all nurses free movement rights, has implemented tight immigration and professional registration policies (Policy+, 2014). Indeed, in 2005, the UK began limiting nurse recruitment to the European Union (EU) countries and only granting work permits to nurses from non-EU countries if National Health Services institutions showed that jobs could not be filled by UK or EU applications. This UK Code of Practice is one of the oldest Codes of Practice in existence (Finnish Medical Society, 2013).

Other countries have initiated or examined various policy responses to reduce outflow, such as requiring nurses to work in their home countries for a certain amount of time after education completion or by charging the nurse a fee to migrate to another country. Another response has been to recognize that outflow cannot be halted if principles of individual freedom are to be upheld, but that the outflow that does occur must be managed and moderated. The "managed migration" initiative being undertaken in the Caribbean, which has provided regional support for addressing the nursing shortage crisis and developed initiatives such as training for export and temporary migration, is one example of a coordinated intervention to minimize the negative effects of outflow while realizing at least some benefit from the process.

US Immigration Policy

Currently, foreign nurses who want to work in the United States must have a valid job offer from an employer, and the employer must obtain Department of Labor approval for that hire. In addition, the employer must file a special petition with the U.S. Citizenship and Immigration Services.

In addition, like most national governments, the US government continues to play a pivotal role in the nurse migration issue by virtue of its ability to issue travel visas. The reality is that a finite number of visas are available and caps exist on how many green cards are issued. Clearly, commercial recruiters and employers would like to see fewer restrictions on nurse migration, but labor certification laws and rules regarding the issuance of visas are complex and ever changing.

Labor certification laws in the United States suggest that under normal circumstances, the Department of Labor is required by law to certify to the Department of State and the Immigration and Naturalization Service (INS) when a foreigner is hired that (1) no US citizens and permanent residents are available or qualified for a given job and (2) the employment of a foreigner will not adversely affect the wages of the concerned profession

(LawBrain, 2010). The main purpose of this legal provision has been to protect the domestic labor market; however, the immigration laws have provided preferential provisions for members of certain professions in the national interest of the United States, and, as a result, the government has created a list of occupations and professions, including nursing, that do not require labor certification. Because nursing has been classified as one of the shortage areas in the US economy, a so-called *blanket waiver* of the labor certification is in place.

In addition, from 1962 to 1989, foreign nurses were regarded as "professionals" under US immigration laws and could therefore seek an H-1 temporary work visa in the United States. In 1989, the Immigration Nursing Relief Act (INRA) created a 5-year pilot program. The INRA stipulated that only health care facilities with "attestations" approved by the Department of Health could obtain H-1A occupation visas to employ nurses on a temporary basis. Consequently, other occupations that formerly fell into the H-1 category became part of the new H-1B category. In addition, in 1990, Congress passed the Immigration and Nationality Act, which is the legal foundation for current immigration policies. In this act, nursing continued to be listed as a shortage area.

In 1999, the Nursing Relief for Disadvantaged Areas Act created H-1C occupational visas, which were perceived largely as an effort to renew the INRA of 1989 but with more restrictions. These temporary visas were created for foreign nurse graduates seeking employment in designated US facilities (serving primarily poor patients in inner cities and some rural areas). This visa classification expired in 2009.

Currently, there are no specific nurse visas available in the United States; however, most foreign nurses apply to work under the H-1B visa for skilled workers (open to individuals from countries other than Canada or Mexico) or the TN North American Free-Trade Agreement (NAFTA) work visa (available only to Canadian and Mexican citizens [U.S. Immigration Support, 2012]). The H-1B is a nonimmigrant visa that allows recruiting of shortage professionals into jobs that require theoretical and practical application of a body of highly specialized knowledge requiring completion of a specific course of higher education (at least a bachelor's degree). Of particular interest is the fact that many RNs do not qualify for the H-1B visa: A Fifth Circuit Court ruling in February 2000 stated that RN hospital jobs do not currently require a bachelor's degree in nursing, regardless of recruiter requirements. Some nurses can still apply for the H-1B status, however, if they have a specialized skill, particularly in intensive care, management, and specialty nursing areas or if US employers can convince immigration officials that specific jobs do meet the H-1B requirement on a case-by-case basis. The H-1B visa has an annual numerical limit "cap" of 65,000 visas each fiscal year. The first 20,000 petitions filed on behalf of beneficiaries with a US master's degree or higher are exempt from the cap (U.S. Citizenship and Immigration Requirements, 2011).

Discussion Point

Does the increased importation of foreign nurses directly or indirectly affect the prevailing wages of domestic RNs?

Still, other foreign nurses have sought employment in the United States in accordance with the NAFTA, enacted in December 1993. NAFTA established a reciprocal trading relationship between the United States, Canada, and Mexico and allowed for a nonimmigrant class of admission exclusively for business and service trade individuals entering the United States.

To complicate the matter further, on July 26, 2003, the U.S. Bureau of Citizenship and Immigration Services ruled that foreign-educated health care professionals, including nurses who are seeking temporary or permanent occupational visas, as well as those who are seeking NAFTA status, must successfully complete a screening program before receiving an occupational visa or permanent (green card) visa. This screening, completed by the CGFNS, includes an assessment of an applicant's education to ensure that it is comparable to that of a nursing graduate in the United States, verification that licenses are valid and unencumbered, successful completion of an English-language proficiency examination, and verification that the nurse has either earned certification by the CGFNS or passed the National Council Licensure Examination for Registered Nurses (NCLEX-RN).

Another way nurses get work visas in the United States has been under the immigrant E3 to I-140 status ("green card" or Alien Registration Receipt Card). Migrant RNs enter into the United States and become permanent residents through petition to the INS. A problem with this visa status is that it does not require labor certification, so the Department of Labor does not have to certify that the wage offered to the nurse is the prevailing wage. However, the law does state that foreign nurses entering under I-140 cannot have a negative effect on domestic wages.

ENSURING COMPETENCY OF FOREIGN NURSES COMMISSION ON GRADUATES OF FOREIGN NURSING SCHOOLS AND THE NCLEX-RN EXAMINATION

Nursing is one of the most highly regulated health professions in the United States, and a license is required to practice in all 50 states and US territories. Before 1977, endorsement and taking the State Board Test Pool Examination (SBTPE) were the two ways for foreign nurses to obtain a license. The SBTPE tested the foreign graduate's English-language proficiency and knowledge of US nursing practice, but, alarmingly, only a small percentage (15% to 20%) of foreign RNs typically passed the NCLEX-RN.

As a result of this high failure rate and a concern for patient safety, the ANA and the NLN, with collaboration from the Department of Labor and the INS, established CGFNS in 1977 as an independent, nonprofit organization. The mission of CGFNS is to serve the global community through programs and services that verify and promote the knowledge-based practice competency of health care professionals (CGFNS, 2014a).

The strategies CGFNS uses to accomplish this mission are to evaluate and test foreign graduates via a certification program before they leave their home countries to ensure that there is a reasonable chance for them to pass the NCLEX-RN needed for licensure in the United States. Through a contract with the NLN, which designed the NCLEX-RN, a CGFNS-qualifying examination was developed. The examination consists of two parts to test the applicant's knowledge of nursing and the English language (both written and oral).

To be eligible to take the examination, RNs must have completed sufficient classroom instruction and clinical practice and hold an initial as well as current license/registration as a first-level general nurse in their country of education (CGFNS, 2014b). In addition, a credentials review of secondary and nursing education, registration, and licensure is required to earn the CGFNS certificate. Earning CGFNS certification meets one of the immigration requirements for securing an occupational visa to work in the United States and helps to meet licensure and NCLEX eligibility requirements in many states (CGFNS, 2014b).

The CGFNS examination, however, should not be mistaken as substitute for the state board licensing examination. Indeed, most states in the United States require foreign nurses to pass the CGFNS certification before they are allowed to take the NCLEX-RN. Of the 5,753 internationally educated nurses who took the NCLEX-RN as first-time test takers in 2014, the pass rate was only 29.13% (NCSBN, 2015). The exam specifications and passing standards are the same for foreign nurses as they are for students taking the NCLEX in the United States.

The NCSBN has also taken steps to make it easier for foreign RNs to take the NCLEX-RN. Until 2005, the NCLEX-RN was offered only in the United States and its territories. In fact, before 2005, the only option foreign nurses had was to earn the CGFNS certificate, secure a job offer from a US employer, and take the NCLEX-RN only after they arrived in the United States with their green cards. Now the exam is offered in numerous countries and nonmember board territories. These locations were selected based on national security, examination security, and similarity with U.S. Intellectual Property and Copyright Laws.

Conclusions

Nurse migration and its associated ethical dilemmas are among the most serious issues facing the nursing profession, and there is little sign that the issue will abate anytime soon. Indeed, Spetz et al. (2014) suggest that the strategy of relying on foreign nurses to attenuate RN shortages will likely continue worldwide.

Clearly, developed countries have an advantage in terms of pull factors to recruit migrant nurses from less-developed countries, and less-developed countries are the ones most likely to suffer the devastating effects of brain drain. One must ask, however, whether this quick-fix solution to the nursing shortage has become too commonplace and too easy. Does it keep recruiter countries from dealing with the issues that led to their shortage in the first place? Does it negatively affect prevailing domestic wages and artificially alter what should be normal supply/demand curves in the health care marketplace? Of even greater concern is the lack of regulatory oversight of contracting with foreign nurses, placing them at risk for unethical, if not illegal, employment practices in their host country.

Delucas (2014) agrees, suggesting that both destination and source countries are challenged by poorly controlled nurse migration. Destination countries must address the ethical implications of aggressive recruitment and their lack of developing a sustainable self-sufficient domestic workforce. Source countries struggle to fund and educate adequate numbers of nurses for domestic needs and migrant replacement.

Some countries and professional nursing organizations are beginning to address these issues. So too are national governments and regulatory agencies in an effort to protect both the migrant nurses and the public those nurses will serve. Delucas (2014) argues passionately, however, that more work must be done to engage nurses at leadership and grassroot levels to establish international treaties regarding foreign nurse migration that work collaboratively for justice and health equity. She suggests that inertia is not an option as nurses must adopt a broader sense of responsibility in addressing global disparities of health and health care and the need to develop a sustainable nursing workforce.

Yet, in the meantime, large numbers of nurses are migrating internationally, and the potentially negative effects of this increasing trend on both the migrant nurse and the donor nation are becoming ever more apparent. Jones and Sherwood (2014) note that "nurse mobility and migration will require nations and health care organizations to continue working to better understand workforce models and the employment, integration, assimilation, and regulation of an international nursing workforce" (p. 62).

For Additional Discussion

1. Are the requirements for foreign nurses to get visas in the United States adequate?
2. Does achieving CGFNS certification and passing the NCLEX-RN examination in the United States assure competency of the foreign nurse graduate?
3. As long as international nurse recruitment is a viable option, will the problems that lead to a nursing shortage in the first place be addressed?
4. Should donor countries develop nurse migration policy efforts that limit human resource exports?
5. How can government and professional nursing organizations work together to ensure that recruitment practices of foreign nurses are both ethical and appropriate?
6. How does the ethical principle of veracity (truth telling) apply to the zealous recruiting efforts of foreign nurses, particularly in developing countries?
7. Is government regulatory oversight of foreign nurse recruitment efforts in conflict with America's value of capitalistic, free enterprise?

References

AcademyHealth. (2008–2012). *About us.* Retrieved January 20, 2015, from http://www.academyhealth.org/About/?navItemNumber=498

Aiken, L. H., Buchan, J., Sochalski, J., Nichols, B., & Powell, M. (2013, December). Trends in international nurse migration. *Health Affairs, 32*(12). Retrieved January 1, 2014, http://content.healthaffairs.org/content/23/3/69.full

FWCanada Inc. (2014, April 3). *Canada: Canada offers registered nurses immigration programs to become permanent residents; No offers of employment necessary.* Montréal, QC: Author. Retrieved January 22, 2015, from http://www.mondaq.com/canada/x/304386/work+visas/Canada+Offers+Registered+Nurses+Immigration+Programs+To+Become+Permanent+Residents+No+Offers+Of+Employment+Necessary

Commission on Graduates of Foreign Nursing Schools. (2014a). *About.* Retrieved January 19, 2015, from http://www.cgfns.org/sections/about/

Commission on Graduates of Foreign Nursing Schools. (2014b). *CGFNS certification program.* Retrieved January 20, 2015, from http://www.cgfns.org/services/certification-program/

Delucas, A. C. (2014). Foreign nurse recruitment: Global risk. *Nursing Ethics, 21*(1), 76–85. Retrieved from http://nej.sagepub.com/content/21/1/76.full.pdf+html

Donkor, N. T., & Andrews, L. D. (2011). 21st century nursing practice in Ghana: Challenges and opportunities. *International Nursing Review, 58*(2), 218–224.

Finnish Medical Society (2013). *Migration: Destination and source countries.* Retrieved January 30, 2014, from http://www.duodecim.fi/kotisivut/sivut.nayta?p_sivu=143597

George, G., & Reardon, C. (2013, May). Preparing for export? Medical and nursing student migration intentions post-qualification in South Africa. *African Journal of Primary Health Care & Family Medicine, 5*(1), 1–9. Retrieved January 31, 2014, from http://www.phcfm.org/index.php/phcfm/article/view/483

George, G., Atujuna, M., & Gow, J. (2013). Migration of South African health workers: The extent to which financial considerations influence internal flows and external movements. *BMC Health Services Research, 13*, 297. Retrieved January 31, 2014, from http://www.ncbi.nlm.nih.gov/pmc/articles/PMC3765273/

Hongyan, L., Wenbo, N., & Junxin, L. (2014, September). The benefits and caveats of international nurse migration. *International Journal of Nursing Sciences, 1*(3), 314–317. Retrieved January 22, 2015, from http://www.sciencedirect.com/science/article/pii/S2352013214000787

International Centre on Nurse Migration. (2014). *About us.* Retrieved January 29, 2015, from http://www.intlnursemigration.org/about/

International Council of Nursing. (2007a). *Position statement: Nurse retention and migration.* Retrieved January 19, 2015, from http://www.icn.ch/images/stories/documents/publications/position_statements/C06_Nurse_Retention_Migration.pdf

International Council of Nurses. (2007b). *Position statement: Ethical nurse recruitment.* Retrieved January 19, 2015, from http://www.icn.ch/images/stories/documents/publications/position_statements/C03_Ethical_Nurse_Recruitment.pdf

International Council of Nurses. (2013). *Who we are.* Retrieved January 19, 2014, from http://www.icn.ch/who-we-are/who-we-are/

Jones, C. B., & Sherwood, G. (2014). The globalization of the nursing workforce: Pulling the pieces together. *Nursing Outlook, 62*(1), 59–63. doi:10.1016/j.outlook.2013.12.005

Kodoth, P. & Jacob, T. K. (2013). *International mobility of nurses from Kerala (India) to the EU: Prospects and challenges with special reference to the Netherlands and Denmark.* CARIM-India Research Report 2013/19. Retrieved November 30, 2014, from http://www.india-eu-migration.eu/media/CARIM-India-2013-19.pdf

LawBrain. (2010, July 13). *Immigration.* Retrieved January 20, 2015, from http://lawbrain.com/wiki/Immigration

Lee, E., & Moon, M. (2013, December). Korean nursing students' intention to migrate abroad. *Nurse Education Today, 33*(12), 1517–1522. Retrieved January 29, 2014, from http://dx.doi.org/10.1016/j.nedt.2013.04.006

Likupe, G. (2013). The skills and brain drain what nurses say. *Journal of Clinical Nursing, 22*(9/10), 1372–1381. doi:10.1111/j.1365-2702.2012.04242.x

Masselink, L. E., & Lee, S. (2013). Government officials' representation of nurses and migration in the Philippines. *Health Policy and Planning, 28*, 90–99. Available online at http://heapol.oxfordjournals.org/content/28/1/90.full.pdf+html

National Council of State Boards of Nursing. (2015). *2014: Number of candidates taking NCLEX examination and percent passing, by type of candidate.* Retrieved January 20, 2015, from https://www.ncsbn.org/Table_of_Pass_Rates_2014.pdf

NZ tightens migration criteria for some overseas nurses. (2014, August–December). *Nursing Review.* Retrieved January 22, 2015, from http://nursingreview.co.nz/news-feed/august-to-december-2014/nz-tightens-migration-criteria-for-some-overseas-nurses/#.VMHCxCzWass

Office for National Statistics (2014, January 17). *Bulgarian and Romanian migration to the UK in 2014.* Retrieved January 22, 2015, from http://www.ons.gov.uk/ons/rel/migration1/migration-statistics-quarterly-report/november-2013/sty-bulgaria-and-romania.html

Office of the United Nations High Commissioner for Human Rights. (1976). *International Covenant on Civil and Political Rights.* Retrieved January 5, 2009, from http://www.ohchr.org/EN/ProfessionalInterest/Pages/CCPR.aspx

Philippines Economy 2014. (2014, January 31). *Economy overview.* Retrieved November 30, 2014, from http://www.theodora.com/wfbcurrent/philippines/philippines_economy.html

Policy+. (2014, March). Nurse migration from the EU: What are the key challenges? *Policy Plus Evidence, Issues, and Opinions in Healthcare,* (42). Retrieved January 20, 2015, from http://www.kcl.ac.uk/nursing/research/nnru/policy/By-Issue-Number/Policy-Issue-42.pdf

Qun, A., & Xiaojing, H. (2014). *Xinhua insight: China's severe nurse shortage continues*. Retrieved November 30, 2014, from http://en.people.cn/90882/8625626.html

Rodis, R. (2013, May 14). *Telltale signs: "Why are there so many Filipino nurses in the US?"* Retrieved November 30, 2014, from http://www.asianweek.com/2013/05/14/telltale-signs-why-are-there-so-many-filipino-nurses-in-the-us/

Silvestri, D. M., Blevins, M., Afzal, A. R., Andrews, B., Derbew, M., Kaur, S., . . . Vermund, S. (2014). Medical and nursing students' intentions to work abroad or in rural areas: A cross-sectional survey in Asia and Africa. *Bulletin of the World Health Organization*, *92*(10), 750–759. doi:10.2471/BLT.14.136051

Spetz, J., Gates, M., & Jones, C. B. (2014). Internationally educated nurses in the United States: Their origins and roles. *Nursing Outlook*, *62*(1), 8–15. doi:10.1016/j.outlook.2013.05.001

United Nations General Assembly. (1948). *The Universal Declaration of Human Rights*. Retrieved April 28, 2012, from http://www.un.org/en/documents/udhr/

United Nations University. (2012, September 19). *Migration, remittances and resilience in Africa.* Retrieved January 28, 2014, from http://unu.edu/publications/articles/migration-remittances-and-resilience-in-africa.html#info

U.S. Citizenship and Immigration Requirements. (2011). H-1B Fiscal Year (FY) 2015 Cap Season. Retrieved January 20, 2015, from http://www.uscis.gov/portal/site/uscis/menuitem.eb1d4c2a3e5b9ac89243c6a7543f6d1a/?vgnextoid=73566811264a3210VgnVCM100000b92ca60aRCRD&vgnextchannel=73566811264a3210VgnVCM100000b92ca60aRCRD

U.S. Immigration Support. (2012). *Your online guide to US visas, green cards and citizenship. Nurse work visa.* Retrieved January 20, 2015, from http://www.usimmigrationsupport.org/nurse-work-visa.html

Wild, V. (2012). Migration and health: Discovering new territory for bioethics. *American Journal of Bioethics*, *12*(9), 11–13.

World Health Organization. (2015). *Task force on migration: Health worker migration policy initiative.* Retrieved January 20, 2015, from http://www.who.int/workforcealliance/about/taskforces/migration/en/

Xu, Y. (2010). Transitioning international nurses: An outlined evidence-based program for acute care settings. *Policy Politics & Nursing Practice, 11*(3), 202–213.

Zander, B., Blümel, M., & Busse, R. (2013). Nurse migration in Europe—Can expectations really be met? Combining qualitative and quantitative data from Germany and eight of its destination and source countries. *International Journal of Nursing Studies*, *50*(2), 210–218. doi:10.1016/j.ijnurstu.2012.11.017

7

Unlicensed Assistive Personnel and the Registered Nurse

Carol J. Huston

ADDITIONAL RESOURCES

Visit thePoint for additional helpful resources

- eBook
- Journal Articles
- WebLinks

CHAPTER OUTLINE

LEARNING OBJECTIVES

The learner will be able to:

1. Identify driving forces leading to the increased use of unlicensed assistive personnel (UAP) beginning in the early 1990s.
2. Name common job titles for UAP.
3. Differentiate between the minimum mandated educational preparation of certified nurse aides (CNAs) and UAP.
4. Analyze current research that explores the effect of increased UAP use on costs and patient outcomes.
5. Discuss how the role of the registered nurse (RN) as delegator has changed with the increased use of UAP.
6. Examine how the role of delegator and supervisor of UAP increases the scope of liability for the RN.
7. Explore strategies for restructuring work environments and clarifying role expectations so that professional nurses spend less time on non-nursing tasks and UAP have role clarity.
8. Identify safeguards that health care organizations can use to increase the likelihood that UAP are used both effectively and appropriately as members of the health care team.
9. Outline current efforts seeking to regulate minimum UAP education and competencies.
10. Discuss factors contributing to both the current and projected shortages of UAP, particularly in long-term care settings.
11. Reflect on the self-confidence and skill that an RN might need to successfully delegate to a UAP.
12. Identify the sources of increased legal liability an RN and his or her employer face when health care institutions allow RNs to work beneath their scope of practice as UAP.

INTRODUCTION

In an effort to contain spiraling health care costs, many health care providers in the 1990s restructured their organizations by eliminating registered nurse (RN) positions and/or by replacing licensed professional nurses with unlicensed assistive personnel (UAP). UAP are unlicensed individuals who provide low-risk, assistive care not requiring the judgment or training of a licensed professional, while working under the direct supervision of an RN. The term includes, but is not limited to, nurse aides, nurse extenders, health care aides, technicians, patient care technicians, orderlies, assistants, and attendants. Although the term UAP will generally be used throughout this chapter, it is noteworthy that in 2007, the American Nurses Association (ANA) stopped using the term UAP and replaced it with *nursing assistive personnel* (NAP), suggesting that many NAP are now licensed or formally recognized in some manner.

Regardless of nomenclature, unlicensed workers are a significant part of the health care landscape and have been for some time. By the late 1990s, hospitals began actively recruiting the RNs who had been let go just a few years before. RNs who lost their jobs, however, were slow to return to the acute-care setting, despite a widespread, worsening nursing shortage. As a result, hospitals again increased their use of UAP early in the 21st century in an effort to supplement their licensed nursing staff.

Both as a result of the restructuring of the 1990s and subsequent nursing shortages, the skill mix in some hospitals still includes a significant percentage of UAP. According to the U.S. Department of Labor, Bureau of Labor Statistics (2014), more than 1.5 million nursing assistants (NAs) and orderlies were employed in the United States in 2012. Twenty six percent of UAP worked in hospitals, 42% worked in skilled nursing facilities, 14% worked in residential care facilities, 4% in home care, and 4% for the government (Bureau of Labor Statistics, 2014).

Several reasons are commonly cited for the increased use of UAP. The primary argument for using UAP instead of licensed personnel is usually cost savings, although the professional nursing shortage may be a contributing factor (Marquis & Huston, 2015). Another widely recognized benefit of using UAP is that they can free professional nurses from tasks and assignments (specifically, non-nursing functions) that can be completed by less well-trained personnel at a lower cost.

So why has the increased use of UAP created so much controversy? The answer is that in many institutions, UAP are not supplements to, but replacements of, professional RN staff. This is of concern because empirical research exists regarding what percentage of the staffing mix can safely be represented by UAP without negatively affecting patient outcomes. In addition, minimum national educational and training requirements have not been established for UAP, and their scope of practice varies from institution to institution. All of these issues raise serious questions as to whether greater use of UAP represents an effective solution to dwindling health care resources or whether it is an economically driven, short-term response that could lead to compromised patient outcomes.

This chapter, however, does not argue for the elimination of UAP. Instead, it addresses what safeguards must be incorporated in the use of UAP so that safe, accessible, and affordable nursing care is possible.

MOTIVATION TO USE UAP

Maximizing RN Time With Patients

UAP can maximize human resources because they free professional nurses from tasks and assignments that do not require independent thinking and professional judgment. This is significant because much of a typical nurse's time is spent on non-nursing tasks and functions. Non-nursing tasks and functions are those routine or standardized activities that can be done by an individual with minimal training and do not require a great deal of individual client assessment, independent thought, or decision making. Examples of non-nursing activities include making a bed, doing vital signs, feeding clients, measuring intakes and outputs, and obtaining a weight or height.

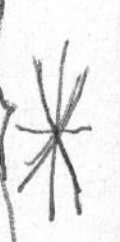

Just how much time is spent by nurses doing non-nursing activities is unclear. Research by Westbrook, Duffield, Li, and Creswick (2011) suggested that nurses spent only 37% of their time with patients. These findings are similar to others reported over the past decade.

Discussion Point

Why are professional RNs still completing so many non-nursing tasks? Are they reluctant to delegate them to ancillary personnel, or are there inadequate support personnel to take on these tasks?

Cost Savings

Cost savings associated with UAP use—the second argument for increased UAP use—are less clear. Studies completed early in the 21st century showed conflicting findings with some suggesting significant cost savings with UAP and others suggesting no cost savings as a result of the costs of supervision, high UAP turnover rates, and medical errors. Current research is limited. Perhaps the most comprehensive meta-analysis of the issue of cost and the use of unlicensed personnel was published by Thungjaroenkul, Cummings, and Embleton (2007). These researchers concluded that the evidence examining the relationships between nurse staffing, hospital costs, and length of stay uses such a variety of methods and definitions that it is difficult to conclude with certainty the results of nurse staffing on cost and length of stay. They suggested that significant reductions in cost might be possible with higher ratios of nursing personnel in hospital settings and that patient costs might be reduced with greater RN staffing as RNs have higher knowledge and skill levels to provide more effective nursing care as well as reduce patient resource consumption. It is this lack of evidence, however, that has led some hospitals to resume reliance on UAP as the primary component of their staffing mix.

Mulrooney (2011) cautions though that there is no general consensus among health care professionals as to what constitutes safe staffing. Instead, she suggests it can be broadly defined as

> *having the appropriate number of staff with a suitable mix of skill levels available at all times to ensure that patient care needs are fulfilled and hazard-free working conditions are maintained. In addition, safe staffing optimally requires the absence of negative consequences and minimal errors consistent with benchmarked data.* (Mulrooney, 2011, para. 6)

EDUCATIONAL REQUIREMENTS FOR UAP

Some monitoring of the regulation, education, and use of UAP has been ongoing since the early 1950s; however, most of this has been for *certified nurse's aides*. The Omnibus Budget Reconciliation Act of 1987 established regulations for the education and certification of nurse's aides (minimum of 75 hours of State-approved theory and practice and successful completion of a competency examination in both areas). A new proposal to increase this education to 80 hours of classroom instruction and 75 hours of supervised clinical experience was introduced in Oregon in 2013 (Buck, 2014).

No federal or community standards have been established, however, for training the more broadly defined UAP. Indeed, the health care industry provides many job opportunities for individuals without specialized training. This does not mean, however, that all UAP are undereducated and unprepared for the roles they have been asked to fill. Indeed, UAP educational levels vary from less than that of a high school graduate to those holding advanced degrees. It does suggest, however, that RNs, in delegating to UAP, must make no assumptions about the educational preparation or training of that UAP. Instead, the RN must carefully assess what skills and knowledge each UAP has or risk increased personal liability for the failure to do so.

The reality is that most UAP training is completed by the employing facility and occurs without formal certification. Formal training programs that do exist are completed at vocational schools and community colleges and typically focus on long-term care, providing certifications only as necessary to meet state requirements. Often, this training is inadequate and does not prepare UAP with the competencies they need to work in a dynamic health care environment, which is very different from that existed even a decade ago. For efficiency and safety, standardized curriculums that address the skill sets needed in the many settings where nurse aides are used should be implemented.

Similar to long-term care, the education and training of UAP in acute-care settings is often inadequate. In fact, there are no required educational standards or guidelines for the use of UAP in acute-care settings. Instead, UAP educational and training requirements for acute-care settings are generally facility based. This is important to remember when UAP transfer from one facility to another because no assumption should be made about UAP competency levels to perform certain tasks, despite their work experience.

Discussion Point

Can an experienced RN accurately assess an individual UAP's "work experience" of patients as a substitute for formal education and training?

UAP SCOPE OF PRACTICE

In some health care agencies, UAP assist with dressing changes, parenteral therapy, urinary catheter insertion, and perform numerous other tasks typically reserved for licensed personnel. The skill assumed by UAP, however, that has garnered the greatest concern, is administering medications. For years, medication administration was considered a professional nursing function, requiring assessment and clinical judgment, but during the past decade, many states granted unlicensed personnel the right to pass medications, particularly in schools, assisted living facilities and correctional institutions.

In addition, *certified medicine aides* have worked in licensed nursing home settings in this country for almost four decades. UAP who administer medications are also known as *unlicensed medication administration personnel*, *medication aides*, or *medication assistant technicians*.

UAP also administer drugs in school settings when a school nurse is not present. It is the position of the National Association of School Nurses that the use of UAP to perform delegated nursing tasks in the school setting is appropriate, however, only if the school nurse is in control of the decision to delegate a health care task and a registered professional nurse conducts the training and supervision of the UAP (National Association of School Nurses, 2014).

As a result, many school nurses and the organizations that represent them are waging a battle to stop the expansion of UAP practice in terms of the drugs they are allowed to administer (eg, currently only licensed school nurses can administer insulin). They argue that the administration of medications is much more than dispensing a pill, handing a student an inhaler, or giving a subcutaneous injection. It requires high-level assessment skills; an understanding of drug actions, interactions, and side effects; and the highly developed critical thinking skills needed to intervene when problems occur. In addition, the practice of nursing clearly requires a license under the Nurse Practice Act.

As a result, numerous law suits have been filed in the last 5 years questioning the use of UAP to administer drugs such as insulin to school children. In fact, in May 2013, the California Supreme Court was asked to make a ruling on whether allowing UAP to administer insulin to school children was unlawful since it sidestepped the Nurse Practice Act (ANA, 2013a,b). The California Nurse Practice Act specifically defines the act of medication administration as a licensed nursing function. The Court ruled that California law does permit trained UAP to administer prescription medications, including insulin, in accordance with written statements of individual students' treating physicians, with parental consent (California Department of Education, 2014). The Supreme Court then remanded the case back to the Court of Appeals to resolve any outstanding claims.

There are those, however, who suggest that the use of UAP to administer drugs to school children is not only appropriate but also essential in today's economic climate with limited resources and increasing health care needs. The American Academy of Pediatrics (AAP), the National Association of School Nurses, and the ANA suggest that trained and supervised UAP, who have the required knowledge, skills, and composure to deliver specific school health services under the guidance of a licensed RN, should be allowed to do so (American Academy of Pediatrics, 2009). The AAP suggests that UAP can provide standardized, routine health services under the supervision of the nurse and on the basis of physician guidance and school nursing assessment of the unique needs of the individual child and the suitability of delegation of specific nursing tasks. Any delegation of nursing duties must be consistent with the requirements of state Nurse Practice Acts, state regulations, and guidelines provided by professional nursing organizations (AAP).

> **Consider This** Many patients given direct care by UAP assume that UAP are licensed nurses. This confusion is promulgated when health care professionals do not include their credentials on their nametags or introduce themselves to patients according to their actual job title.

A similar debate is occurring in hemodialysis clinics and nephrology centers. As of 2014, 22 states allowed dialysis technicians or UAP to administer heparin as ordered to initiate or terminate a hemodialysis treatment (O'Keefe, 2014). In most cases, the express authority for this practice lies in dialysis technician laws or Board of Nursing position statements. With several exceptions, most of these states also permit UAP to administer saline to correct hypotension during hemodialysis. Some states require such duties be under the direct, onsite supervision of an RN or a physician while other states require that administration of heparin or saline by a dialysis technician be pursuant to established facility protocol. In 10 states, the nursing delegation language may permit the RN to delegate IV medication administration through a central line access to UAP. One state, Arizona, permits UAP to administer anticoagulants. O'Keefe (2014) suggests that in the absence of nursing rules that either clearly permit or prohibit the administration of IV medications by UAP, RNs must look to their delegation authority under the state Nurse Practice Act.

The reality, then, is that in many settings, some UAP are performing functions that are within the legal practice of nursing. This may be a violation of the state nursing practice act and poses a possible threat to public safety. Clearly, certain professional responsibilities related to nursing care must never be delegated.

It is critical, then, that the RN never lose sight of his or her ultimate responsibility for ensuring that patients receive appropriate, high-quality care. This means that although the UAP may complete non-nursing functions such as bathing the patient, taking vital signs, and measuring and recording intake and output, it is the RN who must analyze that information using highly developed critical thinking skills and then use the nursing process to see that desired patient outcomes are achieved. Only RNs have the formal authority to practice nursing, and activities that rely on the nursing process or require specialized skill, expert knowledge, or professional judgment should never be delegated.

Case (2013) agrees, noting that "while nursing tasks may be delegated, the licensed nurse's generalist knowledge of patient care indicates that the practice-pervasive functions of assessment, evaluation and nursing judgment must not be delegated" (para. 11). This includes such skills as the initial and ongoing assessment of patients, administering treatments and medications ordered by a licensed prescriber; initiating and coordinating the plan of care; teaching and counseling patients; promoting and maintaining health; and teaching and supervising students.

Regulatory Oversight of UAP

The increased use of UAP, called by some the "deskilling of the nursing workforce," has raised concern among professional organizations, consumers, and legislators alike. In the early 1990s, the ANA took the position that the control and monitoring of assistive personnel in clinical settings should be performed through the use of existing mechanisms that regulate nursing practice. Typically, this includes the State Board of Nursing, institutional policies, and external agency standards.

Legislation has been introduced at the state level to regulate UAP use and scope of practice. Some states have attempted to regulate UAP practice through registration and certification. Others have proposed direct regulation of UAP by passing legislation that requires UAP to be certified by meeting education and competency requirements. Still others require the state boards of nursing or the department of health to register or certify UAP. Thus, regulation by state and jurisdiction vary widely and getting all states to agree to uniform regulations is unlikely.

Discussion Point

Why has the movement to regulate UAP education and training occurred primarily at the state level? Why has there been no national movement to do the same?

Some state boards of nursing have issued recommendations regarding scope of practice for UAP or attempted to delineate the relationship between RNs and UAP. Few states, however, used the ANA or National Council of State Boards of Nursing definitions for delegation, supervision, or assignment. Most states also report that there are no standardized curricula in place for UAP employed in acute-care hospitals. The states have not been able to reach a consensus regarding the education, training, and scope of practice needed for UAP to safely practice either. The end result, then, is that there is no universally accepted scope of practice for UAP.

In addition to existing state regulations regarding UAP education and training, as well as required competencies, many professional nursing organizations have studied the use and effect of UAP and are adopting position statements regarding their use. One national effort to define the scope of practice for UAP was undertaken by the ANA in their delineation of tasks appropriate for UAP practice in the early 1990s. Multiple revisions have followed. In 2007, the ANA suggested six actions that should be taken to create a national and/or state policy agenda about the educational preparation of UAP or NAP and the competencies they should have for safe practice. These are shown in Box 7.1.

In addition, to address the problem, some state boards of nursing have issued task lists for UAP (lists of activities considered to be within the scope of practice for UAP). However, in creating such a list, an unofficial scope of practice is created, and this suggests that such individuals will be performing activities independently. Task lists also suggest that there is no need for

BOX 7.1 American Nurses Association (2007)

Recommendations for a National and/or State Policy Agenda for NAP

1. Recognize that the NAP should never be considered or used as a replacement for RNs or licensed practical nurses.
2. Aggressively promote the understanding that delegation is an integral part of professional nursing practice and not a supervisory act connected to acting on behalf of the employer.
3. Establish recognized competencies for the NAP that will guide the development of a core curriculum.
4. Promote national nursing initiatives to establish criteria and guidelines for the clinical training of the NAP through the use of evidence-based research, preparing the NAP to provide routine care in predictable patient functions.
5. Establish systems for training, certification, registry, and disciplinary monitoring of the NAP.
6. Support continued efforts to implement recommendations related to patient safety and quality and the nursing work environment articulated in reports generated by the Institute of Medicine such as *To Err Is Human: Building a Safer Health System*; *Crossing the Quality Chasm: A New Health System for the 21st Century*; and *Keeping Patients Safe: Transforming the Work Environment of Nurses.*

Source: Excerpted from American Nurses Association. (2007). *Position statement: Registered nurses utilization of nursing assistive personnel in all settings*. Retrieved January 21, 2015, from http://gm6.nursingworld.org/MainMenuCategories/Policy-Advocacy/Positions-and-Resolutions/ANAPositionStatements/Position-Statements-Alphabetically/Registered-Nurses-Utilization-of-Nursing-Assistive-Personnel-in-All-Settings.html

delegation, in that the UAP already has a list of nursing activities that he or she may perform without waiting for the delegation process (Marquis & Huston, 2015).

Yet, despite the efforts by the ANA and state boards of nursing, at the institutional level, most health care organizations interpret regulations broadly, allowing UAP a broader scope of practice than that advocated by professional nursing associations or state boards of nursing. In addition, although some institutions limit the scope of practice for UAP to non-nursing functions, many organizations allow the UAP to perform skills traditionally reserved for the licensed nurse.

Consider This Given the lack of national regulatory standards regarding the scope of practice for UAP, some health care institutions allow UAP to complete tasks traditionally reserved for licensed practitioners.

Jenkins and Joyner (2013) concur that in lieu of regulation of UAP by boards of nursing or government entities, many health care agencies and organizations have developed their own educational standards, role definitions, and scopes of practice for UAP in acute care. In their study of eight hospitals in the Washington, DC, area, all hospitals used UAP in medical-surgical areas to perform basic nursing care functions, such as hygiene and comfort care activities; assisting patients with eating, positioning, and mobility; and monitoring vital signs, intake and output, and blood glucose levels. In addition, the duties of UAP at some hospitals included phlebotomy, intravenous therapy initiation, maintenance and troubleshooting, ECG lead placement, alarm prioritization and response, and production of a rhythm strip. UAP also worked in intensive care units, operating rooms, postanesthesia care, and emergency departments. The researchers concluded that UAP appear to be performing skills and tasks once performed by LPNs. This observation supported the need for increased regulation of the UAP as a significant group of acute-care providers.

UAP AND PATIENT OUTCOMES

Because UAP are often involved in providing direct patient care activities, they directly influence not only the quality of care but also the care recipient's quality of life. A well-trained, caring, and competent UAP then can be a vital and contributing member of the health care team.

Certainly at some point though, given the increasing complexity of health care and the increasing acuity of patient illnesses, there is a maximum representation of UAP in the staffing mix that should not be breached. Those levels have not yet been determined. Considerable evidence does exist, however, that demonstrates a direct link between decreased RN staffing and declines in patient outcomes. Some of these declines in patient outcomes are nurse sensitive and include an increased incidence of patient falls, nosocomial infections, increased physical restraint use, and medication errors (see Chapter 9).

Outcome data also exist regarding the use of UAP to assist with and administer medications. A large survey of school nurses showed that nearly half of them reported medication errors in their schools during the previous year (Host, 2011). A major factor in these medication errors was the use of "unlicensed assistive personnel" such as school secretaries, health aides, teachers, parents, and even students, to administer medications, with UAP being three times more likely to make medication errors than their school nurse counterparts. Host also reported that three quarters of the schools had training programs for their UAP administering medications, but in most cases the training was 2 hours or less in length.

RN LIABILITY FOR SUPERVISION AND DELEGATION OF UAP

Delegation has long been a function of registered nursing, although the scope of delegation and the tasks being delegated have changed dramatically over the last three decades with the increased use of UAP in acute-care settings. As a result, the professional nurse (RN) role changed in many acute-care institutions from one of direct care provider to one requiring delegation of patient care to others.

This role of delegator and supervisor increased the scope of legal liability for the RN. Although there is limited case law involving nursing delegation and supervision, it is generally accepted that the RN is responsible for adequate supervision of the person to whom an assignment has been delegated. Although nurses are not automatically held liable for all acts of negligence on the part of those they supervise, they may be held liable if they were negligent in the supervision of those employees at the time that those employees committed the negligent acts (Marquis & Huston, 2015).

Liability is based on a supervisor's failure to determine which patient needs could safely be assigned to a subordinate or for failing to closely monitor a subordinate who requires such supervision. Experienced nurses have traditionally been expected to work with minimal supervision. The RN who delegates care to another competent RN does not have the same legal obligation to closely supervise that person's work as when the care is delegated to UAP.

Consider This The UAP has no license to lose for "exceeding scope of practice," and nationally established standards to state what the limits should be for UAP in terms of scope of practice do not exist. It is the RN who bears the legal liability for allowing UAP to perform tasks that should be accomplished only by a licensed health care professional.

In assigning tasks to UAP, then, the RN must be aware of the job description, knowledge base, and demonstrated skills of each person. Thus, the need for nurses to have highly developed delegation skills has never been greater than it is today. The ability to use delegation skills appropriately will help to reduce the personal liability associated with supervising and delegating to UAP. It will also ensure that clients' needs are met and their safety is not jeopardized. General principles for RNs to use in delegating to NAP are shown in Box 7.2.

Discussion Point

What happens when the condition of a patient changes? Is the training of UAP adequate to recognize changes in clients' conditions that warrant seeking intervention from the licensed nurse?

In addition, communication between the RN–UAP dyad is a critical factor in direct patient care and thus patient safety. The bottom line is that delegating to UAP is similar to delegating to other types of health care workers. RNs are always accountable for the care given and must be responsible for instructing UAP as to who needs care and when. The UAP should be accountable for knowing how to properly perform their segment of assigned care and for knowing when other workers should be called in for tasks beyond the limits of their knowledge and training. As such, the UAP does bear some personal accountability for their actions, despite the legal doctrine of *respondent superior* (the employer can be held legally liable for the conduct of employees whose actions he or she has a right to direct or control).

Stonehouse (2014) agrees, suggesting that UAP must recognize the responsibility and accountability that exist with the support worker's role. Support workers are responsible for what they choose to do, but equally for that which they choose not to do. In addition, "support workers need to embrace the fact that they, day in and day out, are personally responsible and accountable for delivering care of the highest possible standard and

BOX 7.2 American Nurses Association (2013)

Delegation Principles for RNs Who Work With Nursing Assistive Personnel (NAP)

1. The RN takes accountability and responsibility for all nursing care performed by the RN or an UAP.
2. The RN directs care and determines the appropriate utilization of any assistant involved in providing direct patient care.
3. The RN may delegate components of care but does not delegate the nursing process itself. The practice pervasive functions of assessment, planning, evaluation, and nursing judgment cannot be delegated.
4. The decision of whether or not to delegate or assign is based upon the RN's judgment concerning the condition of the patient, the competence of all members of the nursing team, and the degree of supervision that will be required of the RN if a task is delegated.
5. The RN delegates only those tasks for which she or he believes the other health care worker has the knowledge and skill to perform, taking into consideration training, cultural competence, experience, and facility/agency policies and procedures.
6. The RN individualizes communication regarding the delegation to the nursing assistive personnel and client situation, and the communication should be clear, concise, correct, and complete. The RN verifies comprehension with the nursing assistive personnel and that the assistant accepts the delegation and the responsibility that accompanies it.
7. Communication must be a two-way process. Nursing assistive personnel should have the opportunity to ask questions and/or for clarification of expectations.
8. The RN uses critical thinking and professional judgment when following the Five Rights of Delegation, to be sure that the delegation or assignment is:
   1. The right task
   2. Under the right circumstances
   3. To the right person
   4. With the right directions and communication; and
   5. Under the right supervision and evaluation
9. Chief Nursing Officers are accountable for establishing systems to assess, monitor, verify, and communicate ongoing competence requirements in areas related to delegation.

Source: Excerpted from American Nurses Association, National Council of State Boards of Nursing. (2013b). *Joint statement on delegation.* Retrieved January 22, 2015, from https://www.ncsbn.org/Delegation_joint_statement_NCSBN-ANA.pdf

should be duly proud of this, knowing that the care they deliver is evidence-based and within their scope of practice" (Stonehouse, 2014, p. 513).

Discussion Point

Do most UAP believe that they can be held legally liable and accountable for their actions if they are delegated to do something by an RN that is beyond their scope of practice or training?

REGISTERED NURSES WORKING AS UAP: A LIABILITY ISSUE

It must also be noted that some employers reported hiring new graduate RNs into UAP positions with the recent economic downturn. Many of these transitional employees secured employment in these positions while students in nursing programs. Though this practice provides employment opportunities for new graduate nurses, it does raise several matters of legality. First, these RNs are not able to provide care to the level of their expertise. Instead, they must perform only direct care duties and remain in the scope of practice of an unlicensed person. This violates numerous statutes that govern scope of practice, since these statutes suggest that licensees are held to the level of practice associated with his or her licensure, regardless of employment status. Thus, licensed nurses are held liable to provide care to the level of their existing scope of practice and yet also face risk of charges of negligence or malpractice if they provide care only to the level of the constructs of the assumed position (Boone, 2010). Working then in a capacity beneath the level of licensure appears to greatly increase the potential for legal liability for both the nurse and his or her employer and revocation of license for the nurse.

Boone (2010) also notes that most employers offer few definitive answers about how to address this role discrepancy and, instead, leave these critical decisions to the nurse. He concludes that binding a nurse to the constructs of a job description below their level of licensure not only is an ineffective practice but also subjects both employers and RNs working as UAP to greatly increased risks of legal proceedings.

CREATING A SAFE WORK ENVIRONMENT

There are things that health care organizations can do to increase the likelihood that UAP are used both effectively and appropriately as members of the health care team. First, the organization must have a clearly defined organization structure in which RNs are recognized as leaders of the health care team. This organization structure must facilitate RN evaluation of UAP job performance and encourage UAP accountability to the RN.

Job descriptions must also be developed by health care agencies that clearly define the roles and responsibilities of all categories of caregivers. These descriptions should be consistent with that state's nurse practice legislation, as well as with community standards of care, and should reflect differences between the roles of licensed and unlicensed personnel. Policies should facilitate adequate supervision of UAP by RNs and restrict UAP to simple tasks that can be performed safely. In addition, worker credentials should be readily apparent on the nametags worn by nursing health care personnel.

Second, uniform training and orientation programs for UAP must be established to ensure that preparation is adequate to provide at least minimum standards of safe patient care. These training and orientation programs should be based on clearly defined job descriptions for UAP. In addition, organizational education programs must be developed for all personnel to learn the roles and responsibilities of different categories of caregivers. In addition, to protect their patients and their professional license, RNs must continue to seek current information regarding national efforts to standardize scope of practice for UAP and professional guidelines regarding what can be safely delegated to UAP.

In addition, there must be adequate program development in leadership and delegation skills for RNs before UAP are introduced. Delegation is a learned skill, and much can be done to better prepare RNs for this role. Educational programs that produce graduate nurses must explore the nature of the RN role, with a focus on professional nurse leadership roles, to better prepare them to meet the challenges of working in restructured health care settings. Practicing RNs should have opportunities for continuing education in the principles of delegation and supervision. This will allow them not only to recognize the limitations of UAP scope of practice but also to gain confidence in differentiating between skills requiring licensure and those that do not.

UAP SHORTAGES

Finally, if all the issues related to the education, training, scope of practice, and delegation to UAP are resolved, there may be an even greater problem. There may not be enough UAP to meet future demand. The U.S. Department of Labor, Bureau of Labor Statistics (2014) projects that the need for UAP will grow by 21% (321,000 new jobs) by the year 2022, faster than the average for all occupations, predominantly in response to the long-term care needs of an increasing elderly population. In addition, the Labor Department suggests that hospitals will continue to be pressured to discharge patients as soon as possible as a result of diminishing reimbursement and this will boost admissions to nursing and residential care facilities. Modern medical technology will also drive the demand for UAP because as technology saves and extends more lives, the need for long-term care provided by UAP increases.

The unfortunate reality is that the demand for UAP as direct caregivers is already growing and the population of persons who have traditionally filled these jobs is declining. Indeed, there is a nationwide shortage of well-trained UAP in all settings, and although many states report recruitment and retention of support personnel as a major area of concern, few are actively addressing the situation.

UAP in Long-Term Care Settings

One problem contributing to this shortage is the high turnover rate for UAP, particularly in long-term care. The reasons for this high turnover rate are varied, but long hours, inadequate staffing, the low status of the job, exposure to infectious agents and drug-resistant infections, and the physical and emotional demands of the job contribute to it. In addition, 58% of CNAs employed in nursing home reported a workplace injury in the past year, the majority caused by patient aggression (59.4%) (Rico, 2013).

In addition, Sandvoll, Kristoffersen, and Hauge (2013) suggest that nursing homes are much more complex than most people imagine and that a greater appreciation must be given to the need for UAP to handle a combination of working according to routines and handling unexpected events, as well as attending to the personal requirements of individual patients. The skill needed to address the complexity of these care requirements may go unnoticed or be taken for granted. Rico (2013) agrees, noting that in her study of 3,014 CNAs, that supervisor respect was the only significant predictor of retention for UAP in long-term care settings.

It is also important to note that long-term care facilities, the most common employment site for UAP, are required to meet only minimum government standards for staffing and few facilities are cited, even when understaffing occurs. In addition, federal regulations are out of date and do not reflect new knowledge on safe staffing levels. For example, federal standards require that only one RN be on duty 8 hours every day in a nursing home, regardless of its size or the acuity of its patients. A licensed nurse (LPN/LVN) must be on duty the rest of the time (Zhang, Unruh, & Wan, 2013).

Consider This The brunt of work in long-term care settings typically falls on lowly paid, unlicensed workers who have a tremendous impact on patient satisfaction and the quality of care provided.

Low pay is also an issue. The U.S. Department of Labor, Bureau of Labor Statistics (2014) noted that the median hourly wage of UAP as of 2012 was US$11.73. The median hourly wage for UAP employed in general medical and surgical hospitals is generally higher than in nursing care facilities but pay is low for the work that is required. Indeed, research by Meyer, Raffle, and Ware (2014) found that CNAs cited pay as their primary reason for leaving long-term care, but better pay did not characterize the new jobs these CNAs took.

In addition, few employers provide UAP employer-paid benefits such as health insurance coverage, retirement benefits, or childcare. Furthermore, there are limited career paths or advancement opportunities for UAP who do not want to achieve a licensed job category (eg, LPN, RN), and they often have little direct input into organizational decision making.

Working conditions are also often less than ideal. Because of high UAP turnover and absenteeism, those UAP who do work must often work short-handed, which leads to greater stress. Research by Kalisch and Lee (2014) underscored that job satisfaction for nurse assistants depended primarily upon the number of assistive personnel in the mix of the nursing staff. Indeed, the more work experience the UAP reported, the lower their job satisfaction (Research Study Fuels the Controversy 7.1).

Similarly, Chaudhuri, Yeatts, and Cready (2013) noted emotional exhaustion brought on by occupational fatigue as common for UAP. Too much emotional exhaustion can have a detrimental impact on the UAP including the potential for poor decision making. Positive endorsement from supervisors, as well as more shared governance, where the UAP are exposed to shared decision-making, appear to be strategies for increasing structural empowerment of UAP.

Research Study Fuels the Controversy 7.1

Job Satisfaction for UAP

The aim of this cross-sectional study was to examine the relationship between staffing and job satisfaction of RNs and NAs. The study included 3,523 RNs and 1,012 NAs in 131 patient care units.

Source: Kalisch, B., & Lee, K. H. (2014). Staffing and job satisfaction: Nurses and nursing assistants. *Journal of Nursing Management, 22*(4), 465–471. doi:10.1111/jonm.12012

Study Findings

Hours per patient day was a significant positive predictor for RN job satisfaction after controlling for covariates. For NAs, a lower skill mix was marginally significant with higher job satisfaction. In addition, the more work experience the NAs reported, the lower their job satisfaction. The researchers concluded that adequate staffing levels were essential for RN job satisfaction, whereas NA job satisfaction depended on the number of assistive personnel in the staffing mix. Nursing management implications included reengineering the NA job to make it a more attractive and satisfying career.

Conclusions

The increased use of UAP presents both opportunities and challenges for the American health care system. Clearly, UAP play an increasingly integral role in safe and resource-efficient care delivery in this country (particularly in long-term care settings), and they can be successfully used to augment the health care team. Yet, a lack of clarity about roles and negative perceptions continue to persist (Munn, Tufanaru, & Aromataris, 2013).

As the health care system responds to cost escalation, however, a greater number of unlicensed personnel will be used to provide direct care, and the accountability for outcomes will continue to lie with the professional RN. Thus, "the premise that increasing the numbers of UAP in acute-care settings is a viable alternative to increasing the numbers of RNs is a micro political health issue" (Shearer, 2013, p. 24).

Munn et al. (2013) suggest that policy makers should address the barriers to incorporating UAP into models of care and further ensure they are successfully recognized as a delegated clinical role. Stone and Harahan (2010) agree, suggesting that action is needed on the part of policy makers, providers, and other stakeholders to avert an increasing UAP shortage (particularly in long-term care) and to promote worker retention. They argue that explicit policies should be developed to expand the supply of personnel entering the field, including the

> *creation of financial incentives such as grants to foster greater interest among people considering the long-term care field; scholarships, federal traineeships, and residency programs for people preparing for advanced degrees in long-term care; matching grants to fund administrators in-training programs for people interested in management positions; and loan forgiveness programs for people who commit to long-term care careers.* (p. 113)

The challenge though continues to be to use UAP only to provide personal care needs or nursing tasks that do not require the skill and judgment of the RN. With increasing patient loads and an emerging nursing shortage, many health care organizations and the RNs who work within them will be tempted to allow UAP to perform tasks that should be limited to professional nursing practice. Nurses must remember, however, that the responsibility for assuring that patients are protected and that UAP do not exceed their scope of practice ultimately falls on the RN. When UAP are allowed to encroach into professional nursing care, patients are placed at risk.

In addition, the blurring of the lines between the practice of RNs and UAP makes it nearly impossible for patients to make a distinction between providers. One of the most important roles then for the RN is to be a gatekeeper in assuring that care given by UAP under their supervision is always of high quality. Until answers are found, the likelihood is that UAP will continue to constitute a significant portion of the nursing workforce and the boundary between UAP and RN practice will continue to be blurred.

For Additional Discussion

1. Is cost or the nursing shortage the greater driving force in increased UAP use in acute-care hospitals today?
2. Is institutional training and certification of UAP a precursor to future initiatives for institutional licensure of RNs?
3. Are the cost savings associated with increased UAP use offset by the need for greater supervision by RNs and potential declines in patient outcomes?
4. Should UAP be allowed to administer medications, perform intravenous cannulation, and change sterile dressings?
5. Do you believe that patients typically are aware whether it is the UAP or licensed nurse that is caring for them?
6. How comfortable do you believe most RNs are in the role of delegator to UAP? Do you believe most RNs feel clarity regarding role differentiation between the RN and the UAP?
7. Should the training and certification of UAP fall under the purview of state boards of registered nursing?

References

American Academy of Pediatrics. (2009). *Policy statement—Guidance for the administration of medication in school. Pediatrics. 124*(4), 1244–1125. Retrieved January 22, 2015, from http://pediatrics.aappublications.org/content/124/4/1244.abstract

American Nurses Association. (2013a). *Fact sheet.* Retrieved January 22, 2015, from http://nursingworld.org/DocumentVault/Legal-Action/California-Supreme-Court-May-2013.pdf

American Nurses Association, National Council of State Boards of Nursing. (2013b). *Joint statement on delegation.* Retrieved January 25, 2015, from https://www.ncsbn.org/Delegation_joint_statement_NCSBN-ANA.pdf

Boone, T. W., Sr. (2010). *New nurses working as unlicensed assistive personnel: Nurses may not be able to provide effective care within their scope of practice.* Retrieved June 30, 2011, from Advance Healthcare Network—For Nurses website: http://nursing.advanceweb.com/Student-and-New-Grad-Center/Student-Top-Story/New-Nurses-Working-as-Unlicensed-Assistive-Personnel.aspx

Buck, D. K. (2014). Client need prompts changes to nursing assistant training curriculums and authorized duties. *Oregon Board of Nursing Sentinel, 33*(3), 18–19.

Bureau of Labor Statistics, U.S. Department of Labor. (2014). Nursing assistants and orderlies. In *Occupational Outlook Handbook* (2014–2015 ed.). Washington, DC: Author. Retrieved January 24, 2015, from http://www.bls.gov/ooh/Healthcare/Nursing-assistants.htm

California Department of Education. (2014, December 19). *K.C. Settlement Agreement & Legal Advisory.* Updated November 6, 2013. Retrieved January 22, 2015, from http://www.cde.ca.gov/ls/he/hn/legaladvisory.asp

Case, B. (2013). *Delegation skills.* Retrieved June 20, 2013, from Advance Healthcare Network—For Nurses website: http://nursing.advanceweb.com/Article/Delegation-Skills.aspx

Chaudhuri, T., Yeatts, D. E., & Cready, C. M. (2013). Nurse aide decision making in nursing homes: Factors affecting empowerment. *Journal of Clinical Nursing, 22*(17-18), 2572–2585. doi:10.1111/jocn.12118

Host, P. (2011). *School medication administration: How to make it work for you and your child.* Retrieved June 29, 2011, from http://bipolar.about.com/cs/kids_parents/a/0207_schoolmeds.htm

Jenkins, B., & Joyner, J. (2013). Preparation, roles, and perceived effectiveness of unlicensed assistive personnel. *Journal of Nursing Regulation, 4*(3), 33–40.

Kalisch, B., & Lee, K. H. (2014). Staffing and job satisfaction: Nurses and nursing assistants. *Journal of Nursing Management, 22*(4), 465–471. doi:10.1111/jonm.12012

Marquis, B., & Huston, C. (2015). *Leadership roles and management functions in nursing* (8th ed.). Philadelphia, PA: Lippincott Williams & Wilkins.

Meyer, D., Raffle, H., & Ware, L. J. (2014). The first year: Employment patterns and job perceptions of nursing assistants in a rural setting. *Journal of Nursing Management, 22*(6), 769–778. doi:10.1111/j.1365-2834.2012.01441.x

Mulrooney, G. (2011). A case for improved quality of care through more accurate staffing. Safe staffing legislation, an API Healthcare White Paper. Retrieved July 6, 2011, from http://www.apihealthcare.com/safe_staffing_legislation/

Munn, Z., Tufanaru, C., & Aromataris, E. (2013). Recognition of the health assistant as a delegated clinical role and their inclusion in models of care: A systematic review and meta-synthesis of qualitative evidence. *International Journal of Evidence-Based Healthcare, 11*(1), 3–19. doi:10.1111/j.1744-1609.2012.00304.x

National Association of School Nurses. (2014). *Unlicensed assistive personnel—The role of the school nurse: Position statement.* Revised January 2011. Retrieved January 24, 2015, from http://www.nasn.org/PolicyAdvocacy/PositionPapersandReports/NASNPositionStatementsFullView/tabid/462/ArticleId/116/Unlicensed-Assistive-Personnel-The-Role-of-the-School-Nurse-Revised-2011

O'Keefe, C. (2014). The authority for certain clinical tasks performed by unlicensed patient care technicians and LPNs/LVNs in the hemodialysis setting: A review. *Nephrology Nursing Journal, 41*(3), 247–255.

Rico, J. S. (2013). *Staffing the nation's nursing homes* (Doctoral dissertation, Northeastern University). Available from: CINAHL Plus, Ipswich, MA. Accessed January 25, 2015.

Sandvoll, A. M., Kristoffersen, K., & Hauge, S. (2013). The double embarrassment: Understanding the actions of nursing staff in an unexpected situation. *International Journal of Nursing Practice, 19*(4), 368–373. doi:10.1111/ijn.12086

Shearer, T. (2013). Getting the mix right: Assistants in nursing and skill mix. *Australian Nursing & Midwifery Journal, 21*(5), 24–27.

Stone, R., & Harahan, M. F. (2010). Improving the long-term care workforce serving older adults. *Health Affairs, 29*(1), 109–115.

Stonehouse, D. (2014). Who's responsible and who's accountable? You are! *British Journal of Healthcare Assistants, 8*(10), 511–513.

Thungjaroenkul, P., Cummings, G. C., & Embleton, A. (2007). The impact of nurse staffing on hospital costs and patient length of stay: A systematic review. *Nursing Economic$, 25*(5), 255–265.

Westbrook, J. I., Duffield, C., Li, L., & Creswick, N. J. (2011). How much time do nurses have for patients? A longitudinal study quantifying hospital nurses' patterns of task time distribution and interactions with health professionals. *BMC Health Services Research, 11*, 319. Retrieved January 24, 2015, from http://www.biomedcentral.com/1472-6963/11/319

Zhang, N. J., Unruh, L., & Wan, T. H. (2013). Gaps in nurse staffing and nursing home resident needs. *Nursing Economic$, 31*(6), 289–297.

8

Diversity in the Nursing Workforce

Carol J. Huston

ADDITIONAL RESOURCES

Visit thePoint for additional helpful resources

- eBook
- Journal Articles
- WebLinks

CHAPTER OUTLINE

LEARNING OBJECTIVES

The learner will be able to:

1. Examine the relationship between health disparities and a lack of diversity in the health care workforce.
2. Explore factors leading to the lack of ethnic and gender diversity in nursing.
3. Suggest individual, organizational, and professional strategies to increase ethnic and gender diversity in nursing.
4. Identify common barriers faced in both recruiting and retaining minority students and faculty in higher education.
5. Compare opportunity levels for decision making at senior levels of health care management between racial/ethnic minorities and Whites.
6. Identify at least three professional nursing associations that are directed at serving the needs of a specific racial or ethnic population.
7. Investigate stereotypes of male nurses that both hinder the recruitment and retention of men into nursing and pose socialization and acceptance challenges for them.
8. Compare economic and advancement opportunities for men and women in nursing.
9. Argue for or against the need for affirmative action to bring more men into the nursing profession.
10. Analyze research exploring generational differences in work values and preferences among registered nurses, and explore the challenges inherent in having up to four generations cohabitate in the same profession at the same time.

INTRODUCTION

Diversity has been defined as the differences among groups or between individuals, and it comes in many forms, including age, gender, religion, customs, sexual orientation, physical size, physical and mental capabilities, beliefs, culture, ethnicity, and skin color. Yet, despite increasing diversity (particularly ethnic and cultural) in the United States, the nursing workforce continues to be fairly homogeneous, at least in terms of ethnicity and gender, being White, female, and middle aged.

This lack of ethnic, gender, and generational diversity is a concern not only for the nursing profession but also for its clients since a lack of diversity in the workforce has been linked to health disparities. John Bluford, President and CEO of two-hospital Truman Medical Centers in Kansas City, MO, suggests that "diverse perspectives yield better decisions, and better decisions yield better outcomes" (Selvam, 2013, para. 5). Clearly then, the nursing workforce should be at least as diverse as the population it serves. Indeed, a clamor for greater diversity in the profession continues to occur, and this is readily apparent in a review of the literature.

Discussion Point

For nursing care to be culturally and ethnically sensitive, must it be provided by a culturally and ethnically diverse nursing population?

Phillips and Malone (2014) suggest that as nursing continues to advance health care in the 21st century, the current shift in demographics, coupled with the ongoing disparities in health care and health outcomes, will warrant our ongoing attention and action. The nursing profession, in particular, will be challenged to recruit and retain a culturally diverse workforce that mirrors the nation's change in demographics.

Historically, despite this stated need for and appreciation of the benefits of a diverse health care workforce, efforts to increase the number of minority professionals have not been as successful as hoped. The reasons barriers remain are numerous, but the roots can certainly be found in racism, discrimination, and a lack of commitment to changing the situation.

Consider This Barriers to increasing the number of minority health care professionals include, but are not limited to, racism, discrimination, and a lack of commitment to changing the situation.

This chapter focuses primarily on three aspects of diversity in the nursing workforce: ethnicity, gender, and age (generational factors). Factors leading to the lack of ethnic and gender diversity in nursing are explored, as are individual and organizational strategies to address the problem. (The importation of foreign nurses as a factor in workforce diversity is discussed in Chapter 6.) In addition, the efforts of health care stakeholders, the government, states, and current professional nursing organizations to increase diversity in the profession are examined. Finally, the effect of generational diversity on workers and workplace functioning is presented.

ETHNIC DIVERSITY IN THE UNITED STATES

Demographic data from the U.S. Census Bureau continue to show increased diversification of the US population, a trend that began almost 35 years ago. As of 2013, 62.6% of the population was White, not of Hispanic origin (U.S. Census Bureau, 2013). Hispanics continue to be the largest minority group at 17.1% and are the fastest growing population group. Blacks are the second largest minority group (13.2%), followed by Asians (5.3%), American Indians and Alaska natives (1.2%), and native Hawaiians and other Pacific Islanders (0.2%) (U.S. Census Bureau, 2013). Projections suggest that current minority populations will become the majority by the year 2043 (American Association of Colleges of Nursing [AACN], 2014a).

ETHNIC DIVERSITY IN NURSING

There are significant differences between the ethnic and gender demographics of the US population and those of the nursing workforce in the United States (Table 8.1). Whereas the number of nurses from minority backgrounds continues to rise in the United States, it is considerably lower than the minority representation in the general population.

According to 2013 data from the National Council of State Boards of Nursing and the Forum of State Nursing Workforce Centers, nurses from minority backgrounds represent just 19% of the registered nurse (RN) workforce, with the RN population comprising 83% White, 6% African American, 6% Asian, 3% Hispanic, 1% American

TABLE 8.1 Comparison of US Population and Registered Nurse Workforce in Terms of Ethnicity and Gender

Characteristic	Year 2013 U.S. Census Data (% Representation)	Year 2013 Registered Nurse Workforce (% Representation)
Gender: Male	49.2	9.6
Gender: Female	50.8	90.4
White (non-Hispanic)	62.6	83.0
Black/African American	13.2	6.0
Asian/Native Hawaiian/Pacific Islander	5.5	7.0
American Indian/Alaskan native	1.2	1.0
Hispanic/Latino	17.1	3.0
Persons responding to two or more races	1.7	

Source: American Association of Colleges of Nursing. (2014a). *Fact sheet: Enhancing diversity in the nursing workforce.* Retrieved January 25, 2015, from http://www.aacn.nche.edu/media-relations/diversityFS.pdf; U.S. Census Bureau. (2013). *State and county quick facts.* Retrieved January 24, 2015, from http://quickfacts.census.gov/qfd/states/00000.html

Indian/Alaskan Native, 1% Native Hawaiian/Pacific Islander, and 1% other (with these figures showing only small increases over the past decade) (AACN, 2014a).

Recruiting and Retaining Minority Students into Nursing

Clearly, increasing diversity in the nursing profession must begin with the aggressive recruitment and retention of minority students. The reality is that White students continue to dominate ethnicity on most college campuses in the United States. Only 28.3% of nursing students in entry-level baccalaureate programs in 2012 to 2013 were from minority backgrounds (AACN, 2014a). In addition, about 29.3% of master's students and 27.7% of students in research-focused doctoral programs were from minority backgrounds. These numbers reflect small percentage increases from 2010 to 2011 (1% to 3%), suggesting that while some strides have been made in recruiting and graduating minority nurses, more must be done before equal representation is realized.

Discussion Point

Should more resources (time, energy, money) be devoted to the recruitment of or retention of minority students? Is a two-pronged approach (emphasizing both recruitment and retention) necessary? Why or why not?

The key to recruiting more minority students into nursing is likely creating learning environments that integrate diversity and cultural competence across academic programs and demonstrate an appreciation and respect of minority students themselves. Research by Sedgwick, Oosterbroek, and Ponomar (2014), however, suggests that while undergraduate nursing students quickly learn that RNs, clinical nursing instructors, and peers support the abstract notion of cultural diversity and its inclusion in nursing education in principle, their practices and behaviors often differ. Indeed, minority students often report experiencing bias and discrimination in their interactions with all groups of people involved in their learning Thus, bias and discrimination are often a systems issue at the institutional level as well as a systemic issue, that is, biased and discriminatory behavior is not limited to one particular group.

Consider This While most nurse educators and nursing students support the abstract notion of cultural diversity and its inclusion in nursing education in principle, their practices and behaviors often differ.

To address these concerns, many universities have launched initiatives directed at both the recruitment and retention of these minority students. Melillo, Dowling, Abdallah, Findeisen, and Knight (2013) detailed the implementation of a *Bring Diversity to Nursing* project at the University of Massachusetts that included the promotion of nursing to minority students as a career choice by recruiters at primary, middle, and high schools. The program also provided stipends, scholarships, and educational technologies to assist admitted students in passing the NCLEX. A Coordinator of Diversity Support, advisors, counselors, and tutors provide additional support.

Similarly, Johnson Rowsey, Kneipp, and Woods-Giscombe (2013) described their efforts to develop a program to increase the number of minority students in the baccalaureate nursing program at their university and to prepare them to enroll in doctoral programs within 1 year of graduation. The *Careers beyond the Bedside* program offers undergraduates preentry, academic enrichment, and graduate school preparation activities designed to facilitate careers as nursing faculty educators and researchers.

Unfortunately, positive and nurturing environments for students from underrepresented backgrounds are inadequate in number, and the end result is that many such students either are never presented the opportunity to pursue nursing as a career or fail to receive the necessary support to successfully complete their nursing education

In addition, many experts suggest that recruitment and retention rates are low with underrepresented groups because such groups are at greater risk of being economically disadvantaged, and this, in turn, places them at greater risk of having received an inferior preparatory education. Students who complete their secondary education in economically disadvantaged communities or institutions may have inadequately developed reading, writing, and critical thinking skills and often lack access to advanced preparation in the natural and physical sciences. This makes them less viable as candidates for admission to a nursing program.

Consider This Recruitment and retention of minority nursing students could improve if these students were given solid secondary academic preparation and if the environments in which they are educated were more accepting of and hospitable to students from diverse backgrounds.

For some minority students, it is an inferior secondary education preparation that predisposes them to course and even program failure. In addition, because many minority students are the first in their families to attend college, it might be difficult for family members to understand and be supportive of the challenges of higher education and the rigor of academic coursework. Minority students also tend to experience more difficulty with social adjustment in the college environment, particularly when they are attending a predominantly White institution and a lack of diversity in faculty role models and mentors contribute to their social isolation.

Finances are also often a barrier to minority students, many of whom must work at least part time to subsidize the cost of their college education. To address the need for financial support for individuals from disadvantaged backgrounds, the U.S. Health Resources and Services Administration (HRSA) began offering the *Nursing Workforce Diversity* (NWD) program in 1998. This program provides grants or contracts to projects that provide student stipends or scholarships, stipends for diploma or associate degree nurses to enter a bridge or degree completion program, student scholarships or stipends for accelerated nursing degree programs, preentry preparation, advanced education preparation, and retention activities (HRSA, 2015). To be eligible for an NWD grant, students must come from an educationally or economically disadvantaged background (including students who belong to racial/ethnic minorities underrepresented among nurses) and express an interest in becoming an RN (Rural Assistance Center, 2002–2015). Unfortunately, NWD grant competition was not planned for in fiscal year 2015 because funds were not available (HRSA, 2015).

Consider This It is the retention and graduation of minority students that will begin to change the cultural face of nursing.

A summary of the barriers minority students face in completing their nursing education is shown in Box 8.1.

Minority Nurse Educators

The underrepresentation of minority nurse faculty is well documented. Data from 2012 suggest that only 12.3% of all full-time instructional faculty members in baccalaureate and graduate programs are members of racial/ethnic minority groups, and only 5.4% are male (AACN, 2014a). The fact is that far too few nurses from racial/ethnic minority groups with advanced nursing degrees pursue faculty careers.

In an effort to increase the number of minority nurse scholars, the American Association of Colleges of Nursing (AACN) and the Johnson & Johnson Campaign for Nursing's Future launched a national scholarship program in 2007 to increase the number of nursing faculty

BOX 8.1 Common Barriers for Minority Students in Academic Nursing Programs

1. Inferior academic preparation
2. Financial problems
3. Inadequate social support
4. A lack of mentoring opportunities
5. Inconsistent faculty and institutional support
6. Inadequate numbers of minority faculty role models

from ethnic minority backgrounds (AACN, 2015). This scholarship program supports full-time nursing students in doctoral or master's degree programs, with a preference given to those completing a doctorate. Scholarship recipients must agree to teach in a US school of nursing after completing their advanced degree. Five scholarship recipients are selected annually, with each receiving a US$18,000 scholarship.

Another opportunity to support minority faculty is the HRSA *Minority Faculty Fellowship Program* grants. These program grants provide stipends to educational programs to increase the number of faculty representing racial and ethnic minorities. This stipend provides up to 50% of the faculty salary, which is matched or exceeded by the employing institution. Jacob and Sanchez (2011) describe how the grant was used at the University of Tennessee Health Science Center College of Nursing to recruit, mentor, and support a new Hispanic nursing faculty member.

ETHNIC DIVERSITY IN HEALTH CARE ADMINISTRATION

Based on 2012 data from the Institute for Diversity in Health Management, an affiliate of the American Hospital Association, minorities now make up 14% of hospital C-suite positions (Selvam, 2013). While up significantly from 9% in 2011 and from 2% in the organization's first benchmark survey in 1994, these numbers still fall far short of the 22% of non-Whites in the US population as a whole. This increase is likely due to stepped up efforts to focus on diversity as well as recent retirements of senior-level executives that have created new opportunities.

In addition, only 9% of CEO positions at hospitals and health systems were held by minority populations, the second-lowest percentage of all C-suite positions (Selvam, 2013). Chief financial officers scored lower, at 7%. In addition, minorities held only 16% of chief medical officer positions and 14% of chief operating officer jobs. Not surprisingly, the top role for minority executives was chief diversity officer, at 60% (Selvam, 2013).

David Elgarico, Board Chairman of the Asian Health Care Leaders Association and Executive Director of ancillary services-administration at the University of California at Irvine Medical Center, suggests that the problem is not a lack of highly qualified minority candidates to fill these top jobs (Selvam, 2013). Instead, he argues that "the challenge is some people will pick only people who remind them of themselves or someone you know. They're not consciously aware that this is going on. It's only human nature" (Selvam, 2013, para. 8).

Linda Hill, a professor of business administration at Harvard Business School, agrees, suggesting that many organizations fail to view talented people as potential leaders. This may occur because "'demographic invisibles'—people who, because of their gender, ethnicity, nationality, or even age, don't have access to the tools—the social networks, the fast-track training courses, the stretch assignments—that can prepare them for positions of authority and influence" (Hemp, 2008, p. 125). Hill also suggested that other potential leaders are missed since they are viewed as "'stylistic invisibles'—individuals who don't fit the conventional image of a leader, since they don't exhibit take charge, direction setting behavior" (Hemp, 2008, p. 125). This also may represent cultural differences more than leadership ability.

There is hope, however. Selvam (2013) notes that judging by enrollment in health care management programs, governing boards should be seeing a sharp increase in qualified minority candidates for top management positions. According to the Association of University Programs in Health Administration, about 42% of graduate students in health care management programs nationally were minorities in the 2009 to 2010 academic year (Selvam, 2013). But even more effort is needed; companies need to offer minorities opportunities to shadow senior executives and should recruit at schools with diverse ethnic enrollments. In addition, minority candidates should be offered a battery of internships, residencies, and fellowships to provide the requisite experience highly valued by health care employers (Selvam, 2013).

Marquis and Huston (2015) agree, suggesting that health care organizations must be more open-minded about who health care's future leaders might be and begin to prepare more diverse candidates to be effective leaders. This will require the formal education and training that are a part of most management-development programs, as well as a development of appropriate attitudes through social learning.

Consider This Increasing the number of ethnic minorities in executive health care positions will require an intentional commitment to do so and a well-planned development program that includes the same type of mentoring activities that their White counterparts have long enjoyed and benefited from.

ETHNIC PROFESSIONAL ASSOCIATIONS IN NURSING

There is a professional association for almost every ethnic group in nursing. Several of the many organizations include the National Black Nurses Association, the National Association of Hispanic Nurses, the Philippine Nurses Association, the National Alaska Native American Indian Nurses Association, and the Asian American/Pacific Islander Nurses Association Incorporated. See Box 8.2 for more information on these groups.

Discussion Point

If our goal is to better appreciate and merge cultural and ethnic diversity in nursing, why do culturally and ethnically diverse nurses separate themselves with their own professional nursing organizations?

GENDER DIVERSITY IN NURSING

Diversity goals in nursing are not just directed at ethnicity—they also frequently include increasing the number of men in nursing. Although men have worked as nurses for centuries, just 9.6% of the nation's 3.5 million nurses are men, a percentage that has climbed slowly but steadily since 1980 (AACN, 2014a). There are efforts underway to increase the number of men in nursing. Some suggest that recruitment campaigns are not enough and that affirmative action, similar to the efforts used to increase the number of women in medicine and engineering, will be required before there will be any significant increase in the number of male nurses.

Discussion Point

Affirmative action has been used successfully to increase the presence of some underrepresented minorities in health care. Should the same be done to increase the number of men in nursing?

Yet, despite a call to increase the number of men in nursing, progress in this regard has been slow. Clow, Ricciardelli, and Bartfay (2014) suggest that social isolation (a lack of role models and mentors, lack of peer support); failure to acknowledge and discuss gender differences in expressions of care (eg, physical touch used by men vs. women); sexism (professors and textbooks that refer nurses solely with feminine pronouns; antimale comments in the classroom); suppression of the contributions men have made to the field of nursing (eg, textbooks and nursing programs that ignore the historical role of men in nursing, lectures and textbooks that only portray women as nurses); and media portrayals of male nurses as socially or sexually deviant are part of the problem. In addition, male nonnursing students hold significantly more negative attitudes toward male nurses than female nonnursing students (Clow et al., 2014).

The reality is that most of the public would describe nursing as a female occupation, and young men often report they never even consider a career as a nurse. The media also perpetuates the image of the nurse as female. Many media sources, and even nursing textbooks at times, refer to the comforting caregiver nurse as "she," suggesting that male nurses are unable to demonstrate caring behavior and touch similar to their female counterparts. In addition, male nurses may be stereotyped as effeminate, homosexual, or predatory. These stigmatizing discourses may deter men's entry into nursing. The difficulty of male nurses socializing into what has long

BOX 8.2 Ethnic Professional Associations in Nursing

Support groups and professional associations abound among nurses in the United States. Some of the groups formed to address specific issues related to ethnic diversity in nursing include the following:

National Black Nurses Association

The National Black Nurses Association (NBNA), founded in 1971, represents approximately 150,000 Black nurses from the United States (with 91 chartered chapters nationwide), the Eastern Caribbean nations, and Africa (NBNA, 2014). The mission of the NBNA is to "provide a forum for collective action by African American nurses to represent and provide a forum for black nurses to advocate for and implement strategies to ensure access to the highest quality of health care for persons of color" (NBNA, 2014, para. 4).

National Association of Hispanic Nurses

The National Association of Hispanic Nurses (NAHN) was founded in 1975 by Ildaura Murillo-Rohde and evolved out of the Ad Hoc Committee of the Spanish-Speaking/Spanish Surname Nurses' Caucus, which was formed during the American Nurses Association convention in San Francisco in 1974 (NAHN, 2014). The NAHN is committed to advancing the health in Hispanic communities and to lead, promote, and advocate the educational, professional, and leadership opportunities for Hispanic nurses.

Philippine Nurses Association, Inc.

The mission of the Philippine Nurses Association Inc. (PNA) is to promote professional growth toward the attainment of the highest standards of nursing. Its vision is that by 2030, PNA will be the primary professional association advancing the welfare and development of globally competent Filipino nurses (PNA, 2015).

National Alaska Native American Indian Nurses Association

The National Alaska Native American Indian Nurses Association (NANAINA) was founded on its predecessor organization, the American Indian Nurses Association, and, later, the American Indian Alaska Native Nurses Association. The NANAINA is dedicated to supporting Alaska Native and American Indian students, nurses, and allied health professionals through the development of leadership skills and continuing education. It also advocates for the improvement of health care provided to American Indian and Alaska Native consumers and culturally competent health care (NANAINA, n.d.).

Asian American/Pacific Islander Nurses Association Inc

The Asian American/Pacific Islander Nurses Association Inc. (AAPINA) obtains current statistics and national information on the health status of Asian Americans and Pacific Islanders (APIs), publishes information on fellowship, grants, and meetings for API nurses, represents API nurses on national and federal groups, and participates in the National Coalition of Ethnic Minority Nurse Associations (AAPINA, 2008–2014).

been perceived as a woman's occupation is depicted in Figure 8.1.

Consider This Caregiving is not just a feminine trait.

Clearly, stereotypes that suggest male nurses are less capable of therapeutic caring, compassion, and nurturing than female nurses hurt the profession, as well as society in general. At least partly as a result of these stereotypes, some patients have gender preferences (more commonly female) for their caregivers. This seems to be particularly true for nurses employed in labor and delivery settings.

Brusie (2013) reports that in a 2005 survey of male nurses, less than 1% of male nurses work in obstetrics—the lowest percentage of any field. And as recently as 10 years ago, some states, like California, actually legally banned males from working as nurses on obstetrical floors. (Today, states and hospitals cannot deny a male entry into a nursing profession simply based on his gender.) Court cases have confused the issue further. In some cases, the courts have ruled that female gender is a legitimate qualification for labor and delivery nurses, yet other courts have found these qualifications to be discriminatory.

Wolfenden (2011) suggests that the barring of men from specific areas of practice, combined with the education of nurses being increasingly feminized,

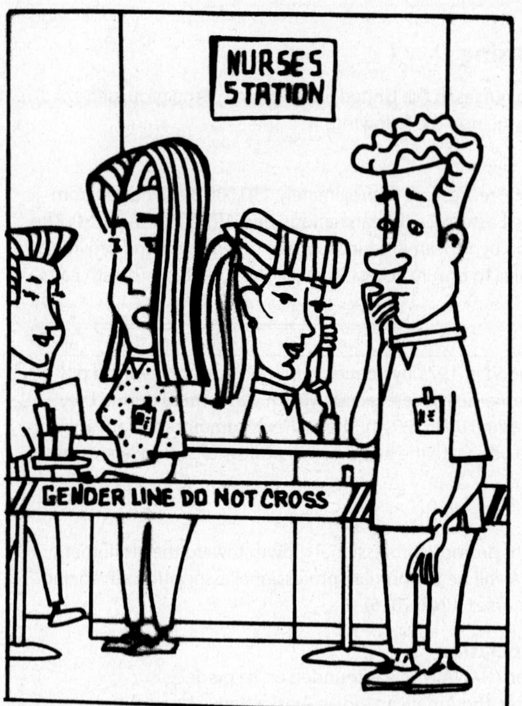

Figure 8.1 Challenges faced by men in nursing. (*Source*: Copyright © 2002, Medzilla, Inc. http://www.medzilla.com. Reprinted with permission.)

marginalizes men in nursing. He suggests that if this trend continues, the result will be fewer men seeking nursing careers, and a gradual erosion of the professional and academic capacity of nursing.

Is There a Male Advantage in Nursing?

Despite the barriers that male nurses face, their minority status may give male nurses advantages in hiring and promotion, unlike women in male-dominated professions. Despite their minority status, men in nursing often rise more rapidly into management positions and earn more money than their female counterparts.

Indeed, Casselman (2013) notes that the average female nurse earned $51,100 in 2011, 16% less than the $60,700 earned by the average man in the same job. Sagon (2013) cites similar statistics in her assertion that for every dollar male nurses earned, female nurses earned 91 cents; in contrast, women earned 77 cents to every dollar men earned across all occupations. Some experts have suggested that the more rapid career trajectory and relative higher pay for male nurses likely reflects the historical trend that more men are employed full time in their career paths, whereas women tend to have career gaps related to childbearing or rearing families and often work fewer hours. However, when looking only at full-time year-round workers, the gap narrows, but it doesn't disappear; female nurses working full-time, year-round earned 9% less than their male counterparts (Casselman, 2013).

Men also appear to have an easier time getting hired into nursing jobs, although the high demand for nurses means unemployment rates are low across categories—less than 2% for RNs, and even lower for more advanced professionals. Among licensed practical nurses, the only category with meaningful levels of unemployment, men had an unemployment rate of 4%, versus 5.1% for women (Casselman, 2013).

In addition, male nurses in the United States hold disproportionately more positions of influence and authority than their female counterparts. McMurry (2011) notes that most of the discrimination and prejudice facing men in female professions emanates from outside those professions and that research has found that men in nursing have been given fair, if not preferential, treatment in hiring and promotion. In fact, McMurry suggests that subtle mechanisms are in place to enhance men's position in the nursing profession and that their minority status often results in advantages that promote rather than hinder their careers.

Consider This Many experts suggest that the power of the profession would be elevated if more men were to become nurses. Yet men in nursing hold a disproportionately large share of the high-income jobs and have higher salaries than their female counterparts.

Why Are Men Leaving Nursing?

Although increased numbers of men are joining the nursing profession, disproportionate numbers of male nurses are also leaving, as compared with female nurses. In fact, new male nurses leave the profession at a much higher rate than female nurse graduates. Wallen, Mor, and Devine (2014) suggest this may be a result of the potentially conflicting social expectations men face when they work in female-dominated professions. A scarcity of male role models and conflicting expectations regarding social approval for men in nursing and the assumption of traditional feminine values related to nurturing and caring accentuate the problem.

Research by Wallen et al. (2014) suggests that the respect nurses receive in general as a profession does mediate these conflicting social expectations for male nurses, and in fact, this respect is a significant factor in determining the job satisfaction and affective commitment of male nurses. Thus, efforts to increase occupational status among all nurses decrease the attrition of all nurses, but male nurses in particular. In addition, interventions aimed at male nurses' gender and professional identities might have positive effects on their professional outcomes. This could be as simple as paying attention to the gender neutrality of language used in job advertisements and internal communication.

In addition, although the literature has been mixed, the majority of nursing studies that examined gender and job dissatisfaction suggested that male nurses are more dissatisfied than their female counterparts. Some experts argue that more men than women leave nursing because nursing still lacks status and therefore nurses are often demeaned by other health professionals. Male nurses may be less willing to tolerate this kind of treatment.

Consider This Recent graduates of the nation's nursing schools are leaving the profession more quickly than their predecessors, with male nurses leaving at a higher rate than their female counterparts.

GENERATIONAL DIVERSITY IN NURSING

Age has become a diversity issue during the last decade. Not surprisingly, each generation has its own way of doing things and seeing the world, which is based upon their shared life experiences (Clipper, 2013). The problem is not that the nursing workforce lacks generational diversity but that typically four generations have not cohabitated at the same time in a profession. This climate offers challenges and opportunities for leaders. Opportunities include having a workforce that more closely resembles the diversity of clients served and the chance for best thinking from different perspectives. The challenges include the complexities that result when productivity and efficiency are dependent upon each team member working together effectively.

According to the 2010 National Sample Survey of Registered Nurses, the average age of an RN in the United States was 47 years, up from 46.8 years in the year 2004 (AACN, 2014b). In addition, according to a 2013 survey conducted by the National Council of State Boards of Nursing and The Forum of State Nursing Workforce Centers, 55% of the RN workforce is age 50 or older. Indeed, nurses over the age of 50 have become the largest segment of the nursing workforce. Given the need to both retain older nurses and to recruit new, young nurses into the field, generational issues must be examined further.

Defining the Generations

The research increasingly suggests that the different generations represented in nursing today may have different attitudes and value systems, which greatly impact the settings in which they work. They may also have significantly different career socialization experiences and expectations regarding their chosen profession and employer. In addition, workplace relationships are often influenced by these generational differences.

Most experts identify four generational groups in today's workforce: the veteran generation (also called the *silent generation*), the baby boomers, Generation X, and Generation Y (also called the *millennials*).

The *veteran generation* is typically recognized as those nurses born between 1925 and 1942. Having lived through several international military conflicts (World War II, the Korean War, and the Vietnam War) and the Great Depression, they are often risk averse (particularly in regard to personal finances), respectful of authority, and supportive of hierarchy. They are also called the *silent generation* because they tend to support the status quo rather than protest or push for rapid change. As a result, these nurses are less likely to question organizational practices and more likely to seek employment in structured settings (Marquis & Huston, 2015). Their work values are traditional, and they are often recognized for their loyalty to their employers.

The *boom generation* (born 1943 to 1960) also displays traditional work values; however, they tend to be more materialistic and present oriented and are thus willing to work long hours at their jobs in an effort to get ahead. Clipper (2013) notes that overall, boomers enjoy work, often make the choice to "live to work," and put in many hours. They are personally gratified when they perform well at work. This is also a very competitive cohort by nature that insists that their work is done to the best of their ability and will often beat deadlines. Nurses born in this generation may be best suited for work that requires flexibility, independent thinking, and creativity.

In contrast, *Generation Xers* (born between 1961 and 1981), a much smaller cohort than the baby boomers who preceded them or the Generation Yers who follow them, may lack the interest in lifetime employment at one place that prior generations have valued, instead valuing greater work-hour flexibility and opportunities for time off. Indeed, Clipper (2013) suggests this generation generally works because it is a necessity. This likely reflects the fact that many individuals born in this generation had both parents working outside their home as they were growing up and they want to put more emphasis on family and leisure time in their own family units. Thus, this generation may be less economically driven than prior generations and may define success differently than the veteran generation or the baby boomers. Generation Xers don't mind working hard, but they typically expect something in return, such as job security, good pay, promotions, and flexible schedules. This group is willing to be a team player if they like the team and enjoy what they are doing (Clipper, 2013).

Generation Y (born 1982 to 1999) represents the first cohort of truly global citizens. They are known for their optimism, self-confidence, relationship orientation, volunteer-mindedness, and social consciousness. This generation has difficulty taking accountability for their actions and work; a poor performance is usually not "their fault." In addition, Clipper (2013) notes that as a whole, millennials don't need their work to define them. They do get bored easily, but are willing to work hard as long as they perceive an equivalent benefit to them personally, such as career advancement or financial rewards. A good performance by this group means that all of the variables are in their favor, the right resources, the right team (no conflict among the team as this group prefers group processes/decisions), and the right reasons to do it. Accountability, however, is sometimes an issue since poor performance is usually not "their fault." They are also technologically savvy, which is why some people call them "digital natives."

Joan M. Kavanagh, Associate Chief Nursing Officer for nursing education and professional development at Cleveland Clinic, notes however, that millennials often "get a bad rap" (Krischke, 2014, para. 3). "They may tend to change jobs more frequently, but much of that has to do with growth and expansion since their work ethic is intense and committed. They also tend to be innovators, entrepreneurs and bold risk takers. While those aren't competencies we may have been looking for in the past, they are certainly competencies that will serve us well in this time of unprecedented change" (Krischke, 2014, para. 3).

Given these attitudinal and value differences, it is not surprising that some workplace conflict results between different generations of workers. The reason for this is that each generation may use its own value system as the measurement tool when comparing themselves to their colleagues (Clipper, 2013). Baby boomers may perceive Generation Y nurses as brash or disrespectful or feel that they come to work with a sense of entitlement. There are differing levels of formality, with the older generations preferring the use of titles and Mr. and Mrs., while the younger generations default to using first names, not only with peers, but with patients and supervisors (Krischke, 2014). Generation X workers also report higher levels of burnout as compared with baby boomers, related to incivility from colleagues and cynicism. In addition, there may also be conflicts related to competencies and strategies for knowledge acquisition.

Although this type of generational diversity poses management challenges, it also provides a variety of perspectives and outlooks that can enhance productivity and result in the generation of new ideas. While the literature often focuses on differences and negative attributes between the generations, particularly for Generations X and Y, a more balanced view is needed. Generational diversity allows patients to receive care from both the most experienced nurses as well as those with the most recent education and likely greater technology expertise.

The key is that nurse leaders must be clear on workplace expectations so that everyone understands the goals, and so that nurses can accept their colleagues' differences in work performance (Clipper, 2013). Thus, an appreciation of differences is fostered while focusing on what the team has in common—such as common goals (Krischke, 2014). In doing so, nurse leaders must foster a culture of inclusivity and encourage their staff to learn and understand the generational differences that are behind the perceptions of work ethic and performance, so that colleagues can appreciate how the attitude and expectation has been formed (Clipper, 2013). This was clearly the case in research completed by Hendricks and Cope (2013) that suggested that valuing the unique contributions of each generation promotes a richer scope of practice and increases the retention of workers (Research Study Fuels the Controversy 8.1).

THE CLAMOR FOR DIVERSITY

While the need for diversity in nursing is not new, the need to successfully address this issue has never been greater. In response, the government, professional organizations, coalitions, and other health care stakeholders have introduced initiatives/funding to address the issue and bring attention to the problem.

Research Study Fuels the Controversy 8.1

What Nurse Managers Need to Know About Generational Diversity

This literature review used the words generational diversity, nurse managers, and workforce from sources dated 2000 to 2012, to assess how personal and generational values differed related to communication, commitment, and compensation and to suggest strategies nurse managers could use to bring cohesion to a diverse workforce.

Source: Hendricks, J. M., & Cope, V. C. (2013). Generational diversity: What nurse managers need to know. *Journal of Advanced Nursing, 69*(3), 717–725. doi:10.1111/j.1365–2648.2012.06079.x

Study Findings

The literature review suggested that an acceptance of generational diversity in the workplace allows a richer scope for practice as the experiences and knowledge of each generation in the nursing environment create an environment of acceptance and harmony, facilitating retention of nurses. Acknowledgment of generational characteristics provides the nurse manager with strategies that focus on mentoring and motivation, communication, the increased use of technology, and the ethics of nursing, to bridge the gap between generations of nurses and to increase nursing workforce cohesion.

For example, the Joint Commission (2008) released a report titled *One Size Does Not Fit All: Meeting the Health Care Needs of Diverse Populations.* This report called on health care organizations to meet the unique cultural and language needs of a diverse population and provided a tool for organizations to use that promotes patient safety and health care quality for all patients. In addition, the Institute of Medicine (IOM, 2010) report *The Future of Nursing* noted that to improve the quality of patient care, more emphasis was needed to make the nursing workforce diverse, particularly in the areas of gender and race.

In 2010, the AACN (2014a) published a new set of competencies and an online faculty tool kit at the culmination of a national initiative funded by The California Endowment titled *Preparing a Culturally Competent Master's and Doctorally-Prepared Nursing Workforce.* Working with an expert advisory group, AACN identified a set of expectations for nurses completing graduate programs and created faculty resources needed to develop nursing expertise in cultural competency. This work complemented a similar project for undergraduate programs that resulted in the publication of the document *Cultural Competency in Baccalaureate Nursing Education* and the posting of an online toolkit for faculty.

In addition, in 2013, AACN and the Robert Wood Johnson Foundation (RWJF) initiated the *Doctoral Advancement in Nursing (DAN) Project* to enhance the number of minority nurses completing PhD and DNP degrees (AACN, 2014a). DAN's expert committee developed a white paper featuring successful student recruitment and retention strategies to be used by schools of nursing; comprehensive approaches to leadership and scholarship development for students; and suggestions for model doctoral curriculum. The DAN project has also created faculty and student tool kits to guide the process of gaining entry into doctoral programs.

In addition, the *American Assembly for Men in Nursing* launched a campaign known as *20 × 20* to make 20% of nursing student enrollment men by the year 2020 (Anderson, 2014). This three-phase campaign was presented at the IOM and Robert Wood Johnson Foundation Future of Nursing Summit in Washington, DC in 2010.

Even state coalitions have joined in the effort. Turk (2014), in detailing efforts in New Mexico to increase diversity in the nursing workforce, noted that the Con Alma Health Foundation received a *Partners Investing in Nursing's Future* grant from the RWJF and Northwest Health Foundation (RWJF, 2011), which allowed for development of strategies for strengthening community and organizational capacity via formation of new connections and partnerships among stakeholders invested in health care and NWD. The New Mexico Institute for Nursing Diversity, Empowerment, and Health Equity was founded as an affinity group of the New Mexico Nurses Association, and is working toward improving the leadership status of Hispanic and other minority nurses and advancing health equity for the citizens of New Mexico.

In addition, many professional nursing organizations have issued position statements or recommendations on diversity. In 1997, the AACN, the national voice for baccalaureate and higher-degree education programs, drafted a position statement that suggests that diversity and inclusion have emerged as central issues for organizations and institutions and that leadership in nursing must respond to these issues by finding ways to accelerate the inclusion of groups, cultures, and ideas that traditionally have been underrepresented in higher education. Moreover, the position statement argues that health care providers and the nursing profession should reflect and value the diversity of the populations and communities they serve.

The ANA also issued a position statement on discrimination and racism in health care in 1998 and stated its commitment to working toward the eradication of discrimination and racism in the profession of nursing, in the education of nurses, in the practice of nursing, and in the organizations in which nurses work. The *ANA Code of Ethics for Nurses* advocates diversity in its assertion that the nurse, in all professional relationships, practices with compassion and respect for the inherent dignity, worth, and uniqueness of every individual, unrestricted by considerations of social or economic status, personal attributes, or the nature of health problems.

The American Organization of Nurse Executives also developed a diversity statement in 2005. This statement suggests that the success of nursing leadership as a profession depends on reflecting the diversity of the communities it serves and that diversity is one of the essential building blocks of a healthful practice/work environment. In contrast, the International Council of Nurses does not have a diversity statement, but rather has embedded *diversity* in its policy and practice. For example, the organization promotes the principles of equal opportunity employment, pay equity, and occupational desegregation.

Conclusions

Projections suggest that current ethnic minorities are likely, in the not too distant future, to become the majority of the US population. This diversity, however, is not reflected in the nursing workforce or in schools of nursing. Similarly, men are underrepresented in nursing, and efforts to increase the number of men in the nursing profession are even fewer than those directed at increasing ethnic diversity. Finally, generational diversity is occurring in all health care organizations; however, few organizations have directly confronted the implications of how to deal with this diversity or examined the impact it has on the quality of care provided.

Diversity, equity, and parity are business imperatives but should also be moral imperatives. Using "change by drift" strategies to address the lack of ethnic and gender diversity in nursing has been ineffective. Chavez and Weisinger (2008) argue that contemporary organizations have likely spent millions of dollars on diversity training that has either failed or resulted in less-than-desired outcomes. Instead, they argued, organizations must create a "culture of diversity" that requires a longer-term relational approach that emphasizes attitudinal and cultural transformation. Thus, energy is not directed at "managing *diversity*"; instead, it is directed toward "managing *for diversity*" to capitalize on the unique perspectives of a diverse workforce. It is clear that proactive, well-thought-out strategies at multiple levels and by multiple parties will be needed before diversity in the nursing profession mirrors that of the public it serves.

For Additional Discussion

1. What are the strongest driving and restraining forces for increasing ethnic diversity in nursing, increasing gender diversity in nursing, and having a multigenerational nursing workforce?
2. Should funding for diversity initiatives come from federal or state governments, or from corporate partnerships?
3. Should the institutions that reap the benefits of a diverse workforce share the costs to make that happen?
4. Should there be different nursing school entry requirements for minority students than for their White counterparts?
5. Is an affirmative action approach needed to increase the number of both men and minorities in the nursing profession?

(continued)

6. Will having more men in nursing raise the status of the profession?
7. What are the potential barriers to having more men in the nursing profession?
8. Why have women been better able to further their numbers in medicine than men have in nursing?
9. How does the use of mentors assist in both the recruitment and the retention of minority (ethnic and gender) nurses?
10. Does a multigenerational nursing workforce improve patient care? If so, how?
11. Which health disparities do you think would be more positively impacted if the nursing workforce was more diverse?

References

American Association of Colleges of Nursing. (2014a). *Fact sheet: Enhancing diversity in the nursing workforce.* Retrieved January 25, 2015, from http://www.aacn.nche.edu/media-relations/diversityFS.pdf

American Association of Colleges of Nursing. (2014b). *Nursing shortage.* Retrieved January 30, 2015, from http://www.aacn.nche.edu/Media/FactSheets/NursingShortage.htm

American Association of Colleges of Nursing. (2015). *Johnson & Johnson/AACN Minority Nurse Faculty Scholars.* Retrieved January 30, 2015, from http://www.aacn.nche.edu/students/scholarships/minority

Anderson, D. (2014). *Man enough: The 20 × 20 choose nursing campaign.* Retrieved January 30, 2015, from Minority Nurse website: http://www.minoritynurse.com/man-enough-20-x-20-choose-nursing-campaign/

Asian American/Pacific Islander Nurses Association, Inc. (2008–2014). *About us.* Retrieved January 30, 2015, from http://www.aapina.org/about-us/

Brusie, C. (2013, September 10). *Would you trust a male nurse during your labor and delivery?* Retrieved January 30, 2015, from http://www.pregnancyandbaby.com/pregnancy-birth/articles/966941/would-you-trust-a-male-nurse-during-your-labor-and-delivery

Casselman, B. (2013, February 25). *Male nurses make more money.* The Wall Street Journal Business. Retrieved January 30, 2015, from http://blogs.wsj.com/economics/2013/02/25/male-nurses-make-more-money/

Chavez, C. I., & Weisinger, J. Y. (2008). Beyond diversity training: A social infusion for cultural inclusion. *Human Resource Management, 47*(2), 331–350.

Clipper, B. (2013). *Generational diversity: Implications for nurse staffing.* Retrieved January 31, 2015, from Advance Healthcare Network—For Nurses website: http://nursing.advanceweb.com/Features/Articles/Generational-Diversity-Implications-for-Nurse-Staffing.aspx

Clow, K. A., Ricciardelli, R., & Bartfay, W. J. (2014). Attitudes and stereotypes of male and female nurses: The influence of social roles and ambivalent sexism. *Canadian Journal of Behavioural Science/Revue Canadienne Des Sciences Du Comportement, 46*(3), 446–455.

Health Resources and Services Administration. (2015). *Nursing workforce diversity (NWD).* Retrieved January 30, 2015, from http://bhpr.hrsa.gov/nursing/grants/nwd.html

Hemp, P. (2008). *Where will we find tomorrow's leaders? A conversation with Linda A. Hill by Paul Hemp.* Harvard Business Review. Retrieved April 28, 2012, from http://hbr.org/2008/01/where-will-we-find-tomorrows-leaders/ar/1

Hendricks, J. M., & Cope, V. C. (2013). Generational diversity: What nurse managers need to know. *Journal of Advanced Nursing, 69*(3), 717–725. doi:10.1111/j.1365-2648.2012.06079.x

Institute of Medicine. (2010, October). *The future of nursing: Leading change, advancing health.* Retrieved January 31, 2015, from http://thefutureofnursing.org/IOM-Report

Jacob, S. R., & Sanchez, Z. V. (2011). The challenge of closing the diversity gap: Development of Hispanic nursing faculty through a health resources and services administration minority faculty fellowship program grant. *Journal of Professional Nursing, 27*(2), 108–113.

Johnson Rowsey, P., Kneipp, S. M., & Woods-Giscombe, C. (2013). Careers beyond the bedside: One approach to develop the ethnic minority nursing faculty pool. *Journal of Nursing Education, 52*(10), 593–596. doi:10.3928/01484834-20130924-01

Joint Commission. (2008). *Patient safety pulse: Joint commission releases report on health care and diversity*. Retrieved August 11, 2008, from https://aphid.csuchico.edu/illiad/illiad.dll?SessionID=O065311247Y&Action=10&Form=75&Value=88871

Krischke, M. M. (2014, May 6). *Generational differences in nursing: Has the work ethic changed?* Retrieved January 31, 2015, from NurseZone.com website: http://www.nursezone.com/Nursing-News-Events/more-news/Generational-Differences-in-Nursing-Has-the-Work-Ethic-Changed_42173.aspx

Marquis, B., & Huston, C. (2015). *Leadership roles and management functions in nursing* (8th ed.). Philadelphia, PA: Lippincott Williams & Wilkins.

McMurry, T. B. (2011). The image of male nurses and nursing leadership mobility. *Nursing Forum, 46*(1), 22–28.

Melillo, K. D., Dowling, J., Abdallah, L., Findeisen, M., & Knight, M. (2013). Bring diversity to nursing: Recruitment, retention, and graduation of nursing students. *Journal of Cultural Diversity, 20*(2), 100–104.

National Alaska Native American Indian Nurses Association. (n.d.). *About us*. Retrieved January 29, 2015, from http://nanainanurses.org/?page_id=124

National Association of Hispanic Nurses. (2014). *About us*. Retrieved January 30, 2015, from http://www.nahnnet.org/AboutNAHN.html

National Black Nurses Association. (2014). *About NBA*. Retrieved January 31, 2015, from http://www.nbna.org/about

Philippine Nurses Association Inc. (2015). *About PNA*. Retrieved January 29, 2015, from http://www.pna-ph.org/about_life.asp

Phillips, J. M., & Malone, B. (2014). Increasing racial/ethnic diversity in nursing to reduce health disparities and achieve health equity. *Public Health Reports, 129*(2), 45–50.

Robert Wood Johnson Foundation. (2011). *Partners Investing in Nursing's Future. Retrieved September 19, 2015, from http://www.rwjf.org/en/library/programs-and-initiatives/P/partners-investing-in-nursing-s-future.html*

Rural Assistance Center. (2002–2015). *Nursing workforce diversity grants*. Retrieved January 30, 2015, from http://www.raconline.org/funding/246

Sagon, C. (2013, March 13). *More men choose nursing—And earn more than women*. AARP Health Talk. Retrieved January 30, 2015, from http://blog.aarp.org/2013/03/12/more-men-choose-nursing-and-earn-more-than-women/

Sedgwick, M., Oosterbroek, T., & Ponomar, V. (2014). "It all depends": How minority nursing students experience belonging during clinical experiences. *Nursing Education Perspectives, 35*(2), 89–93. doi:10.5480/11-707.1

Selvam, A. (2013, May 18). *Making progress: Sustained efforts to increase minority representation in healthcare executive ranks are delivering results, but barriers still remain*. Modern Healthcare. Retrieved January 30, 2015, from http://www.modernhealthcare.com/article/20130518/MAGAZINE/305189958

Turk, L. (2014). Issue: Nursing workforce diversity. *New Mexico Nurse, 59*(2), 8–11.

U.S. Census Bureau. (2013). *State and county quick facts*. Retrieved January 24, 2015, from http://quickfacts.census.gov/qfd/states/00000.html

Wallen, A. S., Mor, S., & Devine, B. A. (2014). It's about respect: Gender-professional identify integration affects male nurses' job attitudes. *Psychology of Men & Masculinity, 15*(3), 305–312.

Wolfenden, J. (2011). Men in nursing. *Internet Journal of Allied Health Sciences & Practice, 9*(2). Retrieved April 29, 2012, from http://ijahsp.nova.edu/articles/Vol9Num2/pdf/Wolfenden.pdf

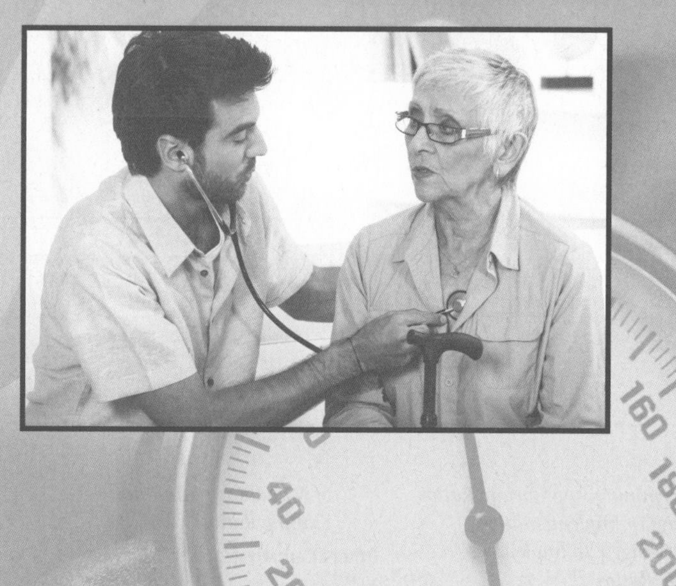

3

Workplace Issues

Mandatory Minimum Staffing Ratios
Are They Needed?

9

Carol J. Huston

ADDITIONAL RESOURCES

Visit thePoint for additional helpful resources

- eBook
- Journal Articles
- WebLinks

CHAPTER OUTLINE

LEARNING OBJECTIVES

The learner will be able to:

1. Explore factors driving legislative mandates for minimum registered nurse (RN) representation in the staffing mix.
2. Summarize current research findings regarding the effect of staffing ratios and staffing mix on patient outcomes.
3. Debate driving and restraining forces for legislating minimum licensed staffing ratios.
4. Assess the efficiency and effectiveness of the processes used by the state of California Department of Health Services to determine initial minimum RN–patient staffing ratios for different types of hospital units.
5. Describe challenges to staffing ratio implementation in California, including the need to define "licensed nurses," legal challenges to the "at all times clause," and strategies directed at delaying or rescinding the mandate altogether.
6. Investigate the movement and/or progress of states other than California to adopt minimum RN staffing ratios.
7. Discuss the effect of the current nursing shortage on the likelihood of successful passage of proposed staffing ratio legislation in states other than California.
8. Argue for or against the appropriateness of the "at all times clause" as part of California's staffing ratio mandate.
9. Assess whether California's 2004 implementation of mandatory minimum RN staffing ratios has met its goals.

(continues on page 125)

10. Identify alternatives to staffing ratio mandates that seek to ensure that staffing resources are adequate to provide safe patient care.
11. Reflect on the staffing ratios used in his or her work setting and assess, using clearly defined criteria, whether they are adequate to provide quality patient care.

INTRODUCTION

For some time now, economics has been the primary driver in dictating changes in the registered nurse (RN) skill mix in hospitals. As a result, the trend early in the first decade of the 21st century was to reduce RNs in the staffing mix and to replace them with less expensive personnel. Empirical research increasingly concludes, however, that the number of RNs in the staffing mix has a direct effect on quality care and, in particular, patient outcomes. In response, legislators, health care providers, and the public are increasingly demanding adequate staffing ratios of RNs in health care settings.

It is noteworthy that the US federal government has established minimum standards for licensed nursing in certified nursing homes but not in acute care hospitals. Several attempts have been made in Congress in the past decade to enact hospital nurse staffing laws; however, none have come close to fruition. Section 42 of the Code of Federal Regulations (42CFR 482.23[b]) does require Medicare-certified hospitals to "have adequate numbers of licensed RNs, licensed practical (vocational) nurses, and other personnel to provide nursing care to all patients as needed"; however, this "nebulous language and failure of Congress to enact a quality nursing care staffing act to date, has left it to the states to ensure that staffing is appropriate to patients' needs" (American Nurses Association [ANA], 2015, para. 3).

As a result, a national (indeed international) movement to examine the need for minimum staffing ratios has begun. Many states in the United States, with the backing of some nursing organizations, have moved toward imposing mandatory licensed staffing requirements, and one state (California) enacted legislation requiring mandatory staffing ratios that affect hospitals and long-term care facilities. In fact, as of 2015, 13 states addressed nurse staffing in hospitals in law/regulations (California, Connecticut, Illinois, Maine, Nevada, New Jersey, New York, Ohio, Oregon, Rhode Island, Texas, Vermont, and Washington) (ANA, 2015). Many of the states that have adopted legislation about staffing originally sought staffing ratio legislation. Seven states (Connecticut, Illinois, Nevada, Ohio, Oregon, Texas, and Washington) now require hospitals to have staffing committees responsible for plans and staffing policy (ANA, 2015).

California is the only state that stipulates in law, regulations for required minimum nurse-to-patient ratios to be maintained at all times by unit. In addition, Massachusetts recently passed a law specific to intensive care units requiring a 1:1 or 1:2 nurse-to-patient ratio, depending on stability of the patient, and Minnesota now requires a Chief Nursing Officer or designee to develop a core staffing plan with input from others (ANA, 2015).

This chapter explores both the driving and the restraining forces for legislatively mandated minimum RN representation in the staffing mix. California's experience, as the first and only state to implement minimum staffing ratios, is detailed, as well as its struggle to define appropriate ratios and implement staffing ratios in an era of limited fiscal and human resources. The chapter concludes by looking at the movement of other states toward the adoption of minimum staffing ratios and strategies that have been suggested as alternatives to mandatory staffing ratios.

Consider This Identifying and maintaining the appropriate number and mix of nursing staff is critical to the delivery of quality patient care (ANA, 2015).

STAFFING RATIOS AND PATIENT OUTCOMES

Linda Aiken, "undoubtedly the most influential researcher in nurse staffing, not only in the United States, but globally," suggests that while most research "has little impact on actual practice, that 20 years of research on the impact of nurse staffing on patient outcomes has made a big difference in the outcomes of patients and nurses, and managerial and clinical practice" (Kerfoot & Douglas, 2013, p. 216). Indeed, hundreds, if not thousands, of studies in the last decade have examined the link between staffing mix and patient outcomes. Many of the studies note a link between the increased representation of RNs in the staffing mix and improved patient outcomes.

Consider This There is wide variation in the skill mix (percentage of licensed to unlicensed workers) and RN-to-patient ratios across the United States.

Few studies, however, have had as much effect on determining safe staffing ratios as two benchmark research studies published in 2002. The first study was the work of Needleman, Buerhaus, Mattke, Stewart, and Zelevinsky (2002). This study of 799 hospitals in 11 states found a higher prevalence of infections, such as pneumonia and urinary tract infections, failure to rescue, and shock or cardiac arrest when the nurses' workload was high.

The second study, which is often cited as the seminal work in support of establishing minimum staffing ratio legislation at the federal or state level, was completed by Aiken, Clarke, Sloane, Sochalski, and Silber (2002). This study of more than 10,000 nurses and 230,000 patients in 168 hospitals concluded that in hospitals with higher patient-to-nurse ratios, surgical patients had a greater likelihood of dying within 30 days of admission. In addition, they experienced increased odds of failure to rescue (mortality following complications). This occurred because the time nurses have for surveillance, early detection, and timely intervention—particularly with patients who are not at high risk but who are vulnerable to other unfavorable outcomes—has a direct effect on patient outcomes.

In addition, the study found that staffing at 6 patients per nurse rather than 4 would result in an additional 2.3 deaths per 1,000 patients and an additional 8.7 deaths per 1,000 patients with complications. Staffing at 8 patients per nurse rather than 6 would incur an additional 2.6 deaths per 1,000 patients and 9.5 deaths per 1,000 patients with complications. Uniformly staffing at 8 patients per nurse rather than 4 was expected to entail 5 excess deaths per 1,000 patients and 18.2 complications per 1,000 patients. In addition, patients had a 31% higher chance of dying within 30 days of admission (Aiken et al., 2002).

Consider This There is compelling evidence to suggest that increasing the number of RNs in the staffing mix leads to safer workplaces for nurses and a higher quality of care for patients.

Within days of the study's release, Aiken's study results were summarized, repeated, and analyzed in detail in almost all relevant public forums and by most professional health care organizations. The message was clear: There was a direct link between nurse-to-patient ratios and mortality rates from preventable complications, and having an inadequate number of RNs places the public at risk.

Discussion Point

Why did the study by Aiken et al. (2002) garner so much national attention in so many public forums? Were the findings significantly different than those of earlier studies? Was it timing? Was it how "the message" was managed?

Over the past 15 years, research sophistication regarding how best to study the relationship between staffing and patient outcomes has increased dramatically. Still, there are issues related to how outcomes are defined, what operational definitions should be used, and who should be counted in nurse staffing. Perhaps that is why more recent research has raised questions about whether RN staffing levels truly do have an impact on patient outcomes. Summaries of select research studies completed in 2013–2014 are shown in Table 9.1. This has made the determination of the optimal nurse-to-patient ratio an ongoing challenge.

ARE MANDATORY MINIMUM STAFFING RATIOS NEEDED?

One proposed solution to Aiken's research findings was the implementation of minimum mandatory RN–patient staffing ratios in acute care hospitals. Numerous articles have appeared in the media attesting to grossly inadequate staffing in hospitals and nursing homes, and professional nursing organizations, such as the ANA, continue to express concern about the effect poor staffing has both on nurses' health and safety and on patient outcomes.

Proponents of mandated minimum staffing ratios argue that minimum staffing ratios are absolutely essential to ensuring that staffing is adequate to promote patient safety and to achieving desired patient outcomes. They also suggest that the use of standardized ratios provides a more consistent approach than acuity-based staffing.

Consider This The bottom line is that minimum staffing ratios would not have been proposed if staffing abuses and the resultant decline in the quality of patient care had not occurred in the past.

Critics, however, suggest that the overall cost of care would increase exponentially if mandatory ratios were imposed nationally and that no guarantee of quality

TABLE 9.1 Selected Recent Research on Nurse Staffing Levels and Patient Clinical Outcomes (2013 to 2014)

Citation	Description
Clark, Saade, Meyers, Frye, and Perlin (2014)	This retrospective analysis of perinatal outcomes in 208,033 women receiving oxytocin for induction or augmentation of labor during 2010 found there was no relation between the frequency of 1:1 nurse-to-patient staffing ratio and improved perinatal outcomes.
Stamp, Flanagan, Gregas, & Shindul-Rothschild (2014)	In this study of California, Massachusetts, and New York hospitals, 6 factors predicted 27.6% of readmissions for patients with heart failure (HF). HF readmissions were lower when nurse staffing was greater and more patients reported receiving discharge information, and among hospitals in California where mandated staffing ratios are in place.
Everhart et al. (2014)	This 54-month (July 2006 to December 2010) longitudinal study of US acute care general hospitals participating in the National Database for Nursing Quality Indicators found that hospitals with higher total nurse staffing and bed size greater than 300 beds were significantly less likely to be categorized in the "consistently high" fall rate group.
Sung-Heui, Kelly, Brewer, & Spencer (2014)	This research using negative binomial regression modeling with hospital- and time-fixed effects from 35 units in 3 hospitals found that rates of patient falls and injury falls were greater with higher temporary registered nurse staffing levels but decreased with greater levels of licensed practical nursing care hours per patient day. Pressure ulcers were not related to any staffing characteristics.
West et al. (2014)	This cross-sectional, retrospective, risk-adjusted observational study, using a merged data set with information on 65 ICUs and 38,168 patients, tested the relationship between staffing and outcomes in UK ICUs. After controlling for patient characteristics and workload, researchers found that higher numbers of nurses per bed were associated with higher survival rates. Further exploration revealed that the number of nurses had the greatest impact on patients at high risk of death.
Spetz, Harless, Herrera, & Mark (2013)	This multivariate analysis of nurse staffing and patient outcomes suggested that significant improvements in patient mortality following a medical or surgical complication occurred when RN staffing was increased. Additional data showed a decrease in pulmonary embolism, deep vein thrombosis, sepsis, and shorter lengths of stay.
Frost & Alexandrou (2013)	This study of elective cardiac patients found that cardiac readmissions declined when nurse staffing levels increased. In addition, inpatient hospital mortality decreased.
Shekelle (2013)	This study suggested that the differences in nurse-to-patient staffing ratios (4:1 vs. 8:1) may have been a factor in the deaths of 4,535 surgical patients (2% of the surgical patient admissions) who died within 30 days of discharge.
Tubbs-Cooley, Cimiotti, Silber, Sloane, & Aiken (2013)	This observational cross-sectional study of readmissions of children in 225 hospitals found that for every one patient increase in a hospital's average pediatric staffing ratio, a medical child's odds of readmission within 15 to 30 days increased by a factor of 1.11, or by 11% (95% CI 1.02 to 1.20) and a surgical child's likelihood of readmission within 15 to 30 days by a factor of 1.48, or by 48% (95% CI 1.27 to 1.73). Children treated in hospitals with pediatric staffing ratios of 1:4 or less were significantly less likely to be readmitted within 15 to 30 days.

improvement or positive outcomes exists with such ratios. In fact, evidence regarding the benefits of staffing ratios is mixed and sometimes contradictory. Mandatory ratios also ignore the education, experience, and skill level of the individual nurse. In addition, there is a risk that staffing may actually decline with ratios because they might be used as the ceiling or as ironclad criteria if institutions are unwilling to make adjustments for patient acuity or RN skill level.

Aiken concurs, suggesting that "It's the legislative mandate aspect that is controversial—not so much the actual focus on safe staffing, or the required staffing levels. Americans tend not to like legislative mandates" (Kerfoot & Douglas, 2013, p. 217).

It is cost, though, that is likely most often cited as a deterrent for implementing minimum staffing ratios. Bobay, Yakusheva, and Weiss (2011) suggested that although increasing RN staffing would likely reduce postdischarge readmissions or emergency department visits, this alternative is not financially attractive to hospitals. Goryakin, Griffiths, and Maben (2011) agree, suggesting that although more intensive nurse staffing is likely associated with better outcomes, it is also more expensive and, therefore, cost effectiveness is not easy to assess. However, in their review of staffing-ratio costs, Goryakin et al. concluded that hiring more RNs, as would be expected under a federal mandatory staffing policy, would likely not create undue financial burdens in the long-term for most urban hospitals. They cautioned, however, that this might not be the case in rural hospitals, and they thus suggested that mandatory staffing policy is better left to the states than to the federal government.

Some researchers, however, have found that increasing RN staffing could have significant cost implications. For example, Clark et al. (2014), in examining the relationship between nurse-to-patient staffing ratios and perinatal outcomes in women receiving oxytocin during labor, noted that adoption of universal 1:1 staffing for this patient population in the United States would result in the need for an additional 27,000 labor nurses at a cost of $1.6 billion. They suggest this cost cannot be justified given the lack of evidence in their research regarding the relationship between nurse-to-patient staffing ratio and improved perinatal outcomes.

Still others argue that it is health care professionals—not legislators or regulators—who understand health care and are best qualified to determine staffing needs, particularly when best practices in staffing are used (Box 9.1). This might be the case, but given that hospitals are no longer exempt from "big business," profit-driven motives, one must question whether what is best for patients can be separated from what is best financially for the institution. Wallace (2013) argues, then, that staffing must always take into account educational preparation, experience, and professional needs, and nurse managers must always evaluate competency levels and critical thinking skills as a basis for staffing to create a safe patient care environment.

CALIFORNIA AS THE PROTOTYPE FOR MANDATORY MINIMUM STAFFING RATIOS

Passing the Legislation

California has had a minimum ratio of licensed nurse-to-patient requirement (Title 22 of the California Code of Regulations) for intensive care and coronary care units for more than three decades; however, no minimums were initially established for other types of acute care units. Given increasing pressure from nursing unions in the state, increasing bad press about poor-quality care, the increased use of unlicensed assistive personnel as direct care providers, and skyrocketing patient loads for licensed nurses in acute care, California stepped forward as the first state in the nation to implement mandatory minimum staffing ratios.

Under Assembly Bill (A.B.) 394 ("Safe Staffing Law"), passed in 1999 and crafted by the California Nurses Association (CNA), all hospitals in California were to comply with the minimum staffing ratios shown in Table 9.2 by January 1, 2004. These ratios, developed by the California Department of Health Services (CDHS) with assistance from the University of California, Davis, represented the maximum number of patients an RN could be assigned to care for, under any circumstance. In addition, this legislation prohibited unlicensed personnel from performing certain procedures such as administering medication, performing venipuncture, providing parenteral or tube feedings, inserting nasogastric tubes, inserting catheters, performing tracheal suctioning, assessing patient conditions, providing patient education, and performing moderately complex laboratory tests.

BOX 9.1 Best Practices for Determining Nurse Staffing Ratios

1. Develop strategies to use when staffing levels are not adequate.
2. Create an internal resource pool for flexibility and census adjustments.
3. Communicate all action plans to staff nurses and administrative stakeholders.
4. Empower staff nurses to identify solutions for staffing decisions and budget.
5. Benchmark staffing ratios annually with other facilities.
6. Correlate staffing with patient outcomes, adverse events, and root causes.
7. Evaluate patient satisfaction feedback.

Source: Nurse staffing ratios. (2013). *AORN Journal, 97*(5), 604–538. doi:10.1016/j.aorn.2013.02.011

TABLE 9.2 Minimum RN Staffing Ratios for Hospitals in California in 2004 and New National Nurses United (NNU) Recommendations for 2015

Unit	Minimum RN–Patient Ratio Required in California in 2004 as a Result of AB 394	Minimum RN–Patient Ratio Recommended by NNU in 2015
Critical care/ICU	1:2	1:2
Neonatal ICU	1:2	1:2
Operating room	1:1	1:1 (plus at least one additional scrub assistant)
Postanesthesia		1:2
Labor and delivery	1:2	1:2
Antepartum	1:4	1:3
Postpartum couplets	1:4	
Combined labor and delivery and postpartum		1:3
Postpartum women only	1:6	1:3
Intermediate-care nursery		1:4
Pediatrics	1:4	1:3
Emergency room (ER)	1:4	1:3
Trauma patient in ER		1:1
ICU patient in ER		1:2
Step-down	1:4 initially; 1:3 as of 2008	1:3
Telemetry		1:3
Medical–surgical	1:6 initially; 1:5 as of 2005	1:4
Oncology	1:5 initially; 1:4 as of 2008	
Coronary care		1:2
Acute respiratory care		1:2
Burn unit		1:2
Other specialty care units		1:4
Psychiatry	1:6	1:4
Rehabilitation		1:5
Skilled nursing facility		1:5

Source: National Nurses United. (2010–2015). *National campaign for safe RN-to-patient staffing ratios.* Retrieved February 1, 2015, from http://www.nationalnursesunited.org/issues/entry/ratios

Determining Appropriate Ratios

Developing draft regulations for minimum staffing ratios was challenging for the CDHS because data were not readily accessible regarding the distribution of nurse staffing in California hospitals, the number of hospitals likely to be affected by the minimum staffing requirements, or the expected costs of this legislation. In addition, the ratios were meant to supplement valid and reliable patient classification systems (PCS), which had been required in California hospitals since 1996. The problem was that although California hospitals had been required to submit their PCS data to the state, there was no standardization and little guidance about what characterized a valid PCS or what criteria should be used in determining the PCS. Therefore, PCS data yielded little, if any, helpful information to the CDHS for determining appropriate ratios.

Discussion Point

The California Healthcare Association advocated the use of PCS as the gold standard for staffing decisions rather than staffing ratios. The CNA argued for the reverse. What motives may have driven these positions?

Cost was also not known. Initial projections by the Public Policy Institute of California suggested that many hospitals in California would experience sharp increases in cost associated with the increase in numbers of licensed staff. At least in part as a result of limited empirical data, proposals received by CDHS suggested a wide range of minimum staffing ratios and even more widely differing estimates of cost. The California Hospital Association (CHA), a hospital trade group representing the interests of nearly 500 hospital and health system members in California at that time, called for a minimum staffing ratio of 1 nurse to 10 patients on medical–surgical units, whereas the unions representing the largest numbers of nurses in the state argued for minimum ratios in medical–surgical units of 1:4. The CNA recommended a 1:3 ratio in medical–surgical units.

Following months of waiting and almost 2 years of wrangling, the final minimum staffing ratios were announced in January 2002 (see Table 9.2). Governor Gray Davis, in a press conference at St. Vincent's Medical Center in Los Angeles, announced that his administration supported a ratio of 1 nurse to every 6 patients in medical–surgical units—twice the number of patients supported by the CNA and 4 fewer than that favored by the CHA. Regulations were released later that spring with 45 days allocated for public comment. Hospitals in California were also required to continue to keep a PCS in place and to staff according to the PCS if it called for a larger number of nurses than the minimum ratios set by the CDHS.

Delays in Implementation

Implementing the ratio legislation proved to be just as difficult as determining what the ratios should be. The first challenge that arose was interpreting the meaning and intent of the legislation's language in regard to what constituted "licensed nurses." Almost immediately, questions were raised about whether the minimum mandatory ratios had to reflect RN representation in the staffing mix or whether licensed vocational/practical nurses (LVNs/LPNs) would meet the requirement.

The CNA argued that the intent of the law was to regulate minimum RN staffing, which inflamed the labor unions representing LVNs. Amid much controversy, the issues were aired at a public hearing before the Department of Health Services in San Francisco, and a determination was provided that the ratios referred to RNs only and that LVNs/LPNs would be authorized to practice only under the direction of licensed RN or physician.

Questions were then raised as to whether hospitals could eliminate or reduce their nonlicensed staff in an effort to save costs, given that the number of RNs would be increased. The CNA argued that the ratios were based on CDHS surveys of existing hospital staffing patterns and that nonlicensed staff should not be cut if safe patient care was to be assured. The state, however, chose not to weigh in, arguing that its position was to regulate minimum RN–patient ratios; as a result, many hospitals immediately began reducing the number of support personnel to offset the increased cost of RN staff, and many RNs were forced to assume nonnursing care tasks.

Finally, the CHA, with the help of State Senator Sam Aanestad, introduced new legislation (A.B. 847) to the California State Senate Health and Human Services committee in April 2003 in an attempt to delay implementation of the 1:5 minimum nurse–patient staffing ratio on medical–surgical units until it could be ascertained that adequate RNs were available to meet the ratios. Opponents of the delay argued that this was simply an effort to preclude implementation of the mandate altogether. The bill failed.

Then the hospitals persuaded Governor Arnold Schwarzenegger to issue an emergency regulation in November 2004 to overturn emergency room ratios and the improved medical–surgical ratios, citing financial crises (Cortez, 2008). In response, the CNA and the National Nurses Organizing Committee (NNOC) launched more than 100 protests against Schwarzenegger, which resulted in a massive grassroots movement and the stinging defeat of four Schwarzenegger-ballot initiatives in a 2005 special election (Cortez, 2008). The emergency regulation was ruled illegal in March 2005 by a state superior court judge and overturned. The judge argued that the financial state of hospitals did not give the state the right to delay implementing the law because the law's intent was to improve patient safety. Hospitals were told to comply immediately.

Still, resistance to staffing ratio implementation continued. Hospitals were accused of encouraging management staff to undermine and avoid compliance with the new RN staffing ratios. Nursing unions responded with threats to close down units with inadequate staffing, to delay elective surgeries, and to wage a public relations campaign to garner public support for the nurses.

The Struggle to Implement the Ratios

Despite these efforts and a pervasive, ongoing resistance to staffing ratio implementation, the staffing ratio mandate did become effective on January 1, 2004. But were hospitals ready and willing to implement these changes? By and large, bigger hospitals in the state were ready to meet the mandate by the time of its implementation. Many smaller hospitals, however, had existing budget deficits and had to seek waivers from the CDHS because of their difficulty in meeting ratios. Waivers were allowed; however, hospitals had to be rural and meet very strict conditions.

Discussion Point

Should small rural hospitals be given waivers for the mandatory staffing ratios? Is this justified by the patient population characteristics, or is it simply an economic incentive to keep these hospitals viable?

The dire predictions about reductions in hospital services increased emergency room diversions, and hospitals in California having to close doors if mandatory staffing ratio legislation passed, never materialized. In fact, most hospitals in California did not have to hire more contracted RNs to comply with the ratios. Nor was there a decrease in skill mix as a result. In fact, nurses from all over the country moved to California for jobs when the staffing ratios legislation passed.

Aiken agrees, noting that the adverse, unintended consequences of mandatory nurse staffing levels, feared before the implementation of mandated staffing ratios, never materialized (Kerfoot & Douglas, 2013). Instead, a large proportion of hospitals continued to have more nurses than required, most nurses reported that their workloads decreased, and when more agency nurses were used, there did not appear to be any negative impacts on quality of care (Kerfoot & Douglas, 2013).

The "At All Times" Clause

Almost immediately after implementation of A.B. 394, legal clarification did become necessary regarding interpretation of the law with regard to ratio coverage "at all times." A ruling by the CDHS blindsided many hospitals in its strict interpretation that ratios had to be maintained at all times, including breaks and lunches. For many hospitals, this meant hiring additional rotating staff to fill in for nurses when they leave the bedside for short periods (breaks, lunch, transporting patients, etc.) or face being noncompliant.

As a result, the CHA filed a lawsuit on December 30, 2003, challenging the ruling and arguing that the "at all times" ruling was impossible to implement. The motion was heard in a Sacramento court on May 14, 2004. In a 10-page ruling issued on May 26, 2004, the judge dismissed the hospital association lawsuit, saying that not adhering to the "at all times" clause would make the nurse-to-patient ratios meaningless. Again, the ruling was an effort to maintain the intent of the law—to protect patients.

Discussion Point

Is an "at all times" ruling necessary to ensure quality health care?

Have RN Staffing and Patient Outcomes Improved in California as a Result of Mandatory Minimum Staffing Ratios?

As of January 1, 2008, California's historic staffing law for RN staffing ratios completed its phase-in period, and almost a decade of data now exist regarding compliance with the staffing ratios, as well as changes in patient outcomes. A synthesis by Donaldson and Shapiro (2010) of 12 studies examining the impact of California's ratios on patient care cost, quality, and outcomes in acute care hospitals revealed that the implementation of minimum nurse-to-patient ratios did reduce the number of patients per licensed nurse and increase the number of worked nursing hours per patient day in hospitals. There were, however, no significant impacts of these improved staffing measures on measures of nursing quality and patient safety indicators across hospitals. Donaldson and Shapiro emphasized, however, that adverse outcomes did not increase despite the increasing patient severity reflected in case mix index and cautiously posited that this finding might actually suggest an impact of ratios in preventing adverse events in the presence of increased patient risk.

In addition, Aiken (2010) and the Center for Health Outcomes and Policy Research at the University of Pennsylvania conducted an independent evaluation of California's mandated nurse staffing requirements. This survey of more than 22,000 RNs, working in 604 hospitals in California and two comparison states without legislation—Pennsylvania and New Jersey—found that overall, nurses in California cared for an average of one patient fewer than nurses in the two comparison states. On medical and surgical units, California hospital nurses each took care of two fewer patients. In terms of patient outcomes, Aiken studied more than 1 million patients who had common surgical procedures in these hospitals in 2006, more than 2 years after mandatory nurse staffing was implemented. She found that California hospitals had significantly lower risk-adjusted mortality and were better at rescuing patients who experienced complications than the comparison states, even after taking into account factors other than differences in nurse staffing.

Similarly, a literature review conducted by Serratt (2013b) suggested mixed results, with three studies finding both positive and negative outcomes and five studies reporting no significant changes in patient outcomes (Research, Fuels the Controversy 9.1). Serratt concluded that some improvements resulted from the implementation of staffing ratios, but the positives were not as significant and widespread as predicted. Another study reported by Serratt (2013a) found an increase in labor costs and some reduction in services with ratio implementation, suggesting a negative financial impact on selected outcomes of California hospitals.

In addition, Munnich (2014) reported that little evidence exists to support the idea that this law was effective in attracting more nurses to the hospital workforce or improving patient outcomes, although nurse-to-patient ratios in medical–surgical units increased substantially following the staffing mandate. Survey data from two nationally representative datasets indicate that the law had no effect on the aggregate number of RNs or the hours they worked in California hospitals, and at most a modest effect on wages. Munnich cautioned that California's experience with minimum nurse staffing legislation may not be generalizable to states considering similar policies in very different hospital markets.

Another literature review by Mark, Harless, Spetz, Reiter, and Pink (2013) also noted mixed results in terms of whether mandatory ratios in California improved patient quality. Although the Agency for Healthcare Research and Quality (AHRQ) reported that its patient safety indicators showed a significant reduction in patient falls, pressure ulcers, and restraint use, conflicting data by California hospitals, Mark et al. found no significant differences to support AHRQ's findings.

Yet, Tellez and Seago (2013) note that nurse satisfaction and nurse retention rates did rise after passage of the California staffing law. The significance is that as the nursing workforce ages and retires; there will be a shortage of experienced nurses to care for the increasing demand for health care put forward by the Affordable Care Act. These facts place pressure on the health care system to care for more patients with fewer nurses. California's staffing legislation is serving to counter mounting pressure.

The answer as to whether mandated ratios have improved care or created new cost burdens for California is still unclear. The CNA says the ratios have improved nurse retention, raised the numbers of qualified nurses willing to work, reduced burnout, and improved morale. Aiken agrees, suggesting that there is very good scientific evidence that staffing improved even in safety-net hospitals that had long had poor staffing (Kerfoot & Douglas, 2013). Aiken also notes that prior to the California

Research Study Fuels the Controversy 9.1

This literature review examined eight studies that examined the impact nurse-to-patient ratios have on the quality and safety of care and patient satisfaction.

Source: Serratt, T. (2013b). California's Nurse-to-Patient Ratios, Part 3. *Journal of Nursing Administration, 43*(11), 581–585.

Study Findings

The findings from the majority of these studies did not support the assumption that increases in nurse staffing would lead to better quality of care, improvements in patient safety, or increased patient satisfaction. However, the number of studies examining these measures was limited, and the outcome measures differed widely, with only four studies utilizing similar measures. The researchers concluded that given these limitations and evidence from earlier studies that found lower nurse staffing levels were associated with higher rates of adverse outcomes, it would be premature to conclude that nurse-to-patient ratios did not improve patient quality, safety, and/or satisfaction. Further studies exploring the relationship between nurse-to-patient ratios and patient outcomes are needed to determine the benefits of this type of staffing regulation on patient-level outcomes.

BOX 9.2 Three General Approaches Recommended by the ANA (2015) to Maintain Sufficient Staffing

1. The formation of nurse-driven staffing committees to create staffing plans that reflect the needs of the patient population and match the skills and experience of the staff.
2. Legislators mandate specific nurse-to-patient ratios in legislation or regulation.
3. Facilities are required to disclose staffing levels to the public and/or a regulatory body.

staffing legislation, all of the blue ribbon committees that looked at safe nurse staffing shied away from establishing specific patient-to-nurse ratios. Thus, communicating with stakeholders and the media was difficult without "a recommended number." "The evidence-based benchmark implemented in California of no more than five patients per nurse on medical and surgical units has become 'the number' against which to evaluate hospital staffing" (Kerfoot & Douglas, 2013, p. 217).

Consider This The answer as to whether mandated ratios have improved care or created new cost burdens for California is still unclear.

OTHER ALTERNATIVES

Efforts are also under way, in both California and the rest of the nation, to explore alternatives to improving nurse staffing that do not require legislated minimum staffing ratios. The reality is that many leading health care and professional nursing organizations do not support the need for legislated minimum staffing ratios. For example, the Joint Commission, one of the most powerful accrediting bodies for hospitals in the United States, has been reluctant to endorse nationally mandated minimum staffing ratios, suggesting that this would not be flexible enough to encompass the diversity represented in hospitals across the United States.

In addition, the ANA does not support fixed nurse–patient ratios. Instead, it advocates a workload system that takes into account the many variables that exist to ensure safe staffing. Instead of staffing ratios, the ANA (2015) has recommended three general approaches to assure sufficient nurse staffing at the state level (Box 9.2). The ANA argues that this type of approach better accommodates changes in patients' needs, available technology, and the preparation and experience of staff. In addition, the ANA argues that what may be established through legislation today as an appropriate minimum nurse-to-patient ratio may be obsolete by the next shift or 2 years from now and that disclosure of staffing plans without evaluation and recourse for inadequate levels are futile.

Aiken also suggests that she is not necessarily an advocate of legislative mandates (Kerfoot & Douglas, 2013). Instead, she argues that there are multiple ways to achieve the objectives that have been achieved in California. She continues to support publicly reported nurse staffing and urges nurses to do the same so that greater transparency regarding hospital staffing can occur. She concludes that "even folks who are not in favor of legislative mandates should open their minds to the evidence that the California legislation did work as intended" and that "it is a mistake for nurses to reject evidence if not to their liking for some reason (Kerfoot & Douglas, 2013, p. 217).

Buchan (2014) agrees, suggesting that research regarding mandated staffing ratios is a "scientific exercise hampered by inadequate research, limited data, disagreement on definitions in differences between organization and health system norms" (para. 1). Indeed, he argues that while proponents may have the best intentions, insufficient quality outcome evidence exists to support the imposition of mandated nurse staffing ratios. Still, he notes that in areas where there are so few nurses that patient care is unsafe, ratios do provide some type of bulwark against further erosion of staffing levels. Ratios then appear to make sense only where management and resources are most inadequate.

Conclusions

The literature suggests that increasing RN representation in the staffing mix improves at least some patient outcomes. What is less clear is what the optimal staffing levels are for various patient populations and when costs associated with staffing mix become unreasonable in terms of attempting to improve patient outcomes. In addition, given the lessons that have already been learned with the "RN/LVN debate" and the "at all times" requirement, more thought must be given to how strictly staffing ratio regulations are to be interpreted and how enforcement can be effective when there are no monetary consequences for breaking rules. In addition, the intermingling roles of state government as a legislator of minimum staffing ratios, compliance officer, disciplinary enforcer, and potential funding source to assist with mandated ratio implementation need further examination and clarification.

Finally, it must be recognized that patient acuity is continuing to rise, and the mandatory minimum staffing ratios adopted in California in 2003 were arguably inadequate just 5 years later, especially when hospitals refused to staff above the ratios when census and acuity call for it (Cortez, 2008). In fact, the CNA and the NNOC proposed even lower ratios as part of the CNA/NNOC's Hospital Patient Protection Act in 2008 and New National Nurses United (NNU) has advocated even lower ratios for 2015 (NNU, 2015) (see Table 9.2). These ratios would pose even greater fiscal and human resource challenges to California hospitals in terms of their implementation.

The implementation and subsequent evaluation of mandatory staffing ratios in California should, however, provide some insight into these ongoing issues that will be helpful to other states that choose to follow in California's footsteps. Clearly, the enactment of California's nurse-to-patient ratio law was far from smooth, and concerns continue about the costs of hiring additional licensed staff, and the need to meet the "at all times" clause.

It is not clear yet whether California has the resources (both human and fiscal) it would need to lower the staffing ratios further. Some of the initial implementation struggles may have been related to the normal issues that arise whenever a new law takes effect; however, the reality is that California has struggled to implement the mandate. The fact that it took 5 years from passage of the legislation to mandated implementation is telling. What is even more telling are the number of hospitals in California that continue to report difficulty in meeting staffing ratio requirements and the pervasive resistance that continues to be a part of its implementation.

For Additional Discussion

1. Given rising patient acuity levels and increased scope of responsibility for RNs, at what point should California reexamine the adequacy of current staffing ratios?
2. In an effort to cut the costs associated with implementing minimum RN staffing ratios, some hospitals eliminated their support staff. Have RNs gained anything when this is the case?
3. Should LVNs be counted to meet minimum mandatory staffing ratio requirements?
4. Is allowing hospitals to determine their staffing needs a little like having the "fox guard the chicken coop"?
5. Does the implementation of mandatory staffing ratios in the midst of a severe national nursing shortage make sense? Why or why not?
6. At what point does cost related to staffing mix become so prohibitive that society will be willing to accept some increase in patient morbidity and mortality?
7. What critical lessons should other states learn from California's experience thus far in implementing mandatory staffing ratios?

References

Aiken, L. (2010). Safety in numbers. *Nursing Standard, 24*(44), 62–63.

Aiken, L. H., Clarke, S. P., Sloane, D., Sochalski, J., & Silber, J. (2002). Effects of nurse-staffing on nurse burnout and job-dissatisfaction and patient deaths. *The Journal of the American Medical Association, 288*, 1987–1993.

American Nurses Association. (2015, February 1). *Nurse staffing plans & ratios*. Retrieved from http://www.nursingworld.org/MainMenuCategories/

Policy-Advocacy/State/Legislative-Agenda-Reports/State-StaffingPlansRatios

Bobay, K. L., Yakusheva, O., & Weiss, M. E. (2011). Outcomes and cost analysis of the impact of unit-level nurse staffing on post-discharge utilization. *Nursing Economic$, 29*(2), 69–87.

Buchan, J. (2014). Getting staffing levels right. *Nursing Standard, 28*(49), 30.

Clark, S. L., Saade, G. A., Meyers, J. A., Frye, D. R., & Perlin, J. B. (2014). The clinical and economic impact of nurse to patient staffing ratios in women receiving intrapartum Oxytocin. *American Journal of Perinatology, 31*(2), 119–123.

Cortez, Z. (2008, January 4). *California's nurse-patient ratio law: Saving lives, reducing the nursing shortage.* Retrieved from California Progress Report Website: http://www.californiaprogressreport.com/2008/01/californias_nur.html

Donaldson, N., & Shapiro, S. (2010). Impact of California mandated acute care hospital nurse staffing ratios: A literature synthesis. *Policy, Politics & Nursing Practice, 11*(3), 184–201.

Everhart, D., Schumacher, J. R., Duncan, R. P., Hall, A. G., Neff, D. F., & Shorr, R. I. (2014). Determinants of hospital fall rate trajectory groups: A longitudinal assessment of nurse staffing and organizational characteristics. *Health Care Management Review, 39*(4), 352–360.

Frost, S., & Alexandrou, A. (2013). Higher nurse staffing levels associated with reductions in unplanned readmissions to intensive care or operating theatre, and in postoperative in-hospital mortality in heart surgery patients. *Evidence-Based Nursing, 16*(2), 62–63.

Goryakin, Y., Griffiths, P., & Maben, J. (2011). Economic evaluation of nurse staffing and nurse substitution in health care: A scoping review. *International Journal of Nursing Studies, 48*(4), 501–512.

Kerfoot, K. M., & Douglas, K. S. (2013). The impact of research on staffing: An interview with Linda Aiken, Part 1. *Nursing Economic$, 31*(5), 216–253.

Mark, B., Harless, D., Spetz, J., Reiter, K., & Pink, G. (2013). California's minimum nurse staffing legislation: Results from a natural experiment. *Health Services Research, 48*(2), 435–454.

Munnich, E. L. (2014). The labor market effects of California's minimum nurse staffing law. *Health Economics, 23*(8), 935–950.

National Nurses United. (2010–2015, February 1). *National campaign for safe RN-to-patient staffing ratios.* Retrieved from http://www.nationalnursesunited.org/issues/entry/ratios

Needleman, J., Buerhaus, P., Mattke, S., Stewart, M., & Zelevinsky, K. (2002). Nurse-staffing levels and the quality of care in hospitals. *The New England Journal of Medicine, 346*, 1715–1722.

Serratt, T. (2013a). California's nurse-to-patient ratios, Part 2: 8 Years later, what do we know about hospital level outcomes? *Journal of Nursing Administration, 43*(10), 549–553.

Serratt, T. (2013b). California's nurse-to-patient ratios, Part 3. *Journal of Nursing Administration, 43*(11), 581–585.

Shekelle, P. (2013). Nurse–patient ratios as a patient safety strategy: A systemic review. *Annals of Internal Medicine, 158*(5 Pt. 2), 404–410.

Spetz, J., Harless, D., Herrera, C., & Mark, B. (2013). Using minimum nurse staffing regulations to measure the relationship between nursing and hospital quality of care. *Medical Care Research and Review, 70*(4), 380–399.

Stamp, K. D., Flanagan, J., Gregas, M., & Shindul-Rothschild, J. (2014). Predictors of excess heart failure readmissions. *Journal of Nursing Care Quality, 29*(2), 115–123.

Sung-Heui, B., Kelly, M., Brewer, C. S., & Spencer, A. (2014). Analysis of nurse staffing and patient outcomes using comprehensive nurse staffing characteristics in acute care nursing units. *Journal of Nursing Care Quality, 29*(4), 318–326.

Tellez, M., & Seago, J. (2013). California nurse staffing law and RN workforce changes. *Nursing Economics, 31*(1), 18–28.

Tubbs-Cooley, H. L., Cimiotti, J. P., Silber, J. H., Sloane, D. M., & Aiken, L. H. (2013). An observational study of nurse staffing ratios and hospital readmission among children admitted for common conditions. *BMJ Quality & Safety, 22*(9), 735–742.

Wallace, B. (2013). Nurse staffing and patient safety: What's your perspective? *Nursing Management, 44*(6), 49–51.

West, E., Barron, D. N., Harrison, D., Rafferty, A. M., Rowan, K., & Sanderson, C. (2014). Nurse staffing, medical staffing and mortality in intensive care: An observational study. *International Journal of Nursing Studies, 51*(5), 781–794.

10

Mandatory Overtime in Nursing

How Much? How Often?

Carol J. Huston

ADDITIONAL RESOURCES

Visit thePoint for additional helpful resources

- eBook
- Journal Articles
- WebLinks

CHAPTER OUTLINE

LEARNING OBJECTIVES

The learner will be able to:

1. Identify the strengths and the limitations of the Fair Labor Standards Act of 1938 in terms of protecting workers against mandatory overtime.
2. Identify how changes to federal overtime rules in the last decade and more recent court rulings have affected traditional "white collar" employees, including salaried nurses in the United States.
3. Investigate current federal and state legislative efforts to regulate overtime limits for nurses.
4. Explore the current extent of mandatory overtime in nursing as identified in the literature.
5. Identify consequences of mandatory overtime in nursing, including fatigue, increased error rates, increased legal liability, threats to the nurse's personal safety, and increased staff turnover rates.
6. Know and understand the provisions of the Nurse Practice Act in his or her state, as well as the position statements or advisory opinions that have been issued by his or her state board of nursing regarding mandatory overtime and patient abandonment.
7. Discuss the limits of the nurse's professional duty, and assess how much risk a professional nurse should assume in fulfilling a professional duty.
8. Reflect on the number of hours he or she can safely work before quality of care is potentially compromised.

INTRODUCTION

One short-term means of dealing with nursing shortages has been to require nurses to work extra shifts, often under threat of "patient abandonment" or punitive measures. *Mandatory overtime*, also called *compulsory* or *forced overtime*, occurs when employees are required to work more hours than are standard (generally 40 hours per week) or risk employer reprisals as a result of their refusal to do so. Mandatory overtime may result from a number of unexpected events such as natural or human-caused disasters, sudden job vacancies, staff absences due to illness, or rapid changes in patient care requirements, or it may be a standard staffing practice.

A review of the literature suggests that the use of mandatory overtime in nursing varies greatly from institution to institution and from state to state. Some health care employers have suggested that nursing shortages are the cause of mandatory overtime in their facilities. The consensus, however, is that working overtime among nurses is a prevalent practice used to control chronic understaffing and a common method used to handle normal variations in the patient census (Bae, 2013). Increasingly, nurses are reporting that mandatory overtime has become standard operating procedure instead of a last resort to short staffing. In fact, in some hospitals, mandatory overtime is routinely used in an effort to keep fewer people on the payroll, as well as to alleviate immediate shortage needs.

Indeed, Bae and Fabry (2014) note that 54% of respondents to the 2008 National Sample Survey of Registered Nurses worked more than 39 hours per week, approximately 200 hours per year more than the average American worker. Furthermore, American nurses are more likely to work 12-hour shifts, leading to concerns about whether there is adequate time for rest and recovery between shifts.

Some nursing specialty units are known, however, to have more mandatory overtime than others, such as the operating room and postanesthesia care units. This occurs as a result of emergent and dynamic patient needs, unpredictable delays in surgical procedures, and significant differences in the efficiency of members of the operating room staff. In an effort to create guidelines for safe practice in the perioperative setting, the Association of Perioperative Registered Nurses (AORN) created a Position Statement on Safe Work/On-Call Practices in 2007 (AORN, 2014). Excerpts from this document are shown in Box 10.1.

Discussion Point

Is mandatory overtime simply part of the work culture in the operating room or postanesthesia care units? Should there be different expectations or rules regarding mandatory overtime in these units?

MANDATORY OVERTIME AS A WAY OF LIFE IN THE UNITED STATES

Although nurses bemoan mandatory overtime in the profession, the reality is that mandatory overtime is not new, nor is it restricted to nursing. Americans typically work more hours and take fewer vacations than workers in other advanced economies. In fact, Miller (2015) calls the United States the "most overworked developed nation in the world." That's because 85.8% of males and 66.5% of females in the United States work more than 40 hours per week. In comparison, Americans work 137 more hours per year than Japanese workers, 260 more hours per year than British workers, and 499 more hours per year than French workers (Miller, 2015). In addition, the United States is the only industrialized country in the world that has no legally mandated annual leave, and in every country except Canada and Japan (and the United States, which averages 13 days per year), workers get at least 20 paid vacation days. In France and Finland, they get 30—an entire month off, paid, every year (Miller, 2015).

Covert (2014) agrees, reporting that the reality of full-time American workers is not a 40-hour workweek; instead, the average full-time worker is putting in 47 hours each week, nearly an extra day's worth of time. While the workweek has been shrinking among all countries, the United States continues to be well above average in how many hours we work each year, and with more worked hours than other developed countries like Australia, Canada, Germany, and the United Kingdom.

For some Americans, hard work may be a badge of honor, or it may be the means to accommodating lifestyles that increasingly require two wage earners in a household. It may also be that Americans are working this hard because they are afraid not to. In the United States, unlike most other countries, employment is *at will*, meaning that employers can dismiss employees

BOX 10.1 Excerpts From the AORN (2014) Position Statement on Perioperative Safe Staffing and On-Call Practices

The AORN, recognizing the potential negative consequences of sleep deprivation and sustained work hours and further recognizing that adequate rest and recuperation periods are essential to patient and perioperative personnel safety, suggests the following strategies:

1. Perioperative registered nurses should not be required to work in direct patient care more than 12 consecutive hours in a 24-hour period and not more than 60 hours in a 7-day period. All work hours (ie, regular hours and call hours worked) should be included in calculating total work hours.
2. The staffing plan should promote quality patient outcomes by using patient acuity and nursing workload guidelines to deliver safe patient care and support a safe work environment. The plan should identify strategies for cost-effective and efficient staffing priorities without compromising perioperative patient safety and outcomes.
3. The perioperative staffing plan should include provisions for unplanned, urgent, or emergent procedures and how to provide care for patients when procedures run over the scheduled time.
4. Arrangements should be made, in relation to the hours worked, to relieve a perioperative registered nurse who has worked on-call during his or her off shift and who is scheduled to work the following shift to accommodate an adequate off-duty recuperation period.
5. On-call staffing plans should be based on strategies that minimize extended work hours, allow for adequate recuperation, and retain the perioperative RN as circulator.
6. Perioperative nurse managers should determine both direct and indirect care patient caregivers for the unit. Additionally, productive and nonproductive time should be considered.

Source: Association of Perioperative Registered Nurses. (2014). *AORN Position statement on perioperative safe staffing and on-call practices.* Retrieved February 3, 2015, from http://www.aornjournal.org/article/S0001-2092%2813%2901302-1/abstract

for any reason (aside from those of gender, race, age, or disability) or for no reason at all. Thus, employees who refuse to work overtime can lose their jobs or face other reprisals.

Nurses argue, however, that mandatory overtime in nursing is not comparable with mandatory overtime in other fields because the consequences of being overly fatigued for the nurse may literally have life-and-death consequences. Proponents of mandatory overtime argue that it is an economic reality, given how limited labor health care resources are, particularly in light of the international nursing shortage. The problem is that both positions are correct.

Consider This Many nurses report a dramatic increase in the use of mandatory overtime to solve staffing problems and fear potential consequences for safety and quality of care for their patients.

This chapter defines mandatory overtime, examines the extent of its use in nursing, and discusses the consequences of mandatory overtime in nursing as identified in the literature.

LEGISLATING MANDATORY OVERTIME

The Fair Labor Standards Act

The definition of what constitutes overtime in the United States or how it should be calculated has historically varied from state to state and from industry to industry. There are, however, national standards in terms of the *Fair Labor Standards Act* (FLSA) of 1938. This act, which regulates overtime, does not impose limits on overtime hours, or prohibit dismissal or any other sanction for declining overtime work. It does, however, require that payroll employees (those who are not "exempt" from the overtime requirements of the FLSA) be paid an overtime premium of at least one-and-a-half times the regular rate of pay for each hour worked more than 40 in a week (U.S. Department of Labor, n.d.).

Consider This Labor laws such as the FLSA need to be amended to protect workers against excessive work hours and mandatory overtime and to protect the public from the dangers of an overburdened, stressed workforce.

The FLSA does, however, contain language that permits the health care industry to use a different overtime standard than the 40-hour workweek since scheduling occurs 24 hours a day, 365 days a year. Historically, this overtime standard required that hospitals and residential care facilities pay overtime after either 8 hours in a day or 80 hours in a 14-day pay period. It also permits employees to work more than 40 hours in a week and not be paid overtime provided they do not work more than 8 hours in a shift or if they work fewer than 40 hours in the next week. Employers are permitted to use both the 40-hour and the 80-hour standards in the same facility, depending on the scheduling patterns for employees, but they must use one standard for individual employees, and it must be applied consistently.

Recent Changes to Federal Overtime Rules

There have been changes, however, to the federal overtime rules in the last decade or so. Some changes, which became effective in 2004, defined exemptions from the FLSA for what were traditionally called "white-collar" employees. The new rules increased the amount of money employees could earn before they were no longer eligible to receive overtime pay; however, employees who directed and supervised two or more other full-time employees fell under the executive exemption. Similarly, the new rules excluded from the FLSA employees who had the authority to hire, fire, and promote employees or if their primary duties involved the performance of office or nonmanual work and the exercise of discretion and independent judgment.

Almost immediately, nursing leaders expressed concern that the language in the new rules opened the door for employer attempts to reclassify nurses as exempt from overtime protections historically given to workers under the FLSA. This occurred because under the new regulations, "learned professionals" earning fairly low salaries (anything above US$455 per week) could not earn overtime pay.

Nurses met the criteria of *learned professional*, which is defined in part as employees who perform work that requires advanced knowledge (work that is predominantly intellectual in character and that includes work requiring the consistent exercise of discretion and judgment) (U.S. Department of Labor, n.d.). In addition, the learned professional must have advanced knowledge in a field of science or learning, and the advanced knowledge must be customarily acquired by a prolonged course of specialized intellectual instruction.

Concerns about the exemption of health care workers from protection under the FLSA were borne out in a June 2007 Supreme Court ruling that the U.S. Department of Labor had acted appropriately in denying FLSA protection to 10 home care workers even when employed by large, third-party home care agencies (Dawson, 2007). In the case of *Long Island Care at Home, LTD. versus Coke*, "the Court ruled that Ms. Evelyn Coke, a home care aide from Queens, New York, deserved neither overtime pay nor minimum wage, although she was frequently asked to work up to 70 hours per week" (Dawson, 2007, para. 1). This ruling occurred because of an exemption to the FLSA that applies to companions and housekeepers who work in the homes of their clients. On October 7, 2014, however, the United States Department of Labor announced that it would delay enforcement of its new rules designed to narrow the companionship exemption for home care workers under the FLSA, previously scheduled to begin January 1, 2015 (Mullett, 2015). The new rules extend minimum wage and overtime protections to direct care workers, which are the same protections provided to most US workers, including those who perform the same work in nursing homes.

In addition, it is important to note that nurses are eligible for overtime pay and protection under the FLSA if they are classified by employers as hourly—not salaried—employees, because salaried employees are not eligible for overtime. Thus, salaried employees and nurses who are considered to be exempt under the FLSA have virtually no rights under these new overtime rules. They are entitled only to their base salary, less deductions, by law and may be held to whatever schedule an employer demands because there are no restrictions on mandatory overtime in the FLSA.

In early 2014, President Obama issued an Executive Order to the Secretary of Labor to update the regulations regarding overtime exemptions and increase the overtime exemption salary (McBrayer, McGinnis, Leslie, & Kirkland, PLLC, 2015). The White House cited the erosion of the 40-hour workweek coupled with the failure to update the salary threshold to keep current with inflation as grounds for the order. The proposed rulemaking was to take place in November of 2014 but had not occurred as of early 2015. What is expected is that the current salary exemption of $23,000 annually (or $455 a week) is expected to at least double. That means that an entire swath of employees who make between $23,000 a year and $56,000 a year will now be subject to overtime pay requirements, regardless of their duties.

McBrayer, McGinnis, Leslie, & Kirkland, PLLC (2015) also note that employers should also plan for the exemption for executive, administrative, or professional roles to become somewhat more constricted, as many commentators feel that regulations regarding these roles might start to track similar regulations in other states. Those states have a minimum threshold for the amount of an employee's time that must be performed in a "white collar" role to continue to be exempt.

Legislating Limits on Nursing Overtime

Despite multiple efforts over the last decade to introduce national legislation directed at prohibiting employers from requiring licensed health care employees to work more than 8 hours in a single workday or 80 hours in any 14-day work period—except in the case of a natural disaster or declaration of emergency by federal, state, or local government officials—no such legislation has been passed.

States are, however, increasingly taking a role in both defining mandatory overtime and putting limits to its use. Every nurse should know and understand the provisions of the Nurse Practice Act in his or her state, as well as the position statements or advisory opinions that have been issued by the state board of nursing on mandatory overtime and patient abandonment.

Discussion Point

What position statement or advisory opinion has your state board of nursing issued regarding mandatory overtime and patient abandonment? Do you feel that it is adequate to protect both nurses and patients from unsafe working conditions?

In addition, the ANA has added the mandatory overtime issue to its Nationwide State Legislative Agenda, supporting the enactment of mandatory overtime legislation by state legislatures and the attention to such issues by regulatory agencies. As of December 2014, 14 states had restrictions in law on the use of mandatory overtime for nurses (Alaska, Connecticut, Illinois, Maryland, Massachusetts, Minnesota, New Hampshire, New York, Oregon, Pennsylvania, Rhode Island, Texas, Washington, and West Virginia) and 2 by including such provisions in regulations (California and Missouri) (ANA, 2015b).

Alaska passed mandatory overtime restrictions for nurses in health care settings in 2010 (became effective in 2011) preceded by Texas in 2009. In Alaska, the law states that a registered nurse or licensed practical nurse in a health care facility who is not employed in a federal or tribal facility may not be required or coerced, directly or indirectly, to work beyond his or her agreed-upon regular shift or accept overtime if in the judgment of the nurse, the overtime would jeopardize patient or employee safety ("Mandatory Overtime Limitations," 2014). In addition, the nurse cannot work more than 14 consecutive hours except under very specific conditions such as a nurse voluntarily working overtime on an aircraft in use for medical transport or a nurse participating in the performance of a medical procedure that has begun but not completed. On-call time is not counted in the 14 hours unless the nurse is actually called back into work ("Mandatory Overtime Limitations," 2014).

Pennsylvania enacted the Prohibition of Excessive Overtime in Health Care Act (HB 834) in October 2008. This law states that a health care facility could not require an employee to work in excess of an agreed to, predetermined, and regularly scheduled daily work shift unless there was an unforeseeable declared national, state, or municipal emergency or a catastrophic event that was unpredictable or unavoidable and that substantially affects or increases the need for health care services (ANA, 2015c). This law did not preclude employees from voluntarily accepting overtime, and it did not apply to those workers compensated for "on call" time.

New York also enacted legislation in 2008 prohibiting health care employers (excluding home care facilities) from forcing nurses to work overtime, except during health care disasters that increased the need for health care personnel unexpectedly or when a health care employer determined that there was an emergency and had made a good faith effort to have overtime covered on a voluntary basis (ANA, 2015c). Another exception included an ongoing medical or surgical procedure in which the nurse is actively engaged, such as in surgery, and whose continued presence through completion is essential to the health and safety of the patient (ANA, 2015c).

Although the New York legislation provides a good example of how states can reduce the risk of mandatory overtime for nurses, it should be noted that the New York Nurses Association first proposed legislation to ban mandatory overtime in 2000. Eight years were required to gain enough support from patient advocacy groups and other unions that represent nurses.

Minnesota also successfully passed legislation in 2007 that prohibited nurses from being required to work more than a "normal work period," meaning 12 or fewer consecutive hours, consistent with their predetermined work shift, but again excludes an emergency (ANA, 2015c):

> *The definition of emergency refers to a period when replacement staff are not able to report for duty for the next shift or increase patient need, because of unusual, unpredictable, or unforeseen circumstances such as, but not limited to, an act of terrorism, a disease outbreak, adverse weather conditions, or natural disasters which impact the continuity of patient care.* (para. 5)

Similar legislation became effective in New Hampshire in 2008. This legislation prohibited an employer from disciplining or removing any right, benefit, or privilege of a registered nurse, licensed practical nurse, or licensed nursing assistant for refusing to work more than 12 consecutive hours, except under specific circumstances, such as those identified in the New York and Minnesota legislation (ANA, 2015c). A nurse might be disciplined for refusing to work mandatory overtime in these situations.

Research conducted by Bae and Yoon (2014) found that mandatory overtime and consecutive work hour regulations were significantly associated with 3.9 percentage-point decreases in the likelihood of working mandatory overtime and 11.5 percentage-point decreases in the likelihood of working more than 40 hours per week, respectively. Having such policies then appears to be an effective regulatory tool for reducing long work hours for nurses.

THE CONSEQUENCES OF MANDATORY OVERTIME

Research on the effects of overtime has largely focused on studies of individuals working scheduled 12-hour shifts. However, when staff *plan* to work 12-hour shifts or additional shifts on a volunteer basis, they are more likely to get plenty of rest immediately before working the extended shift. Overtime mandated by an employer, however, occurs with little or no prior notice, so higher levels of fatigue may occur. In addition, many nurses report working far more than 12 hours when mandatory overtime is involved.

How long can nurses work safely? Given the variability in each situation, there is no one answer to this question. There is little doubt, however, that after a certain point of protracted work time, fatigue becomes a factor and the likelihood of errors, near errors, mistakes, and lapses in judgment increases.

Other industries, such as airlines and trucking, have recognized this for years and have limited the hours employees in these industries can work without breaks. The ANA authored a position statement in 2006, arguing that nursing employers should do the same by ensuring that sufficient system resources exist to (1) provide the individual registered nurse in all roles and settings with a work schedule that provides for adequate rest and recuperation between scheduled work and (2) provide sufficient compensation and appropriate staffing systems that foster a safe and healthful environment in which the registered nurse does not feel compelled to seek supplemental income through overtime, extra shifts, and other practices that contribute to worker fatigue (ANA, 2006).

Consider This Federal regulations have used transportation laws to place limits on the amount of time that can safely be worked in aviation and trucking. It seems appropriate that Congress needs to go beyond the FLSA and at least examine the need to create safety parameters around mandatory overtime in nursing.

The reality, however, is that mandatory overtime is very much a part of contemporary nursing practice, and the literature increasingly suggests that fatigue can result in a whole host of negative consequences including occupational injury, illness, burnout, reduced quality of care, and errors. For example, research conducted by Bae (2013) found that mandatory overtime and working on call increased the odds of nurse injuries. In addition, verbal abuse was significantly more likely to be reported for nurses who worked mandatory overtime (Research Study Fuels the Controversy 10.1).

Similarly, Griffiths et al. (2014) found that nurses working for ≥12 hours were more likely to report poor or failing patient safety, poor/fair quality of care, and more care activities left undone. The researchers concluded that policies to adopt a 12-hour nursing shift pattern should proceed with caution and that use of overtime to mitigate staffing shortages or increase flexibility may also incur additional risk to quality.

These findings echo those of Chen, Davis, Daraiseh, Pan, and Davis (2014), who concluded that nurses working 12-hour shifts experienced a moderate to high

Research Study Fuels the Controversy 10.1

The Impact of Work Schedule on Occupational Injury and Illness

The purpose of this cross-sectional study incorporating data from staff RNs working in hospitals in North Carolina and West Virginia was to examine the relationship between the presence of mandatory nurse overtime regulations and nurse injuries and adverse patient events. In addition, the study examined the mediating effect of nurse overtime on the relationship between the regulations and outcomes after controlling for other nurse work characteristics.

Source: Bae, S. (2013). Presence of nurse mandatory overtime regulations and nurse and patient outcomes. *Nursing Economic$, 31*(2), 59–89.

Study Findings

From the sample, 15.6% of the RNs worked mandatory overtime (either paid or unpaid), while 34.1% worked voluntary overtime (either paid or unpaid) in a typical week. About 32% of RNs worked on-call hours (either paid or unpaid). When all types of overtime are considered, 60.1% of RNs worked at least one type of overtime among mandatory, voluntary, and on-call. About 16% of nurses actually worked more than 40 hours in a typical week.

Among nurse injuries, verbal abuse (56.6%) and bruises or contusions (49.7%) were the two most frequently experienced nurse injuries. In total, 79.2% of nurses experienced one of those injuries during the prior month. In regard to adverse patient events, medication errors (44.5%) and patient falls (38.2%) were the most frequently reported adverse patient events by nurses. Sixty-one percent of nurses perceived that patients in their unit experienced one of these adverse events during their hospital stay.

After controlling for work settings, workload, and nurse educational level, the mandatory nurse overtime regulation did not have any relationship with nurse injuries. The results did suggest, however, that working mandatory overtime and on-call increased the odds of nurse injuries. Verbal abuse was significantly more likely to be reported for nurses who worked mandatory overtime. The variable of any nurse injuries showed a significant association with working on-call hours as well.

level of acute fatigue and moderate levels of chronic fatigue and intershift recovery. Fatigue and recovery levels differed by the interaction between hospital and unit after controlling for individual factors. Lack of regular exercise and older age were associated with higher acute fatigue.

In addition, a literature review by Bae and Fabry (2014) found that 21 nurse outcome measures and 19 patient outcome measures correlated with work hours and overtime. These findings suggested that the positive relationships between working long hours and adverse outcomes to the nurses are strong, although more evidence is needed.

These findings reinforce those of a report of the Board on Health Care Services and the Institute of Medicine, *Keeping Patients Safe: Transforming the Work Environment of Nurses*, which said that nurses' long working hours pose a serious threat to patient safety. In fact, the report argued that "limiting the number of hours worked per day and consecutive days of work by nursing staff, as is done in other safety-sensitive industries, is a fundamental safety precaution" (PA Nurses Also Address, 2007, para. 3). Similarly, Marquis and Huston (2015) argued that certain minimum criteria should always be met for safe staffing. These criteria are shown in Box 10.2.

Discussion Point

How many hours can the typical nurse work before she or he might be considered unsafe? How much individual leeway is feasible in making this determination?

Discussion Point

Is increasing the use of mandatory overtime perpetuating the nursing shortage? Do you think nurses who no longer work in nursing roles would be more apt to return to work if they felt they had more control over the hours they worked (mandatory overtime was banned)?

BOX 10.2 Minimum Criteria for Staffing Decisions

- Decisions made must meet state and federal labor laws and organizational policies.
- Staff must not be demoralized or excessively fatigued by frequent or extended overtime requests.
- Long-term as well as short-term solutions to staffing shortages must be sought.
- Patient care must not be jeopardized.

Source: Marquis, B., & Huston, C. (2015). *Leadership roles and management functions* (8th ed.). Philadelphia, PA: Lippincott Williams & Wilkins.

PROFESSIONAL DUTY AND CONSCIENCE

Mandatory overtime and patient abandonment must also be examined in terms of professional duty. A *professional duty* is the direct result of others having welfare rights, such as the right to safe care. Because people have a right to such care, nurses have an associated duty to ensure that they accept patient care assignments only if they are mentally and physically able to provide, at minimum, safe care.

The problem is that there is great variability in terms of how many hours a nurse can work and still provide competent safe care. For example, the practice of mandatory overtime is grounded in the commitment to prevent harm to patients by guaranteeing adequate nurse–patient ratios, yet the overfatigued nurse may pose even greater risk of harm to patients by agreeing to work. The ANA (2014) agrees, suggesting that regardless of the number of hours worked, each registered nurse has an ethical responsibility to carefully consider his/her level of fatigue when deciding to accept any assignment extending beyond the regularly scheduled work day or week. The ANA concludes that registered nurses are responsible for negotiating or even rejecting a work assignment that compromises the availability of sufficient time for sleep and recovery from work. The amount of recovery time necessary depends on the amount of work, including regularly scheduled shifts and mandatory or voluntary overtime.

Discussion Point

Who bears the risk or the consequences of risk when an overworked nurse makes errors that contribute to patient harm?

What happens when the nurse determines that he or she must refuse to work additional hours because of safety concerns related to level of fatigue? Saying no to a desperate employer, especially when the fear that short staffing may compromise patient safety, is likely much harder than it sounds. Indeed, moral dilemmas abound when health care providers feel they must refuse a patient care assignment.

When this occurs, some nurses feel compelled to file their refusal to work as a *conscientious objection.* The purpose of conscientious objection is to protect the rights of employees who refuse to participate in procedures on the basis of conscience. The issue of whether a nurse can refuse mandatory overtime on the basis of conscience, however, has limited case law precedent.

The ANA's (2015a) *Code of Ethics*, newly revised in 2015, might also be helpful to some nurses in resolving potential ethical conflicts between their professional duty to provide care and conscience, or the realization that providing such care may actually place patients at risk for harm. The *Code of Ethics*, however, might actually potentiate the dilemma because it states that nurses should care for all people in need without discrimination. The problem is that it also says that the nurse is to maintain conditions of employment that are conducive to high-quality nursing care.

The ANA also recommends a Bill of Rights as a tool for dialogue to resolve concerns that nurses may have about work environments that might not support professional practice. The Bill of Rights was actually conceived to support nurses in an array of workplace situations, including mandatory overtime, and suggests that nurses must bring these workplace issues to the attention of employers to meet their responsibilities to their patients and to themselves (ANA, 2015d).

Patient Abandonment

One of the most common reasons nurses cite for working mandatory overtime is the threat that refusal to do so could be construed as *patient abandonment*, a charge that can result in loss of licensure. Therefore, many nurses believe that they have no choice when confronted by a request for overtime, despite the fact that they might be working a shift in excess of 12 hours.

Consider This In some facilities, nurses are being threatened with dismissal or with the charge of patient abandonment if they refuse to accept overtime.

Despite this perception, the ANA does not support the forced overtime of nurses, and their position is that a nurse should not be held accountable for patient abandonment if the nurse turned down an assignment that could be unsafe to patients or self. In fact, generally speaking, most state boards of nursing suggest that refusal to work mandatory overtime is not patient abandonment; in a situation in which a nurse has accepted a patient or assignment, the nurse must simply notify the supervisor that he or she is leaving and report off to another nurse.

Usually, however, nurses have less likelihood of losing their license or being reprimanded if an assignment (mandatory overtime) is never accepted in the first place than if the assignment is accepted and then the nurse changes his or her mind. This is because accepting the assignment suggests that a nurse–patient relationship has been established. Thus, patient abandonment is more likely when the nurse accepts a patient assignment and then ceases to provide nursing care without appropriately transferring the responsibility for the patient to another professional nurse. This then becomes a form of negligence in nursing since the termination of the provider–patient relationship was unilateral, despite the patient's continued need for care (What Nurses Should Know, 2013).

In addition, boards of nursing in several states have developed clear statements differentiating patient abandonment from *employer abandonment*. Typically, these statements define *employment abandonment* as nurses leaving their places of work to avoid injury to patients or to themselves.

This definition is similar to language used by the Maryland Board of Registered Nursing (BRN) in defining patient abandonment; however, the Maryland BRN (2011) suggested that there are many variables to be examined in determining whether patient abandonment has actually occurred. The definition of patient abandonment and these variables are shown in Box 10.3.

Consider This Although boards of nursing often rule that refusing mandatory overtime is not patient abandonment and thus is not cause for loss of licensure, they have no jurisdiction over employment and contract issues. Refusing to work mandatory overtime may still result in termination of a nurse's employment.

In addition, the Vermont Board of Nursing (2014) has identified examples of situations that may constitute abandonment. These are shown in Box 10.4.

UNIONS AND MANDATORY OVERTIME

Because collective bargaining agreements can require greater protections beyond those outlined in the FLSA, the position of most collective bargaining agents is that the practice of mandatory overtime should be eliminated entirely. However, there are differences among union contracts, and the strategies used by unions to reduce mandatory overtime vary greatly.

The American Federation of Teachers (AFT, n.d.) has been on record since 1990, calling for a ban on mandatory overtime through a twofold approach—legislation and contract language: At the federal level, AFT is working with legislators to require facilities receiving Medicare funding to stop mandating overtime and notes that on-call time should be treated as work time. In addition, many local unions have negotiated contract language limiting the practice of mandatory overtime.

The Service Employees International Union (SEIU) has also consistently spoken out against mandatory overtime. In addition, the SEIU, in partnership with the Nurse Alliance, created an Overtime Report Form for nurses, union or nonunion, to document mandatory or pressured overtime.

Similarly, the American Federation of State, County and Municipal Employees (AFSCME) is also working to eliminate mandatory overtime, suggesting that an increasing prevalence of hospitals that use mandatory overtime do so as a routine staffing solution (AFSCME, 2015). AFSCME suggests that "presumably, hospital administrators believe that the imposition of mandatory overtime will save money by limiting recruitment and

BOX 10.3 The Link Between Nurse–Patient Relationships and Patient Abandonment as Outlined by the Maryland Board of Registered Nursing

Abandonment occurs when a licensed nurse terminates the nurse–patient relationship without reasonable notification to the nursing supervisor for the continuation of the patient's care.

The nurse–patient relationship begins when responsibility for nursing care of a patient is accepted by the nurse. Nursing management is accountable for assessing the capabilities of personnel and delegating responsibility or assigning nursing care functions to personnel qualified to assume such responsibility or to perform such functions.

The Variables That Need To Be Examined in Each Alleged Incident of Abandonment Include But Are Not Limited To

1. What were the licensee's assigned responsibilities for what time frame? What was the clinical setting and resources available to the licensee?
2. Was there an exchange of responsibility from one licensee to another? When did the exchange occur, that is, shift report and so on?
3. What was the time frame of the incident, that is, time licensee arrived, time of exchange of responsibility, and the like?
4. What was the communication process, that is, whom did the licensee inform of his or her intent to leave, and was it lateral, upward, downward, and so forth?
5. What are the facility's policies, terms of employment, and/or job description regarding the licensee and call-in, refusal to accept an assignment, reassignment to another unit, mandatory overtime, and the like?
6. What is the pattern of practice/events for the licensee and the pattern of management for the unit/facility, that is, is the event of a single isolated occurrence, or is it one event in a series of events?
7. What were the issues/reasons why the licensee could not accept an assignment, continue an assignment, or extend an original assignment, and so forth?

Source: Maryland Board of Registered Nursing. (2011, July 1–Last updated). *Abandonment*. Retrieved September 3, 2015, from http://mbon.maryland.gov/Pages/practice-abandonment.aspx

BOX 10.4 Sample Situations That Might Constitute Patient Abandonment

- Leaving the patient care area without transferring responsibility for patient care to an authorized person
- Remaining unavailable for patient care for a period of time such that patient care may be compromised due to lack of available qualified staff
- Inattention or insufficient observation or contact with a patient
- Sleeping while on duty without the approval of a supervisor in accordance with written facility policy
- Failing to timely notify a supervisor or employer if the licensee will not initiate or complete an assignment where the licensee is the sole provider of care
- For the APRN, terminating the nurse–patient relationship without providing reasonable notification to the patient and resources for continuity of care

Source: Vermont Board of Nursing. (2014). Vermont Board of Nursing position statement on abandonment. *Vermont Nurse Connection, 17*(4), 9.

benefit expenses. However, multiple studies have shown mandatory overtime to be perhaps the single worst practice to emerge from the era of downsizing and managed care" (para. 1) and that indeed, it often generates very large costs, even if sometimes unaccounted for, in the form of increased turnover, lower productivity, longer patient stays, and higher rates of treatment errors that in turn necessitate more extended and costly solutions.

Conclusions

In the end, the mandatory overtime dilemma, like so many in nursing, comes down to a conflict regarding how best to use limited resources (fiscal and human) to provide safe, quality health care. Most nurses and administrators can agree on two goals: (1) staffing should be at least minimally adequate to assure that all patients receive safe care and (2) nursing staff should not be placed at personal or legal risk to provide that care.

The problem is that the onus is on management to ensure that there is appropriate staffing, and most health care institutions state that there simply are not enough resources to meet the first goal without jeopardizing the second. Clearly, more alternatives such as shift bidding and pay enhancement programs need to be explored. Neither health care administrators nor nurses should have to choose between meeting the needs of patients and meeting the needs of nurses.

The bottom line is that workers should have the right to refuse overtime without fear of repercussion, especially when staffing shortages and mandated overtime are the norm and not the exception. Unfortunately, as long as nursing shortages exist, mandatory overtime will continue to be used as a means of meeting minimum staffing needs.

For Additional Discussion

1. How does the presence of a collective bargaining agreement affect a hospital's ability to require mandatory overtime? How much power do unions have in negotiating this aspect of working conditions?
2. Would passage of a national ban on mandatory overtime tie the hands of hospitals to assure that staffing is at least minimally adequate during periods of acute nursing shortages?
3. Does the use of mandatory overtime really save hospitals money in terms of recruitment and benefits?
4. How do the rates of mandatory overtime in nursing compare with those in other professions?
5. Are other nonnursing health care professionals at risk for loss of licensure if they are found guilty of patient abandonment?
6. Are charges of patient abandonment legally and morally appropriate if a nurse works his or her required shift but refuses to stay and work longer?
7. Given the severity and scope of the nursing shortage, what is the likelihood that mandatory staffing will continue to be used for both emergency and routine staffing needs?

References

American Federation of State, County and Municipal Employees, AFL–CIO. (2015). *Worst practices: Mandatory overtime.* Retrieved February 3, 2015, from http://www.afscme.org/news/publications/health-care/solving-the-nursing-shortage/worst-practices-mandatory-overtime

American Federation of Teachers. (n.d.). *Mandatory overtime.* Retrieved February 4, 2015, from http://www.aft.org/healthcare/mandatory-overtime

American Nurses Association. (2006). *Position statements: Assuring patient safety: The employers' role in promoting healthy nursing work hours for registered nurses in all roles and settings.* Retrieved February 5, 2015, from http://www.nursingworld.org/MainMenuCategories/Policy-Advocacy/Positions-and-Resolutions/ANAPositionStatements/Archives/AssuringPatientSafety.pdf

American Nurses Association (2014, September 10). *Position statement: Addressing nurse fatigue to promote safety and health: Joint responsibilities of registered nurses and employers to reduce risks.* Retrieved February 3, 2015, from Nursing World Website: http://www.nursingworld.org/MainMenuCategories/Policy-Advocacy/Positions-and-Resolutions/ANAPosition

Statements/Position-Statements-Alphabetically/Addressing-Nurse-Fatigue-to-Promote-Safety-and-Health.html

American Nurses Association. (2015a). *Code of ethics for nurses with interpretive statements*. Silver Springs, MD: Nurse Books.Org.

American Nurses Association. (2015b). *Mandatory overtime*. Retrieved February 4, 2015, from Nursing World Website: http://www.nursingworld.org/MainMenuCategories/Policy-Advocacy/State/Legislative-Agenda-Reports/MandatoryOvertime

American Nurses Association. (2015c). *Mandatory overtime: Summary of state approaches*. Updated March 7, 2011. Retrieved February 4, 2015, from Nursing World Website: http://www.nursingworld.org/MainMenuCategories/Policy-Advocacy/State/Legislative-Agenda-Reports/MandatoryOvertime/Mandatory-Overtime-Summary-of-State-Approaches.html

American Nurses Association (2015d). *Nurses' bill of rights*. Retrieved September 2, 2015, from http://nursingworld.org/NursesBillofRights

Association of Perioperative Registered Nurses. (2014). *AORN Position statement on perioperative safe staffing and on-call practices*. Retrieved February 3, 2015, from http://www.aornjournal.org/article/S0001-2092%2813%2901302-1/abstract

Bae, S. (2013). Presence of nurse mandatory overtime regulations and nurse and patient outcomes. *Nursing Economic$, 31*(2), 59–89.

Bae, S., & Fabry, D. (2014). Assessing the relationships between nurse work hours/overtime and nurse and patient outcomes: Systematic literature review. *Nursing Outlook, 62*(2), 138–156.

Bae, S., & Yoon, J. (2014). Impact of states' nurse work hour regulations on overtime practices and work hours among registered nurses. *Health Services Research, 49*(5), 1638–1658.

Chen, J., Davis, K. G., Daraiseh, N. M., Pan, W., & Davis, L. S. (2014). Fatigue and recovery in 12-hour dayshift hospital nurses. *Journal of Nursing Management, 22*(5), 593–603.

Covert, B. (2014, September 2). *The truth about the 40-hour workweek: It's actually 47 hours long*. Think Progress. Retrieved February 5, 2015, from http://thinkprogress.org/economy/2014/09/02/3477937/workweek/

Dawson, S. L. (2007). Taking a cue from the Supreme court. *Nursing Homes: Long Term Care Management, 56*(10), 8–10.

Griffiths, P., Dall'Ora, C., Simon, M., Ball, J., Lindqvist, R., Rafferty, A., & Aiken, L. H. (2014). Nurses' shift length and overtime working in 12 European countries: The association with perceived quality of care and patient safety. *Medical Care, 52*(11), 975–981.

Mandatory overtime limitations for nurses. (2014). *The Alaska Nurse, 64*(4), 9.

Marquis, B., & Huston, C. (2015). *Leadership roles and management functions in nursing: Theory and application* (8th ed.). Philadelphia, PA: Lippincott Williams & Wilkins.

Maryland Board of Registered Nursing. (2011, July 01). *Abandonment*. Retrieved September 2, 2015, from http://mbon.maryland.gov/Pages/practice-abandonment.aspx

McBrayer, McGinnis, Leslie, & Kirkland, PLLC. (2015, February 2). *What employers can (probably) expect from the FLSA overtime exemption (yet to be) proposed rules*. Retrieved February 4, 2015, from http://www.natlawreview.com/article/what-employers-can-probably-expect-flsa-overtime-exemption-yet-to-be-proposed-rules

Miller, G. E. (2015, January 17). *The U.S. is the most overworked developed nation in the world—When do we draw the line?* Retrieved February 5, 2015, from 20SomethingFinance.com Website: http://20somethingfinance.com/american-hours-worked-productivity-vacation/

Mullett, N. (2015). *Fair labor standards act update regarding home care workers*. Kalamazoo, MI: Kreis Enderle. Retrieved February 4, 2015, from http://www.kreisenderle.com/news/fair-labor-standards-act-update-regarding-home-care-workers/

PA nurses also address mandatory overtime [Abstract]. (2007). *American Nurse, 39*(3), 4.

U.S. Department of Labor. (n.d.). *Overtime pay*. Retrieved February 4, 2015, from http://www.dol.gov/dol/topic/wages/overtimepay.htm

Vermont Board of Nursing. (2014). Vermont board of nursing position statement on abandonment. *Vermont Nurse Connection, 17*(4), 9.

What nurses should know about patient care abandonment and negligence. (2013, October 10). Retrieved February 3, 2015, from http://www.nursetogether.com/what-every-nurse-should-know-about-patient

11

Violence in Nursing
The Expectations and the Reality

Charmaine Hockley

ADDITIONAL RESOURCES

Visit thePoint for additional helpful resources

- eBook
- Journal Articles
- WebLinks

CHAPTER OUTLINE

LEARNING OBJECTIVES

The learner will be able to:

1. Identify common terms used to describe workplace violence, including violence, bullying, conflict, and "personality clash."
2. Explore the prevalence of workplace violence in nursing as compared with other professions.
3. Recognize workplace violence as an individual, national, and global problem.
4. Differentiate among the different categories of violence in the health care sector, generally, and nursing, specifically.
5. Compare the incidence, most frequent types, and common consequences of workplace violence.
6. Analyze common reasons that nurses are reluctant to report workplace violence.
7. Recognize potential long-term consequences of workplace violence, including physical, emotional, and financial repercussions.
8. Delineate specific strategies that can be undertaken by individuals, employers, organizations, and governments to reduce workplace violence.
9. Integrate ethical, legal, and human rights as guides for developing best practices to guard against and respond to workplace violence.
10. Reflect on personal behaviors or attitude that might create a threatening workplace environment for others.

INTRODUCTION

Violence in nursing continues to be one of the major professional issues facing nurses in the 21st century. After the slow acceptance in the 1990s that violence in nursing was occurring, research has evolved rapidly. Until recently, research has focused on the nature and extent of bullying. This was important work. We now have a good understanding of the nature of violence in nursing and that it is not rare or confined to a single setting but is experienced by nurses in a wide variety of geographical locations and service areas. Research has shown that nurses can be targeted by other nurses, or by other health professionals, patients, visitors, or strangers. In other words, the violence that nurses experience may occur wherever they may live or work, or whatever position they may hold.

This chapter moves beyond an understanding of the nature and extent of workplace violence by introducing different perspectives that have the potential to reduce the violence nurses experience. However, it is important to reflect on what is meant by violence in nursing, the language that is used to describe this behavior, and the types of violence that nurses experience. Therefore, this chapter begins by providing an overview of violence nurses experience followed by important legal and ethical considerations in addressing this behavior. In addition, the integration of studies undertaken to add to the knowledge of violence in nursing is discussed within an ethical, legal, and human rights framework.

Discussion Point

Is it likely that violence in nursing is multidetermined and rarely, if ever, due to a single factor?

WHAT IS VIOLENCE IN NURSING?

Over the years, violence in nursing has often been a difficult concept to grasp, partly because of people's misunderstanding of what the term violence implies, as well as because of the language used to describe this behavior. The language issues often derive from a reluctance to expand the meaning of violence to being more than a physical act, or from an erroneous perception that violence does not happen in nursing. Furthermore, when people consider violence, they often ignore the nonphysical aspects, such as the emotional, financial, and psychological harm, that are experienced by many people who are abused.

Another reason violence in nursing is often misunderstood is the lack of an agreed upon definition. One possible reason for this misunderstanding is that other terms such as horizontal violence, lateral violence, bullying, and mobbing are used interchangeably when discussing violence in nursing.

Not having an agreed definition and using different terms to describe violence in nursing often makes meaningful discussion difficult. For example, some authors base their definitions on the context they are studying. One Australian study of nurses' and midwives' experiences of occupational violence and aggression clearly differentiated these two concepts by classifying the patient's behavior as violence and colleagues' behavior as bullying (Farrell & Shafiei, 2012).

One advantage of this broader and expanded view of violence in nursing is that nurses as a whole now have a wider appreciation of this phenomenon. However, it is now apparent that it is not only the targeted person who is affected by these inappropriate behaviors in the workplace but also their colleagues, line managers, bystanders, and other personnel who are required to address these issues in the workplace. Their concerns can potentially also have negative effects on their own work performance, health, and safety.

Discussion Point

What would be the advantages and disadvantages of responding to violent situations as a bystander? Would the "Good Samaritan" rule apply in these situations?

Terminology

Historically, different countries have used different terms to describe this violent behavior. For example, the nursing literature in the United States led the way by referring to this behavior as horizontal violence. Although the term horizontal violence continues to be referred to (Iheduru-Anderson, 2014), it appears to have been overtaken by the use of constructs such as abusive conduct, lateral violence, bullying, and incivility (American Nurses Association [ANA], 2015; Todaro-Franceschi, 2014; Walsh & Magley, 2014).

In Europe, the preferred term has been mobbing, and in the United Kingdom, the literature refers to this behavior as bullying. Although the Australian nursing literature initially used the term horizontal violence or occupational violence in nursing, bullying became the term of choice during the 1990s. However, since then other terms are continually being introduced. In Australia, there is no uniformity in the terminology used in Federal and State legislation. For example, at the state level, in The South Australian Work Health and Safety Act 2012, use of "inappropriate behaviors" has replaced the term "bullying." At the Federal level, the term "bullying" has been used in their amended Fair Work Act to introduce antibullying legislation (Commonwealth Fair Work Amendment Act 2013 [No. 73, 2013]—Schedule 3, 789fd).

The term workplace violence has gradually become the preferred term in many countries, particularly since the release of papers from internationally recognized organizations such as the International Council of Nurses (ICN), the World Health Organization, the Honor Society of Nursing, Sigma Theta Tau International, and the United Kingdom (UK) Royal College of Nursing.

Theory

The theory underpinning violence in nursing has generally received less attention than the practical manifestation of this behavior. One of the earliest references is from Roberts (1983), who, in examining horizontal violence, argued compellingly that some of the salient aspects of nursing subculture and behaviors came within the framework of oppression theory. Since then, different theoretical frameworks have been proposed to explain inappropriate workplace behaviors (for example, Clarke, 2015).

According to Branch, Ramsay, and Barker (2013), "many challenges remain, particularly in relation to its theoretical foundations and efficacy of prevention and management strategies" (p. 280). Theory-based research has the ongoing potential to considerably reduce the amount of violence experienced by nurses by assisting them to develop informed strategies to manage the violent behavior.

RESEARCHING VIOLENCE IN NURSING

An Expanding Global Perspective

In recent years, violence in nursing has been researched from very different geographical locations, for example, the United States (Sharp, 2015), Slovenia (Kvas & Seljak, 2014), and Uganda (Mulago, 2014), to name a few. There continues to be interest in nursing areas such as midwifery (Esfahani & Shahbazi, 2014), mental health (Flannery, Wyshak, & Flannery, 2014), and aged care (Rodwell & Demir, 2014). Research into the incidence and costs of workplace violence experienced by nurses from patients and patient visitors is specifically being explored (Speroni, Fitch, Dawson, Dugan, & Atherton, 2014). Violence in tertiary institutions in student–faculty relationships has also continued to gain interest with a particular focus on incivility in clinical practice (Babenko-Mould & Laschinger, 2014; Opperman, 2014). Recently, there has been a renewed and growing interest in workplace violence within a sexual context and domestic violence (DV) in the workplace.

Consider This Do you consider sexual harassment a workplace violence issue?

NEW PERSPECTIVES: DOMESTIC VIOLENCE IN THE WORKPLACE

DV is a pervasive problem, and yet, there has been limited contemporary research undertaken to explore the impact that it has in the workplace, on nurses, and other health professionals. In addition, persons who identify themselves with the gay, lesbian, bisexual, transsexual, queer, or intersex population, culturally and linguistically diverse communities, and abused men are often reluctant to discuss their experiences.

There is the possibility that some of the DV victims may be a patient or a work colleague. How all nurses react to working and supporting patients/colleagues who are, or have experienced, DV is under-researched. Even less is known about how nurses manage themselves or each other following a DV homicide of a patient or colleague.

Human Rights Response: Domestic Violence

It is a basic human right to work in a safe and healthy workplace, no matter where the person works, the work performed, or the position held. For more than a decade, various researchers have stated that workplace violence is a human rights issue. However, it is not an area that is well recognized as a process to be considered when addressing violence in nursing, particularly DV in the workplace.

In Australia, it was estimated that around one in six female workers has experienced or is currently experiencing violence (Australian Bureau of Statistics, 2005). According to the Australian Human Rights Commission (AHRC), this means that "a significant number of Australian workplaces will be impacted by women's experiences of DV, which can significantly undermine the working lives of both victims and survivors" (AHRC, 2014).

In Australia, "Domestic violence is the leading cause of death and injury in women under 45, with more than one woman murdered by her current or former partner every week... The Easter period marked the deaths of six women and children in a single week" (Malone & Phillips, 2014). These murdered women are of working age, and some could have been nurses.

In the United States, DV became a human rights issue in *Jessica Lenahan (Gonzales) v. United States* through the Inter-American Commission on Human Rights. This was the first case brought by a survivor of DV against the United States before an international human rights tribunal (American Civil Liberties Union, 2014).

Consider This Do you consider DV a workplace violence issue?

TYPES OF VIOLENCE IN NURSING

Nurses experience different forms of violence, often depending on the location, the service provided, and the perpetrator. Moreover, what one person considers as a harmful experience another may not. Therefore, every person's experience with, or perceptions about, violence are unique to that person. However, it is possible to categorize the different types of violence that nurses might experience.

Who are the Victims?

Although the true extent of violence in nursing is considered to be greater than the statistics indicate, studies show that violence against female nurses is greater than that against male nurses. Compared with the experiences of female nurses, there is a dearth of research into male nurses and their experiences. Studies into violence against men in other contexts tend to focus on rites of initiation of apprentices, college fraternity rites of passage (hazing), and armed service "bastardization" practices. However, the question of whether violence against male nurses is an outcome of the same forces identified in studies into violence between female nurses is open to further research. Because the statistics show that men are often the major perpetrators of violence in society and in the workplace (except possibly for internal violence in nursing, that is, violence that comes from within the organization), the very fear that some male nurses may experience violence could also create more violent incidents in the workplace, generating a recurring cycle of violence.

Box 11.1 lists eight basic categories specific to nursing. Boxes 11.2 and 11.3 expand upon the nonphysical and physical aspects of violence in nursing. Box 11.4 lists the potential factors leading to patient–nurse violence, and Box 11.5 lists the signs to look for in aggressive and violent behavior.

Nurses working in different locations and settings could have different issues to address compared with those working in a large metropolitan hospital setting, for example, home nursing, rural and remote nursing, working alone, night duty, and nurse researchers, to name a few (see Box 11.6).

Potential Violence

A violent person can take their aggression out on any objects near at hand. As well as those outlined in

BOX 11.1 Typology of Violence in Nursing

1. Nurse-to-nurse violence (horizontal violence, lateral violence)
2. Patient-to-nurse violence (including visitors)
3. Organization-to-nurse violence (vertical down violence)
4. External perpetrators (strangers, criminal intent)
5. Third-party violence (colleagues/family members and significant others)
6. Impact of mass trauma or natural disasters on nurses (terrorism, wars, earthquakes, tornadoes, tsunamis)
7. Nurse-to-patient violence
8. Personal violence (eg, domestic violence, family violence, interpersonal violence)

BOX 11.2 Types of Nonphysical Violence Involving Nurses

- Being uncivil, such as exhibiting rudeness, impoliteness, and silence
- Condoning improper behavior by being unsupportive and uncooperative
- Setting someone up for failure, imposing ideas, taking someone's ideas, undermining, embarrassing someone
- Exhibiting threatening behavior—making someone feel intimidated, threatened, or fearful
- Spreading rumors, making defamatory online statements, improperly taking credit, assigning blame or fault
- Stalking
- Defaming
- Cyber bullying

BOX 11.3 Types of Physical Violence Involving Nurses (Predominantly by Patients, Families, and Visitors)

Nonphysical

Verbal: For Example

- Swearing
- Yelling
- Shouting
- Making threats
- Calling names

Nonverbal: For Example

- Invading personal space
- Threatening gestures
- Constant eye contact
- Facial features such as scowling, frowning

Physical

- Hitting/punching/pinching/kicking/scratching/spitting
- Combat devices such as walking sticks, knives, knuckle dusters, baseball bats, guns, chemical sprays
- Sexual assault/rape
- Assault
- Homicide

BOX 11.4 Potential Factors Leading to Patient–Nurse Violence

- Negative attitude of staff toward patients
- Certain staff are prone to being assaulted
- Limited time to communicate
- Some nurses appear to have an aggressive approach
- Nurses are increasingly forced to act in controlling ways because of institutional pressures

BOX 11.5 Signs to Look For

Does the patient:

- Indicate a heightened level of anxiety or depression?
- Have hostile or aggressive body language?
- Complain about the provision of services?
- Refuse to cooperate?
- Display suicidal tendencies or cries for help?
- Have rapid breathing, clenched fists/teeth, appear restless, or talk loudly?
- Swear excessively or use sexually explicit language?
- Make verbal threats?
- Show noncompliance with requests?

BOX 11.6 What to Do in Different Contexts

- Policies and procedures should reflect the location and setting nurses work in.
- There are some aspects of a policy that would be the same wherever you may work or live, for example, stay calm and don't panic; if you are unable to remove yourself from the situation, attempt to defuse the situation.
- There may be some aspects that are different, for example if a home/community nurse, leave as quickly as possible—suggest you have something for the client in your car.
- When working alone, have the police/emergency numbers entered on your cell phone speed dial.

Box 11.3, Box 11.7 expands on objects that may be used as potential weapons or become property damage through frustration and aggression.

Discussion Point

Case Study

Two nurses entered a psychiatric patient's room to give the patient medication. They assisted the patient to sit up, and the patient was initially co-operative. Suddenly, the patient punched one of the nurses, then grabbed the nurse's hair. The coworker got the patient to let go of the injured nurse's hair, and the two nurses *then left the patient's room.*

Source: http://www2.worksafebc.com/Publications/Incidents-Topic.asp?ReportID=36693

It is important for nurses to be observant and remain alert, particularly if the patient has a history of violent behavior.

Homicide Statistics in Hospitals

Although homicides and nonfatal assaults are rare, they are not isolated occurrences, and in some instances, for example assaults on health care workers, occur four times more frequently than assaults in the private sector industries (Kelen, Catlett, Kubit, & Yu-Hsiang, 2012). Kelen et al. (2012), in this "groundbreaking" study, investigated 154 hospital-related shootings in 40 US states, in 148 different hospital settings, resulting in 235 injured or dead victims. Box 11.8 shows the locations of the shootings, followed by Boxes 11.9 and 11.10 expanding on the shooters' rationale and victim roles.

The above results show shootings are relatively infrequent compared with the other forms of violence experienced by nurses in the workplace. Nurses can be targeted by perpetrators who often have a grudge, and they in turn become victims themselves (n = 106/45%). From these data, it appears that physicians are more at risk than nurses. A shooting at the Johns Hopkins Hospital in 2010 was reported as follows:

> *A gunman upset over news about his mother's medical condition opened fire inside Baltimore's Johns Hopkins Hospital Thursday morning, wounding a doctor before fatally shooting his mom and then turning the gun on himself* (Freidman, 2010).

BOX 11.7 Potential Weapons/Damaged Property

- Chairs/tables/furniture
- Equipment in treatment rooms, scissors, scalpel, chemicals, and fire extinguishers
- Equipment located in wards (bed pans/urinals/IV stands)
- Equipment that are sharp or blunt
- Telephones, computers

BOX 11.8 The Location Where Shootings Occurred in Hospital Settings

Location	Number, *n* = 154	Percentage
Emergency Dept (ED)	31	20
Non-ED	41	27
Other (eg, pharmacy)	19	12
TOTAL INSIDE	**91**	**59**
Parking lot	35	23
Other	28	18
TOTAL OUTSIDE	**63**	**41**

Source: Kelen, G. D., Catlett, C. L., Kubit, J. G., & Yu-Hsiang, H. (2012). Hospital-based shootings in the United States: 2000 to 2011. *Annals of Emergency Medicine, 60*(6), 790–798.

BOX 11.9 Rationale for Shootings Occurring in Health Care Settings

Rationale for Shooting	Victims, *n* = 235	Percentage
Determined shooter with a grudge or revenge	55	23
Suicide	50	21
Euthanizing an ill relative	33	14
Escape attempt	36	15
Other	61	26

Source: Kelen, G. D., Catlett, C. L., Kubit, J. G., & Yu-Hsiang, H. (2012). Hospital-based shootings in the United States: 2000 to 2011. *Annals of Emergency Medicine, 60*(6), 790–798.

Kelen (2014), at a symposium designed to assist health care providers and staff to better prepare for and react to an "active shooter," stated:

> *If you are a doctor or nurse and there is an armed person firing a weapon on your floor, what should you do if you have patients who can't run, hide or fight? ... The appropriate actions of frontline staff members not trained in law enforcement are undefined.*

In summary, of the 106 perpetrators who died as reported in the Kelen et al. (2012) study, 24 were in the

BOX 11.10 Victims of Shootings Occurring in Health Care Settings

Victims	*N* = 235	Percentage
Physicians	8	3
Nurses	12	5
Pharmacists	4	2
Other	24	10
Total number of hospital employees	**48**	**20**
The perpetrator	106	45
Patients	31	13
Others	50	22
Total number of hospital nonemployees	**187**	**80**

Source: Kelen, G. D., Catlett, C. L., Kubit, J. G., & Yu-Hsiang, H. (2012). Hospital-based shootings in the United States: 2000 to 2011. *Annals of Emergency Medicine, 60*(6), 790–798.

ED, 36 were outside ED, and 46 were in other locations. These horrific events must have had a traumatic effect on all those who were involved or who witnessed these events. Furthermore, to be placed in a situation described by Kelen et al. (2012), creates the potential for long-term health and mental issues, such as posttraumatic stress disorder.

Discussion Point

Do you agree or disagree with the following statement:
Is there a relationship between patients' violent behaviors and the environment they are in?

ADDRESSING VIOLENCE IN NURSING

Violence in nursing is an emotive phenomenon to all involved. It can affect families and other service providers as well as those who are being targeted. Even strangers can be victims of violence in the workplace, often because they are in the wrong place at the wrong time.

However, there is the belief among some nurses that reporting incidents of violent behavior may attract retribution (Franklin & Chadwick, 2013) or will make no difference (Canadian Centre for Occupational Health and Safety, 2014a; Kvas & Seljak, 2014; United States Department of Labor, Occupational Safety & Health Administration, n.d.; Varney, 2014). It is difficult to understand why this view remains despite research, education, legislation, and other strategies that explain and inform nurses that this behavior is not acceptable (Davis, Landon, & Brothers, 2015).

Discussion Point

Should a patient be charged with assault if they threaten and/or cause physical harm to a nurse in the workplace?
Would you feel the same if the perpetrator was one of your colleagues?
Should nurses take civil action against patients or work colleagues that attack them?

Legislative Response

Many countries have legislation that specifically focuses on workplace violence and consider this behavior as an occupational health and safety hazard. Invariably, there is a statutory responsibility to meet standards, provide training and education, as well as requiring reports relating to workplace injuries or deaths.

United States of America

Under the US Occupational Safety and Health Act (1970) (OSH Act), employers are responsible for providing safe and healthful workplaces for their employees. The role of the Occupational Safety and Health Administration (OSHA) is to ensure these conditions for all workers by setting and enforcing standards, as well as providing training, education, and assistance (OSHA, 2004).

The OSHA investigates and reports on events leading to injuries and death. For example, in 2013, "workplace violence, including assaults and suicide accounted for 17 per cent of all work related fatal occupational injuries" (United States Department of Labor, U.S. Bureau of Labor Statistics, 2014). Preliminary 2013 work-related homicides data show that "... The most frequent type of assailant in work-related homicides involving women was a relative or domestic partner" (U.S. Department of Labor, U.S. Bureau of Labor Statistics, 2014). It is not possible to separate how many of these victims are nurses, but the research into violence in nursing would indicate that nurses and/or their coworkers and patients could be victims.

New bills are continually being introduced in various states of the United States to promote antibullying behavior. In 2014, it was reported that "26 [US] states have introduced antibullying bills that seek to prohibit mistreatment in the workplace. None of these bills have yet to be passed" (Melnick, 2014). In January 2015, California Assembly Bill 2053 amended California's mandatory sexual harassment prevention training statute—AB 1825—and requires "prevention of abusive conduct" to be included as a component of the training (California Assembly Bill 2053, n.d.).

Canada

Most of Canada's Occupational Health and Safety (OHS) legislation includes a "general duty provision," which requires employers to take all reasonable precautions for the protection of their employees (Canadian Centre for Occupational Health and Safety, 2014b). Within the Canadian OHS legislation is a due diligence clause, which means "that employers shall take all reasonable precautions, under the particular circumstances, to prevent injuries or accidents in the workplace. This duty also applies to situations that are not addressed elsewhere in the occupational health and safety legislation" (Canadian Centre for Occupational Health & Safety, 2014b).

Australia

Australia has made significant changes to its Federal and State legislation relating to inappropriate workplace behaviors and bullying in recent years. Federal antibullying laws came into effect from 1 January 2014 under the Commonwealth Fair Work Act (2009), which requires that bullying behavior must be repeated over a period of time and that this behavior creates a risk to health and safety to be actionable. The amendments created changes in terminology—"employee" has become "worker." The concept of "worker" has broadened and covers more workplace relationships, such as employees, contractors, subcontractors, volunteers, and students gaining work experience. This group of "workers" will be able to make an application if they consider they are experiencing workplace bullying (Commonwealth Fair Work Amendment Act 2013 [No. 73, 2013]—Schedule 3, 789fd).

Nurses Legislation

Similar to California Nurses Practice Act, in Australia, the Commonwealth Nurses Act gives the Australian Health Professional Registering Agency legislative power for the registration of nurses. In general, a typical registering agency's role is to endorse professional standards and ensure that the highest standards are achieved and maintained. Disciplinary powers can range from requiring mediation and education to addressing the problem (eg, managing aggressiveness), to requiring registration restrictions, and in very severe cases, the power to deregister/revoke license (for example, Australian Health Practitioners Registration Authority, 2014; Texas Board of Nursing, 2014).

Discussion Point

Are registering bodies and statutory legislation an effective approach to addressing violence in nursing?

Discussion Point

Why should professional nursing bodies have a role in addressing violence in nursing and promoting antibullying behavior?

Professional Response

The three main ethical, legal, and human rights principles that apply to nurses are that they (1) should do no harm, (2) have a duty of care to persons in their care, and (3) have the rights to work in a safe and healthy environment. The legal requirements of nurses may vary, but they must consider the consequences of their actions to ensure that they have not breached their legal, ethical, and human rights obligations toward their colleagues as well as to those in their care. For example, from an individual perspective, nurses must be aware of the laws that relate to negligence, defamation, discrimination, assault, and homicide.

Respect for each other is one of the guiding principles of most contemporary codes of ethics. For example, the ICN (2012) Code of Ethics states that "The nurse sustains a collaborative and respectful relationship with co-workers in nursing and other fields; ... The nurse takes appropriate action to support and guide co-workers to advance ethical conduct."

In 2014, the *Blueprint for 21st century Nursing Ethics: Report of the National Nursing Summit* was released. Responding to the outcome of this Summit, in 2015, the American Nurses Association (ANA) celebrated the Year of Ethics by introducing the first revision of the Code of Ethics for Nurses since 2001 (ANA, 2015). The new code consists of nine provisions. Provision 5.4 of the ANA Code of Ethics with interpretive statements states:

> *1.4 Preservation of Integrity*
>
> *Verbal and other forms of abuse by patients, family members, or co-workers are also threats; nurses must be treated with respect and need never tolerate abuse.* (p. 20)

Nurses have an ethical, a legal, and a human right to work in a safe and healthy environment. The conundrum when discussing violence in nursing is society's perception of nurses compared with the reporting of violence in nursing. In 2013, "82 per cent of Americans rated nurses' honesty and ethical standards as 'very high' or 'high,' a full 12 per cent points above any other profession" (ANA, 2014). The perception of nurses in Australia (Roy Morgan Image of Professions Survey, 2014) is similar to that identified in the USA, Canada, and Britain (Angus Reid Public Opinion, 2012).

Discussion Point

1. Is it an ethical dilemma for you if mandatory reporting of inappropriate workplace behaviors was required?
2. Would your opinion change if the perpetrator was a colleague?

Research Study Fuels the Controversy 11.1

What Do Nurses and Midwives Value about Their Jobs?

The aim of this study was to examine nurses' and midwives' (n = 990) preferences for the characteristics of their work. To design effective policies to recruit and retain nurses it was imperative to understand "(i) the range of factors that influence job choices; (ii) which factors are most important and are amenable to policy and (iii) how these factors vary across different types of staff and contexts" (p. 31). The discrete choice experiment method used is a survey-based technique that presents respondents with alternative job packages that vary across job characteristics, and respondents choose the job package they prefer.

Source: Scott, A., Witt, J., Duffield, C., & Kalb, G. (2015, January). What do nurses and midwives value about their jobs? Results from a discrete choice experiment. *Journal Health Services Research Policy, 20*(1), 31–38.

Study Findings

The researchers found evidence that the most highly valued results were autonomy, working hours, and processes to deal with violence and bullying. Results showed that nurses and midwives respectively would be willing to forgo 19% and 16% of their annual income for adequate autonomy and adequate processes to deal with violence and bullying, compared to poor autonomy and poor processes for violence and bullying. They would need to be paid an additional 24% to increase their working hours by 10% ($73 per hour [2008]). Job characteristics that were less important were shift work, nurse-to-patient ratios, and public or private sector work.

It could be anticipated that the violence and bullying nurses are experiencing would be reflected in their patient care. It is well established that workplace violence and bullying has a significant effect on staff morale, and results in greater turnover, less job satisfaction, anxiety, depression, self-harm, suicide, and homicide (see Research Study Fuels the Controversy 11.1).

And yet a Spanish study (Galián-Muñoz, Ruiz-Hernández, Llor-Esteban, & López-García, 2014) reported that the relationship between patient's physical violence and nursing staff burnout had no effects on their job satisfaction. It appears that the profession is able to maintain a strict boundary such that the violence nurses experience is not reflected in their patient care.

Organizational Response

In most advanced societies, organizations have a legal and moral duty of care to their employees. Through OHS legislation, organizations can proactively address violence in nursing through policies and procedures, education, and training, as well as by having an organizational culture that does not condone this behavior.

An Australian study (Farrell, Shafiei, & Chan, 2014) reported that the measures to control risks and to prevent and manage occupational violence showed that there was at times a wide difference between what the respondents considered of highest importance for safe systems to prevent and manage occupational violence and what was offered in the workplace. Twenty-six items were listed in this Australian study (Farrell et al., 2014). Boxes 11.11 and 11.12 summarize the staff's ranking of safety process following patient- and visitor-initiated violence at work and the realities of the organizations.

Discussion Point

What would be your highest and lowest priority in your workplace taking into consideration what is already in place?

Have your current workplace strategies been successful in reducing violent behavior?

Have your current workplace strategies been successful for improving safety in the workplace?

Individual Response

Addressing, preventing, and protecting self and others is as much an individual responsibility as it is an organizational one. An individual responsibility often overlaps with an organizational response. Nevertheless, it is expected that individual nurses are familiar with their legal, ethical, and human rights responsibility as well as the workplace policies and procedures. Novice nurses are at high risk of bullying victimization within 2 years of starting nursing practice (Grubb, Gillespie, Brown, Shay, & Montoya, 2014). Student nurses, for example, may be taken by surprise when a patient

BOX 11.11 Staff's Perception of Top Five Priorities

	High Importance (%)	Present at Workplace (%)
Training and awareness in emergency response procedures	88	85
Appropriate physical environment for safe care	87	83
Appropriate staff skill mix to provide safe care	82	69
Adequate external security lighting	81	72
Effective duress alarm and communication systems	80	68

Source: Farrell, G. A., Shafiei, T., & Chan, S-P. (2014, February). Patient and visitor assault on nurses and midwives: An exploratory study of employer 'protective' factors. *International Journal of Mental Health Nursing, 23*(1), 88–96.

BOX 11.12 Staff's Perception of Lowest Five Priorities

	Lowest Importance (%)	Present at Workplace (%)
Minimal hiding spots	57	42
Personal protective equipment (eg, personal duress alarms)	65	56
Appropriately designed retreat when needed (eg, escape doors)	67	54
24-hour onsite security guards in workplace	64	54
Appropriately located CCTV at entrances/exits, car parks, and other areas	66	51

Source: Farrell, G. A., Shafiei, T., & Chan, S-P. (2014, February). Patient and visitor assault on nurses and midwives: An exploratory study of employer 'protective' factors. *International Journal of Mental Health Nursing, 23*(1), 88–96.

becomes violent. Workplace violence literature shows that education and training, including appropriate communication skills to de-escalate the violent behavior, aggression management skills, and a supportive workplace environment are key factors in minimizing the risk. Box 11.13 lists internal factors to manage violent behavior followed by Boxes 11.14 and 11.15 that expand upon on how to manage these behaviors.

Discussion Point

Does your workplace have a critical incident policy? If not, why not?
Does your workplace conduct critical incident drills and evaluate the responses to identify if policy is still relevant and easy to follow?
If so, what did you learn from this drill?

Reaction to Aggressive Behavior

Nurses and others (coworkers, security staff, cleaners, etc.) who have been involved in a critical incident should be involved in the debriefing exercise. Each person may react differently to a particularly stressful situation. These feelings may range from anger and frustration to anxiety, guilt, or embarrassment. Some may have a physical reaction such as vomiting, sweating, or shaking uncontrollably. Psychological long-term reactions may include sleeplessness, fear of returning to work, and reliving the event. It is important for the individual as well as the organization that these reactions are recognized and managed quickly after the incident to reduce the risk of psychological harm.

Consider This Is there a debriefing process after a critical incident in your workplace?
If so, has it been evaluated for its success or otherwise?

BOX 11.13 Internal Factors

- Reviewing workplace policies and procedures
- Attending education, training, and staff development programs
- Undertaking evaluation of policies and procedures, etc.
- Identifying and initiating research projects

BOX 11.14 Work Practice Strategies

- Ensure that patients with a history and likelihood of violence are identified beforehand with, for example, having a "red flag" in their records.
- Minimize the risk of violence by ensuring that patients are appropriately placed in organizations with experienced and trained staff within those organizations.
- Obtain a current medical report from the referral agency, a general practitioner, psychologist, and/or psychiatrist.
- Each nursing workplace should have their own specific code (eg, Code Black/Blue/Red) that will identify that a person is at risk. Activating this code sets in place an emergency response from a team that has been trained in dealing with these situations.

BOX 11.15 External Factors

- Being aware of relevant legislation, for example, Work, Health & Safety
- Maintaining knowledge of state/province registering body, for example, discipline, complaints, and disciplinary action
- Reviewing literature on policies and procedures relating to aggression/violence—nationally/internationally
- Active member of professional organizations
- Attending conferences, networking

Conclusions

As discussed throughout this chapter, studies have consistently shown that violence in nursing continues to be a major issue within the nursing profession. Studies show that there is a consistency about the prevalence rate of workplace violence. In the past decade there has been a growth in the political, professional, and legislative awareness of workplace violence, particularly in the health sector. This growth has been national and international. The whole phenomenon has become a part of everyday discourse. Social media has played a role in modern society, providing greater opportunities for public awareness while at the same time offering a platform for bullying behavior.

There has been a growing interest in violence in nursing as researchers have become increasingly aware that this phenomenon is not only an individual or organizational problem but also a public health and human rights issue. Although many changes have been made to minimize this unconscionable behavior in the health care culture and environment, much more work is needed. Current evidence continues to highlight the need for more research and a better understanding of the strategies required to address violence in nursing.

Recent research has added to the violence in nursing debate proposing if certain behaviors should be considered workplace violence issues. Two examples are sexual violence (Strauss, 2014) and DV. In many countries, sexual violence, which may be an umbrella term to cover sexual harassment/sexual assault/sexual abuse including rape, has been addressed with legislation and in some instances by a criminal code. Therefore, it could be debated if this behavior should be included in violence in the workplace. There has also been increasing interest in the transition of violent behavior from the home into the workplace including specifically DV, family violence, and more generally interpersonal violence. Future areas for research could be to study how and to what extent patient care is influenced by the violence nurses experience in the workplace as well as the impact of terrorism and other extremely violent incidents in health care institutions and agencies. It is vital not only to have a better understanding of this phenomenon but also how to be prepared for violent situations.

For Additional Discussion

1. What are the behavioral differences between workplace bullying, a "personality clash," and a workplace conflict of interest?
2. Can workplace bullying occur on one occasion?
3. Should there be a clear distinction made between the terms and outcomes of workplace bullying, horizontal violence, mobbing, and workplace violence when developing policies and procedures?
4. Is it possible to reach a zero violence culture within nursing?
5. Should risk management strategies relating to inappropriate behaviors in the workplace be included in student nurses curriculum?
6. Why is it necessary to have specific antibullying legislation when there is current occupational health and safety legislation and civil and criminal laws already in place?
7. How do you prevent the "code of silence" by nursing staff after an aggressive incident?
8. Do you consider the employee assistance programs the appropriate strategy in lieu of an internal debriefing session?
9. Is there a time when violent behavior is acceptable in the workplace?
10. Should nurses be trained to use taser guns in a workplace environment?
11. Should nurses be trained to use guns in a workplace environment?

References

American Civil Liberties Union. (2014). *Jessica Gonzales v. U.S.A.* Retrieved December 11, 2014, from https://www.aclu.org/human-rights-womens-rights/jessica-gonzales-v-usa

American Nurses Association. (2014). *Nurses retain top spot as most ethical.* Retrieved December 4, 2014, from http://www.theamericannurse.org/index.php/2014/03/03/nurses-retain-top-spot-as-most-ethical/

American Nurses Association. (2015). *Code of ethics for nurses with interpretive statements.* Retrieved January 17, 2015, from http://www.nursingworld.org/MainMenuCategories/EthicsStandards/CodeofEthicsforNurses/Code-of-Ethics-For-Nurses.html

Angus Reid Public Opinion. (2012). *Nurses, doctors are most respected jobs in Canada, U.S. and Britain.* Retrieved November 5, 2014, from http://www.angusreidglobal.com/wp-content/uploads/2012/09/2012.10.02_Professions.pdf

Australian Bureau of Statistics. (2005). *4906.0—Personal safety, Australia, 2005 (Reissue).* Retrieved December 9, 2014, from www.abs.gov.au/AUSSTATS/abs@.nsf/Lookup/4906.0Main+Features12005%20(Reissue)?OpenDocument

Australian Health Practitioners Registration Authority. (2014). *Tribunal reprimands, disqualifies nurse and cancels registration.* Retrieved December 11, 2014, from http://www.ahpra.gov.au/News/2014-12-01-media-release.aspx

Australian Human Rights Commission. (2014). *Fact sheet: Domestic and family violence—A workplace issue, a discrimination issue.* Retrieved December 9, 2014, from https://www.humanrights.gov.au/publications/fact-sheet-domestic-and-family-violence-workplace-issue-discrimination-issue

Babenko-Mould, Y., & Laschinger, H. K. S. (2014, October). Effects of incivility in clinical practice settings on nursing student burnout. *International Journal of Nursing Education Scholarship, 11*(1), 145–154.

Branch, S., Ramsay, S., & Barker, M. (2013). Workplace bullying, mobbing and general harassment: A review. *International Journal of Management Reviews, 15*, 280–299.

California Assembly Bill 2053. (n.d.). *Bill analysis.* Retrieved December 11, 2014, from http://www.leginfo.ca.gov/pub/13-14/bill/asm/ab_2051-2100/ab_2053_cfa_20140509_113346_asm_floor.html

Canadian Centre for Occupational Health & Safety. (2014a). *Bullying is not a part of the job.* Retrieved November 30, 2014, from http://www.ccohs.ca/products/posters/bullying.html

Canadian Centre for Occupational Health & Safety. (2014b). *Violence in the workplace.* Retrieved December 2, 2014, from http://www.ccohs.ca/oshanswers/psychosocial/violence.html#_1_8

Clarke, P. N. (2015). Nursing science: An answer to lateral violence? *Nursing Science Quarterly, 28*(1), 34–35.

Commonwealth Fair Work Act. (2009). Retrieved September 19, 2015, from http://www.austlii.edu.au/au/legis/cth/consol_act/fwa2009114/

Commonwealth Fair Work Amendment Act 2013 (No. 73, 2013)—Schedule 3, 789fd. Retrieved November 7, 2014, from http://www.austlii.edu.au/au/legis/cth/num_act/fwaa2013194/sch3.html

Davis, C., Landon, D., & Brothers, K. (2015). Safety alert: Protecting yourself and others from violence. *Nursing, 45*(1), 55–59.

Esfahani, A. N., & Shahbazi, G. (2014, July–August). Workplace bullying in nursing: The case of Azerbaijan province, Iran. *Iranian Journal of Nursing & Midwifery Research, 19*(4), 409–415.

Farrell, G. A., & Shafiei, T. (2012). Workplace aggression, including bullying in nursing and midwifery: A descriptive survey (the SWAB study). *International Journal of Nursing Studies, 49*(11), 1423–1431.

Farrell, G. A., Shafiei, T., & Chan. S-P. (2014, February). Patient and visitor assault on nurses and midwives: An exploratory study of employer 'protective' factors. *International Journal of Mental Health Nursing, 23*(1), 88–96.

Flannery, R. B., Jr., Wyshak, G., & Flannery, G. J. (2014, December). Characteristics of international staff victims of psychiatric patient assaults: Review of published findings, 2000–2012. *Psychiatric Quarterly, 85*(4), 397–404.

Franklin, N., & Chadwick, S. (2013, October). The impact of workplace bullying in nursing. *Australasian College of Health Service Management Member e-newsletter.* Retrieved December 1, 2014, from http://www.achsm.org.au/about-us/e-newsletter/1-October-2013---Member-enewsletter.html

Freidman, E. (2010, September 10). Johns Hopkins hospital: Gunman shoots doctor, then kills self and mother. *ABC News.* Retrieved December 10, 2014, from http://abcnews.go.com/US/shooting-inside-baltimores-johns-hopkins-hospital/story?id=11654462

Galián-Muñoz, I., Ruiz-Hernández, J. A., Llor-Esteban, B., & López-García, C. (2014). User violence and nursing staff burnout: The modulating role of job satisfaction [published online ahead of print on November 11, 2014]. *Journal Interpersonal Violence.* pii:0886260514555367.

Grubb, P., Gillespie, G., Brown, K., Shay, A., & Montoya, K. (2014). *Qualitative evaluation of a role play bullying simulation.* Presented at the Fourth International Conference on violence in the health sector: Towards safety, security and wellbeing for all, Miami, FL.

Iheduru-Anderson, K. (2014, July). Educating senior nursing students to stop lateral violence in nursing. *Australian Nursing & Midwifery Journal, 22*(1), 15.

International Council of Nurses. (2012). *The ICN Code of ethics for nurses.* Retrieved December 2, 2014, from http://www.icn.ch/images/stories/documents/about/icncode_english.pdf

Kelen, G. D., Catlett, C. L., Kubit, J. G., & Yu-Hsiang, H. (2012). Hospital-based shootings in the United States: 2000 to 2011. *Annals of Emergency Medicine, 60*(6), 790–798.

Kelen, G. D. (2014, March 6). *Johns Hopkins to host national symposium on hospital shootings.* University News, Health, Politics+Society. Retrieved January 19, 2015, from http://hub.jhu.edu/2014/03/06/active-shooter-in-hospital-settings-symposium

Kvas, A., & Seljak, J. (2014). Unreported workplace violence in nursing. *International Nursing Review, 61*(3), 344-351.

Malone, U., & Phillips, J. (2014, 6 May). Domestic violence of epidemic proportions a 'national emergency': Campaign groups. *ABC News.* Retrieved November 28, 2014, from http://www.abc.net.au/news/2014-05-05/domestic-violence-reaches-epidemic-proportions/5426214

Melnick, R. (2014, August 13). Understanding workplace-bullying legislation. *Employment & Labor Relations Law.* Retrieved September 19, 2015 from http://apps.americanbar.org/litigation/committees/employment/articles/summer2014-0814-understanding-workplace-bullying-legislation.html

Mulago, M. M. (2014). *Safety and security in Africa.* Presented at the Fourth International Conference on violence in the health sector: Towards safety, security and wellbeing for all, Miami, FL.

Occupational Safety and Health Act. (1970). Retrieved September 19, 2015 from http://www.dol.gov/compliance/laws/comp-osha.htm

Occupational Safety and Health Administration. (2004). *Guidelines for preventing workplace violence for health care & social service workers*. Retrieved December 4, 2014, from http://www.osha.gov/Publications/osha3148.pdf

Opperman, C. (2014). *The pebble effect: Stopping incivility in clinical environments*. Sigma Theta Tau International Research Congress, Hong Kong, July 24–28. Retrieved December 4, 2014, from http://www.nursinglibrary.org/vhl/handle/10755/335145

Roberts, S. (1983). Oppressed group behavior: Implications for nursing. *Advances in Nursing Science, 5*(4), 21–30.

Rodwell, J., & Demir, D. (2014, March). Addressing workplace violence among nurses who care for the elderly. *Journal of Nursing Administration, 44*(3), 152–157.

Roy Morgan Image of Professions Survey 2014—Nurses still most highly regarded—Followed by doctors, pharmacists & high court judges. (2014). Retrieved November 30, 2014, from http://www.roymorgan.com/findings/5531-image-of-professions-2014-201404110537

Sharp, M. T. (2015, February). Workplace violence: Assessing risk, promoting safety. *Nursing Made Incredibly Easy*! *13*(1), 42–49.

Speroni, K., Fitch, T., Dawson, E., Dugan, L., & Atherton, M. (2014). Incidence and cost of nurse workplace violence perpetrated by hospital patients or patient visitors. *Journal of Emergency Nursing, 40*(3), 218–228.

Strauss, S. (2014). Is it bullying or sexual harassment. *Minnesota Women's Press*. Retrieved November 11, 2014, from http://www.womenspress.com/main.asp?SectionID=2&SubSectionID=692&ArticleID=4118

Texas Board of Nursing. (2014). *Notice of disciplinary action*. Retrieved December 11, 2014, from https://www.bon.state.tx.us/discipline_and_complaints_disciplinary_action_042014.asp

Todaro-Franceschi, V. (2014, July). Are you being bullied or are you a bully? *New Jersey Nurse, 44*(3), 6.

United States Department of Labor, Occupational Health & Safety Administration. (n.d). *Safety & health topics*. Retrieved November 30, 2014, from https://www.osha.gov/SLTC/workplaceviolence/index.html

United States Department of Labor, U.S. Bureau of Labor Statistics. (2014). *Workplace injury, illness and fatality statistics*. Retrieved December 10, 2014, from https://www.osha.gov/oshstats/work.html

Varney, J. (2014). Nurses believe speaking up about workplace violence will make no difference. *Nursing Standard, 29*(5), 17.

Walsh, B. M., & Magley, V. J. (2014). An empirical investigation of the relationship among forms of workplace mistreatment. *Violence and Victims, 29*(2), 363–379.

Work Health and Safety Act 2012 (SA). Retrieved December 8, 2014, from http://www.legislation.sa.gov.au/LZ/C/A/WORK%20HEALTH%20AND%20SAFETY%20ACT%202012/CURRENT/2012.40.UN.PDF

12

The Use of Social Media in Nursing
Pitfalls and Opportunities

Perry M. Gee[1]

ADDITIONAL RESOURCES

Visit thePoint for additional helpful resources
- eBook
- Journal Articles
- WebLinks

CHAPTER OUTLINE

LEARNING OBJECTIVES

The learner will be able to:

1. Define social media and social networking.
2. Identify the different types of software platforms used for social media.
3. Analyze how social media can be effectively used by the professional nurse.
4. Explore how patients and caregivers are using social media for self-management support of illness.
5. Identify the challenges nurses may encounter when using social media.
6. Review the standards and guidelines for safe and effective use of social media by the registered nurse.

[1] I would like to acknowledge Idaho State University nursing career path intern Samantha Fullmer for her assistance in researching references to support this chapter.

INTRODUCTION

What an exciting time to be a nurse! Health care in America is changing—with the Affordable Care Act, the Institute of Medicine's Future of Nursing Report, state action coalitions, patient-centered care, and the *democratization* of health information and knowledge, the nurses role is evolving. At the center of this nursing evolution is social media. *Social media* is a method for nurses to share and transmit information as well as knowledge to a far-reaching audience; *social networking* is the process of engaging with that audience using social media. This chapter will focus on the nurses' role with both social media and social networking in practice, administration, education, research, as well as consumers who are using the tools for self-management support and health promotion.

Among all health care consumers and caregivers (including nurses), the use of social media is rapidly on the rise (Box 12.1). Social media is becoming ubiquitous in society and certainly among patients, caregivers, and their health care provider teams. Nurses who are interacting with patients are encountering social media every day and the nurses' understanding of this phenomenon is imperative for patient teaching and the promotion of health. In fact, social media is starting to play a central role in patient engagement and has potential to improve health outcomes. Patients are using social media to learn about health conditions and treatments, to connect with other patients, to update family members and caregivers, and to communicate with members of the health care team.

Consider This Social media has tremendous power. Many political analysts attribute the success of the 2011 Egyptian Revolution to the use of Facebook and Twitter by the citizens of Egypt.

Nurses are becoming very savvy users of social media for (1) enhancing their own knowledge; (2) affecting health care policy; (3) promoting of causes and to raising money; (4) staying connected to other nurses; (5) participating in professional organizations; (6) informing patients, caregivers, and the public; (7) communicating with patients and colleagues; (8) research; and just to relax and have fun. This chapter will explore the important role of social media for nursing, both now and in the future, and then provide some tools for nurses to successfully navigate this exciting new technology. We will also discuss some of the pitfalls of social media and how the nurses can protect themselves from the drawbacks of participating in this vast new environment. We will begin this chapter with an overview of the different types of social media.

Discussion Point

Are there appropriate times for the nurse to use social media in the clinical setting?

TYPES OF SOCIAL MEDIA AND HOW IT CAN BE USED FOR NURSING

Social media is currently made up of several kinds of software platforms. Each platform has unique strengths and it is not unusual to combine different platform types into one social media experience. For instance, a single site may contain both social networking and sharing of media (photos, videos, etc.). Let us now identify the most often used forms of social media.

BOX 12.1 Social Media Use 2014

- Multiplatform use is on the rise: 52% of online adults now use two or more social media sites, a significant increase from 2013, when it stood at 42% of Internet users.
- For the first time, more than half of all online adults 65 and older (56%) use Facebook. This represents 31% of all seniors.
- For the first time, roughly half of Internet-using young adults ages 18 to 29 (53%) use Instagram. And half of all Instagram users (49%) use the site daily.
- For the first time, the share of Internet users with college educations using LinkedIn reached 50%.
- Women dominate Pinterest: 42% of online women now use the platform, compared with 13% of online men.

Source: Duggan, M., Ellison, N. B., Lampe, C., Lenhart, A., & Madden, M. (2015). *Social media update 2014: While Facebook remains the most popular site, other platforms see higher rates of growth.* Washington, DC: Pew Internet & American Life Project.

Social Networks

Social networks are supported by software that allows individuals to connect and share with others. Social networks can take several forms and the focus can range from personal relationships to professional relationships and everything in-between. Other names sometimes used for social networks are virtual networks, virtual communities, or online communities, Note the use of the term "community"; this social media platform gives others access to communities or groups of people outside their geographic boundaries. This access may promote engagement with a nurse in a rural area who wants to have a relationship with other nurses who have similar interests. These online communities may also provide a supportive environment for a person with a chronic illness who can learn about self-care management activities.

The most used social network is Facebook. Facebook currently has over 1.4 billion active users worldwide. Close to a billion people log into Facebook every day! Even without access to a personal computer, people worldwide use Facebook every day using mobile smartphones. A smartphone or mobile phone is a cellular telephone with expanded capabilities like email, calendar functions, and access to the Internet using browser software. People in very remote parts of the earth are using smartphones for networking, accessing health care information, and social networking on sites like Facebook or Instagram. People with similar interests can use Facebook *groups* or *pages* to communicate and engage with peers. There are currently over 620 million individual groups on Facebook and many of those groups are devoted to nursing interests or health care.

To illustrate, nurses in the most remote counties in far Northern California have developed a group to network and stay connected to the current issues in nursing care using a Facebook group. This group was easy to develop taking 5 minutes or less to build. The group is free to join and members were invited by word of mouth and through email. As of today the group is very active and has over 400 members. Members of the Northern California Professional Nurse Network (www.Facebook.com/groups/101668026599850/) have used the group to find jobs, to get advice on furthering education, to share best practice, and to promote community health initiatives. Most nursing organizations have groups or pages in Facebook to communicate and share information with members and people who are interested in the groups. To illustrate, simply check out the American Association of Critical-Care Nurses page at www.Facebook.com/aacnface.

Social networking groups in Facebook can be open to the public or "closed" and only open by invitation. The regulation and access to these groups is controlled by the group or page administrator through settings in the software application. Patients or health care consumers also use social networking groups in Facebook. For example, www.Facebook.com/groups/100425715503/ is a Facebook group where caregivers of children with severe food allergies and asthma can go to get health information that may impact their children. Social networking is one of the most powerful and used components of social media and can be an important for the professional nurse and the patient.

Discussion Point

It is common for nursing students to set up private Facebook groups for discussion of school-related issues. If negative postings appear in the group about curriculum, faculty, or clinical sites, what can be done to keep the discussion from getting out-of-hand or inappropriate?

Social Bookmarking Sites

Bookmarking sites are a way nurses can search, organize, individualize, and comment with lists of Internet bookmarks or links to Web pages of interest. There are several popular social bookmarking sites including Digg.com, Reddit, and Stumbleupon. Stumbleupon has a great listing of pages organized for nursing (www.stumbleupon.com/interest/nursing). Individuals can go to social bookmarking sites and comment on individual links and even critique a site. This may provide a valuable tool for nurses to rapidly find sites important to their areas of interest or the needs of their patients.

Social News

Similar to social bookmarking, *Social news* has links to news links on the Internet that is organized, posted, and voted upon with the most popular news links appearing at the top of the list. The social news site Reddit (www.reddit.com/) helps users find top relevant news articles in nursing by going to the site and performing a search on the word "nursing." Conducting this type of search yields top news storied voted to be of interest to nursing. Social news sites are another good method for nurses to rapidly stay apprised to what is happening in the world of nursing and health care.

Media Sharing

Media Sharing is a software platform where users can share photos and/or videos and these sites may also have user profiles and other social components. YouTube is the most used form of media sharing. In addition to sharing videos, users can log in, comment, or vote on the videos and see a profile of the person who posted the video. YouTube has over one billion users and every day hundreds of millions of videos are uploaded to YouTube. There are thousands of good videos related to nursing and health care on YouTube that are free to view and provide a great opportunity for educating nurses. For example, the nurse educator Michael Linares has a YouTube channel (www.YouTube.com/results?search_query=simple+nursing) called Simple Nursing where there are dozens of educational videos geared for nursing students as well as seasoned nurses who need a refresher on nearly any clinical topic. Nurse educators can create videos related to any subject area, upload that video to YouTube, and send a link to student who can access the video from any computer or smartphone worldwide. Nurses may also want to take advantage of these educational videos when illustrating treatments or procedures to patients and/or their caregivers. Media sharing is a great way to stay current in nursing and to visually share knowledge with others.

Discussion Point

What is the responsibility of the nurse who observes a YouTube or other media-sharing site that contains a video of a nursing procedure that would be considered unsafe or even potentially dangerous to patients?

Microblogging

Microblogging is a social media platform where users can post short comments and links to their "wall" and where others can view or follow the comments. Twitter (Twitter.com) is far and away the most popular microblogging site on the Internet. There are over 600 million Twitter users worldwide and people send out over 58 million "Tweets" (comments on Twitter) every day. Thousands of nurses have Twitter accounts and so do schools of nursing, nursing organizations, hospitals, governmental health organizations, and patients. Twitter users Tweet out messages that are limited to 140 characters or less. In addition to messages, users can send out photos, links to websites, and links to other media like videos. Users have a Twitter "handle" or name that starts with the @ symbol. For example, the nursing school at John Hopkins has a handle of @JHUNursing. Hashtags are used in microblogs like Twitter to bring conversations about the same topic together so people can view the topics and compare ideas. A hashtag is preceded by the pound "#" sign and the word or phrases are listed without spaces following this symbol. So if one wanted to start a conversation about homecare nursing, a hashtag "#homecarenursing" could be created to keep the conversation together in one easily searched location. A search using #homecarenursing in the media sharing/microblogging site Instagram yields a list of images related to homecare nursing posted by others who used the same hashtag.

Virtual Worlds

Virtual worlds are computer-generated simulated settings where the user can manipulate the elements of the environment and interact in the environment using an avatar. Users may be able to interact with others in the environment, learn in the environment, and even purchase goods and services in the environment. Nursing has successfully used virtual worlds to educate nursing students in public health and even a simulated birthing center. The University of Delaware has the Te Wāhi Whānau—the birth place in SecondLife, which is an example of a virtual setting where nurses can simulate a training experience working as a nurse in a birthing center. A movie of this virtual center can be seen at http://youtu.be/Kw-KL-lCesE.

Wikis

A *Wiki* allows multiple users to post Internet-based content, modify content, and create online communities. The largest and most popular Wiki is of course Wikipedia (www.wikipedia.org). Wikipedia is essentially a Web-based encyclopedia that is dynamic and has an open structure that can be authored or corrected by users. Wikihealth.com is a wiki site devoted to health care and wellness issues and might be a good site for nurses and patients to access when looking for health resources. While there is excellent content throughout

Wikipedia, due to its open-source nature, the nurse must carefully evaluate the clinical and evidence-based content to assure its accuracy and currency.

Blogs

Blogs or (Weblogs) are a place where individuals can write comments or forums about the topic of their choice. Typically users are focused on one specific topic area, for example, public health nursing. Blogs may also promote discussion or engagement and can be developed for free using many software platforms; WordPress is one example (wordpress.org). There are many excellent nursing blogs where professionals may go and observe and interact with nurses who choose to post comments.

A well-known and award-winning nursing blog is RTConnections (blog.rtconnections.com/). Dr. Renee Thompson has developed a blog devoted to professional nursing subjects and highlights current and future nursing issues. She is especially passionate about the problem of nurse bullying and frequently "blogs" about solutions for this troublesome condition. Keith Carson is another well-known nurse blogger. He is the co-host of RN.FM Radio, which is an online radio station devoted to the field of nursing and Nurse Keith has a blog called the Digital Doorway where he posts comments weekly about issues important to the nursing profession (digitaldoorway.blogspot.com/).

Consider This Blogging can be an easy, immediate, and free way for nurses to share their important messages. The most popular blog in the world, The Huffington Post, receives over 110 million visits per month! Consider setting up your own free blog today, for example, www.blog.com, www.blogger.com, or others.

SOCIAL MEDIA USE BY PATIENTS (HOW NURSES CAN SUPPORT PATIENTS)

Like nurses health care consumers (patients and/or caregivers) are rapidly adopting social media. With all the different types of social media available to patients, Nyongesa, Munguti, Omondi, and Mokua (2014) suggest that there is an opportunity for nurses to provide guidance. When nurses have a strong understanding of the social media tools available, they can then educate patients and caregivers in their selection and use. For instance, a new model for chronic illness self-managed support has been developed utilizing social media and other eHealth tools. The Enhanced Chronic Care Model (eCCM) augments the traditional supportive "community" for a person with chronic illness by providing an "eCommunity" or online community using social networking (Gee, Greenwood, Paterniti, Ward, & Miller, in press). The eCCM also promotes the role of nurses and providers in helping patients choose a social network and to train them on effective participation in the group that will help promote self-management goals.

Patients are already quite active using technology for self-management support, and in fact about 80% of adults have sought health information on the Internet, including 62% of adults with a chronic illness. Of that group, 75% of those who have chronic illness and who were surveyed stated that their most recent Internet encounter affected decisions about the self-management of their condition (Fox, 2006, 2007; Fox & Purchell, 2010). Patients are already seeking and sharing health information on the Internet through blogs, wikis, microblogging, media sharing, and through social networking.

The Rise of the e-Patient

There is a new and powerful movement of engaged patients using social media to seek care and help others with their illness. People who are empowered, engaged, educated, and informed are sometimes known as *e-Patients* (Gee et al., 2012). E-patients are consumers of health care or providers of care for those who are ill and who actively use social media to (1) seek out the most current evidence for care; (2) engage others who are ill or caregivers of the ill for care advice and knowledge; and (3) use the *collaborative wisdom* provided by a social network of others who are also ill (Gee et al., 2012; Greenwood, 2015). E-patients are expert at using social media to manage complex health conditions and nurses can learn from their success (Fox, 2008). With both patients and providers using social media, the opportunity exists to better coordinate care and collaborate together using the collective wisdom of both the provider world and the patient community (Gee et al., 2012; Timimi, 2013). At this time most of the research related to patients using social media has been descriptive and there have only been a small number of randomized controlled trials (Hamm et al., 2013). The opportunity exists for more rigorous research and for research focusing on health outcomes (Korda & Itani, 2013).

Consider This The most notable and arguably the leader of the e-patient movement is Mr. Dave deBonkart a.k.a. "e-Patient Dave." Mr. deBonkart travels the world speaking at health care–related conferences advocating for the role of the e-patient. Watch a TED talk delivered by e-Patient Dave—keep a hanky handy—www.ted.com/talks/dave_debronkart_meet_e_patient_dave.

Facebook has been used extensively by patients wanting to connect with others for help, advice, and social support. For instance, people with diabetes are using the Facebook platform for asking questions about their condition, the sharing of information, and for other health promotion activities (Greene, Choudhry, Kilabuk, & Shrank, 2011). The informed e-patient may arrive at the health care setting with substantial knowledge about their own health condition, possibly even more than the nurse or other members of the provider team. The challenge for the nurse is to find a way to evaluate the e-patient's knowledge and then to work together as a proactive team member with the patient to meet the individual's health care goals.

Given the propensity of adolescents and young adults to use social media, greater opportunities exist for health care professionals to use these sites to educate the e-patients of the future. Research by Yonker, Zan, Scirica, Jethwani, and Kinane (2015) supports this idea (Research Study Fuels the Controversy 12.1).

Virtual Health Communities That Are Consumer Centered

Many patients all over the world are using social media, specifically social networking in the form of a virtual online community, to find information and support for their health conditions. Many people with rare diseases have historically been isolated and have had very limited access to pertinent health information. Now, these same people with rare conditions can find support for their disorders using social media. To illustrate, a site devoted to the parents of children with clubfoot can seek information and communicate with the parents and caregivers of children who have the same condition (Oprescu, Campo, Lowe, Andsager, & Morcuende, 2013). In a similar situation, people with primary biliary cirrhosis can find self-management information and social support from others with the same disease at a site (pbcers.org/) devoted to that rare condition (Lasker, Sogolow, & Sharim, 2005).

Research Study Fuels the Controversy 12.1

Social Media and Health Care for Adolescents and Young Adults

Adolescents and younger adults are the most active groups of social media users. This group of individuals is also the fastest adopters of wireless and mobile technologies, for example, mobile or smartphones. This is also a time in a person's life when many life-long health habits are formulated. Social media may have an impact on the health choices of the adolescent or younger adult. This study was a systematic review of the social media literature related to positive health outcomes among adolescents and younger adults.

Source: Yonker, L. M., Zan, S., Scirica, C. V., Jethwani, K., & Kinane, T. B. (2015). "Friending" teens: Systematic review of social media in adolescent and young adult health care. *Journal of Medical Internet Research, 17*(1), e4. doi:10.2196/jmir:3692

Study Findings

This systematic review focused on the social media and adolescent health papers published between 2002 and 2013. The authors used keywords related to social media, health, and adolescents/young adults. Because they found so few studies related to adolescents under the age of 18 in their first pass with the literature, they included the young adult group (18 to 25 year old) to obtain a larger number of results. Ultimately they identified 87 articles that met their inclusion criteria and found that 75 were observational and only 12 were interventional studies. The common health problems studied in this group of papers were sexual behaviors, alcohol tobacco or drug use, mental health issues, and general health. Overall, the papers focused on how young people use social media and less on how social media can affect health. These findings identified a significant need for more focused studies on health and social media and highlighted the importance of using sound methodologies in conducting such research. Opportunities exist for high-quality nursing research for this important group of social media users.

Britt Johnson a.k.a. the "@HurtBlogger" who at the young age of 29 has lived for 22 years in chronic pain has a website and blog devoted to those living with chronic pain (www.thehurtblogger.com). Britt recently used microblogging (Twitter) to complete what she called the *#ChronicLife* experiment where she tweeted her feelings, pain level, self-management activities, diet, sleep, and other activities of daily living for 48 hours to raise awareness of what it is like to live with chronic pain. People with diabetes who speak either English or Spanish language are using discussions in the online community *TuDiabetes* (http://www.tudiabetes.org/) to track adverse events with blood glucose monitoring equipment (Mandl et al., 2014). Members of that same diabetes online community have also successfully used the social networking site for the self-surveillance of hypoglycemia among members of the group (Weitzman, Kelemen, Quinn, Eggleston, & Mandl, 2013). In their recent paper, Betton and Tomlinson (2013) found that people with mental illness can feel less isolated and provide peer support for one another with the use of social networking for engagement. There is no end to the types of health conditions or demographic makeup of people who can be helped with virtual health communities.

Discussion Point

Is there a role for the professional registered nurse in virtual health communities or would nursing involvement in the group change the dynamics? What about the nurse who is also a patient and wants to join a virtual health community? What should we disclose?

Patients are also participating in research regarding their condition using social media. The social networking site *PatientsLikeMe* (www.patientslikeme.com) is a location where patients and caregivers can join groups of others with their same conditions. The community also ranks the best treatments for specific conditions and allows users to participate in research about things like symptom management should they choose to partake. The *Society of Participatory Medicine* (participatorymedicine.org) is a place where patients, providers, and health researchers can come together using social media to explore treatment options and support health conditions using the collective wisdom of the group.

The Nurse's Role

To help patients traverse the world of these new Web-based platforms, nurses can become familiar with some of the major social media outlets for patients and steer them to those resources. Nurses should develop the skills to educate patients and caregivers on the use of social media. Nurses ought to routinely assess and see if their patients are good candidates for using social media to support their conditions, then develop an education plan around these assessment findings (Box 12.2).

Nurses must also consider if their patients have access to broadband technologies that support the social media tools being discussed. A *digital divide* is the situation where consumers do not have access to the Internet or social media tools. The older adult, the poor, the rural, and some underrepresented groups have less access to the broadband Internet technology and have fewer computers in their homes (Chou, Hunt, Beckjord, Moser, & Hesse, 2009). People who live in rural areas make up the majority of those who have not accessed the Internet for the past year. Additionally the majority

BOX 12.2 Potential Patient Education Topics Related to Social Media

- The pros and cons of using social media
- How to choose an appropriate social media for specific health conditions
- The type of hardware, software, and networking needed to participate in social media
- How to join a social network
- How to navigate the individual sites
- How to maintain one's privacy on social media
- How to verify if information is credible
- How to protect one's self from scams
- How to formulate a message in a blog or microblog
- How to ask for help from an online community

of Americans who do not use or have access to the Internet live in rural areas or on American Indian lands (Stenberg et al., 2009).

Discussion Point

Should nurses routinely include assessment of social media use and broadband Internet access when taking a history and physical? Should the homecare nurse be trained to do basic troubleshooting with a patient's home networking equipment?

Consider This Nurses are excellent at troubleshooting very complicated and potentially life-threatening health care–related technologies, for example, IV pumps, cardiac and hemodynamic monitors, defibrillators, pacemakers, etc. Should registered nurses be trained to troubleshoot basic home-networking and broadband systems used in the patient's home?

Cell phones, smartphones, tablet computers, and other mobile devices are ways individuals affected by a digital divide are gaining access to the Internet and the health care system. In fact nearly six out of every seven of the inhabitants of the planet Earth have a cellular or mobile phone (PricewaterhouseCoopers, 2012). Homes where the incomes are less than $30,000 a year have the same smartphone adoption rate as the general population (Smith, 2011). African and Hispanic Americans have the highest rate of adoption of smartphone users. Forty four percent of African and Hispanic American adults have adopted smartphones as compared to only 30% among Caucasians (Schroeder, Hix, Dean, Fiordelisi, & Thorpe, 2011; Smith, 2011). These numbers show it is possible to provide mobile access to social media even though patients may not have home computers with traditional Internet access. Older Americans are also adopting mobile technologies at a rapid pace. Nearly 70% of those over age 65 now use a cell phone and this number is up 12% since the year 2010 (Zickuhr & Madden, 2012). Nurses should advocate for broadband or Internet access for their patients and make it part of the assessment process to evaluate Web access and individuals ability to obtain these services.

PITFALLS OF SOCIAL MEDIA AND NURSING

Social media may prove to be a major factor in encouraging patient engagement and in improving health care. However, social media can also be unpredictable, dangerous, and harmful. As nurses we must advocate and protect our patients as they use social media. As professionals it is imperative for registered nurses to follow ethical and professional standards as we use this new media platform.

Social media can literally expose nurses and/or their patients to access of billions of individuals on the Internet. And while this open access may offer endless opportunities, it can also open people to serious breaches in privacy and exposure to Internet predators and criminals who take advantage of users of the medium. One problem with social media is the environment allows users to remain anonymous (Korda & Itani, 2013). The nurse or patient may believe they are interacting with a highly trained professional or a caring friend and find the individuals are not who they say they are. Patients may encounter a social media environment that reports to offer a "cure" for their conditions and nurses may find a group of "experts" who claim to have new standards for nursing care; social media sites need to be carefully analyzed to determine if they are legitimate. This analysis may be an excellent opportunity for the professional nurse to act in an advocacy and education role for their patients.

Nurses from students to veteran professionals have been negatively impacted by the interaction with social media. Many times the nurse has just unintentionally revealed personally identifiable patient information or revealed patient information in an environment they believed was safe and private. The privacy laws of the Health Insurance Portability and Accountability Act (HIPAA) equally apply to the world of social media. As a case in point, a young nursing student was being romantically pursued by one of her patients in the hospital. Later in the shift the patient was discharged and somehow managed to pass a note expressing his affections to the student. Disturbed by the letter the student wanted to share the note with her classmates in a "private" social media platform. The student scanned a digital image of the note and posted the document to the group; unfortunately, the image of the note also contained the patient's full name. Within hours of the image being posted in the "private" Web location it somehow ended up on a public Facebook page where the patient saw the note and reported the HIPAA infraction to the hospital. The hospital, nursing school, and individual nursing student all suffered serious consequences because of this unintentional breach by the student. This story highlights many concerns with social media starting first with the notion that just because something says it is private does not mean it will remain private. **As a rule**, assume anything you post in social media can and will be viewed by all. This is an especially important rule for the nurse to follow.

Discussion Point

What should the nurse do if they witness a posting with patient identifiable information on a social media site? What if they live in a different community or even state?

Nurses can face personal liability for inappropriate use of social media. In fact according to the National Council of State Boards of Nursing (NCSBN) the majority of states have sanctioned registered nurses due to complaints of social media abuse (National Council of State Boards of Nursing, 2011). The majority of the infractions are due to nurses violating privacy laws and exposing identifiable patient information. The NCSBN has been working with the American Nurses Association and developed a comprehensive whitepaper highlighting the appropriate and inappropriate use of social media by the professional nurse (www.ncsbn.org/Social_Media.pdf) (Boxes 12.3 and 12.4).

The literature suggests avoiding the invitation of patients to be "friends" in social media sites. And while some health care providers are known to interact with patients using social media, the standard practice at this time is to keep personal and professional use of

BOX 12.3 National Council of State Boards of Nursing Implications for Inappropriate Use of Social Media

Instances of inappropriate use of social and electronic media may be reported to the Board of Nursing (BON). The laws outlining the basis for disciplinary action by a BON vary between jurisdictions. Depending on the laws of a jurisdiction, a BON may investigate reports of inappropriate disclosures on social media by a nurse on the grounds of:

- Unprofessional conduct
- Unethical conduct
- Moral turpitude
- Mismanagement of patient records
- Revealing a privileged communication
- Breach of confidentiality

If the allegations are found to be true, the nurse may face disciplinary action by the BON, including a reprimand or sanction, assessment of a monetary fine, or temporary or permanent loss of licensure.

Source: National Council of State Boards of Nursing. (2011). *White paper: A nurse's guide to the use of social media*. Chicago, IL: Author.

BOX 12.4 American Nurses Association's Principles for Social Networking

1. Nurses must not transmit or place online individually identifiable patient information.
2. Nurses must observe ethically prescribed professional patient—nurse boundaries.
3. Nurses should understand that patients, colleagues, institutions, and employers may view postings.
4. Nurses should take advantage of privacy settings and seek to separate personal and professional information online.
5. Nurses should bring content that could harm a patient's privacy, rights, or welfare to the attention of appropriate authorities.
6. Nurses should participate in developing institutional policies governing online conduct.

Source: American Nurses Association. (2011). ANA's *principles for social networking and the nurse*. Silver Spring, MD: Author.

these platforms separated by clear boundaries (Barry & Hardiker, 2012). Rubolino-Gallego, Hedden, and Gonzolez (2012) recommend that nurse practitioners resist the temptation to accept patients as "friends" on social media sites. They also note that social media is a forum where dissatisfied or even only disappointed patients may harm the practitioner's reputation; this damage may be difficult or even impossible to correct. Patients may use social media to give the nurse practitioner bad scores for quality or care, length of the visit, cleanliness of the office, friendliness of the office staff, and even what the nurse is wearing. One disgruntled patient can use social media to cause significant damage to the nurse's reputation of ability to recruit new patients. This concern holds true for health care businesses or even hospitals. It is prudent for practitioners and health care businesses to routinely examine their Web presence for negative comments from customers.

Discussion Point

Is there ever a time the nurse or other health care provider would want to be social media "friends" with one or more of their patients?

Consider This Some nurse entrepreneurs successfully use social media to stay connected with their patients and inform them of the latest treatments and services available. Consider a nurse-run laser and skin rejuvenation clinic "The Disappearing Act" that uses a Facebook page to apprise clients of the latest advancements and upcoming events www.facebook.com/Disappearing.Act.Laser.

Nurse leaders with a high local or national profile need to realize that participation in social media may be great for the promotion of a cause; however, it may also open the individual to personal scrutiny. Recently the nurse leader of a large health care professional organization was viciously and personally attacked for several days in the microblog *Twitter* for a personal photo that was found on a public social media site. The photo was of the professionally dressed and physically fit nurse leader holding a cake that had been presented at a party. This photo was then attached to a tweet and exposed to the Internet to degrade the leader and identify the leader as a hypocrite who was promoting unhealthy eating. The innocent photo caused several days of grief and inhibited the nurse leader from promoting the intended national health agenda. Nurse leaders who use social media on a large scale may need to develop a "thick skin" and prepare to occasionally be attacked using the Internet platform (Marshall, 2015).

More and more employers are looking at social media as part of the hiring process. In a survey completed in 2009, 45% of employers were using social media sites to screen for potential employees (Haefner, 2009). For nursing leadership positions, using the Internet is commonplace for human resource specialists, recruiters, or hiring managers to review a candidate's profile in the social media professional site *LinkedIn* (www.LinkedIn.com). The professional registered nurse will want to carefully use online platforms and consider steps to evaluate and tidy up their current social media presence. Strategies for keeping a positive social media image and avoiding problems with social media are shown in Boxes 12.5 and 12.6.

SOCIAL MEDIA IN PROFESSIONAL NURSING PRACTICE

While the social media environment does contain some risks, carefully utilized Web-based platforms can potentially enhance practice, education, and research. Nurses will need to carefully consider their use of social media as a tool and develop knowledge and expertise in its implementation.

Social Media in Nursing Practice

Clinically practicing nurses need to be familiar with these new media so they can incorporate these tools into their practice. In public and population health, social media has a strong presence in surveillance of disease. Public health experts have used social media and an analysis of the content of consumer's messages in social networking and blogs to identify the rising incidence in diabetes (Eggleston & Weitzman, 2014). At an even more detailed level, algorithms have been developed and used to identify the differences between "chatter" about the flu and actual incidence of the flu (Broniatowski, Paul, & Dredze, 2013). Both Google and the CDC evaluate Internet searches and social media comments to accurately track to detect outbreaks and incidence of the flu at state and national levels (www.google.org/flutrends/us/#US).

BOX 12.5 Keeping a Positive Social Media Image

Five tips for nurse job seekers to keep a positive image online:

1. **Clean up digital dirt before you begin your job search.** Remove any photos, content, and links that can work against you in an employer's eyes.
2. **Consider creating your own professional group** on sites like Facebook or BrightFuse.com. It's a great way to establish relationships with leaders, recruiters, and potential referrals.
3. **Keep gripes offline.** Keep the content you post focused on positive things, whether it's related to professional or personal information. Make sure to highlight specific accomplishments inside and outside of work.
4. **Be selective about whom you accept as friends.** Don't forget others can see your friends when they search for you. Monitor comments made by others and consider using the "block comments" feature. Even better, set your profile to "private" so only designated friends can view it.
5. **If you're still employed, don't mention your job search** in your Tweets or status updates. There are multiple examples of people who have gotten fired as a result of doing this. In addition, a potential employer might assume that if you're willing to search for a new job on your current company's time, why wouldn't you do so on theirs?

Source: Haefner, R. (2009). *More employers screening candidates via social networking sites: Five tips for creating a positive online image.* Retrieved February 1, 2015, from http://www.careerbuilder.com/Article/CB-1337-Interview-Tips-More-Employers-Screening-Candidates-via-Social-Networking-Sites/

BOX 12.6 How to Avoid Problems Using Social Media

It is important to recognize that instances of inappropriate use of social media can and do occur, but with awareness and caution, nurses can avoid inadvertently disclosing confidential or private information about patients. The following guidelines are intended to minimize the risks of using social media:

- First and foremost, nurses must recognize that they have an ethical and legal obligation to maintain patient privacy and confidentiality at all times.
- Nurses are strictly prohibited from transmitting by way of any electronic media any patient-related image. In addition, nurses are restricted from transmitting any information that may be reasonably anticipated to violate patient rights to confidentiality or privacy, or otherwise degrade or embarrass the patient.
- Do not share, post, or otherwise disseminate any information, including images, about a patient or information gained in the nurse–patient relationship with anyone unless there is a patient care related need to disclose the information or other legal obligation to do so.
- Do not identify patients by name or post or publish information that may lead to the identification of a patient. Limiting access to postings through privacy settings is not sufficient to ensure privacy.
- Do not refer to patients in a disparaging manner, even if the patient is not identified.
- Do not take photos or videos of patients on personal devices, including cell phones. Follow employer policies for taking photographs or video of patients for treatment or other legitimate purposes using employer-provided devices.
- Maintain professional boundaries in the use of electronic media. Like in-person relationships, the nurse has the obligation to establish, communicate, and enforce professional boundaries with patients in the online environment. Use caution when having online social contact with patients or former patients. Online contact with patients or former patients blurs the distinction between a professional and personal relationship. The fact that a patient may initiate contact with the nurse does not permit the nurse to engage in a personal relationship with the patient.
- Consult employer policies or an appropriate leader within the organization for guidance regarding work-related postings.
- Promptly report any identified breach of confidentiality or privacy.
- Be aware of and comply with employer policies regarding use of employer-owned computers, cameras, and other electronic devices and use of personal devices in the workplace.
- Do not make disparaging remarks about employers or coworkers. Do not make threatening, harassing, profane, obscene, sexually explicit, racially derogatory, homophobic, or other offensive comments.
- Do not post content or otherwise speak on behalf of the employer unless authorized to do so and follow all applicable policies of the employer.

Source: National Council of State Boards of Nursing. (2011). *White paper: A nurse's guide to the use of social media.* Chicago, IL:Author.

In addition to surveillance, nurses can use social media to promote self-management for patients with chronic illness. For instance, a person with hypertension can be steered to a social network to meet others with high blood pressure for social support on the self-management of their condition. An online health community has been shown to increase empowerment, self-management, and social support among chronically ill adults (Barak, Boniel-Nissim, & Suler, 2008; Shaw & Johnson, 2011; van Uden-Kraan, Drossaert, Taal, Seydel, & van de Laar, 2009). The opportunity exists for nurses working with patients and caregivers of people with chronic illness to guide them in using social media for engagement and support. Nurses who work with those with chronic illness may want to begin to explore health issue–specific social media resources, evaluate the offerings, catalog a list of resources, and make those resources available to patients.

Discussion Point

If the nurse were asked by a patient or caregiver "what would be some good social media resources" for the person with a specific condition, where would the nurse go to find these tools?

To help the nurse who is new to using social media, the American Nurses Association (2011) maintains a Web site that is a *Social Networking Principles Took Kit* where one can find a variety of resources for the registered nurse (www.nursingworld.org/socialnetworkingtoolkit.aspx). Nurses who are part of the policy development process in their organization may want to inform themselves on social media issues and generate unit-based or facility policies to guide nurses new to the organization.

Social Media in Nursing Education

Social media provides an excellent platform for training nurses, patients, and other providers (Lipp, Davis, Peter, & Davies, 2014). Nurses in the large academic medical center or in the very remote part of the country can have access to the exact same clinical reference materials. For the practicing clinical nurse there are thousands of videos devoted to nursing skills and the management of illness. Nurse educators can use YouTube to store and distribute videos to students or the nursing profession in general. Nurse educators can explore the available videos for a specific skill or management of a particular condition and share that content with students without having to take the time to research and develop the content. Students can learn from a variety of nurses and see care accomplished using a range of different methods. One caution, faculty and educators need to carefully review the available audio and video contents to be sure the materials are safe, appropriate, and evidenced based.

Faculty or nurse researchers can use the free online media tool SurveyMonkey (www.surveymonkey.com/) for education in the classroom, scheduling of meetings, or obtaining survey results (Drake & Leander, 2013). Faculty or their nurse educators can use microblogging hashtags to keep topics grouped and organize their online classroom content (Schmitt, Sims-Giddens, & Booth, 2012). Social media tools like blogs, microblogs, and virtual worlds offer a wide variety of methods for students to interact with their local cohort or with students literally anywhere on the planet.

Consider This Social media is a way to be "present" and even participate at a professional conference or symposium without even attending. During the 2013 Stanford MedicineX conference that is devoted to patients, providers and researchers who are interested in technology, social media, and health promotion; 3,576 individual conference participants sent out nearly 8,900 Tweets (microblogs) per day and totaled over 27,000 conversations for the entire conference. The Tweets were real-time informing interested persons all over the globe (medicinex.stanford.edu).

Social Media in Nursing Research

To date, there has been paucity of significant research in social media and nursing. The opportunity exists to examine how these new technologies can be used to augment health care, professional nursing, and how nurses can support patients and their use of social media (Grajales, Sheps, Ho, Novak-Lauscher, & Eysenbach, 2014). Chretien and Kind (2013) suggest that the use of social media by nurses can help facilitate a faster transition of research evidence into clinical practice. We are starting to see patients participating in the research process using social media with the surveillance of hypoglycemia among members of an online community and with research available to members of the site patientslikeme (Weitzman et al., 2013). And last, social media sites afford the nurse researcher opportunities to connect with colleagues with similar nursing research interests using sites like ResearchGate (www.researchgate.net/home.Home.html) where scientists can share ideas and research literature.

Conclusions

If properly harnessed, social media is a powerful tool for professional nursing practice and patient support. Nurses need to add an understanding of these new Web-based platforms to their knowledge base and nursing education is duty-bound to deliberately add social media all levels of curriculum. As part of the patient advocate role, nurses must learn these tools and be prepared to guide patients who are new to social media and those who are experienced in using these platforms. We can also keep in mind that millions of health care consumers and/or their caregivers are already using social media effectively, and as nurses we can take this occasion to learn about this dynamic platform from our patients. We must also note that an opportunity exists for nurses to conduct research with all forms of social media and that we can use this platform to rapidly disseminate new evidence to the nursing domain.

Social media does come with inherent risks for both nurses and patients. Nurses must review the ANA *Scope and Standards of Practice* (www.nursingworld.org/scopeandstandardsofpractice) and *Code of Ethics for Nurses* (www.nursingworld.org/codeofethics) resources and critically apply this content to the use of social media; the rules are the same; however, the reach and magnitude of the consequences of poor decisions are greatly amplified. Social media comes with pitfalls and opportunities for both nurses and patients. Now is the opportunity for nursing to embrace this new and exciting platform and use the social media tools to improve our profession and the health of our communities.

For Additional Discussion

1. What are three components of social media, and how can they be used by the professional nurse?
2. How might social media be used to promote major nursing initiatives, for example, *IOM: Future of Nursing* recommendations? Give some examples.
3. How do the HIPAA requirements apply to the various types of social media? Are there differences in the legal consequences for a social media breach of confidentiality?
4. What are some examples of using social media for the person with a chronic illness? What is the nurses' role?
5. What is the digital divide and how can we as nurses assess the impact of the digital divide related to social media use by our patients?
6. Can you describe two resources available for nurses to explore when considering the implementation of social media projects or interventions?
7. As our population ages what are some considerations for social media use with the older adult?

References

American Nurses Association. (2011). *ANA's principles for social networking and the nurse.* Silver Spring, MD: American Nurses Association.

Barak, A., Boniel-Nissim, M., & Suler, J. (2008). Fostering empowerment in online support groups. *Computers in Human Behavior, 24*(5), 1867–1883.

Barry, J., & Hardiker, N. R. (2012). Advancing nursing practice through social media: A global perspective. *Online Journal of Issues in Nursing, 17*(3), 1–11.

Betton, V., & Tomlinson, V. (2013). *Benefits of social media for nurses and service users.* Retrieved February 1, 2015, from http://www.nursingtimes.net/nursing-practice/specialisms/educators/benefits-of-social-media-for-nurses-and-service-users/5060041.article

Broniatowski, D. A., Paul, M. J., & Dredze, M. (2013). National and local influenza surveillance through Twitter: An analysis of the 2012–2013 influenza epidemic. *PLoS One, 8*(12), e83672. doi:10.1371/journal.pone.0083672

Chou, W. Y., Hunt, Y. M., Beckjord, E. B., Moser, R. P., & Hesse, B. W. (2009). Social media use in the

United States: Implications for health communication. *Journal of Medical Internet Research, 11*(4), e48. doi:10.2196/jmir.1249

Chretien, K. C., & Kind, T. (2013). Social media and clinical care: Ethical, professional, and social implications. *Circulation, 127*(13), 1413–1421. doi:10.1161/CIRCULATIONAHA.112.128017

Drake, M. A., & Leander, S. A. (2013). Nursing students and Ning: Using social networking to teach public health/community nursing in 11 baccalaureate nursing programs. *Nursing Education Perspectives, 34*(4), 270–272.

Eggleston, E. M., & Weitzman, E. R. (2014). Innovative uses of electronic health records and social media for public health surveillance. *Current Diabetes Reports, 14*(3), 468. doi:10.1007/s11892-013-0468-7

Fox, S. (2006). *Online health search 2006.* Washington, DC: Pew Internet & American Life Project.

Fox, S. (2007). *E-patients with a disability or chronic disease.* Washington, DC: Pew Internet & American Life Project.

Fox, S. (2008). *The engaged e-patient population: People turn to the Internet for health information when the stakes are high and the connection fast.* Washington, DC: Pew Research Center.

Fox, S., & Purchell, K. (2010). *Chronic disease and the Internet.* Washington, DC: Pew Internet & American Life Project.

Gee, P. M., Greenwood, D. A., Kim, K. K., Perez, S. L., Staggers, N., & Devon, H. A. (2012). Exploration of the e-patient phenomenon in nursing informatics. *Nursing Outlook, 60*(4), e9–e16. doi:10.1016/j.outlook.2011.11.005

Gee, P. M., Greenwood, D. A., Paterniti, D. A., Ward, D., & Miller, L. M. S. (in press). The e-health enhanced chronic care model: A theory derivation approach. *Journal of Medical Internet Research, 17*(4), e86. doi:10.2196/jmir.4067

Grajales, F. J., III, Sheps, S., Ho, K., Novak-Lauscher, H., & Eysenbach, G. (2014). Social media: A review and tutorial of applications in medicine and health care. *Journal of Medical Internet Research, 16*(2), e13. doi:10.2196/jmir.2912

Greene, J. A., Choudhry, N. K., Kilabuk, E., & Shrank, W. H. (2011). Online social networking by patients with diabetes: A qualitative evaluation of communication with Facebook. *Journal of General Internal Medicine, 26*(3), 287–292. doi:10.1007/s11606-010-1526-3

Greenwood, D. A. (2015). *Collaborative wisdom: Remote monitoring technology facilitates e-patient and diabetes educator engagement.* Paper presented at the American Telemedicine Association 20th Annual Meeting, Los Angeles, CA.

Haefner, R. (2009). *More employers screening candidates via social networking sites: Five tips for creating a positive online image.* Retrieved September 5, 2015, from http://advice.careerbuilder.com/?q=More+employers+screening+candidates+via+social+networking+sites%3A+Five+tips

Hamm, M. P., Chisholm, A., Shulhan, J., Milne, A., Scott, S. D., Given, L. M., & Hartling, L. (2013). Social media use among patients and caregivers: a scoping review. *BMJ Open, 3*(5). doi:10.1136/bmjopen-2013-002819

Korda, H., & Itani, Z. (2013). Harnessing social media for health promotion and behavior change. *Health Promotion Practice, 14*(1), 15–23. doi:10.1177/1524839911405850

Lasker, J. N., Sogolow, E. D., & Sharim, R. R. (2005). The role of an online community for people with a rare disease: Content analysis of messages posted on a primary biliary cirrhosis mailinglist. *Journal of Medical Internet Research, 7*(1), e10. doi:10.2196/jmir.7.1.e10

Lipp, A., Davis, R. E., Peter, R., & Davies, J. S. (2014). The use of social media among health care professionals within an online postgraduate diabetes diploma course. *Practical Diabetes, 31*(1), 14a–17a.

Mandl, K. D., McNabb, M., Marks, N., Weitzman, E. R., Kelemen, S., Eggleston, E. M., & Quinn, M. (2014). Participatory surveillance of diabetes device safety: A social media-based complement to traditional FDA reporting. *Journal of the American Medical Informatics Association, 21*(4), 687–691. doi:10.1136/amiajnl-2013-002127

Marshall, K. (2015). *Embrace your online nemesis.* Retrieved from Vitae, The Chronicle of Higher Education Website: https://chroniclevitae.com/news/895-embrace-your-online-nemesis?cid=VTEVPMSED1

National Council of State Boards of Nursing. (2011). *White paper: A nurse's guide to the use of social media.* Chicago, IL: Author.

Nyongesa, H., Munguti, C., Omondi, C., & Mokua, W. (2014). Harnessing the power of social media in optimizing health outcomes. *The Pan African Medical Journal, 18,* 290. doi:10.11604/pamj.2014.18.290.4634

Oprescu, F., Campo, S., Lowe, J., Andsager, J., & Morcuende, J. A. (2013). Online information exchanges for parents of children with a rare health condition: Key findings from an online support community. *Journal of Medical Internet Research, 15*(1), e16. doi:10.2196/jmir.2423

PricewaterhouseCoopers. (2012). *Emerging mHealth: Paths for growth*. New York, NY: Author.

Rubolino-Gallego, M., Hedden, A. Z., & Gonzolez, S. (2012). *Social media for NPs & PAs*. Retrieved February 1, 2015, from http://nurse-practitioners-and-physician-assistants.advanceweb.com/Columns/Career-Coach/Social-media-for-NPs-PAs-Approach-with-caution-2.aspx

Schmitt, T. L., Sims-Giddens, S. S., & Booth, R. G. (2012). Social media use in nursing. *The Online Journal of Issues in Nursing, 17*(3), 1–13. doi:10.3912/OJIN.Vol17No03Man02

Schroeder, D. G., Hix, B., Dean, D., Fiordelisi, V., & Thorpe, K. (2011). *Improving the health of Hispanics using mobile technology: A roadmap to reach and impact America's fastest growing population*. Roswell, GA: HolaDoctor & 3CInteractive.

Shaw, R. J., & Johnson, C. M. (2011). Health information seeking and social media use on the Internet among people with diabetes. *Online Journal of Public Health Informatics, 3*(1). doi:10.5210/ojphi.v3i1.3561

Smith, A. (2011). *35% of American adults own a smartphone*. Washington, DC: Pew Internet & American Life Project.

Stenberg, P., Morehart, M., Vogel, S., Cromartie, J., Breneman, V., & Brown, D. (2009). *Broadband Internet's value for rural America (Economic Research Service, Trans.)*. Washington, DC: United States Department of Agriculture.

Timimi, F. K. (2013). The shape of digital engagement: Health care and social media. *The Journal of Ambulatory Care Management, 36*(3), 187–192. doi:10.1097/JAC.0b013e3182965512

van Uden-Kraan, C. F., Drossaert, C. H., Taal, E., Seydel, E. R., & van de Laar, M. A. (2009). Participation in online patient support groups endorses patients' empowerment. *Patient Education and Counseling, 74*(1), 61–69. doi:10.1016/j.pec.2008.07.044

Weitzman, E. R., Kelemen, S., Quinn, M., Eggleston, E. M., & Mandl, K. D. (2013). Participatory surveillance of hypoglycemia and harms in an online social network. *JAMA Internal Medicine, 173*(5), 345–351. doi:10.1001/jamainternmed.2013.2512

Yonker, L. M., Zan, S., Scirica, C. V., Jethwani, K., & Kinane, T. B. (2015). "Friending" teens: Systematic review of social media in adolescent and young adult health care. *Journal of Medical Internet Research, 17*(1), e4. doi:10.2196/jmir:3692

Zickuhr, K., & Madden, M. (2012). *Older adults and Internet use: For the first time, half of adults ages 65 and older are online*. Washington, DC: Pew Internet & American Life Project.

13

Medical Errors
An Ongoing Threat to Quality Health Care

Carol J. Huston

ADDITIONAL RESOURCES

Visit thePoint for additional helpful resources
- eBook
- Journal Articles
- WebLinks

CHAPTER OUTLINE

LEARNING OBJECTIVES

The learner will be able to:

1. Differentiate among the terms medical error, medication error, and adverse event.
2. Describe highly publicized patient cases from the mid- to the late 1990s as well as seminal research studies that brought national attention to the problem of medical errors in the United States.
3. Identify current research studies examining the scope, common causes, and financial/human costs of medical errors in the United States.
4. Summarize key findings of the 1999 Institute of Medicine (IOM) report *To Err Is Human*, as well as the multipronged approach identified by the IOM to address the problem of medical errors in the United States.
5. Identify national committees and groups formed as a result of governmental or legislative intervention to address the problem of medical errors.
6. Describe the intent and impact of Medicare's Pay for Performance initiatives, as well as Medicare's 2008 decision to no longer reimburse health care providers for care needed as the result of "never events" or other preventable errors.

(continues on page 180)

7. Differentiate between workplaces that emphasize a "culture of blame" and those that seek to provide a "just culture" or a "culture of safety management."
8. Identify the meaning of a six-sigma error failure rate and determine how error rates in health care compare with other industries such as banking and the airlines.
9. Analyze the effect of the medical liability system on systematic efforts to uncover and learn from mistakes that are made in health care.
10. Differentiate among the three evidence-based standards identified by Leapfrog as having the greatest potential to reduce medical errors: computerized physician order entry, evidence-based hospital referral (EHR), and intensive care unit (ICU) physician staffing.
11. Track current federal and state legislative efforts that encourage the voluntary reporting of health care errors by affording confidentiality protections for such reports.
12. Review current research to determine whether organizational, governmental, and national efforts to reduce the incidence of medical errors in the United States have resulted in desired outcomes.
13. Reflect on the likelihood that he or she would self-report his or her medical errors to his or her employer, as well as to the involved patients and families.

INTRODUCTION

Quality health care has emerged as a critically important yet underachieved goal in the United States. Among the most significant threats to achieving quality health care are the scope and prevalence of medical errors. Indeed, preventable medical errors are now the third highest cause of death in the United States—following heart disease and cancer, claiming the lives of 400,000 Americans every year (Bramhall, 2015).

Indeed, Kliff (2015) points out that medical errors kill more people than car crashes or new disease outbreaks. They also kill more people annually than breast cancer, AIDS, plane crashes, or drug overdoses. "Those left dead as a result of their medical care could fill an average-sized Major League Baseball stadium—sometimes twice over" (Kliff, 2015, p. 2). Kliff goes on to note that "something like 2 to 3 percent of people who go into the hospital are going to have some pretty severe harm as a result" and that "Australian studies suggest the rate might be as high as 12 percent. The harder you look, and the more you study the issue, the more errors you find" (p. 2).

Consider This In Minnesota alone, in 2014, 98 patients were seriously injured and another 13 patients died as a result of medical errors. Falls, pressure ulcers, and wrong-site surgeries declined, but other errors increased, including incorrectly placed catheters and feeding tubes. On 20 occasions, facilities lost irreplaceable patient lab specimens including colon polyps, placentas, and gall bladders (Benson, 2015).

Surprisingly though, the problem of medical errors did not receive nationwide attention in the United States until several highly publicized cases between the late 1990s and early 2000s. One such case involved Betsy Lehman, a *Boston Globe* reporter who died following chemotherapy administration errors. The news media jumped on the story because it demonstrated repeated widespread communication and dispensing errors, despite multiple safeguards in place to keep them from happening.

Libby Zion's case occurred about this same time. Zion, an 18-year-old, died 8 hours after entering a New York emergency department with seemingly minor complaints of fever and earache. Her death from drug interactions brought attention both to the all-too-narrow range between effective and toxic doses of some drugs and the danger of drug–drug interactions, even when all drugs are administered in doses that are considered safe when administered individually. The case also brought attention to the lack of supervision of residents and interns in the United States, as well as the excessive work hours forced on them and the errors that occur as a result.

There was also the story of Willie King, a diabetic man from Tampa, Florida, who had the wrong leg amputated. This case, which became known as the "wrong leg" case, captured the collective dread of wrong-site surgery, but it is a medical error that occurs too frequently as a result of the symmetry of the human body.

Finally, there was the story of Lewis Blackman, a healthy, gifted 15-year-old, who slowly bled to death after undergoing a minor surgical procedure at a major university medical center. Despite multiple warning signs, those caring for him repeatedly missed signs and symptoms that he was bleeding internally from a perforated ulcer.

Discussion Point

Do you believe that the public considers itself to be at risk for harm when receiving health care? Do you personally know someone who has been harmed by a medical error?

Perhaps, it was the clustering of these high-profile cases that made Americans stop and look at the problem of medical errors, or maybe it was just time to do so. The result was that an unprecedented number of seminal research studies delving into medical errors were undertaken over the past 15 to 20 years to discover how many errors were occurring, what was causing them, and what their financial and human costs were.

The results have been disconcerting, to say the least. Most studies have highlighted multiple concerns about quality of care, including high rates of provider-induced injury, unnecessary care, and inappropriate care. Many studies found the number of errors in health care to be unacceptably high. The seminal study of this time, *To Err Is Human*, published in 1999 by the Institute of Medicine (IOM), a congressionally chartered independent organization, provided evidence that the public was highly vulnerable to human error in US health care institutions, an arena in which many thought they were safe.

In addition, unlike most health care research, which generally receives little if any national press, medical error research findings in the late 1990s were published and analyzed in almost every media forum in the country. Consumers were barraged with study findings suggesting that the quality of health care was inadequate and that medical errors were a significant problem leading to increased morbidity and mortality.

Discussion Point

Do you believe that the quality of health care has declined in the last few decades, or is it simply better monitored and more openly reported today?

As a result, consumers, providers, and legislators stepped forward to voice their concerns and to demand, at minimum, a safer health care system. The government listened and directed providers to reexamine how quality health care was provided, measured, and monitored so that cultures of safety could be developed in all health care organizations.

This chapter examines seminal and current research on medical errors, medication errors, and adverse events, as well as the directives that emerged as a result of their findings. Mechanisms for achieving four goals put forth by the IOM as part of *To Err Is Human* are identified. Finally, strategies for creating a culture of safety management in health care are identified, as are the challenges of changing a system that all too often focuses on individual errors rather than on the need to make system-wide changes.

DEFINING TERMS: MEDICAL ERRORS, MEDICATION ERRORS, AND ADVERSE EVENTS

In reviewing the literature on medical errors, medication errors, and adverse events in health care, it is helpful to first define common terms. *Medical errors* are defined by the *Encyclopedia of Surgery* (2015) as adverse events that could be prevented given the current state of medical knowledge. In addition, the Quality Interagency Coordination Task Force (QuIC) suggests that medical errors are "the failure of a planned action to be completed as intended or the use of a wrong plan to achieve an aim. Errors can include problems in practice, products, procedures, and systems" (Encyclopedia of Surgery, 2015, para. 3).

Medication errors are the most common type of medical error and are a significant cause of preventable adverse events. *Medication errors* are defined by the National Coordinating Council for Medication Error Reporting and Prevention (NCC MERP) as follows:

> *Any preventable event that may cause or lead to inappropriate medication use or patient harm while the medication is in the control of the health care professional, patient, or consumer. Such events may be related to professional practice, health care products, procedures, and systems, including prescribing; order communication; product labeling, packaging, and nomenclature; compounding; dispensing; distribution; administration; education; monitoring; and use.* (NCC MERP, 2015, para. 1)

Finally, *adverse events* are defined as adverse changes in health that occur as a result of treatment. When medications are involved, these are known as *adverse drug events.*

SEMINAL RESEARCH ON MEDICAL ERRORS: 1990 TO 2000

The last decade of the 20th century was marked by a rapid increase in research on medical errors. One of the earliest large-scale studies suggesting that medical errors were a significant problem in health care was published by Brennan et al. (1991) in *The New England Journal of Medicine*. This benchmark study involved more than 30,000 hospitalized patients in New York State. Nearly 5 of every 100 patients suffered an adverse event caused by a medical error of omission or commission. Of these adverse events, approximately one in four involved negligence. The overwhelming majority of iatrogenic occurrences, however, resulted from organization, system, or process failures. This study, extrapolated to the national population, suggested that 1.3 million people were injured each year in hospitals; of that number, 180,000 would die from those injuries. Providing additional cause for alarm, the report suggested that most of those injuries were actually preventable.

Leape et al. (1991) also reported that drug complications represented 19% of these adverse events and that 45% of these adverse events were caused by medical errors. In this study, 30% of the individuals with drug-related injuries died.

In another study, Leape (1994) reported that the average intensive care unit (ICU) patient experienced almost two errors per day. One of five of these errors was potentially serious or fatal. In fact, this translates into a level of proficiency of approximately 99%, which seems reasonable. However, if performance levels of 99.9%—substantially better than those found in the ICU by Leape—were applied to the airline and banking industries, it would equate to two dangerous landings per day at Chicago's O'Hare International Airport, or 32,000 checks deducted hourly from the wrong account (Leape, 1994).

> **Consider This** The safety record in health care is a far cry from the enviable record of the similarly complex aviation industry.

Another seminal study in the late 1990s involving medical errors was completed by Thomas et al. (1999). Their research, based on a chart review of 14,732 medical records from 28 hospitals in Colorado and Utah, found that 265 of 459 (57%) adverse events were preventable. The total cost of adverse events was US$661,889,000, with preventable adverse events costing an additional US$308,382,000. In addition, the study estimated the national costs of all preventable adverse events to be just under US$17 billion (in 1996 dollars).

A more recent study by Van Den Bos et al. (2011) suggests these costs were relatively unchanged a decade later with the annual cost of measurable medical errors that harm patients being US$17.1 billion in 2008. Similarly, Mallow, Pandya, Horblyuk, and Haplan (2013), using 2009 data from the Premier Hospital Database, found there were 3,466,596 total inpatient visits in 2009. Of these, 1,230,836 (36%) occurred in people aged ≥65. The prevalence rate was 49 medical errors per 1,000 inpatient visits in the general cohort and 79 medical errors per 1,000 inpatient visits for the elderly cohort. The top 10 medical errors accounted for more than 80% of the total in the general cohort and the 65+ cohort. The most costly medical error for the general population was postoperative infection ($569,287,000). Pressure ulcers were most costly ($347,166,257) in the elderly population.

To Err Is Human

Many of the studies done in the 1990s laid the foundation for what is perhaps the best known and largest study ever done on the quality of health care: *To Err Is Human* (Kohn, Corrigan, & Donaldson, 2000). This report, which represented a compilation of more than 30 studies completed by the IOM, found the following:

- At least 44,000 Americans die each year as a result of medical errors, and the number may be as high as 98,000.
- Even when using the lower estimate, deaths due to medical errors could be considered the eighth-leading cause of death in 1999.
- More people die in a given year as a result of medical errors than from motor vehicle accidents, breast cancer, or AIDS.

The IOM study also examined the types of errors that were occurring. Many of the adverse events were associated with the use of pharmaceutical agents and were potentially preventable. Medication errors alone, both in and out of the hospital, were estimated to account for more than 7,000 deaths in 1993, and one of every 854 inpatient hospital deaths was the result of a medication error. Children experienced harmful medication errors three times more often than adults (5.7% of medication orders for pediatric patients), and the rate was higher yet for neonates in the neonatal ICU. In addition, ICU patients suffered more life-threatening medication errors than any other patient population.

Consider This Pediatric patients are at even greater risk for medication errors than the general population because of weight-based dosing calculations and the misreading of decimal points.

Within a short time of the IOM report's release, some people began to question the numbers, asking whether the problem of medical errors could be as serious as it seemed. The first study to reliably confirm the IOM figures was a 2004 study by the health care ratings company HealthGrades (2004). This study looked at 3 years of Medicare data in all 50 states and Washington, DC, and reported that approximately 1.14 million patient safety incidents (PSIs) occurred among the 37 million hospitalizations in the Medicare population for the study period. The most commonly occurring PSIs were failure to rescue, decubitus ulcer, and postoperative sepsis.

Of the total 323,993 deaths among Medicare patients who developed one or more PSIs, 263,864, or 81%, of these deaths were directly attributable to the incidents (HealthGrades, 2004). In addition, one in every four Medicare patients who were hospitalized from 2000 to 2002 and experienced a PSI died. Perhaps most startling, however, was the conclusion that the United States loses more lives to PSIs every 6 months than it did in the entire Vietnam War. This also equates to three fully loaded jumbo jets crashing every other day for the last 5 years. Finally, the study noted that if the Centers for Disease Control and Prevention's annual list of leading causes of death included medical errors, it would show up as number six, ahead of diabetes, pneumonia, Alzheimer's disease, and renal disease (HealthGrades, 2004).

Additional reports since that time have repeatedly confirmed that the figures suggested in *To Err Is Human* were underreported. Indeed, recent study findings released by Patient Safety America suggested that up to 400,000 patients die each year as the result of medical errors (MacDonald, 2013). The lead researcher concluded that

> *There was much debate after the IOM report about the accuracy of its estimates. In a sense, it does not matter whether the deaths of 100,000, 200,000 or 400,000 Americans each year are associated with preventable adverse events in hospitals. Any of the estimates demands assertive action on the part of providers, legislators and people who will one day become patients.* (MacDonald, 2013, para. 6)

Discussion Point

Is the US public aware of the prevalence of medical errors? If not, what could be done to galvanize them to take action?

The Response to the Institute of Medicine Report

Within weeks of the release of *To Err Is Human*, the Senate held its first hearings on the issue, and additional hearings were conducted by committees of both the House of Representatives and the Senate. Local, state, and national leaders, as well as private and public sector leaders, took immediate action. The significance of the IOM report as a catalyst for change cannot be overstated.

That said, however, it is important to note that the problems of medical errors and patient safety were not completely unrecognized before *To Err Is Human* was published. Perhaps the most significant aspect of the IOM study was that it summarized the high human cost of medical errors in language that was understandable by the general public. In addition, previously, an assumption was made that most patient injuries were the result of negligence, incompetence, or corporate greed. The IOM report indicated, however, that errors are simply a part of the human condition and that the health care system needed to be redesigned so that fewer errors would occur.

As a result of these findings, the IOM recommended a national goal of reducing the number of medical errors by 50% over 5 years (Kohn et al., 2000). To that end, it outlined a four-pronged approach to reducing medical mistakes nationwide (Box 13.1). The strategies needed to achieve this national goal and attend to each of the four approaches are numerous, however, and only a few are detailed in this chapter.

WORKING TO ACHIEVE THE INSTITUTE OF MEDICINE GOALS

The first of the IOM's four-pronged approach to reducing medical errors was to "establish a national focus to create leadership, research, tools, and protocols to enhance the knowledge base about safety" (Kohn et al., 2000, p. 6). The second was to "raise standards and expectations for improvements in safety through the actions of oversight organizations, group purchasers, and professional groups" (Kohn et al., 2000, p. 6). Work to

BOX 13.1 The IOM's Four-Pronged Approach to Reducing Medical Mistakes Nationwide

- Establish a national focus to create leadership, research, tools, and protocols to enhance the knowledge base about safety.
- Identify and learn from medical errors through both mandatory and voluntary reporting systems.
- Raise standards and expectations for improvements in safety through the actions of oversight organizations, group purchasers, and professional groups.
- Implement safe practices at the delivery level.

Source: Kohn, L. T., Corrigan, J. M., & Donaldson, M. S. (Eds.). (2000). Executive summary. In *To err is human: Building a safer health system* (pp. 1–6). Retrieved May 20, 2012, from https://www.premierinc.com/safety/topics/patient_safety/downloads/01_exsum-iom_1toerr.pdf

achieve both of these goals began almost immediately after the IOM report was published. Indeed, a number of national committees and groups were formed as a result of governmental or legislative intervention. Some of the committees, groups, and legislative efforts spearheading the task to reduce medical errors are outlined here.

Quality Interagency Coordination Task Force

The QuIC Task Force was established by President Bill Clinton in 1998 to coordinate federal agencies that provided health care services. In December 1999, the task force began to evaluate the IOM recommendations and develop strategies for identifying threats to patient safety and reducing medical errors.

The final report, *Doing What Counts for Patient Safety: Federal Actions to Reduce Medical Errors and Their Impact*, was delivered to the president in February 2000. The report proposed taking strong action on all of the IOM recommendations to reduce errors, implementing a system of public accountability, developing a robust knowledge base about medical errors, and changing the culture in health care organizations to promote the recognition of errors and improvement in patient safety.

The National Forum for Health Care Quality Measurement and Reporting

Consistent with the QuIC's recommendations, the National Forum for Health Care Quality Measurement and Reporting was launched by Vice President Al Gore in 2000. Known as the National Quality Forum (NQF), it is a broad-based, private, not-for-profit body that establishes standard quality measurement tools to help people better ensure the delivery of quality services. The mission of the NQF is to lead collaboration to improve health and health care quality through measurement (NQF, 2015a, para. 1).

Since its inception, the NQF has endorsed hundreds of performance measures and practices, and many more are either in the early stages of development or moving through the NQF endorsement process. NQF was also the first to create a list of 27 *serious reportable events* (SREs), a list that was expanded to 28 events in 2006 (NQF, 2015c). In 2011, the NQF board approved for endorsement a list of 29 SREs in health care (Box 13.2). Of the events, 25 were updated from their earlier endorsement in 2006 and 4 new events were added to the list.

In addition, the NQF board of directors approved expansion of their mission in 2008 to include working in partnership with other leadership organizations to establish national priorities and goals for performance measurement and public reporting. The first draft of their core set of national priorities was created in 2008. The National Quality Strategy as of 2015 in terms of aims, priorities, and levers is shown in Box 13.3.

Finally, the NQF was identified as the consensus-based entity for implementation of the Affordable Care Act (ACA; launched in late 2011), including convening a multistakeholder group to provide annual input to the Department of Health and Human Services on the development of a National Quality Strategy (NQF, 2015b). The resultant National Priorities Partnership includes representatives from 52 major national organizations representing public and private sector stakeholder groups in a forum that balances the interests of consumers, purchasers, health plans, clinicians, providers, communities, states, and suppliers (NQF, 2015b).

BOX 13.2 Serious Reportable Events in Health Care (NQF 2011 Update)

1. Surgical or invasive procedure events
   - Surgery or other invasive procedure performed on the wrong site
   - Surgery or other invasive procedure performed on the wrong patient
   - Wrong surgical or other invasive procedure performed on a patient
   - Unintended retention of a foreign object in a patient after surgery or other invasive procedure
   - Intraoperative or immediately postoperative/postprocedure death in an ASA Class 1 patient
2. Product or device events
   - Patient death or serious injury associated with the use of contaminated drugs, devices, or biologics provided by the health care setting
   - Patient death or serious injury associated with the use or function of a device in patient care, in which the device is used or functions other than as intended
   - Patient death or serious injury associated with intravascular air embolism that occurs while being cared for in a health care setting
3. Patient protection events
   - Discharge or release of a patient/resident of any age, who is unable to make decisions, to other than an authorized person
   - Patient death or serious injury associated with patient elopement (disappearance)
   - Patient suicide, attempted suicide, or self-harm that results in serious injury, while being cared for in a health care setting
4. Care management events
   - Patient death or serious injury associated with a medication error (eg, errors involving the wrong drug, wrong dose, wrong patient, wrong time, wrong rate, wrong preparation, or wrong route of administration)
   - Patient death or serious injury associated with unsafe administration of blood products
   - Maternal death or serious injury associated with labor or delivery in a low-risk pregnancy while being cared for in a health care setting
   - (NEW) Death or serious injury of a neonate associated with labor or delivery in a low-risk pregnancy
   - Patient death or serious injury associated with a fall while being cared for in a health care setting
   - Any Stage 3, Stage 4, and unstageable pressure ulcers acquired after admission/presentation to a health care setting
   - Artificial insemination with the wrong donor sperm or wrong egg
   - (NEW) Patient death or serious injury resulting from the irretrievable loss of an irreplaceable biological specimen
   - (NEW) Patient death or serious injury resulting from failure to follow up or communicate laboratory, pathology, or radiology test results
5. Environmental events
   - Patient or staff death or serious injury associated with an electric shock in the course of a patient care process in a health care setting
   - Any incident in which systems designated for oxygen or other gas to be delivered to a patient contains no gas, the wrong gas, or is contaminated by toxic substances
   - Patient or staff death or serious injury associated with a burn incurred from any source in the course of a patient care process in a health care setting
   - Patient death or serious injury associated with the use of physical restraints or bedrails while being cared for in a health care setting
6. Radiologic events
   - (NEW) Death or serious injury of a patient or staff associated with the introduction of a metallic object into the magnetic resonance imaging area
7. Potential criminal events
   - Any instance of care ordered by or provided by someone impersonating a physician, nurse, pharmacist, or other licensed health care provider
   - Abduction of a patient/resident of any age
   - Sexual abuse/assault on a patient or staff member within or on the grounds of a health care setting
   - Death or serious injury of a patient or staff member resulting from a physical assault (ie, battery) that occurs within or on the grounds of a health care setting

Source: National Quality Forum. (2015c). *List of SREs*. Retrieved March 21, 2015, from http://www.qualityforum.org/Topics/SREs/List_of_SREs.aspx

BOX 13.3 The National Quality Strategy (2015): Aims, Priorities, and Levers

Aims

These aims guide and assess local, state, and national efforts to improve health and the quality of health care.

- *Better Care*: Improve the overall quality, by making health care more patient-centered, reliable, accessible, and safe.
- *Healthy People/Healthy Communities*: Improve the health of the US population by supporting proven interventions to address behavioral, social, and environmental determinants of health in addition to delivering higher-quality care.
- *Affordable Care:* Reduce the cost of quality health care for individuals, families, employers, and government.

Priorities

The National Quality Strategy focuses on six priorities:

1. Making care safer by reducing harm caused in the delivery of care.
2. Ensuring that each person and family is engaged as partners in their care.
3. Promoting effective communication and coordination of care.
4. Promoting the most effective prevention and treatment practices for the leading causes of mortality, starting with cardiovascular disease.
5. Working with communities to promote wide use of best practices to enable healthy living.
6. Making quality care more affordable for individuals, families, employers, and governments by developing and spreading new health care delivery models.

Levers

Each of the nine National Quality Strategy levers represents a core business function, resource, and/or action that stakeholders can use to align to the strategy.

- Public Reporting: Compare treatment results, costs, and patient experience for consumers.
- Learning and Technical Assistance: Foster learning environments that offer training, resources, tools, and guidance to help organizations achieve quality improvement goals.
- Certification, Accreditation, and Regulation: Adopt or adhere to approaches to meet safety and quality standards.
- Consumer Incentives and Benefit Designs: Help consumers adopt healthy behaviors and make informed decisions.
- Payment: Reward and incentivize providers to deliver high-quality, patient-centered care.
- Health Information Technology: Improve communication, transparency, and efficiency for better coordinated health and health care.
- Innovation and Diffusion: Foster innovation in health care quality improvement, and facilitate rapid adoption within and across organizations and communities.
- Workforce Development: Invest in people to prepare the next generation of health care professionals and support lifelong learning for providers.

Source: National Quality Strategy. (2015). *About the National Quality Strategy (NQS).* Retrieved March 21, 2015, from http://www.ahrq.gov/workingforquality/about.htm#aims

The National Patient Safety Foundation

The National Patient Safety Foundation (NPSF) was also formed in response to the IOM report. The mission of the NPSF, as amended in 2003, is to partner with patients and families, the health care community, and key stakeholders to advance patient safety and health care workforce safety and disseminate strategies to prevent harm (NPSF, 2015).

The Joint Commission

New organizations were not the only ones that responded to the recommendations of the IOM. The Joint Commission, in existence since 1951, accredits hospitals, long-term care facilities, psychiatric facilities, ambulatory care programs, and home health operations.

The Joint Commission's National Patient Safety Goals, implemented in January 2003, set forth clear, evidence-based recommendations to focus health care organizations on significant documented safety problems. These goals are updated annually for ambulatory care settings, behavioral health settings, hospitals, home care disease-specific care, laboratories, home-based care, and office-based surgery. The goals for hospitals in 2015 are shown in Box 13.4.

The Joint Commission also maintains one of the nation's most comprehensive databases of sentinel (serious adverse) events by health care professionals and their

BOX 13.4 Joint Commission 2015 National Patient Safety Goals for Hospitals

1. Improve the accuracy of patient identification.
2. Improve the effectiveness of communication among caregivers.
3. Improve the safety of using medications.
4. Reduce the harm associated with clinical alarm systems.
5. Reduce the risk of health care–associated infections.
6. The hospital identifies safety risks inherent in its patient population.

Source: Joint Commission. (2015). *National patient safety goals effective January 1, 2015.* Retrieved March 21, 2015, from http://www.jointcommission.org/assets/1/6/2015_NPSG_HAP.pdf

underlying causes. A *sentinel event* is defined by the Joint Commission (2015a) as "a Patient Safety Event (not primarily related to the natural course of the patient's illness or underlying condition), that results in either death, permanent harm, or severe temporary harm and intervention required to sustain life" (para. 2). Such events are called *sentinel* because they signal the need for immediate investigation and response. Information from the Joint Commission sentinel database is regularly shared with accredited organizations to help them take appropriate steps to prevent medical errors.

Another Joint Commission priority is the development of a *root cause analysis* with a plan of correction for the errors that do occur. The Joint Commission's (2015b) Sentinel Event Policy provides that organizations that are either voluntarily reporting a sentinel event or responding to the Joint Commission's inquiry about a sentinel event submit their related root cause analysis and action plan electronically to the Joint Commission whenever such events occur. The sentinel event data are then reviewed, and recommendations are made. The Joint Commission defends the confidentiality of the information, if necessary, in court.

Similarly, some organizations use a *failure mode and effects analysis* to examine all possible failures in a design—including sequencing of events, actual and potential risk, points of vulnerability, and areas for improvement (American Society for Quality, n.d.).

Consider This National legislation designed to keep such error analyses confidential is a critical but still-unrealized step. This discourages error reporting.

Centers for Medicare and Medicaid Services

The Centers for Medicare and Medicaid Services (CMS), formerly the Health Care Financing Administration, also plays an active role in setting standards and measuring quality of health care. With the introduction of the Medicare Quality Initiatives in November 2001, a new era of public reporting on quality began. These diverse initiatives encouraged the public reporting of quality measures for nursing homes, home health agencies, hospitals, and kidney dialysis facilities. These data are then made available to consumers on the Medicare website to assist them in making health care choices or decisions.

Medicare also established *pay for performance* (P4P), also known as *quality-based purchasing,* in the middle of the first decade of the 21st century. Because research conducted in the past decade has suggested little relationship between quality of care provided and the cost of that care, P4P initiatives were created to align payment and quality incentives and to reduce costs through improved quality and efficiency.

As part of P4P, the Physician Quality Reporting Initiative (PQRI), which was launched in 2007, allowed for payments to eligible professionals who satisfactorily reported quality information to Medicare on at least 3 of 74 individual quality measures on 80% of the cases from July 1, 2007 through December 31, 2007. Those who met the criteria for submitting quality data were eligible to earn a lump-sum incentive payment equivalent to 1.5% of their total estimated allowable charges for Medicare Part B Physician Fee Schedule (American Academy of Orthopaedic Surgeons, 1995–2015).

The Medicare Improvements for Patients and Providers Act of 2008 made the PQRI program permanent, with incentive payments increased to 2.0% and authorized through 2010. There were 153 individual quality measures and 7 measure groups for reporting under the program in 2009. For 2010, there were 175 individual measures and 13 measure groups (American Academy of Orthopaedic Surgeons, 1995–2015).

With the introduction of the ACA in 2011, the PQRI was changed to the Physician Quality Reporting System (PQRS) and incentive payments of 1.0% were established for successfully reporting the current 190 individual PQRS measures. An additional 0.5% incentive payment is possible for providers who qualify for or maintain board certification status, participate in a maintenance of certification program, and successfully complete a qualified maintenance of certification program practice assessment (American Academy of Orthopaedic Surgeons, 1995–2015).

Critics of the P4P incentive system suggest, however, that the system has failed to yield the desired results. They state this has occurred for many reasons including a focus on provider improvement and not achievement, the risk adjustment of provider scores supposedly being imprecise or even inapplicable to certain pay-for-performance metrics, sample sizes being small resulting in too few patients who are eligible to be scored for a given metric, and patients being treated often by multiple physicians ("Pay-for-Performance," 2011).

Discussion Point

Should it be necessary to pay health care professionals bonuses to submit quality information?

Also, as part of the ACA, CMS has now instituted hospital value-based purchasing. In this program, participating hospitals are paid for inpatient acute care services based on the quality of care, not just quantity of the services they provide. The program uses the hospital quality data reporting infrastructure developed for the Hospital Inpatient Quality Reporting Program, which was authorized by Section 501(b) of the Medicare Prescription Drug, Improvement, and Modernization Act of 2003 (CMS, 2014).

In addition, in an effort to reduce the number of preventable medical errors, including *never events* (errors that should never happen, such as removing the wrong limb in surgery, leaving a foreign object inside a patient during surgery, or sending a baby home with the wrong parents), Medicare announced that effective October 1, 2008, it would no longer pay for care that was required as a result of eight specific preventable errors or never events (Box 13.5). Medicaid followed suit in 2011.

In 2008, Medicare also stopped reimbursing hospitals for treating conditions, infections, or illnesses that were acquired in the hospital, and for any readmissions associated with treating those hospital-acquired conditions. The ACA extended the ruling to Medicaid in 2011 by prohibiting states from making Medicaid payments to providers for conditions that are deemed "reasonably preventable." Private insurance companies are following suit. These new policies require hospitals to maintain meticulous documentation about what conditions are present on admission to differentiate between preexisting conditions and those that are acquired during the hospital stay.

Consider This Although few organizations would argue against the benefits of well-developed and well-implemented quality control programs, quality control in health care organizations has evolved primarily from external effects and not as a voluntary monitoring effort.

Discussion Point

Should public or private insurance plans refuse to pay for care that is extended as a result of medical errors?

BOX 13.5 Eight "Never Errors" That Were No Longer Paid for by Medicare as of October 1, 2008

1. Pressure ulcers
2. Preventable injuries such as fractures, dislocations, and burns
3. Catheter-associated urinary tract infections
4. Vascular catheter–associated infections
5. Certain surgical-site infections
6. Objects mistakenly left inside surgical patients
7. Air emboli
8. Blood incompatibility reactions

Institute for Health Care Improvement

The Institute for Healthcare Improvement (IHI), established in the late 1980s by Donald Berwick, is an independent not-for-profit organization focused on improvement capability; person- and family-centered care; patient safety; quality, cost, and value; and the triple aim for populations (improve care, improve population health, and reduce costs per capita; IHI, 2015). During the annual National Forum on Quality Improvement in Health Care conference, the IHI highlights evidence-based best practices in an effort to more rapidly translate research into practice. In addition, IHI maintains disciplined research and development processes and prototyping projects to pursue health care quality improvements. In addition, IHI has facilitated further research, adaptation, and adoption of quality improvement strategies such as rapid response teams and medication reconciliation at health care institutions worldwide.

Quality and Safety Education for Nurses Project

The Quality and Safety Education for Nurses (QSEN) project (funded by Robert Wood Johnson Foundation) began in 2005 with the goal of preparing future nurses who will have the knowledge, skills, and attitudes (KSAs) necessary to continuously improve the quality and safety of the health care systems within which they work (QSEN Institute, 2014). When nurses have these KSAs, they are better able to identify potential errors and intervene before errors occur.

HEALTH CARE REPORT CARDS

In response to the demand for objective measures of quality, including the number and type of medical errors, many health plans, health care providers, employer purchasing groups, consumer information organizations, and state governments have begun to formulate health care quality report cards. Most states have laws requiring providers to report some type of data. The Agency for Healthcare Research and Quality is also exploring the development of a report card for the nation's health care delivery system, and the National Committee for Quality Assurance's Health Plan Report Card lets an individual create a health plan report card online. In addition, CMS released a proposed rule in June 2011 that would make Medicare information regarding provider cost and quality available to certain organizations.

It is important to remember, however, that many report cards do not contain information about the quality of care rendered by specific clinics, group practices, or physicians in a health plan's network. In addition, most report cards focus on service utilization data and patient satisfaction ratings and have minimal data regarding medical errors. Critics of health care report cards also point out that health plans may receive conflicting ratings on different report cards. This results from using different performance measures, as well as how each report card pools and evaluates individual factors. Report cards might also not be readily accessible or might be difficult for the average consumer to understand. Still, there is no doubt that consumers want more access to meaningful quality-of-care information and it is apparent that such data, which have long been kept secret, are now becoming public.

CREATING A CULTURE OF SAFETY MANAGEMENT

In response to public forces and professional concerns, patient safety has become one of the nation's most pressing challenges and a mandate for every health care organization. Indeed, the final recommendation of the IOM report was to implement safe practices at the delivery level. The strategies that have been recommended to achieve this goal are overwhelming both in scope and quantity.

Strategies discussed in this chapter include the "six-sigma" approach (a customer-based management philosophy) to error management; the mandatory/voluntary reporting of errors; attempts to increase confidentiality of reporting to reduce the fear of legal liability for reporting errors that do occur; the Leapfrog recommendations; the use of bar coding; a change in organizational cultures from that of "individual blame" to error identification and system modification; and the development of patient safety solutions by the World Health Organization's (WHO) World Alliance for Patient Safety.

> **Consider This** Because quality health care is a complex phenomenon, the factors contributing to quality in health care are as varied as the strategies needed to achieve this elusive goal.

A Six-Sigma Approach

One approach that has been taken to create a culture of safety management at the institutional level has been the implementation of the "six-sigma" approach. *Sigma* is a statistical measurement that reflects how well a product or process is performing. Higher sigma values indicate better performance. Historically, the health care industry has been comfortable striving for three-sigma processes (all data points fall within three standard deviations) in terms of health care quality instead of six. This is one reason why health care has more errors than the banking and airline industries, in which achieving six sigmas is the expectation. Organizations aim for this lofty target by carefully applying six-sigma methodology to every aspect of a particular product or process.

Discussion Point

Should the health care industry be willing to accept higher error rates than the banking or airline industries? Why or why not? Is the public willing to do so?

Discussion Point

Is a six-sigma failure rate a reasonable goal for all health care organizations? Should some health care organizations be expected to have higher failure (defect) rates than others? What variables might affect an organization's ability to achieve this goal?

Mandatory Reporting of Errors

The third prong of the IOM's four-pronged approach to creating a safer health care system is "to identify and learn from medical errors through both mandatory and voluntary reporting systems" (Kohn et al., 2000, p. 6). To accomplish this, the IOM report recommended developing a mandatory reporting system for medical errors and adverse events at both the state and national levels.

State mandates for reporting medical errors and adverse events have been slow to materialize, although as of 2014, at least 26 states required hospitals and/or other medical facilities to report serious medical errors (Jordan, 2014) and some states also have reporting mandates that apply only to specific types of error, such as hospital-acquired infections. It is important to note that the IOM report did suggest, in addition to mandatory reporting, that more options be created for limited voluntary reporting systems in all 50 states. The IOM also recommended that more research be conducted on how best to develop voluntary reporting systems that complement proposed mandatory reporting systems.

Increased mandatory and voluntary reporting must also occur at the institutional level, as well as by individual providers. As a result, the IOM report suggested that mandatory adverse event reporting should initially be required of hospitals and eventually of other institutional and ambulatory care delivery facilities. This was the impetus for the subsequent Joint Commission action for sentinel event reporting as part of the accreditation process.

Yet, even when error rates are reported, there is some question as to the accuracy of the reported data. Many hospitals rely on incident reporting as their key quality and safety measure, despite widespread acknowledgment that many errors go unreported (Macquarie University, 2015). Indeed, a recent comparative study of two hospitals in Australia found no relationship between the number of reported medication incidents and the "actual" rate of prescribing and medication administration errors observed (Macquarie University, 2015). The hospital with the higher number of incident reports had lower "actual" prescribing errors and vice versa. Thus, in this instance, the higher number of medication incidents actually reported reflected a lower patient risk (Research Study Fuels the Controversy 13.1).

It is difficult, however, to enforce greater disclosure and reporting at the individual provider level. Ethical and professional guidelines suggest that providers have a responsibility to disclose medical errors. Yet, the literature continues to suggest that this does not happen because of fear of legal suits or disciplinary measures by employers. The ironic part is that full disclosure after errors occur often reduces the likelihood of legal suit or the extent of patient retribution.

Discussion Point

Do you believe that error disclosure rates differ between nurses and physicians? If so, which professional group is more likely to disclose errors and why?

Perhaps, this failure to disclose medical errors is a major contributor to the disconnect that exists between consumers' perceptions of the quality of their health care and the actual quality provided. Even consumers who are aware of medical error statistics often report that they believe medical errors to be a problem but believe that such errors will not happen to them because they trust and believe in their health care provider.

Research Study Fuels the Controversy 13.1

A comparative study at two Australian hospitals suggests that hospitals' incident data have significant shortcomings, especially as the basis for monitoring safety over time and between sites. The researchers reviewed 3,291 patient records to identify prescribing errors (eg, wrong drug, dose, or strength) and evidence of their detection by staff. Errors during the administration of medications to patients were identified from a direct observational study of 180 nurses administering 7,451 medications to 1,397 patients across the two hospitals.

Source: Macquarie University. (2015, March 23). *Medication error reporting not indicative of patient safety.* Retrieved March 24, 2015, from Medical Xpress Website: http://medicalxpress.com/news/2015-03-medication-error-indicative-patient-safety.html

Study Findings

The study found no relationship between the number of reported medication incidents and the "actual" rate of prescribing and medication administration errors observed. The hospital with the higher number of incident reports had lower "actual" prescribing errors and vice versa. The researchers concluded that using the frequency of medication incident reports of errors to compare patient risk or performance quality within or between hospitals is unreliable. New approaches including data mining of electronic clinical information systems are required to support more effective medication error detection and to provide the data needed to develop safer practices.

Discussion Point

Do you consider the care you receive from your primary care provider to be of high quality? Are your perceptions subjective, or do you have objective data to back up your impression? Have you actively searched for such data on your primary care provider?

Legal Liability and Medical Error Reporting

If quality health care is to be achieved, the medical liability system and our litigious society must be recognized as potential barriers to systematic efforts to uncover and learn from mistakes that are made in health care. One recommendation of the IOM panel was to encourage learning about safety from cross-institutional reporting systems for errors. This reporting is inhibited by fears that such data will be discovered in liability lawsuits.

Discussion Point

Have you ever encouraged a family member, friend, or colleague to seek compensation for medical errors? If so, do you think this was the most appropriate means of redress?

The provision of stronger confidentiality protections likely would improve the voluntary sharing of data. In 2002, the Patient Safety Improvement Act was introduced in the House of Representatives. This bill provided legal protections for medical error reporting, stating that error information voluntarily submitted to patient safety organizations could not be subpoenaed or used in legal discovery. It also generally required that the information be treated as confidential. After multiple revisions, the final legislation, called the Patient Safety and Quality Improvement Act of 2005, was signed into law by President George W. Bush in July 2005.

Federal legislation has also been proposed to protect the voluntary reporting of ordinary injuries and "near misses"—errors that did not cause harm this time but easily could the next time. This would be like what is done in aviation, in which near misses are confidentially reported and can be analyzed by anyone.

Discussion Point

Given the known incidence of medical errors and adverse events that result in patient injury and the challenges inherent in tracking errors that have already been made, how difficult will it be to track "near misses?" What resources would be needed to accomplish this goal?

Leapfrog Group

The Leapfrog Group is a conglomeration of non-health care *Fortune 500* leaders dedicated to reducing preventable medical mistakes and improving the quality and affordability of health care (Leapfrog Group, 2015a). The group has advised the health care industry that big leaps in patient safety and customer value can occur if specific evidence-based standards are implemented, including (1) computerized physician (or prescriber) order entry (CPOE), (2) evidence-based hospital referral (EHR), and (3) ICU physician staffing (IPS).

CPOE is a promising technology that allows physicians to enter orders into a computer instead of handwriting them:

> *Recent research shows that if this Leapfrog practice was implemented in all urban hospitals in the U.S., we could prevent as many as 3 million serious medication errors each year. Studies have also shown that CPOE reduces length of stay; reduces repeat tests; reduces turnaround times for laboratory, pharmacy and radiology requests; as well as delivering cost savings.* (Leapfrog Group, 2015c, para. 1)

EHR involves making sure that patients with high-risk conditions are treated at hospitals whose characteristics are associated with better outcomes. Indeed, HealthGrades' (2015) analysis found that, if all hospitals as a group, from 2011 to 2013, performed similarly to hospitals achieving HealthGrades 2015 America's 100 Best Hospitals Award, 172,626 lives could potentially have been saved. For patients treated in hospitals achieving HealthGrades 2015 America's 100 Best Hospitals Award, there was roughly a 26.4% lower risk of dying than if the patients were treated in hospitals that did not receive this recognition, as measured across 19 rated conditions and procedures where mortality is the outcome.

IPS considers the level of training of ICU medical personnel. Evidence suggests that quality of care in hospital ICUs is strongly influenced by whether "intensivists" (those familiar with ICU complications) are providing care and how the staff is organized (Leapfrog Group, 2015b). "Mortality rates are significantly lower in hospitals with ICUs managed exclusively by board-certified intensivists. Research has shown that in ICUs where intensivists manage or comanage all patients versus low intensity there is a 30% reduction in hospital mortality and a 40% reduction in ICU mortality" (Leapfrog Group, 2015b, para. 1).

Bar Coding Medications

In addition, Leapfrog has endorsed the use of bar coding to reduce point-of-care medication errors. Per a US Food and Drug Administration (FDA) rule adopted in April 2004, all prescription and over-the-counter medications used in hospitals must contain a national drug code number. The FDA suggested that a barcode system, coupled with a CPOE system, would greatly enhance the ability of all health care workers to follow the "five rights" of medication administration—that the *right* person receives the *right* drug, in the *right* dose, via the *right* route, at the *right* administration time.

In addition, the Joint Commission originally proposed in its 2005 National Patient Safety Goals and Requirements that accredited organizations would have to implement barcode technology to identify patients and match them to their medications or other treatments by January 2007. Because of implementation concerns, especially in terms of costs, this proposal was abandoned by the Joint Commission in July 2004.

Patient Safety Solutions

Recognizing that health care errors affect at least one in every 10 patients around the world, the WHO's World Alliance for Patient Safety and the Collaborating Centre packaged nine effective solutions, called *patient safety solutions,* to reduce such errors. A patient safety solution was defined as any system design or intervention that has demonstrated the ability to prevent or mitigate patient harm stemming from the processes of health care and is based on interventions and actions that have reduced problems related to patient safety in some countries (WHO, 2015). The priority program areas related to patient safety in 2015 are shown in Box 13.6.

Consider This Sadly, from 2010 through 2012, there were 266,813 serious potentially preventable patient safety events among Medicare patients in US hospitals. If during this same time period, all hospitals had performed at the same level as Patient Safety Excellence Award recipients, Medicare patients in US hospitals may have stayed as many as 352,754 fewer days in the hospital by avoiding potentially preventable patient safety events (Business Wire, 2014).

Promoting Just Cultures

Perhaps though, the most significant change that must occur before a nationwide culture of safety management can exist is that organizational cultures must be

BOX 13.6 World Health Organization's Global Patient Safety Challenges (2015)

1. *Clean Care is Safer Care* (focuses on health care–associated infection and hand hygiene in health care)
2. *Safe Surgery Saves Lives* (prioritizes the use of surgery checklists at three phases of an operation: before the induction of anesthesia ["sign in"], before the incision of the skin ["time out"], and before the patient leaves the operating room ["sign out"])
3. *Patients for Patient Safety* (builds a paneled, global network of patients and patient organizations to champion patient safety)
4. *Research for Patient Safety* (undertakes global prevalence studies of adverse effects and is developing a rapid assessment tool for use in developing countries)
5. *International Patient Safety Classification* (aims to define, harmonize, and group patient safety concepts into an internationally agreed classification)
6. *Reporting and Learning* (aims to generate best practice guidelines for existing and new reporting systems, and facilitate early learning from information available)
7. *Solutions for Patient Safety* (interventions and actions that prevent patient safety problems recurring and thus reduce risk to patients)
8. *The High 5s initiative* (spreads best practice for change in organizational, team, and clinical practices to improve patient safety)
9. *Technology for Patient Safety* (focuses on the opportunities to harness new technologies to improve patient safety)
10. *Knowledge Management* (work with Member States and partners to gather and share knowledge on patient safety developments globally)
11. *Eliminating Central Line–Associated Bloodstream Infections*
12. *Education for Safer Care* (develop a curricular guide for medical students as well as other resources)
13. *Safety Prize* (international award for excellence in the field of patient safety that will act as a driver for change and improvement)
14. Medical Checklists

Source: World Health Organization. (2015). *WHO Patient Safety—Programme areas*. Retrieved March 22, 2015, from http://www.who.int/patientsafety/about/programmes/en/

created that remove blame from the individual and instead focus on how the organization can be modified to reduce the likelihood of such errors occurring in the future. Cultures where voluntary reporting is encouraged and constructive feedback is given to those who self-report are often called "just cultures." Just cultures will be needed to encourage voluntary reporting and reduce the prevalence of errors. Just cultures exhibit "giving constructive feedback and critical analysis in skillful ways, during assessments based on facts, and having respect for the complexity of the situation" (p. 14). This type of intervention encourages people to reveal the errors they have made so that the organization can learn from them. In addition, the just culture philosophy suggests rewarding staff who report errors or near-errors to help them overcome the fear of reporting (Gaskill, 2008).

Clearly, a punitive approach to medical errors is not productive, and errors will not be reported if workers fear the consequences. Employees and patients need to feel comfortable and without fear of personal risk in reporting hazards that can affect patient safety.

Consider This Ignoring the problem of medical errors, denying their existence, or blaming the individuals involved in the processes does nothing to eliminate the underlying problems.

Conclusions

Medical errors are not the only indicator of quality of care. They are, however, a pervasive problem in the current health care system and one of the greatest threats to quality health care. Nurses are uniquely positioned to identify, interrupt, and correct medical errors and to minimize preventable adverse outcomes. Only recently, however, have their error-recovery strategies been described.

Efforts to reduce medical errors, however, over the last decade have not resulted in the achievement of desired outcomes. There is a plethora of current studies that suggest that the health care system continues to be riddled with errors and that patient and worker safety is compromised. Yet, movement toward the IOM goals is occurring. It is likely that there has never been another time when the public, providers, and government have worked together so closely to achieve a shared health care goal.

Much, however, remains to be done. Sustained public interest will be needed to create the momentum necessary to systematically change the health care system in a way that reduces patients' vulnerability to medical errors. In addition, although there has been a great deal of talk about using a systems approach to address the problem of medical errors, there has not been much discussion regarding exactly how this integration is to be accomplished. The bottom line is that significant and continuous reform of the health care system will be needed before the problem of medical errors shows any resolution.

For Additional Discussion

1. If cost containment and quality goals conflict, which do you think will take precedence in health care organizations today?
2. Why do so many providers, despite stated dissatisfaction levels, state that they feel helpless about reducing medical errors and improving the quality of health care?
3. Why have quality control efforts in health care organizations evolved primarily from external requirements and not as voluntary monitoring efforts?
4. Where does individual provider responsibility and accountability begin and end in a culture in which medical errors are recognized as being a failure of the system?
5. How common is it that medical error documentation is used against employees as part of the performance appraisal process? If so, does this discourage reporting?
6. Does the average consumer have access to and an accurate understanding of health care report cards?
7. Given that most individuals can quickly identify medical errors that have happened to them, a friend, or a family member, why does the US public seem so reluctant to accept that medical errors constitute a threat to the quality of their health care?
8. Has your fear of legal liability ever influenced your decision to report a medical error?

References

American Academy of Orthopaedic Surgeons. (1995–2015). *Physician quality reporting system (PQRS)*. Retrieved March 20, 2015, from http://www.aaos.org/research/committee/evidence/pqri_info.asp

American Society for Quality. (n.d.). *Quality tools: Failure mode effects analysis (FMEA)*. Retrieved March 21, 2015, from http://asq.org/learn-about-quality/process-analysis-tools/overview/fmea.html

Benson, L. (2015, February 26). Minnesota struggles to reduce medical errors. *MPR News*. Retrieved March 22, 2015, from http://www.mprnews.org/story/2015/02/26/medical-errors

Bramhall, S. J. (2015, January 4). Are doctors serious about reducing medical errors? *Veterans Today*. Retrieved March 22, 2015, from http://www.veteranstoday.com/2015/01/04/are-doctors-serious-about-reducing-medical-errors/

Brennan, T. A., Leape, L. L., Laird, N. M., Hebert, L., Localio, A. R., Lawthers, A. G., . . . Hiatt, H. H. (1991). Incidence of adverse events and negligence in hospitalized patients: Results of the Harvard Medical Practice Study 1. *The New England Journal of Medicine, 324*(6), 370–376.

Business Wire. (2014, June 17). *HealthGrades recognizes 2014 Patient Safety Excellence Award™ recipients.*

Retrieved March 21, 2015, from http://www.businesswire.com/news/home/20140617005517/en/Healthgrades-Recognizes-2014-Patient-Safety-Excellence-Award%E2%84%A2#.VQxUnU10y70

Centers for Medicare and Medicaid Services. (2014, December 18). *Hospital Value-Based Purchasing.* Retrieved March 21, 2015, from http://www.cms.gov/Medicare/Quality-Initiatives-Patient-Assessment-Instruments/hospital-value-based-purchasing/index.html

Encyclopedia of Surgery. (2015). *Medical errors: Introduction and definitions.* Retrieved March 21, 2015, from http://www.surgeryencyclopedia.com/La-Pa/Medical-Errors.html

Gaskill, M. (2008). Learning from mistakes: "Just culture" is replacing blame in some California hospitals. *NurseWeek (California), 21*(8), 14–15.

HealthGrades. (2004). *HealthGrades quality study: Patient safety in American hospitals.* Retrieved August 15, 2008, from http://www.providersedge.com/ehdocs/ehr_articles/Patient_Safety_in_American_Hospitals-2004.pdf

HealthGrades. (2015, February 24). *HealthGrades announces America's Best Hospitals™ for 2015.* Retrieved March 26, 2015, from http://www.healthgrades.com/about/press-room/healthgrades-announces-americas-best-hospitals-for-2015

Institute for Healthcare Improvement. (2015). *About IHI.* Retrieved March 21, 2015, from http://www.ihi.org/about/pages/default.aspx

Joint Commission. (2015a). *Sentinel event.* Retrieved March 21, 2015, from http://www.jointcommission.org/sentinel_event.aspx

Joint Commission. (2015b). *Sentinel event policy and procedures.* Retrieved March 21, 2015, from http://www.jointcommission.org/Sentinel_Event_Policy_and_Procedures/

Jordan, E. (2014, April 24). *Iowa doesn't require reports of medical errors.* Retrieved March 24, 2015, from http://www.kcrg.com/news/local/Iowa-Doesnt-require-reports-of-medical-errors-120932484.html

Kliff, S. (2015, January 29). *Medical errors in America kill more people than AIDS or drug overdoses. Here's why.* Retrieved March 26, 2015, from http://www.vox.com/2015/1/29/7878731/medical-errors-statistics

Kohn, L. T., Corrigan, J. M., & Donaldson, M. S. (Eds.). (2000). Executive summary. In *To err is human: Building a safer health system* (pp. 1–6). Retrieved May 20, 2012, from http://www.nap.edu/openbook.php?record_id=9728&page=1

Leape, L. L. (1994). Error in medicine. *Journal of the American Medical Association, 272*(23), 1851–1857.

Leape, L. L., Brennan, T. A., Laird, N., Lawthers, A. G., Localio, A. R., Barnes, B. A., . . . Hiatt, H. (1991). The nature of adverse events in hospitalized patients: Results of the Harvard Medical Practice Study II. *New England Journal of Medicine, 324*(6), 377–384.

Leapfrog Group. (2015a). *About Leapfrog.* Retrieved March 21, 2015, from http://www.leapfroggroup.org/

Leapfrog Group. (2015b). *ICU physician staffing.* Retrieved November 6, 2011, from http://www.leapfroggroup.org/for_hospitals/leapfrog_hospital_survey_copy/leapfrog_safety_practices/icu_physician_staffing

Leapfrog Group. (2015c). *Computerized physician order entry.* Retrieved March 21, 2015, from http://www.leapfroggroup.org/for_hospitals/leapfrog_hospital_survey_copy/leapfrog_safety_practices/cpoe

MacDonald, I. (2013, September 20). Hospital medical errors now the third leading cause of death in the U.S.: New study highlights the fact that estimates in 'To Err is Human' report were low. *FierceHealthcare.* Retrieved March 27, 2015, from http://www.fiercehealthcare.com/story/hospital-medical-errors-third-leading-cause-death-dispute-to-err-is-human-report/2013-09-20

Macquarie University. (2015, March 23). *Medication error reporting not indicative of patient safety.* Retrieved March 24, 2015, from Medical Xpress Website: http://medicalxpress.com/news/2015-03-medication-error-indicative-patient-safety.html

Mallow, P. J., Pandya, B., Horblyuk, R., & Haplan, H. S. (2013, December). Prevalence and cost of hospital medical errors in the general and elderly United States populations. *Journal of Medical Economics, 16*(12), 1367–1378.

National Coordinating Council for Medication Error Reporting and Prevention. (2015). *About medication errors.* Retrieved March 21, 2015, from http://www.nccmerp.org/aboutMedErrors.html

National Patient Safety Foundation. (2015). *About us.* Retrieved March 20, 2015, from http://www.npsf.org/?page=aboutus

National Quality Forum. (2015a). *Mission and vision.* Retrieved March 20, 2015, from http://www.qualityforum.org/About_NQF/Mission_and_Vision.aspx

National Quality Forum. (2015b). *NQF national priorities partnership.* Retrieved March 21, 2015, from http://www.qualityforum.org/npp/

National Quality Forum. (2015c). *List of SREs*. Retrieved March 21, 2015, from http://www.qualityforum.org/Topics/SREs/List_of_SREs.aspx

National Quality Strategy. (2015). *About the National Quality Strategy (NQS)*. Retrieved March 21, 2015, from http://www.ahrq.gov/workingforquality/about.htm#aims

Pay-for-performance: An overview. (2011). *Healthcare Economist*. Retrieved March 26, 2015, from http://healthcare-economist.com/2011/01/20/pay-for-performance-an-overview/

QSEN Institute. (2014). *Project overview*. Case Western Reserve University. Retrieved March 22, 2015, from http://qsen.org/about-qsen/project-overview/

Thomas, E. J., Studdert, D. M., Newhouse, J. P., Zbar, B. I. W., Howard, K. M., Williams, E. J., & Brennan, T. A. (1999). Costs of medical injuries in Colorado and Utah in 1992. *Inquiry, 36*(3), 255–264.

Van Den Bos, J., Rustagi, K., Gray, T., Halford, M., Ziemkiewicz, E., & Shreve, J. (2011). The $17.1 billion problem: The annual cost of measurable errors. *Health Affairs, 30*(4), 596–603.

World Health Organization. (2015). *World alliance for patient safety*. Retrieved March 22, 2015, from http://www.who.int/patientsafety/worldalliance/en/

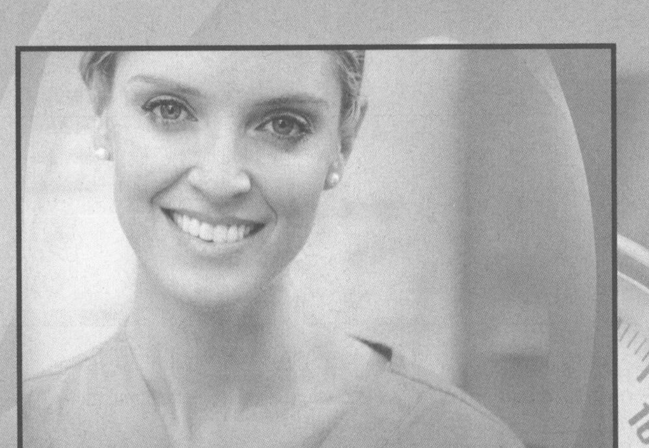

4

Nursing Education Issues

14

Using Simulation to Teach Nurses

Sherry D. Fox and Rebekah Damazo

ADDITIONAL RESOURCES

Visit thePoint for additional helpful resources

- eBook
- Journal Articles
- WebLinks

CHAPTER OUTLINE

LEARNING OBJECTIVES

The learner will be able to:

1. Describe the evolution of simulation technology used in teaching nurses from the late 1990s to the present.
2. Analyze the potential impact of simulation technology on nursing education's ability to produce graduates prepared for current workforce demands, despite inadequate numbers of nursing faculty and inadequate clinical placement sites for nursing students.
3. Explore how the use of simulation as an adjunct to clinical nursing education can mitigate or reduce provider errors and improve patient outcomes.
4. Identify how strategies such as debriefing and guided reflection can be used to stimulate collaborative dialogue and problem solving in simulated learning experiences.
5. Explore common challenges associated with using simulation to teach nurses, including cost, time constraints, and educators who are unprepared for teaching with simulation.
6. Review and summarize the current literature regarding the effect of simulated learning on the achievement of desired learner outcomes.
7. Consider the strengths and limitations of high-fidelity patient simulators as a replacement for traditional acute care clinical experience in nursing education.
8. Explore the likelihood that certifying and licensing boards will look to simulation as one way to validate the initial and ongoing competency of health care professionals.
9. Consider whether simulation could be used more effectively as a supplement to basic nursing education or ongoing continuing education of health care professionals.

INTRODUCTION

Nurses the world over are familiar with the use of simulation for skills training. Most nurses began their exposure to clinical nursing cloistered in a skills lab, with static mannequins on which they practiced positioning, turning, dressings, and inserting various tubes. The skill of injections was often practiced first on oranges, gel pads, or even classmates before the student approached the real patient. Despite such rehearsals, the approach to the real patient was fraught with uncertainty, anxiety, and exposure to multiple contextual elements for which the skills lab did not prepare the student. The practice of nursing was, in fact, *practice*. Nursing education has recently begun a revolution that brings "practice" out of the patient realm, and into simulation settings.

Many a wary patient has watched as a novice anxiously "practiced" some skill or assessment in the real world with varying degrees of success. The student is usually totally focused on the skill, barely able to interact with the patient or the environment. The pressure is compounded because hospitals are narrowing the ways in which students can participate in the health care setting. Some hospitals are severely limiting students' abilities to give medications or participate in procedures due to stringent oversight from accrediting bodies.

The skills needed to meet real-world demands cannot be easily rehearsed in traditional skills labs, with static mannequins such as the ubiquitous "Mrs. Chase," a life-sized doll created over 100 years ago for nursing students' practice (Rizzolo, 2014), and perhaps languishing still in many nursing skills labs. Beyond the necessary psychomotor skills are the skills of clinical reasoning and decision making—picking up appropriate cues, making necessary assessments, and coming to appropriate conclusions about what the patient needs in a dynamic, fast-paced setting. Rehearsal and practice are essential for development of competence (Fisher & King, 2013).

Nurse educators have tried to expand the scope of isolated skills lab practice by introducing computer vignettes, case studies, role playing, and other modalities, with positive results, but these teaching methods invariably lack many aspects of reality and interactivity for the student. Conversely, the real clinical setting lacks aspects of predictability and control in terms of the environment for learning. The instructor cannot ensure that each student attains the same, or even similar, experiences, resulting in highly variable learning outcomes. McNelis et al. (2014) suggested that students in real clinical settings often experience missed opportunities for learning. Inconsistencies in clinical experiences result in variable learning opportunities that provide inadequate measures for clinical progress and learning. Observations of students in a pediatric clinical setting revealed significant amounts of "unengaged" time where students fill time "to the best of their abilities" with activities they can control, such as talking with patients, family, and each other. In contrast, observations of simulation laboratory provide a structured learning environment for students to develop skills not available in the clinical setting (Pauly-O'Neill, Prion, & Nguyen, 2013).

These unmet needs were the impetus for the proliferation of high-fidelity patient simulators in the late 1990s and first decade of the 21st century. Technology innovations have provided new practice tools that include wireless, computer-driven mannequins with lifelike features. Human patient simulation technology offers new possibilities for engaging student nurses in realistic patient scenarios with time to reflect and receive feedback to enhance learning. This chapter describes the emergence of sophisticated simulators as a tool for teaching nurses, provides the rationale for their use, and outlines the challenges inherent in determining how to incorporate simulation into nursing education. In addition, it presents preliminary outcomes of simulation use, as well as examples of emerging applications for staff training and competency assessment and regulatory trends.

THE EMERGENCE OF HIGH-FIDELITY PATIENT SIMULATORS

Within the last decade, the proliferation of high-fidelity patient simulators has set the stage for a revolution in how students are taught. Practicing nurses have also been affected as employers seek to develop and evaluate competency (Decker, Utterback, Thomas, Mitchell, & Sportsman, 2011). Patient simulators are full-sized, computerized mannequins that can be programmed to respond in realistic ways. They can provide dynamic assessment data in real time, display programmed signs and symptoms, and respond to nursing actions.

These sophisticated mannequins evolved from low-technology mannequins and task trainers (such as cardiopulmonary resuscitation [CPR] mannequins and intravenous [IV] arms) as computer technology advanced. Human patient simulators are categorized as "high-fidelity" simulation, compared with the "lower fidelity" of task trainers (mannequins that have limited capabilities, designed for specific tasks, such as pelvic models and IV arms) and static mannequins. Fidelity refers to the degree of realism.

In the 1980s, sophisticated simulators were in use for training anesthesiologists and military personnel. However, the costs of such early versions of patient simulators were prohibitive for most schools of nursing. As the industry has grown and the array of products has expanded, patient simulators are within affordable ranges for many nursing schools and hospital systems and are now an accepted, almost essential technological adjunct for nursing education in the 21st century.

A recent survey of 1,729 prelicensure RN programs in the United States explored the current use of simulators (Hayden, 2010). Eighty-seven percent of those who responded use simulation. The majority of programs use simulation in five or more clinical courses, with an evident trend of incorporating simulation throughout nursing curricula. Kardong-Edgren (2009) asserted, "In nursing education, simulation has become an essential instructional method" (p. e161). An international survey of simulation users (members of the International Nursing Association for Clinical Simulation and Learning [INACSL]) confirmed that nursing educators worldwide are adopting simulation strategies (Gore, Van Gele, Ravert, & Mabire, 2012).

Capabilities of Patient Simulators

High-fidelity mannequins can be programmed to display selected signs and symptoms and to respond to the actions of the learner. The student can listen to preprogrammed heart, lung, and bowel sounds, can assess pulses at anatomically correct sites, can visualize respirations and pupil responses, and can observe displays of physiologic parameters such as the electrocardiogram, blood pressure, hemodynamic wave forms, pulse oximetry, and temperature on a simulated patient monitor. These parameters can all change in a preprogrammed pattern or under the control of a skilled operator. The simulators can be preprogrammed to speak or to respond through operator voices.

Simulation is an educational strategy that allows realistic reproduction of aspects of real health care settings and patient events, which are designed by or under the control of the instructor. Students participate in the simulation scenario just as they would in the actual setting. Students interact with the mannequin, make physical assessments, monitor physiologic parameters, and observe the programmed trajectory of an episode. The student's interventions can affect the "patient's" course, for better or worse. All of the student's actions can be recorded for later reflection and debriefing, and may be observed by peers to stimulate collaborative dialogue and problem solving. Possibly the most powerful component of simulations is the *debriefing*, which is a requisite at the completion of a scenario (Dreifuerst, Horton-Deutsch, & Henao, 2014). Debriefing, guided by a skilled educator, can produce insightful reflection on the events, help students to analyze and explain the reasoning behind actions, and facilitate the exploration of alternative approaches. The instructor is able to determine gaps in knowledge or misguided assumptions. Research supports debriefing as a key component in the learning that occurs with simulation (Shinnick, Woo, Horwich, & Steadman, 2011a). Mariani, Cantrell, Meakim, Prieto, and Dreifuerst (2013) asserted that debriefing can be effective in helping students gain insight and clinical reasoning skills through reflection, thinking about their actions, and even beyond their actions. Shinnick et al. (2011a) determined through a two-group repeated measures design experiment that debriefing was a necessary component for knowledge acquisition after hands-on simulation.

Discussion Point

Following a critical patient incident, what type of discussion ensues in your clinical setting? Who provides input? What type of record is available to trace the actions that occurred (or were omitted)? (One example might be a debriefing session following a "code.")

Discussion Point

Think of a clinical occurrence in which you felt unprepared to handle the situation. What type of practice or rehearsal could have prepared you better?

SIMULATION AND HEALTH CARE QUALITY

Nursing educators in academia, as well as in staff development, face challenges on many fronts in preparing and maintaining a well-educated, competent nursing workforce that is adequate in numbers and in appropriate skills to meet today's health care demands. Above all, the consumer of health care wants assurances that today's nurses are competent and that the care provided is safe and free from errors and omissions that can lead to prolonged illness or death.

The landmark Institute of Medicine (IOM) report *To Err Is Human* promoted simulation training as one way to prevent and mitigate errors (Kohn, Corrigan, & Donaldson, 2000). In simulation related to crisis management, "small groups that work together—whether in the operating room, intensive care unit, or emergency department—learn to respond to a crisis in an efficient, effective, and coordinated manner" (pp. 176, 177). The report proposed the development of simulation technology, although it cautioned that simulation for interdisciplinary teams to practice interpersonal and technical skills with meaningful feedback and reinforcement would be a great challenge. Since this report, simulation technology and its implementation have made great strides in the area of simulation training for the professions and for interprofessional teams. Transformational changes in the safety culture can be observed with team training when the work environment supports the learning of new behavior (Jones, Skinner, High, & Reiter-Palmon, 2013). Simulation has established effectiveness as a technique to train students and practicing nurses for new procedures, communication, processes, and techniques (Aebersold & Tschannen, 2013).

Medical errors continue to headline health care morbidity and mortality reports. Despite decades of research and scientific discovery, patients still experience harmful events with alarming frequency. Recent estimates are that as many as 440,000 deaths occur in hospitals each year due to preventable errors, roughly one sixth of all hospital deaths (James, 2013). The magnitude of the problem poses greater urgency to find solutions to increase patient safety.

Simulation has become an important component of efforts to meet quality and safety. The Quality and Safety Education for Nurses (QSEN) project redefined the competencies that support patient safety: patient-centered care, teamwork and collaboration, evidence-based practice, quality improvement, safety, and informatics. The QSEN project outlined the "knowledge, skills and attitudes" that will change how nurses practice (Cronenwett et al., 2007). National nursing education curricula standards now include QSEN competencies. Simulation is an excellent platform to reflect on behaviors, improve competencies, and establish a new mindset for patient safety (Sherwood & Zomorodi, 2014). A team from the University of San Francisco observed students in both clinical and simulation experiences, and concluded that "work needs to be done" to include all QSEN-related knowledge and skills into prelicensure clinical rotations (Pauly-O'Neill et al., 2013). Through simulation, nurses can practice skills repeatedly, until they can be completed safely. Simulation can provide an environment that mimics the real clinical setting, incorporating the typical distractions that lead to errors.

Teams can practice safe and effective communication (Reising & Hensel, 2014). Strouse (2010) advocated requiring staff to participate in multidisciplinary simulated learning experiences to reinforce principles of effective teamwork and communication. Nurses represent the largest group of health care professionals and, while accreditation standards for all levels of nursing education include a requirement for interprofessional education (National League for Nursing Accreditation Commission [NLNAC], 2011), integration into student learning activities remains piecemeal. Simulated clinical environments are able to provide interactive interprofessional education and practice experiences for nursing students and health professionals teams that may be missing in some programs (National League for Nursing Interprofessional Education Collaborative, 2011). Traditional educational boundaries are removed when simulation is used to incorporate interprofessional practice (Tofil et al., 2014).

Team Strategies and Tools to Enhance Performance and Patient Safety (TeamSTEPPS) is a federally funded initiative by the AHRQ, designed to improve patient safety through effective teamwork and communication. Online resources provide free access to a comprehensive set of ready-to-use materials and a training curriculum to successfully integrate teamwork principles into any health care system. Simulation methods are offered as a powerful component of TeamSTEPPS (Agency for Healthcare Research and Quality, n.d.). Research findings indicate that the TeamSTEPPS methods applied in simulation-based team training had significant benefit in improving nurse confidence in, and performance of teamwork skills in recognizing and managing early warning signs of failure to rescue, as compared with case study review methods (Harvey, Echols, Clark, & Lee, 2014).

NEW GRADUATE NURSE READINESS

Even with the best efforts of nursing academia to produce competent graduates, nursing educators know that a new graduate, at best, is a novice nurse, lacking confidence and competence in many areas. It is generally acknowledged that a transition period is needed to acclimate the new nurse to the practice arena, with nurse residencies becoming more necessary and popular. The practice arena is often fast-paced and chaotic, plagued by rapid turnover, and staff shortages. Experienced nurses have their hands full meeting the needs of high-acuity patients. The nurse who is not well practiced is at risk of making serious errors in omission and commission. Compounding the problem, new nurses are often hired directly into settings demanding high-level competencies, without the luxury of practice experience in lower-acuity settings. Not surprisingly, there is a gap between the competence achieved by completing a nursing program and passing NCLEX, and the competence desired by practice settings.

Specific competencies that comprise the gap between academic preparation and practice expectations were identified in an ambitious survey of frontline nurse managers who work with new graduates by Berkow, Virkstis, Stewart, and Conway (2009). In an iterative process with experts, a list of 36 competencies were derived as essential, and as a starting point for establishing shared goals between academia and practice. The competencies were grouped into the categories of *clinical knowledge, technical skills, critical thinking, communication, professionalism, and management of responsibilities.* These competencies formed the basis of the survey, sent to 53,000 frontline nurse leaders. Respondents (5,700) comprised 11% of the sample. Only about 25% were completely satisfied with new graduate performance, and more than 25% were somewhat dissatisfied or worse. Satisfaction with new graduate performance reached the 50% level on only two competencies—"utilization of information technologies" and "rapport with patients and families." The competencies from the broader categories were widely distributed across the satisfaction levels, so there is no one category that engenders satisfaction. The competencies for the category *management of responsibilities* all fell into the lowest tier of satisfaction—encompassing skills such as taking initiative, tracking multiple responsibilities, and delegation—all skills requiring clinical practice.

Landmark research by Benner, Sutphen, Leonard, and Day (2010) summarized the profound changes in 21st-century nursing, showcasing the significant gap between current practice and the education of nurses preparing them for practice. They called for radical changes in nursing education and the pedagogies involved. One recommendation for pedagogy change is keeping the student focused on the patient's experience, through unfolding cases, such as simulation scenarios; such teaching strategies will require resources to assist faculty to develop and implement effective clinical simulation exercises. Furthermore, Benner et al. recommended the addition of competency assessments throughout the educational path, as well as with the NCLEX-RN examination, and again following a 1-year postlicensure residency, using simulation.

Ironside, McNelis, and Ebright (2014) completed a comprehensive study examining faculty and student expectations of clinical practice. Investigators noted that "faculty interactions with students predominantly focused on determining if students were completing assigned work in a timely manner and appropriately documenting care provided." The researchers interviewed faculty and stated expectations did not meet intentions or practice reality as both faculty and students focused on completing tasks and time management and not on higher-level skills and problem solving. Students assumed that "doing more tasks" improved their education and ensured success. This study proposes that the focus on task completion dominates clinical experiences, and may often even be at odds with students' learning in practice settings.

Fortunately, the "perfect storm" of health care chaos and increased demands on nursing educators is crossing paths with the recent revolution in high-technology patient simulators. Simultaneously, as production and market competition grow, these simulators are becoming priced at levels that make them more affordable. The planned integration of patient simulators in nursing, for academic education as well as for staff development, is one major avenue to producing higher levels of competency and safe practice for nursing. Several nurse residency programs report the effectiveness of such programs that incorporated simulation along with structured support of new graduates (Beyea, Slattery, & von Reyn, 2010; Everett-Thomas et al., 2014; Goode, Lynn, McElroy, Bednash, & Murray, 2013; Rhodes, et al., 2013). Zigmont et al. (2015) reported positive outcomes, significant cost savings, and improved transition to practice with a new nurse orientation program that included simulation-based learning.

BENEFITS OF SIMULATION FOR NURSING EDUCATION

When supervising students in actual clinical practice, an instructor's vigilance is spread over many students and many patients. However, with simulation, the instructor can observe every step the student makes, allowing for many teachable moments and the possibility of coaching to correct fallacies of judgment and erroneous actions. In addition, simulations can expose students to rare events that they do not commonly see in the practice setting—events where competent performance is critical but rarely possible without practice opportunities.

With simulation, faculty can ensure that all students have exposure to specific critical learning experiences, providing more uniformity in student experience. Critical events that occur infrequently, such as cardiac arrest, can be practiced repeatedly in simulation, allowing for competent performance in the real setting. Moreover, the rapid assessment of patient deterioration and the advanced decision making needed to prevent the actual cardiac arrest are expert skills that need ongoing rehearsal and reinforcement, which students and novice nurses usually do not receive. On-the-job training is not the ideal place to develop such critical competencies. Nor are students in clinical practice always able to see the outcomes of care, or the effects of errors in the limits of the clinical shift. Simulation allows students to experience the full consequences of their decisions, even to the point of the "death" of their "patients," which can profoundly affect the students' learning and retention of what they have learned.

The level of difficulty in simulation can be adapted for the student level. Simulators are differentiated according to the complexity needed for specific objectives. For example, anesthesiology training and advanced military training for casualty management involve highly complex simulators with advanced capabilities. However, the standard mannequins in use in most schools of nursing can be programmed for simple to advanced scenarios by manipulating one or more parameters to the level of difficulty. A novice student may have to respond to a simple declining blood pressure, whereas an advanced student may be dealing with a plummeting oxygen saturation, apparent respiratory distress, tachycardia, pharmacological effects, and distressed family members.

Beyond uses in teaching assessment and providing realistic skills practice, scenarios can be developed and validated to provide for the development of critical thinking and clinical decision making and can be used for competency evaluation. The ability for nurse educators to be able to observe a complete set of actions, question a student's line of thinking, and provide guidance when the student fails to notice or incorporate important cues is a powerful teaching adjunct, allowing for many more of the precious "teachable moments" valued by faculty.

Simulations can be designed for team practice, enhancing collaboration, and improving team communication skills. Simulations that provide for interdisciplinary training, including the full array of roles in a patient care scenario, are becoming an important part of staff development. Health care professionals are predominantly trained in their individual disciplines, yet they must be able to come together as teams, with little or no interdisciplinary training. Simulation can provide the common ground for health care teams to learn how to function as teams (Kenaszchuk, MacMillan, van Soeren, & Reeves, 2011). Patient safety requires highly organized systems of care, yet the training of the individuals who comprise the teams has been neglected. The IOM report *To Err Is Human* emphasized the need for team training using simulation (Kohn et al., 2000).

DISADVANTAGES OF SIMULATION

The use of patient simulators may not be a total panacea for educators. Initial costs for the acquisition of the simulators are prohibitive for many programs. New wireless high-fidelity simulators cost US$40,000 to US$90,000 and have an expected shelf life of around 3 years. More basic models are available but are rapidly being replaced with wireless models with improved reality features such as blinking eyes and the ability to measure values using real-world equipment. Models that sense and respond to medications and have other sophisticated features necessary for anesthesiology or military training can cost as much as US$250,000. Institutions must augment their traditional equipment budgets to accommodate this emerging technology. Beyond the initial investment in high-fidelity mannequins, ongoing considerations of space, technician support, and faculty training mandate continuing expenses (Frick, Swoboda, Mansukhani, & Jeffries, 2014).

The number of students who can work with the simulators at one time is limited, and students require intensive faculty involvement, which is often more time-consuming than regular clinical supervision for a group of students. Traditional student-to-faculty ratios may need to be evaluated as simulation users become more knowledgeable about the most effective use of simulation time schedules. Faculty may need to rethink the "8-hour" student shift and replace it with shorter, more frequent training days.

Perhaps the most significant barrier to the use of simulation is the need for well-trained faculty who can devise the best uses of simulation within specific curricula. All too often, expensive simulators are purchased but not effectively used, lacking a champion who can bring about the extensive curricular planning and faculty training needed. It is not uncommon for expensive mannequins to lie dormant in their shipping crates long after their arrival. Seasoned educators may find the technology interface daunting (Taplay, Jack, Baxter, Kevin, & Martin, 2015). Despite the availability of predeveloped scenarios for nursing education, nursing faculty will have their own priorities and will desire modifications that must be programmed into the computer. The availability of skilled technicians who can assist with the computer interface removes one of the major faculty hurdles but poses additional costs.

Students may feel put on the spot and experience anxiety, especially when being observed by faculty and peers. However, as simulation has become more prevalent, most studies show high student satisfaction with this learning methodology. Though some students may report increased anxiety, others experience less anxiety (Research Study Fuels the Controversy 14.1).

Discussion Point

1. Do you consider the viewpoint of Diener and Hobbs compelling?
2. If you have experienced simulation, do you feel that caring can develop within the context of an artificial environment, such as simulation?
3. State regulatory nursing boards often determine the percentage of clinical time that can be used for simulation, with ranges of 10% to 50%. What do you think would be the ideal balance between simulation experience and actual clinical practice?

Although it is important to note the cautionary views on simulation, it is noteworthy that those who are using and evaluating simulation are passionate champions of this rapidly advancing field. Today's simulation is not focused on isolated skill building. It builds on a skills foundation and requires students to acquire cognitive and affective skills and to develop clinical judgment.

Research Study Fuels the Controversy 14.1

Can Simulation Develop Caring in Nursing Students?

Diener and Hobbs (2012) raised concerns about the ability of "technology-driven robotic devices to form and cultivate caring behaviors, or sufficiently develop interactive nurse-client communication necessary in the context of nursing." They raised the question of whether students can learn to care in simulated settings, without the reciprocity involved in actual human relationships. They proposed that "unless time is spent with human beings in even the earliest stages of nursing education, transpersonal caring relationships do not have space to develop." They challenged nurse educators to integrate technology wisely within a caring curriculum.

Source: Diener, E., & Hobbs, N. (2012). Simulating care: Technology-mediated learning in twenty-first century nursing education. *Nursing Forum, 47*(1), 34–38.

Study Findings

Eggenberger, Keller, Chase, and Payne (2012) developed a tool to measure caring in the nursing simulation environment. The Caring Efficacy Scale-Simulation Student Version (CES-SSV) and Caring Efficacy Scale-Simulation Faculty Version (CES-SFV) were developed and applied in a correlational study to compare student self-ratings with faculty ratings. The rating scales were applied in a scenario that included a family member in a simulated cardiac arrest. Fifty-seven students participated and completed self-ratings, which were correlated with two independent faculty raters. The tools were shown to have excellent reliability and interrater reliability and show promise for being able to reliably measure caring attributes of nursing students. Studies using this tool may be able to answer the question of whether simulation can help to develop caring behaviors.

Source: Eggenberger, R., Keller, K., Chase, S., & Payne, L. (2012). A quantitative approach to evaluating caring in nursing simulation. *Nursing Education Perspectives, 33*(6), 406–409.

In many areas, students are required or encouraged to practice in a team of health professionals, building competencies essential for working within teams. Research is steadily accumulating to inform educators on outcomes and methods in applying simulation.

RESEARCH ON SIMULATION OUTCOMES

Agencies that have instituted simulation training are usually very positive about their outcomes. However, research on simulation outcomes for nursing is in its infancy. Much of the literature is of a developmental nature, describing programs and processes but not evaluating outcomes. Is there evidence that these expensive programs lead to better learning than traditional teaching strategies? Schools of medicine, training in anesthesiology, and the military have been using sophisticated patient simulators for a long time and have performed studies on the effect on learning, lending extensive credibility to simulation training methods, but less data are available for nursing.

Nursing Student Perceptions of Simulation

Many of the studies performed in nursing have focused on how acceptable this mode of learning is to students and their satisfaction levels. In general, this mode of learning is very well received by students. Foronda, Liu, and Bauman (2013) synthesized research findings on evaluation of simulation in undergraduate nursing education, in 101 research articles published between 2007 and 2012. Five predominant themes were found in the outcomes: confidence/self-efficacy, satisfaction, anxiety/stress, skills/knowledge, and interdisciplinary experiences. Much of the evaluation focused on learner self-report. Confidence/self-efficacy improved with simulation, and students were satisfied with simulation as a mode for learning and skills/knowledge acquisition (including communication). Students viewed interdisciplinary experiences as positive. Mixed results were found related to anxiety/stress, with the majority of studies finding simulation caused anxiety or stress, but others indicating that simulation led to decreased stress/anxiety. Similar results were found by Mould, White, and Gallagher (2011) in a senior critical care course. Confidence and competence improved, and the simulations were seen as enjoyable. Hsu, Chang, and Hsieh (2015) found overwhelmingly greater satisfaction with simulation-based learning compared with traditional classroom lectures.

Students who participated in a study by Kaddoura (2010) commented that they were able to sharpen their leadership skills, improve teamwork, and practice effective communication as part of the simulation experience. Students reported that they believed their real ICU patients were safer because they learned how to deal with similar situations in simulation. They also expressed value in learning from each other when a collaborative approach is used in which classmates observe and contribute to each other's scenarios (Hober & Bonnel, 2014).

Learning Outcomes With Simulation

Perhaps most relevant to educators is the degree to which simulation experiences actually contribute to learning outcomes. Most of those who use simulation believe in the value of simulation for improving learning outcomes. The research literature is rapidly growing; however, research findings are not definitive. The majority of studies report qualitative data; many of those that have a quantitative focus use weak designs and small sample sizes, lack valid and reliable measurement tools, and present limited details on methodology (Lapkin, Levett-Jones, Bellchambers, & Fernandez, 2010; Shinnick, Woo, & Mentes, 2011b).

Several recent systematic reviews of research on simulation have attempted to determine the actual impact of simulation on outcomes (Cant & Cooper, 2009; Harder, 2010; Lapkin et al., 2010; Shinnick et al., 2011b). The majority reported an increase in students' clinical skills using simulation compared with other teaching methods. None found that clinical skills *decreased* in the simulation groups. Several reported increases in students' perceived self-confidence and competence. Harder (2010) concluded that the evidence supports using simulation as a teaching tool despite many gaps and limitations in simulation research. Lapkin et al. (2010) found support for the use of human patient simulators to significantly improve knowledge acquisition, critical thinking, and the ability to identify deteriorating patients. Shinnick et al. (2011b) concluded that the literature shows that students like simulation and that self-efficacy improves with simulation. However, they found no evidence that simulation impacts students' ability to use critical thinking. They assert that, lacking solid research evidence, the efforts to integrate simulation into nursing education may be wasted. Common to these reviews were concerns about study limitations, including lack of formal evaluation tools with good reliability and validity; lack of uniform measures of outcomes, weak study designs, and small sample sizes.

A large and more recent review study looked specifically at the learning outcomes construct (based on the NLN/Jeffries Simulation Framework) (O'Donnell, Decker, Howard, Levett-Jones, & Miller, 2014). Subcomponents of the learning outcomes construct include skills performance, learning satisfaction, knowledge/learner, critical thinking/clinical judgment, and self-confidence/self-efficacy. The reviewers concluded that, overall, students and faculty are highly satisfied with simulation as a learning modality. Outcomes of learning or knowledge gain were less clear-cut, due to self-report measures, weak instruments, and lack of control of extraneous variables. Similarly, growth in critical thinking or clinical judgment was also hard to quantify, lacking clear definitions and sound measures of these concepts and small sample sizes. Self-confidence measures were similarly lacking, typically relying on self-report or anecdotes. The challenges for simulation research will be to measure retention and transferability of learning, and the addition of other important learning outcomes to the NLN/Jeffries framework, including transferability to clinical practice, improved communication, clinical performance, professional behaviors, and clinical outcomes.

A common theme in evaluation of simulation outcomes is lack of suitable evaluation tools to effectively measure outcomes. Kardong-Edgren, Adamson, and Fitzgerald (2010) reinforced the call for reliable and valid instruments to measure simulation learning outcomes. They surveyed available instruments and concluded that only four tools currently come close to addressing cognitive, psychomotor, and affective learning domains. They advocated reuse of existing tools, with emphasis on establishment of reliability and validity in multiple venues, to expand the science of simulation research. A follow-up to the original survey revealed that studies using the predominant evaluation tools continue, along with the development of new tools (Adamson, Kardong-Edgren, & Willhaus, 2013). However, despite some progress, most instruments focus on learner reactions to simulation and to cognitive learning, the "low-hanging fruit of simulation evaluation." They challenged researchers to progress to higher levels of evaluation that will gauge actual behavior change in practice and ultimately improved patient outcomes (Research Study Fuels the Controversy 14.2).

Research Study Fuels the Controversy 14.2

The growth of simulation, along with limitations on clinical placements for students, has led nursing programs to request state board permissions to use simulation as a replacement for some traditional clinical experience hours (Hayden, Smiley, & Gross, 2014b). Research to date has not provided the strong evidence needed for state board policy decisions. The National Council of State Boards of Nursing commissioned a large-scale, randomized, controlled study to examine the impact of simulation (Hayden, Smiley, Alexander, Kardong-Edgren, & Jeffries, 2014a). Ten prelicensure programs were recruited, and randomized into one of three study groups: Control group (traditional clinical experience with no more than 10% simulation; 25% group (25% of clinical hours replaced by simulation); 50% group (50% of clinical hours replaced by simulation). The study followed 666 students, from the first clinical nursing course, through graduation, and for the first 6 months of clinical practice. Outcomes measured included knowledge, clinical competency, critical thinking, and readiness for practice. Standardized ATI tests, NCLEX pass rates, and surveys of students, clinical preceptors/instructors, and managers (using established scales with validity/reliability measures) provided the data, at defined measurement intervals.

Source: Hayden, J. K., Smiley, R. A., Alexander, M., Kardong-Edgren, S., & Jeffries, P. R. (2014a). The NCSBN National Simulation Study: A longitudinal, randomized, controlled study replacing clinical hours with simulation in prelicensure nursing education. *Journal of Nursing Regulation, 5* (Suppl. 2), C1–S64.

Study Findings

There were no statistically significant differences in clinical competency, nursing knowledge, or NCLEX pass rates among the three study groups. Likewise, for the first 6 months of practice, there were no differences in manager ratings of clinical competency or readiness for practice. The researchers concluded that the results provide "substantial evidence that substituting high-quality simulation experiences for up to half of traditional clinical hours produces comparable end-of-program educational outcomes and new graduates that are ready for clinical practice" (p. S3).

SIMULATION FOR PRACTICE SETTINGS

Patient simulators are not relegated only to academic settings for the initial training of nursing students. Simulation has been used to test new procedures before bringing them to the patient bedside, training individuals and teams for specific advanced skills in specialty settings, for orienting new nurses and performance evaluations.

Dartmouth-Hitchcock Medical Center initiated a nurse residency program using human patient simulation to address issues related to the orientation time required for new graduates to become competent and to feel confident (Beyea, von Reyn, & Slattery, 2007). A 12-week program was developed, with didactic courses, weekly simulation experiences, and clinical time with a preceptor. At the end of the residency, the nurses were evaluated with simulations designed to assess competence. The program resulted in a markedly reduced time for orientation, with the program participants able to take full patient assignments. Participants were better prepared for skills. The simulation experiences allowed early identification of areas in which participants needed remediation or more guidance. The residents improved in self-rated confidence, competence, and readiness for independent practice. An overwhelming majority of the participants were positive about the simulation experiences. Further outcomes from this continued project reinforced the value of the simulation-based residency program as a "powerful and effective strategy" (Beyea et al., 2010, p. e174). Recruitment and retention improved markedly. Nurse residents experienced significant improvement in perceived confidence, competence, and readiness for practice.

Stefanski and Rossler (2009) developed a critical care orientation program for new graduates, with positive outcomes in perceived confidence of the new nurses. Kaddoura (2010) explored the use of simulation to develop critical thinking skills for graduates on critical care units. Participants reported that they were more confident in dealing with critical situations, and simulation helped to develop their critical thinking skills. A systematic review of the effectiveness of simulation in critical care found only one study met inclusion criteria (Jansson, Kaariainen, & Kyngas, 2013). That study demonstrated that simulation led to a significant improvement in medication error rates, when compared with didactic lectures, with the results persisting after 2 to 3 months.

Many institutions have incorporated simulation training into critical care settings, and it is projected to play a prominent role in critical care education as several critical care organizations are exploring the technology (Alinier & Platt, 2013). Simulation is seen as useful for numerous activities in critical care, including technical and nontechnical (communication) skills, competency-based assessment, performance feedback, crisis resource management, and assessment of team performance.

The use of patient simulators in actual clinical environments—in situ simulation—is growing as well. A recent review of 29 publications summarized how in situ simulation is being used (Rosen, Hunt, Pronovost, Federowicz, & Weaver, 2012). The operating room was predominant (30%), followed by labor and delivery (15%), emergency department (15%), and intensive care (7%). However, nine other settings were using simulation as well. All of the settings included multidisciplinary teams, with objectives that included teamwork competency, but many included objectives focused on procedural skills, decision making, and orientation, as well as identifying system issues and hazards. As a relatively new development, research on in situ simulation is not well developed, but it has the potential to be a powerful learning strategy (Rosen et al., 2012). It is likely that more settings will adopt simulation methods, impacting the practicing nurse in many health care settings.

SIMULATION ADOPTION: DRIVING AND RESTRAINING FORCES

Resistance to change in education and the desire to protect traditional education practices have been identified as major barriers to the success of simulation. These challenges require leadership support and cultural readiness to overcome. Most simulation centers, faculty champions, and students are positive about the future of simulation education. Some centers project a 55% growth in the next 5 years with supporting funding. Learners are the "driving force" behind simulation education and programs will adjust to increased demand with larger centers and programs. Educators will need to change their vision from individualized teacher-centered programs to team-based training. At the same time, simulation centers will rely on collaboration to develop the funding support, faculty training, and changing policies that will surround growing simulation programs. The financial commitment to support curricular integration, simulation technology, and the supporting infrastructure is substantial. While the potential exists for simulation methods to improve health professions education and expand to other areas of promise—such as faculty development and patient safety—simulation suffers from a lack of substantial financial support. Sustainable funding is a potential barrier and important factor that will contribute to the future growth of simulation education (Qayumi et al., 2014).

REGULATORY TRENDS RECOGNIZE THE VALUE OF SIMULATIONS

Regulatory boards are challenged to determine competence standards for initial and continued licensure for health professions. In 2010, the NCSBN took on this challenge and convened the National Simulation Study (Hayden et al., 2014a) (see Research Study Fuels the Controversy 14.2). Led by investigator Jennifer Hayden, the study examined whether or not simulation could be substituted for traditional clinical hours for prelicensure nursing students. The study followed 666 prelicensure nursing students from entry through graduation. This study is considered groundbreaking research that demonstrated the role regulatory boards can play in supporting education and curriculum development. By funding this quality research on simulation education, the NCSBN was able to demonstrate that there is no statistical difference between traditional groups and those with a high percentage of simulated clinical experiences in the areas of critical thinking, clinical competency, and readiness for practice as rated by managers at intervals of the first 6 months of practice.

Benner et al. (2010) asserted that nursing licensure must be based on competency evaluation that extends far beyond the current multiple-choice NCLEX. They advocated a three-part performance assessment, beginning with the last year of nursing school, a second for licensure, and a third on completion of a 1-year postlicensure residency. Simulation would provide the method for these assessments.

The Accreditation Council for Graduate Medical Education (ACGME) and the American Board of Medical Specialties (ABMS) both have embraced simulation as one of a variety of tools that can assist in determining practitioner competency (Decker et al., 2011). The American Academy of Pediatrics (AAP) steering committee on Neonatal Resuscitation Programs (NRPs) announced its commitment to base newborn resuscitation on the best evidence-based science available. With that in mind, AAP incorporates practice on an infant simulator as part of its NRP (Perlman et al., 2010).

As part of heightened emergency preparedness efforts, the U.S. Department of Health and Human Services, together with the Joint Commission on the Accreditation of Healthcare Organizations and other agencies, is extending disaster training to the inpatient bedside environment. High-fidelity human patient simulators are used for training in disaster and terrorism response and treatment, as well as in patient safety and other issues raised in the IOM report *To Err Is Human* (Scott et al., 2012).

Recent outbreaks ranging from measles to Ebola put the spotlight on the need for simulation training that includes real-time training for infectious disease outbreaks. Hospitals in New York demonstrated that simulation practice could produce measurable improvement in early disease recognition and response, as well as provide opportunity for practice to develop dexterity in donning and doffing protective isolation garb (Sutherland & Perez, 2014).

STANDARDS FOR SIMULATION

The rapid growth of simulation technology has been accompanied by practice standards to guide appropriate implementation of simulation. The INASCL developed the first evidence-based standards on simulation (Borum, 2013). The initial set of standards and the recently revised standards have attained widespread adoption, and guide research projects. Additional standards are under development, to guide simulation design, interprofessional simulations, and simulation research. The guidance of these standards is likely to produce higher quality and more effective simulation efforts, with more predictable outcomes (Box 14.1).

SIMULATION CERTIFICATION FOR SIMULATION EDUCATORS

The Society for Simulation in Healthcare (SSH) is the premier organization representing health care professionals, educators, scientists, and advocates of simulation methodologies. SSH has always had the goal of improved performance and reduction in errors in patient care. In 2012, SSH launched a certification program for educators that is consistent with its mission. Though voluntary, simulation educators from around the world have taken the SSH Educator Certification exam and have received the title CHSE (Certified Healthcare Simulation Educator). The exam was developed through the work of a variety of individuals from varying specialties and was developed to

BOX 14.1 INACSL Standards of Best Practice: Simulation^{SM} Standards I to VII

Standard I: Terminology

Consistent terminology provides guidance and clear communication and reflects shared values in simulation experiences, research, and publications. Knowledge and ideas are clearly communicated with consistent terminology to advance the science of simulation (Meakim et al., 2013).

Standard II: Professional Integrity of Participant(s)

The simulation learning, assessment, and evaluation environments will be areas where mutual respect among participants and facilitator(s) is expected and supported. As such, it is essential to provide clear expectations for the attitudes and behaviors of simulation participants. Professional integrity related to confidentiality of the performances, scenario content, and participant experience is required during and after any simulation. Confidentiality is expected in live, recorded, or virtual simulation experiences (Gloe et al., 2013).

Standard III: Participant Objectives

All simulation-based learning experiences begin with development of clearly written participant objectives, which are available prior to the experience (Lioce et al., 2013).

Standard IV: Facilitation

Multiple methods of facilitation are available, and use of a specific method is dependent on the learning needs of the participant(s) and the expected outcomes (Franklin et al., 2013).

Standard V: Facilitator

A proficient facilitator is required to manage the complexity of all aspects of simulation. The facilitator has specific simulation education provided by formal coursework, continuing education offerings, and targeted work with an experienced mentor (Boese et al., 2013).

Standard VI: The Debriefing Process

All simulation-based learning experiences should include a planned debriefing session aimed toward promoting reflective thinking (Decker et al., 2013).

Standard VII: Participant Assessment and Evaluation

In a simulation-based experience, formative assessment or summative evaluation can be used (Sando et al., 2013).

Source: INACSL Standards of Best Practice: Simulation^{SM}. (2013). Retrieved from http://www.inacsl.org/i4a/pages/index.cfm?pageid=3407

recognize simulation educators. As a follow-up to this exam two other certifications have become available. The CHSE-A designation is an advanced certification that involves a body of work in simulation that is submitted as a digital portfolio. The CHSOS (Certified Healthcare Simulation Operation Specialist) is a certification exam offered to simulation operation specialists, previously referred to as simulation technologists. Certification in Healthcare Simulation—as in other certified specialties—provides a quality indicator for the role of simulation educator. Maintaining credible standards for simulation education requires professional accountability. Certification promotes continuous learning and contributes to quality. It is important to support clinical certification that will encourage high standards in simulation education. SSH provides a learning blueprint, practice exam, and sample materials for educators interested in applying for certification (SSH, 2015).

SIMULATION IN CONTINUING EDUCATION FOR NURSES

All licensed professions require ongoing education to maintain and expand the competency needed in a dynamic health care system. Yet traditional methods of continuing education are under scrutiny. Typical education for license renewal includes attendance at lectures or commercial self-study packages. There is little evidence that lectures endured for continuing education requirements actually improve practice (see Chapter 22). A Cochrane review of studies involving over 11,000 health professionals concluded that while didactic meetings may have a small effect on professional practice, they are not likely to change complex behaviors (Forsetlund et al., 2009). Simulation-based continuing education holds the promise of leading to longer-lasting performance change, as objective assessments are incorporated (Dow, Salas, & Mazmanian, 2012). Simulation-based continuing education is seen as one potential solution to an ongoing debate about how best to ensure meaningful professional development among certified registered nurse anesthetists (Zambricki, Horowitz, Blumenreich, & Fallacaro, 2015). Though no changes in registered nurse licensure requirements are in the offing, efforts to improve professional practice through simulation education will likely continue.

National and international trends ensure that students, nurse educators, and practicing nurses will encounter high-fidelity human patient simulators in their career pathways (Research Study Fuels the Controversy 14.3). While there are debates about the actual outcomes, and the extent of the role of simulation, simulation is an educational strategy that continues to gain momentum.

Conclusions

The advance of technology in health care is relentless; simulation brings significant technological change to nursing education as well. Regardless of how nurses were initially educated, all nurses can anticipate exposure to simulation technology, whether as students or new graduates, in orienting to new roles or specialties, for demonstrating ongoing competency, and even for continuing education. Nurses in staff development or responsible for training nurses for specialty settings will need to consider simulation as a teaching and competency assessment strategy. In a profession that requires

Research Study Fuels the Controversy 14.3

Is It Ethical to Train Nurses *Without* the Use of Simulation?

Given expanding simulation technology, which allows for much greater demonstration of competency before entering the real patient care setting, is it ethical to continue to educate students *without* simulation? Decker (2007) discussed the educational ethics related to the use of patient simulators as a means to provide realistic training for students without endangering patients versus traditional clinical learning experiences in which patients are subjected to the ministrations of inexperienced students.

Source: Decker, S. (2007). Simulations: Education and ethics. In P. Jeffries (Ed.), *Simulation in nursing education: From conceptualization to evaluation* (pp. 11–19). New York, NY: National League for Nursing.

Study Findings

Discussing ethical principles of justice, autonomy, beneficence, nonmaleficence, veracity, and compassion, Decker presented examples of how simulation training might lead to more ethical care for patients. For example, Decker asked, "Are nurse educators and other healthcare professionals demonstrating compassion when they allow students to perform procedures for the first time on clients instead of first providing students with simulated experiences?" (p. 16). Decker raised questions for nursing faculty to consider regarding their obligation to ensure nursing student competencies before engaging in patient care, in light of the looming opportunities presented by patient simulators. She posed a need for a change in the culture of nursing education, related to use of simulation. The study below presents a picture of some nurse educators' viewpoints related to student learning.

Nursing educators in the United Kingdom ($n = 19$) were interviewed regarding the use of patients in nursing education, in light of the development of simulation opportunities. Overwhelmingly, the nurse educators supported the view that students need to participate with patients in order to become well-qualified nurses. The historical view of how nurses have always been trained predominated. Although informed patient consent was seen as important, it was deemed secondary to the need for training safe nurses, which requires patient care experience. The authors concluded that using patients for training nurses is probably ethical, as long as the patient is fully informed. They also recommended appropriate use of viable alternatives to the traditional learning environment (eg simulation).

Source: Torrance, C., Mansell, I., & Wilson, C. (2012). Learning objects? Nurse educators' views on using patients for students learning: Ethics and consent. *Education for Health, 25*(2), 92–96.

For Additional Discussion

1. Consider your first skill applied to a real patient, such as giving an injection or starting an IV line. How confident were you of your skill? How anxious were you? How much of your anxiety was transmitted to the patient? Would simulation practice have improved your confidence and decreased your anxiety?
2. Reflect on a crisis situation in patient care that you had to solve quickly on your own. Would prior simulation practice have helped you in your ability to anticipate and critically analyze the situation? Why or why not?
3. Consider a clinical situation in which you experienced profound learning, something you will never forget. Is there a way to replicate that situation through simulation so that others could experience the same learning? Why or why not?
4. Simulation has been faulted for not being totally realistic. Which factors in patient care can readily be incorporated into simulation? Which cannot?
5. Consider the anxiety experienced by students in a simulation who are being observed by faculty and peers. In the clinical setting, is there more or less anxiety when you are uncertain of your actions and are being observed by patients, family, nurses, physicians, and others?
6. When a student approaches a patient procedure, is it ethical to ask for the patient's consent without fully disclosing the student's qualifications to perform the procedure?
7. In comparing traditional models of nursing education—skills labs followed by clinical practice—with simulation prior to clinical practice:
   a. Which model provides for greater patient safety?
   b. Which model provides for the greatest security for the patient?
   c. Which model provides for the greatest confidence building for students?

lifelong learning, the question of how best to learn new competencies is partially answered by the promise of simulation. Although research still needs to be done on how much simulation should be used, and how much it can impact actual nurse performance and patient outcomes, the rapid growth of this field indicates that simulation is likely here to stay as a mainstay of health care professional training.

References

Adamson, K., Kardong-Edgren, S., & Willhaus, J. (2013). An updated review of published simulation evaluation instruments. *Clinical Simulation in Nursing, 9*, e393–e400.

Aebersold, M., & Tschannen, D. (2013). Simulation in nursing practice: The impact on patient care. *The Online Journal of Issues in Nursing, 18*(2), 6. doi:10.3912/OJIN.Vol18No02Man06

Agency for Healthcare Research and Quality. (n.d.). *About team STEPPS*. Retrieved from http://www.ahrq.gov/professionals/education/curriculum-tools/teamstepps/index.html

Alinier, G., & Platt, A. (2013). International overview of high-level simulation education initiatives in relation to critical care. *British Association of Critical Care Nurses, 19*(1), 42–49.

Benner, P., Sutphen, M., Leonard, V., & Day, L. (2010). *Educating nurses: A call for radical transformation*. San Francisco, CA: Jossey-Bass.

Berkow, S., Virkstis, K., Steward, J., & Conway, L. (2009). Assessing new graduate nurse performance. *Nurse Educator, 34*(1), 17–22.

Beyea, S. C., von Reyn, L., & Slattery, M. (2007). A nurse residency program for competency development using human patient simulation. *Journal for Nurses in Staff Development, 23*(7), 77–82.

Beyea, S., Slattery, M., & von Reyn, L. (2010). Outcomes of a simulation-based nurse residency program. *Clinical Simulation in Nursing, 6*(5), e169–e175.

Boese, T., Cato, M., Gonzalez, L., Jones, A., Kennedy, K., Reese, C., . . . Borum, J. (2013). Standards of best practice: Simulation Standard V: Facilitator. *Clinical*

Simulation in Nursing, 9(6 Suppl.), S22–S25. doi:10.1016/j.ecns.2013.04.010

Borum, J. (2013). Introduction: Standard revisions. *Clinical Simulation in Nursing, 9*(6 Suppl.), S1. doi:10.1016/j.ecns.2013.05.009

Cant, R., & Cooper, S. (2009). Simulation-based learning in nurse education: Systematic review. *Journal of Advanced Nursing, 66*(1), 3–15.

Cronenwett, L., Sherwood, G., Barnsteiner, J., Disch, J., Johnson, J., Mitchell, P., . . . Warren, J. (2007). Quality and safety education for nursing. *Nursing Outlook, 55*(3), 122–131.

Decker, S. (2007). Simulations: Education and ethics. In P. Jeffries (Ed.), *Simulation in nursing education: From conceptualization to evaluation* (pp. 11–19). New York, NY: National League for Nursing.

Decker, S., Fey, M., Sideras, S., Caballero, S., Rockstraw, L., Boese, T., . . . Borum, J. (2013). Standards of best practice: Simulation Standard VI: The debriefing process. *Clinical Simulation in Nursing, 9*(6S), S27–S29. doi:10.1016/j.ecns.2013.04.008.

Decker, S., Utterback, V., Thomas, M., Mitchell, M., & Sportsman, S. (2011). Assessing continued competency through simulation: A call to action. *Nursing Education Perspectives, 32*(2), 120–125.

Diener, E., & Hobbs, N. (2012). Simulating care: Technology-mediated learning in twenty-first century nursing education. *Nursing Forum, 47*(1), 34–38.

Dow, A., Salas, E., & Mazmanian, P. (2012). Improving quality in systems of care: Solving complicated challenges with simulation-based continuing professional development. *Journal of Continuing Education in the Health Professions, 32*(4), 230–235.

Dreifuerst, K., Horton-Deutsch, S., & Henao, H. (2014). Meaningful debriefing and other approaches. In P. Jeffries (Ed.), *Clinical simulations in nursing education: Advanced concepts, trends, and opportunities* (pp. 44–57). Philadelphia, PA: Wolters Kluwer Health/Lippincott Williams and Wilkins.

Eggenberger, R., Keller, K., Chase, S., & Payne, L. (2012). A quantitative approach to evaluating caring in nursing simulation. *Nursing Education Perspectives, 33*(6), 406–409.

Everett-Thomas, R., Valdes, B., Valdes, G., Shekhter, I., Fitzpatrick, M., Rosen, L., . . . Birnbach, D. (2014). Using simulation technology to identify gaps between education and practice among new graduate nurses. *Journal of Continuing Education for Nurses, 46*(1), 34–40.

Fisher, D., & King, L. (2013). An integrative literature review on preparing nursing students through simulation to recognize and respond to the deteriorating patient. *Journal of Advanced Nursing, 69*(11), 2375–2388. doi:10.1111/jan.12174

Foronda, C., Liu, S., & Bauman, E. (2013). Evaluation of simulation in undergraduate nurse education: An integrative review. *Clinical Simulation in Nursing,* 9(10), e409–e416. doi:10.1016/j.ecns.2012.11.003.

Forsetlund, L., Bjorndal, A., Rashidian, A., Jamtvedt, G., O'Brien, M. A., Wolf, F. M., . . . Oxman, A. D. (2009). Continuing education meetings and workshops: Effects on professional practice and health care outcomes. *The Cochrane Database of Systematic Reviews,* (2), CD003030. doi:10.1002/14651858.CD003030.pub2

Franklin, A., Boese, T., Gloe, D., Lioce, L., Decker, S., Sando, C., . . . Borum, J. (2013). Standards of best practice: Simulation Standard IV: Facilitation. *Clinical Simulation in Nursing, 9*(6 Suppl.), S19–S21. doi:10.1016/j.ecns.2013.04.011.

Frick, K., Swoboda, S., Mansukhani, K., & Jefffries, P. (2014). An economic model for clinical simulation in prelicensure nursing programs. *Journal of Nursing Regulation, 5*(3), 9–13.

Gloe, D., Sando, C., Franklin, A., Boese, T., Decker, S., Lioce, L., . . . Borum, J. (2013). Standards of best practice: Simulation standard II: Professional integrity of participant(s). *Clinical Simulation in Nursing, 9* (6 Suppl.), S12–S14. doi:10.1016/j.ecns.2013.04.004.

Goode, C., Lynn, M., McElroy, D., Bednash, G., & Murray, B. (2013). Lessons learned form 10 years of research on a post-baccalaureate nurse residency program. *Journal of Nursing Administration, 43*(2),73–79.

Gore, R., Van Gele, P., Ravert, P., & Mabire, C. (2012). A 2010 survey of the INACSL membership about simulation use. *Clinical Simulation in Nursing, 8*(4), e125–e133.

Harder, N. (2010). Use of simulation in teaching and learning in health sciences: A systematic review. *Journal of Nursing Education, 49*(1), 23–28.

Harvey, E., Echols, S., Clark, R., & Lee, E. (2014). Comparison of two teamSTEPPS training methods on nurse failure-to-rescue performance. *Clinical Simulation in Nursing, 10*(2), e57–e64. doi:10.1016/j.ecns.2013.08.006.

Hayden, J. (2010). Use of simulation in nursing education: National survey results. *Journal of Nursing Regulation, 1*(3), 52–57.

Hayden, J. K., Smiley, R. A., Alexander, M., Kardong-Edgren, S., & Jeffries, P. R. (2014a). The NCSBN National Simulation study: A longitudinal, randomized, controlled study replacing clinical hours with simulation in prelicensure nursing education. *Journal of Nursing Regulation, 5*(Suppl. 2), S4–S64.

Hayden, J. K., Smiley, R. A., & Gross, L. (2014b). Simulation in nursing education: Current regulations and practices. *Journal of Nursing Regulation, 5*(2), 25–30.

Hober, C., & Bonnel, W. (2014). Student perceptions of the observer role in high-fidelity simulation. *Clinical Simulation in Nursing, 10*(10), 507–514. doi:10.1016/j.ecns.2014.07.008

Hsu, L., Chang, W., & Hsieh, S. (2015). The effects of scenario-based simulation course training on nurses' communication competence and self-efficacy: A randomized controlled trial. *Journal of Professional Nursing, 31*(1), 37–49.

Ironside, P., McNelis, A., & Ebright, P. (2014). Clinical education in nursing: Rethinking learning in practice settings. *Nursing Outlook, 62*(3), 185–191. doi:10.1016/j.outlook.2013.12.004

James, J. T. (2013). A new, evidence-based estimate of patient harms associated with hospital care. *Journal of Patient Safety, 9*(3), 122–128.

Jansson, M., Kaariainen, M., & Kyngas, H. (2013). Effectiveness of simulation-based education in critical care nurses' continuing education: A systematic review. *Clinical Simulation in Nursing, 9*(9), e355–e360. doi:10.1016/j.ecns.2012.07.003

Jones, K., Skinner, A., High, R., & Reiter-Palmon, R. (2013). A theory-driven, longitudinal evaluation of the impact of team training on safety culture in 24 hospitals. *BMJ Quality and Safety, 22*(5), 394–404.

Kaddoura, M. (2010). New graduate nurses' perceptions of the effects of clinical simulation on their critical thinking, learning, and confidence. *Journal of Continuing Education in Nursing, 41*(11), 506–515.

Kardong-Edgren, S. (2009). A letter to nursing program administrators about simulation. *Clinical Simulation in Nursing, 5*, e161–e162.

Kardong-Edgren, S., Adamson, K., & Fitzgerald, C. (2010). A review of currently published evaluation instruments for human patient simulation. *Clinical Simulation in Nursing, 6*, e25–e35.

Kenaszchuk, C., MacMillan, K., van Soeren, M., & Reeves, S. (2011). Interprofessional simulated learning: Short-term associations between simulation and interprofessional collaboration. *BMC Medicine, 9*, 29. Retrieved from http://biomedcentral.com/1741-7015/9/29

Kohn, L., Corrigan, J., & Donaldson, M. (Eds.). (2000). *To err is human: Building a safer health system.* Washington, DC: National Academy Press.

Lapkin, S., Levett-Jones, T., Bellchambers, H., & Fernandez, H. (2010). Effectiveness of patient simulation manikins in teaching clinical reasoning skills to undergraduate nursing students: A systematic review. *Clinical Simulation in Nursing, 6*, e207–e222.

Lioce, L., Reed, C., Lemon, D., King, M., Martinez, P., Franklin, A., . . . Borum, J. (2013). Standards of best practice: Simulation standard II: Participant objectives. *Clinical Simulation in Nursing, 9*(6 Suppl.), S15–S18. doi:10.1016/j.ecns.2013.04.005.

Mariani, B., Cantrell, M. A., Meakim, C., Prieto, P., & Dreifuerst, K. (2013). Structured debriefing and students' clinical judgment abilities in simulation. *Clinical Simulation in Nursing, 9*(5), e147–e155. doi:10.1016/j.ecns.2011.11.009. Retrieved from http://www.sciencedirect.com/science/article/pii/S1876139911002660

McNelis, A. M., Ironside, P. M., Ebright, P. R., Dreifuerst, K. T., Zvonar, S. E., & Conner, S. C. (2014). Learning nursing practice: A multisite, multimethod investigation of clinical education. *Journal of Nursing Regulation, 4*(4), 30–35.

Meakim, C., Boese, T., Decker, S., Franklin, A., Gloe, D., Lioce, L., . . . Borum, J. (2013). Standards of best practice: Simulation Standard I: Terminology. *Clinical Simulation in Nursing, 9*(6 Suppl.), S3–S11. doi:10.1016/j.ecns.2013.04.001.

Mould, J., White, H., & Gallagher, R. (2011). Evaluation of a critical care simulation series for undergraduate nursing students. *Contemporary Nurse, 38*(1/2), 189–190.

National League for Nursing Accreditation Commission. (2011). *NLNAC Accreditation Manual.* Atlanta, GA: Author.

National League for Nursing Interprofessional Education Collaborative. (2011). *A nursing perspective on simulation and Interprofessional Education (IPE): A report from the National League for Nursing's Think Tank on using simulation as an enabling strategy for IPE.* Retrieved from http://www.nln.org/docs/default-source/professional-development-programs/a-nursing-perspective-on-simulation-%28ipe-nln-invitational-think-tank-report,-2011%29-pdf.pdf?sfvrsn=0

O'Donnell, J., Decker, S., Howard, V., Levett-Jones, T., & Miller, C. (2014). NLN/Jeffries simulation framework state of the science project: Simulation learning outcomes. *Clinical Simulation in Nursing, 10*(7), 373–382. doi:10.1016/j.ecns.2014.06.004.

Pauly-O'Neill, S., Prion, S., & Nguyen, H. (2013). Comparison of Quality and Safety Education for

Nurses (QSEN)-Related student experiences during pediatric clinical and simulation rotations. *Journal of Nursing Education, 52*(9), 534–538. doi:10.3928/01484834-20130819-02

Perlman, J., Wyllie, J., Kattwinkel, J., Atkins, D., Chameides, L., Goldsmith, J., . . . Valaph, S. (2010). Special Report—Neonatal resuscitation: 2010 international consensus on cardiopulmonary resuscitation and emergency cardiovascular care science with treatment recommendations. *Pediatrics, 129*(5), e1319–e1344. Retrieved February 16, 2014, from http://pediatrics.aappublications.org/content/126/5/e1319.full.pdf+html?sid=8ce05eda-19b8-4f26-9d3c-c773d796fe06

Qayumi, K., Pachev, G., Zheng, B., Ziv, A., Koval, V., Badiei, S., & Cheng, A. (2014). Status of simulation in health care education: an international survey. *Advances in Medical Education and Practice, 5*, 457–467. doi:10.2147/AMEP.S65451

Reising, D., & Hensel, D. (2014). Clinical simulations focused on patient safety. In P. Jeffries (Ed.), *Clinical simulations in nursing education: Advanced concepts, trends, and opportunities* (pp. 22–43). Philadelphia, PA: Wolters Kluwer Health/Lippincott Williams and Wilkins.

Rhodes, C., Radziewicz, R., Amato, S., Bowden, V., Hazel, C., McClendon, S., . . . McNett, M. (2013). Registered nurse perceptions after implementation of a nurse residency program. *The Journal of Nursing Administration, 43*(10), 524–529.

Rizzolo, M. (2014). History and evolution of simulations: From oranges to avatars. In P. Jeffries (Ed.), *Clinical simulations in nursing education: Advanced concepts, trends, and opportunities* (pp. 1–8). Philadelphia, PA: Wolters Kluwer Health/Lippincott Williams and Wilkins.

Rosen, M., Hunt, E., Pronovost, P., Federowicz, M., & Weaver, S. (2012). In situ simulation in continuing education for the health care professions: A systematic review. *Journal of Continuing Education in the Health Professions, 32*(4), 243–254.

Sando, C., Coggins, R., Meakim, C., Franklin, A., Gloe, D., Boese, T., . . . Borum, J. (2013). Standards of best practice: Simulation Standard VII: Participant assessment and evaluation. *Clinical Simulation in Nursing,* 9(6S), S30–S32. doi:10.1016/j.ecns.2013.04.007

Scott, L. A., Maddux, P. T., Schnellmann, J., Hayes, L., Tolley, J., & Wahlquist, A. (2012). High fidelity multi-actor emergency preparedness training for patient care providers. *American Journal of Disaster Medicine, 7*(3), 175–188.

Sherwood, G., & Zomorodi, M. (2014). A new mindset for quality and safety: The QSEN competencies redefine nurses' roles in practice. *Nephrology Nursing Journal, 41*(1), 15–22, 72.

Shinnick, M. A., Woo, M., Horwich, T. B., & Steadman, R. (2011a). Debriefing: The most important component in simulation? *Clinical Simulation in Nursing, 7*, e105–e111.

Shinnick, M. A., Woo, M., & Mentes, J. (2011b). Human patient simulation: State of the science in prelicensure nursing education. *Journal of Nursing Education, 50*(2), 65–72.

Society for Simulation in Healthcare. (2015). *CHSE: Transform simulation education, get certified!* Retrieved from http://www.ssih.org/Certification/CHSE

Stefanski, R., & Rossler, K. (2009). Preparing the novice critical care nurse: A community-wide collaboration using the benefits of simulation. *Journal of Continuing Education in Nursing, 40*(10), 443–451.

Strouse, A. (2010). Multidisciplinary simulation centers: Promoting safe practice. *Clinical Simulation in Nursing, 6*(4), e139–e142.

Sutherland, A., & Perez, C. (2014, October 8). NYC hospitals prepared to treat Ebola: Officials. *New York Post*. Retrieved February 16, 2014, from http://nypost.com/2014/10/08/nyc-hospitals-prepared-to-treat-ebola-officials/

Taplay, K., Jack, S., Baxter, P., Kevin, E., & Martin, L. (2015). The process of adopting and incorporating simulation into undergraduate nursing curricula: A grounded theory study. *Journal of Professional Nursing, 31*(1), 26–36.

Tofil, N. M., Morris, J. L., Peterson, D. T., Watts, P., Epps, C., Harrington, K. F., . . . White, M. L. (2014). Interprofessional simulation training improves knowledge and teamwork in nursing and medical students during internal medicine clerkship. *Journal of Hospital Medicine, 9*, 189–192. doi:10.1002/jhm.2126

Zambricki, C., Horowitz, J., Blumenreich, G., & Fallacaro, M. (2015). Recertifying the professional nurse anesthetist: A call for national dialogue. *AANA Journal, 83*(1), 7–14.

Zigmont, J., Wade, A., Edwards, T., Hayes, K., Mitchell, J., & Oocumma, N. (2015). Utilization of experiential learning, and the learning outcomes model reduces RN orientation time by more than 35%. *Clinical Simulation in Nursing, 11*(2), 79–94. doi:10.1016/j.ecns.2014.11.001.

15

Can Clinical Reasoning Be Taught?

Keith Rischer

ADDITIONAL RESOURCES

Visit thePoint for additional helpful resources

- eBook
- Journal Articles
- WebLinks

CHAPTER OUTLINE

LEARNING OBJECTIVES

The learner will be able to:

1. Identify the changes that are required in nursing education to best prepare students for clinical practice.
2. Describe the key components of clinical reasoning.
3. Differentiate between critical thinking and clinical reasoning.
4. Distinguish clinical reasoning from clinical judgment.
5. Explain how clinical reasoning is utilized to make a correct clinical judgment.
6. Discuss what is meant by the term "failure to rescue."
7. Explain how clinical reasoning can decrease the incidence of "failure to rescue" when a patient experiences a complication.
8. Explore how clinical reasoning benefits student learning and can improve patient outcomes.
9. List the 12 questions that identify the steps of a clinical reasoning a nurse uses in practice.
10. Identify the four steps that are required by the nurse to make a clinical judgment.
11. Explore how reflection can guide the development of clinical judgment.

Portions of this chapter have been excerpted from Rischer, K. (2015). *Think like a nurse: Practical preparation for professional practice* (2nd ed.). Minneapolis, MN: KeithRN.

INTRODUCTION

Nursing education is in need of radical transformation because the current structure of nursing education is not adequate to prepare students for clinical practice. This includes the ability of the nurse to clinically reason by thinking in action and reasoning as a situation changes, recognizing and then responding appropriately to a patient's deteriorating condition (Benner, Sutphen, Leonard, & Day, 2010). As a result, patients whose deaths could have been prevented have died as a result of failure to rescue by the nurse (Clarke & Aiken, 2003). To realize this needed transformation in nursing education, and facilitate patient rescue by graduate nurses in the clinical setting, elements of clinical reasoning that include noticing crucial changes in patient status and evaluating the response need to be leveled throughout the curriculum (Russell, Geist, & Maffett, 2013).

Although clinical reasoning is an essential component of nurse thinking that requires clinical experience to develop (Benner, 1984), can it be effectively taught in nursing education? This question will be explored as well as how the need for comprehensive transformation in nursing education must be realized to strengthen student understanding of clinical reasoning. Clinical reasoning will then be defined and broken down to deepen understanding of this nurse thinking skill and how clinical reasoning is required to make a correct clinical judgment. Tools that students can use to apply and develop clinical reasoning in both the classroom and clinical settings will be presented. Finally, barriers to integrate clinical reasoning in nursing education will be discussed.

NURSING EDUCATION: IN NEED OF RADICAL TRANSFORMATION

Is nursing education currently prepared to integrate the emphasis of clinical reasoning effectively into the curriculum so it can be taught and emphasized? Based on the findings of educational research conducted by the Carnegie Foundation and led by preeminent nurse educator/researcher Patricia Benner, there are numerous barriers that must be addressed to integrate clinical reasoning and bring needed change. The conclusion of this work was published in 2010 and was titled *Educating Nurses: A Call for Radical Transformation* and was a wake-up call to challenge the current status quo in nursing education. *Educating Nurses: A Call for Radical Transformation* defined the problem and came to the conclusion that nursing education needs to be radically transformed by contextualizing classroom content to the clinical setting, integrating and bringing clinical realities to the classroom, and emphasizing clinical reasoning (Benner et al., 2010). To prepare the way for the successful integration of clinical reasoning into the curriculum so that it can be effectively taught, the following barriers need to be dealt with:

- Content overload and saturation
- Fragmented student learning
- Education–practice gap
- Emphasis on critical thinking over clinical reasoning.

Consider This Nursing education is not adequately preparing students for the realities of clinical practice.

Content Overload and Saturation

The growing amount of content that students are expected to master in nursing education is a barrier to student learning and mastery of content. del Bueno (2005) recognized the correlation between too much content and the inability of new nurses to translate knowledge to the bedside.

> "*The author believes that a highly probable cause (inability to translate knowledge to the bedside) is the emphasis on teaching more and more content in the nursing education curricula rather than a focus on use of or application of knowledge. A look at the size and plethora of nursing textbooks supports this conclusion*". (p. 281)

Nursing curriculum and slide presentations in the classroom tend to be additive, as new information and new research findings are incorporated. Instead of removing and reworking current content, faculty simply add more (Benner et al. 2010; Tanner, 2004). Benner (1984) identified that a characteristic of novice student nurses is that all content is seen as relevant and as a result, they are unable to differentiate between what is most and least important to practice. The consequence of an ever-growing amount of content is that novice students get a superficial learning of a broad amount of subject matter that they attempt to master, but lack the deep learning of what is most important to practice.

As a result, novice nurses work diligently to learn and memorize content that they may rarely or never see in clinical practice. It is important that nurse educators use the lens of clinical practice to filter ever-growing amounts of content in the nursing curriculum by emphasizing and identifying which content is most important for students to learn so they can put their energy into acquiring a mastery over what is most important to clinical practice. When the most important content is then oriented toward practice and particular situations that students will likely experience, an optimum learning environment is created that will maximize student learning. To see this realized, it is imperative that nurse educators decrease the emphasis on learning outcomes, and instead create classrooms that become rich learning environments for relevant, experiential learning (Handwerker, 2012).

Discussion Point

How do you feel with the amount of content you are expected to master in your program? Is it realistic from your perspective?

Fragmented Student Learning

One of the observations of the Carnegie Foundation's research (Benner et al., 2010) was that the content in most classrooms was presented to students abstractly with little to no contextualization to practice. This resulted in fragmented, superficial learning that hinders the ability to apply essential content and make correct clinical judgments in practice. Classroom learning consisted primarily of classroom lectures using slide presentations that did not engage student learners. Little dialogue took place between faculty and students, and some faculty limited questions so they could "cover the content" (Benner et al., 2010).

The current classroom/clinical divide directly impacts the ability of students to develop clinical salience (Benner et al., 2010). Student learning is maximized when clinical realities are integrated into theory content. Students must be prepared to assimilate knowledge and think in action in order to establish nursing care priorities. Separating these two essential components of nursing education hinders the ability to transfer knowledge and skills that students must master for clinical practice. Integrating classroom and clinical learning with innovative and creative teaching strategies into a seamless whole where students are able to use and apply knowledge is required for practice in the classroom setting (Benner et al., 2010).

A false assumption that faculty make is that abstract learning devoid of context translates to application in the clinical setting by students. Instead, there must be ongoing dialogue between classroom content and clinical practice so students can readily apply learning to the bedside. Content presented in the classroom requires a clinical "hook" of contextualization to clinical practice so students can readily recognize its importance and how this knowledge is used by the nurse, as well as develop a sense of salience about what is most and least important in the clinical setting. To develop this salience, students must be able to use and apply knowledge and then have opportunities to practice this outside the context of direct patient care (Benner et al., 2010). Activities that require students to apply, analyze, and synthesize knowledge in the context of patient scenarios can help develop clinical reasoning that leads to a sound nursing judgment.

Discussion Point

How is the content in your program consistently contextualized to the bedside so you are able to recognize how important it is to clinical practice?

Education–Practice Gap

A major finding of the research presented in *Educating Nurses* was "that a significant gap exists between today's nursing practice and the education for that practice… the quality of nursing education must be uniformly higher" (Benner et al., 2010, p. 4). This gap is currently significant. To bridge this gap, the classroom must teach for salience and guide student development of clinical reasoning as well as emphasize application of content and guide the development of clinical judgment (Glynn, 2012). Integration between classroom and clinical is a must (Handwerker, 2012) because expert nursing involves an "ongoing dialogue between information and practice" (Benner et al., 2010, p. 14).

Fragmented student learning contributes to the education–practice gap when the student is unable to provide safe patient care because he or she is unable to translate classroom content to the bedside and has not deeply understood the rationale for basic nursing interventions in the clinical setting. In one study, only 35% of new nurse graduates met basic expectations of making a correct clinical judgment and were unable to translate knowledge and theory to the bedside (del Bueno, 2005).

Consider This What would be the implications for the medical profession if only 35% of residents were able to meet entry-level expectations of clinical judgment? Would this be acceptable?

del Bueno (2005) detailed the struggles that graduate nurses encountered to make correct clinical judgments. For example, incorrect rationales made by graduate nurses included the importance of straining urine for the size and number of ketones and that an elevated BUN/creatinine indicated liver problems. When the "why" or rationale is integrated into theory content or a specific skill, the bigger picture becomes apparent and its relevance to students becomes apparent, thus closing the education–practice gap. A key component of clinical reasoning is related to the ability to provide a rationale for all that the nurse does in practice (Gonzol & Newby, 2013).

NANDA-I (international), and its taxonomy of 205 nursing diagnostic statements that represent a nursing diagnosis, is traditionally situated in Step 2 of the nursing process, where the nurse must make a diagnosis after completing the first step of assessment. This taxonomy has been the primary way to establish a nursing priority in the clinical setting as well as written care plans for over 30 years in nursing education. But this emphasis may increase the prevalence of "failure to rescue" by the nurse in practice.

del Bueno (2005) identified a relationship between the use of NANDA-I nursing diagnostic statements and the nurses' inability to readily recognize a change of status. del Bueno (2005) found that new nurses were unable to exercise correct clinical judgment at a basic level to "rescue" (identify the problem and then intervene) their patient in a simulated scenario due in part to the inappropriate use of NANDA-I nursing diagnostic statements to make them "fit" when there was a change in status (del Bueno, 2005).

For example, when a patient had a condition change consistent with a stroke, the nurse used the NANDA-I statement "alteration in sensory perception" or "alteration in nutrition." In another patient having symptoms consistent with a myocardial infarction, the nurse used "activity intolerance related to pain." del Bueno (2005) summarizes her research findings with the following statement, "Many inexperienced RN's also attempt to use a nursing diagnosis for the problem focus. Whatever the original intent for its use the results are at best cumbersome and at worst risible" (p. 280).

Another consideration that questions the current emphasis and relevance of NANDA-I nursing diagnostic statements in nursing education is that the NCLEX licensure examination does not require the candidate to use NANDA-I nursing diagnostic statements to identify the nursing priority. Instead, the NCLEX emphasizes the principles of clinical reasoning that include the ability to grasp the essence of the scenario on each question, recognize what clinical data are relevant, and make a correct clinical judgment. In care plans used by electronic medical records, NANDA-I taxonomy is not typically used to establish care priorities. Instead, a problem-based approach to establishing nursing priorities that are based on body systems throughout the care plan is utilized instead.

Discussion Point

What NANDA-I nursing diagnostic statements do you find most relevant to establish patient care priorities? Do you struggle to sometimes make a statement "fit" your patient's care priority?

Emphasis on Critical Thinking Over Clinical Reasoning

Critical thinking has historically been emphasized in nursing education to describe the multiple ways of thinking that are required by the professional nurse. Critical thinking needs to be clearly defined so that it can be seen in its proper context as just one of the ways that a nurse situates knowledge to the bedside. Critical thinking in and of itself is unable to guide students in the usage of practical knowledge in a particular clinical situation. Instead, clinical reasoning needs to be emphasized as an essential nurse thinking skill that is distinct from critical thinking. Critical thinking must be de-emphasized yet still retained in nursing education (Benner et al., 2010).

The current usage and emphasis of critical thinking in nursing education is also hindered by an inability to clearly define what it consists of. Depending on the textbook, there are significant interpretations about how it should be defined. The inability to concretely define critical thinking and the resultant ambiguity of how it is defined may make it difficult for novice nursing students to integrate critical thinking into their practice. Alfaro-LeFevre (2013) recognizes this dilemma of the numerous constructs of critical thinking:

> *"Critical thinking is a complex process that changes depending on context–what you're trying to accomplish.* **For this reason there is no one right definition**

> **for critical thinking.** *Many authors (including me) develop their own descriptions to complement and clarify someone else's…to analyze it and decide what it means to you rather than simply memorizing someone else's words.*
>
> (p. 7, emphasis in original)

Critical Thinking Defined

Potter and Perry (2009) define critical thinking as "a commitment to think clearly, precisely, and accurately and to act on what you know about a situation" (p. 216). This definition is concrete and recognizes the importance of accuracy and making a correct clinical judgment as well as the importance of application of knowledge to the bedside where it matters most. This reinforces the essence of applied clinical reasoning and emphasizes accuracy in utilizing nursing process so that patient outcomes are improved by implementing needed rescue when warranted.

Discussion Point

What critical thinking skills do you currently utilize when caring for patients? What skills could you incorporate to strengthen your ability to critically think?

WHAT IS CLINICAL REASONING?

Patients do not stay static. Students must be able to think on their feet and recognize the nursing priority when the status of their patient changes, and be skilled in early recognition and management if this occurs (Shoulders, Follett, & Eason, 2014). In one study, students were able to identify relevant clinical data in a simulation, but struggled with how to interpret the data and then respond (Lasater, Johnson, Ravert, & Rink, 2014). Students must be given numerous opportunities to think in action and be able to transfer classroom learning to the bedside. To think like a nurse, students must understand and then incorporate clinical reasoning into their practice. Nurse educators have a responsibility to ensure that every student has clinical reasoning skills before they graduate (Jensen, 2013).

To deeply understand and then apply clinical reasoning to the bedside, it must first be concretely defined. Clinical reasoning describes the way a nurse reflectively thinks about their thinking, uses nursing knowledge to quickly review and analyze clinical data, evaluate the relevance of this clinical data, and then formulate a judgment that leads to action (Koharchik, Caputi, Robb, & Culleiton, 2015). Another way to define clinical reasoning is that it is the ability of the nurse to think in action and reason as a situation changes over time by capturing and understanding the significance of clinical trajectories and grasping the essence of the current clinical situation (Benner et al., 2010). The nurse must be able to focus and filter clinical data in order to recognize what is most and least important so the nurse can identify if an actual problem is present (Benner, Hooper-Kyriakidis, & Stannard, 2011).

The essence of clinical reasoning and how it can be situated to bedside practice consists of four components. These components are:

- Priority setting
- Rationale for nursing interventions
- Grasp the essence of the clinical situation
- Identify and trend relevant clinical data (Benner et al., 2010).

Priority Setting

For the novice nursing student, the challenge of establishing nursing care priorities is that all tasks and priorities seem to be of equal significance (Benner, 1984). Priority setting is one of the most difficult skills for students to master (Russell et al., 2013). Knowing which interventions are a priority is not always readily apparent to students. A novice nurse has difficulty seeing the big picture and identifying what is clinically significant. Novice nurses are also task-oriented and focus on the tasks that need to be done, not necessarily what is most important (Benner, 1982). Student nurses require guidance and instruction to identify care priorities in the clinical setting. Using the A, B, C's of nursing priority setting (airway, breathing, circulation) is one way to guide priority setting in the clinical setting by the nurse.

Another common example of priority setting in the clinical setting is to identify which of the patients that a student has will be seen first. Principles to guide the development of this essential clinical reasoning skill in students are shown in Box 15.1.

Rationale Required

Students must be able to understand and state the rationale of everything that is done in the clinical setting. When the scientific rationale or "why" is understood

BOX 15.1 Principles to Guide the Development of Clinical Reasoning Skills in Students

- **How old is the patient?** The older the patient, the higher the risk of him or her developing complications. Therefore, if all considerations are equal, the oldest patient should be seen first.
- **When were they admitted?** The more recent the day of admission, the more likely they are to be higher acuity and at risk for a change of status. Therefore, if all considerations are equal, see the most recently admitted patient first.
- **When did they have surgery?** The more recent the day of surgery, the higher the acuity and risk of a change of status. Therefore, if all considerations are equal, see the most recent surgical patient first.
- **How many body systems are involved?** Chronic renal failure patients are an excellent example of patients who typically have multiple body system derangements because of the systemic metabolic changes influenced by renal disease. If medical complexity is present, such patients should be seen first.

and integrated with all that a nurse does in practice, the big picture is realized, and clinical reasoning is realized (Gonzol & Newby, 2013). It is only when deep knowledge of the most important content has been understood that the student is able to apply, analyze, and see the relevance of clinical data in the context of patient care (Olson, 2000).

Grasp the Essence of the Situation

Grasping the essence of the current clinical situation is an essential component of clinical reasoning (Benner et al., 2010). In nursing practice, it means being able to identify the most significant aspect of the current clinical situation. It also involves the ability to break down the patient and their current needs to the lowest common denominator of what is needed and what must be done to advance the plan of care. Essence is developed by seeing patients with similar problems and the patterns that are seen with the typical chief complaint, nursing assessments, vital signs, lab values, and expected medical treatment. Grasping the essence of the patient care problem does require time and clinical experience, and is another aspect of clinical reasoning that can be guided by an experienced nurse to develop this sense of salience in the clinical setting.

Identify and Trend Relevant Clinical Data

Identifying the most important clinical data and trending them by comparing them with the most recent is an essential component of clinical reasoning and thinking like a nurse in practice (Benner et al., 2010). But since students tend to see all clinical data as relevant, they will have difficulty sorting out the least from the most important (Benner, 1984). To "rescue" a patient with a change in status, the nurse must be able to recognize subtle changes in a patient's condition over time. Because students have limited clinical experience, they are unable to grasp the essence of the clinical scenario without guidance. It is the early changes in a patient's status that are subtle and, therefore, must be recognized before a problem progresses and an adverse outcome results. In addition to trending vital signs and nursing assessment data, evaluation of nursing interventions and laboratory values must also be consistently compared and trended.

"Five Rights" of Clinical Reasoning

Although nursing education has 5 to 10 rights of safe medication administration that students must memorize to safely administer medications, there are also "five rights" of clinical reasoning, as shown in Box 15.2 (Levett-Jones et al., 2010). These 5 rights are another way to teach the essence of clinical reasoning, and are an easy acronym to guide nurse thinking in the clinical setting.

Discussion Point

Think of a clinical situation when the status of your patient changed. Which one of these "rights" could have prepared you to handle this more effectively?

BENEFITS OF CLINICAL REASONING

Emphasizing and integrating clinical reasoning will not only benefit and improve student learning, but will also translate to better outcomes for the patients that students will care for in practice. To consistently make safe and correct clinical judgments, the nurse must be able to use knowledge, integrate nursing processes, think critically, and use clinical reasoning to make a correct clinical judgment. If a nurse is unable to clinically reason, it

BOX 15.2 "Five Rights" of Clinical Reasoning

- **RIGHT Cues.** Cues are the clinical data that are collected and clustered by the nurse. Recognizing the relevance of clinical data and applying it to the patient is the essence of this "right." Missing or not identifying early cues that allow a complication to progress is an example of "failure to rescue" by the nurse when this "right" is not exercised in practice.
- **RIGHT Patient.** This "right" refers to the ability of the nurse to identify a patient who is at high risk for developing a potential complication. The nurse must be able to recognize that an 18-year-old with an appendectomy is not as likely to develop a complication as a patient with the same problem who is 88! Patients who are susceptible hosts due to chemotherapy, radiation, or medications such as prednisone also fall under this "right" as patients at risk.
- **RIGHT Time.** This refers to the timeliness of identifying a change of status. Recognizing early signs of a complication and then initiating nursing interventions at the right time and in the right sequence is imperative to prevent an adverse outcome. "Failure to rescue" occurs not only by not recognizing a complication that develops, but also when nursing/medical interventions start too late.
- **RIGHT Action.** Once a clinical judgment is made, the right action or intervention must be initiated. Clinical data that suggest a potential complication must be acted upon. The consequences of an incorrect clinical judgment can make the difference between life and death. In one study, one half of patients who had cardiac arrests on the floor of a hospital had clinical signs of deterioration 24 hours before the arrest. These signs were NOT recognized and then acted upon by the nurse (Thompson et al., 2008).
- **RIGHT Reason.** The right reason refers to understanding the rationale of everything that is done in practice. To do this consistently, the nurse must be able to apply key aspects of clinical reasoning, which include grasping the essence of the current situation to put the clinical puzzle together.

will lead to an incorrect clinical judgment. When clinical reasoning is integrated and deeply understood by students, it will result in the following benefits.

Improved Student Learning

Patricia Benner's novice-to-expert framework of professional progression details how nurses progress and develop skills and understanding of patient care over time. The five levels of nurse proficiency in practice that Benner identified are novice, advanced beginner, competent, proficient, and expert (Benner, 1984). The relevance of Benner's framework is that it establishes definite steps and levels of clinical progression and the characteristics of nursing practice at each level of proficiency.

A student novice nurse with little to no clinical experience will be a concrete/textbook learner who sees everything as relevant and important to know in both the classroom and clinical settings. Students at this level are also task-oriented and focused on the tasks that need to be completed instead of the thinking that is required for practice (Benner, 1984). Because of a lack of clinical experience, novice nurses are unable to expect or recognize variations from textbook content in practice and readily identify nursing priorities. To develop clinical reasoning and the ability to make correct clinical judgments, clinical experience with patient care is required (Benner, 1984). When the components of clinical reasoning are emphasized, student learning is maximized as a deep knowledge of this essential content and its relevance to clinical practice accrue to the student.

As students progress through the final year of the nursing program, they are at the advanced beginner stage. At this level, they will begin to recognize exceptions to concrete textbook content, and see certain clinical data as relevant because of their limited clinical experience, but they will continue to have difficulty recognizing nursing priorities (Benner, 1984). The ability to recognize what clinical data are relevant and to identify nursing priorities is also an essential component of clinical reasoning. When this weakness of nursing students is recognized as a result of their lack of clinical experience, nurse educators can help develop and strengthen clinical reasoning by having students reflect while in the clinical setting on the following questions while providing care:

- What clinical data are relevant?
- What is the nursing priority?

By emphasizing the importance of identifying relevant clinical data and correct nursing priorities, the essence of clinical reasoning can begin to be situated in a way that students can recognize why it is salient to practice so it can be further developed as they progress through the program.

Improved Patient Outcomes

The ability of the nurse to exercise sound judgment is imperative to clinical practice because correct decisions made by the nurse directly impact patient outcomes (Cappelletti, Engel, & Prentice, 2014). In one study, the majority of new RN graduates were unable to translate knowledge to practice, and only 35% were able to meet entry expectations for clinical judgment (del Bueno, 2005). Because nursing is a practice-based profession, content that is taught must be readily applicable to the bedside of every patient the nurse cares for. The nurse must then be able to take this knowledge and use it to clinically reason and to establish nursing priorities. The inability of a nurse to use knowledge and clinically reason to recognize the significance of a change in status to save a patient's life is known as "failure to rescue," and could lead to the development of an adverse outcome that could result in patient harm, injury, or even death. Failure to rescue is based on the premise that although some deaths are unavoidable, many patient deaths could be prevented (Clarke & Aiken, 2003). In many cases, clinical deterioration began up to 24 hours before emergency intervention was required (Felton, 2012).

Consider This Since a nurse is at the patient's bedside 24/7, a complication that goes unrecognized until it is too late will lead to the death of the patient that could have been prevented.

Just as a lifeguard continually and vigilantly scans the water for signs of a struggling swimmer, the nurse, in order to rescue a patient from a deteriorating change of status, must also be vigilant to look for the patient who may be developing a change in status, by clinically reasoning. This is practically done by continually assessing, trending all clinical data, and assessing for early signs and symptoms of a potential complication. An experienced nurse anticipates potential problems, recognizes the significance of clinical cues, and practices proactively to prevent a patient problem from progressing (Levett-Jones et al., 2010).

Novice nurses with limited clinical experience are particularly vulnerable to failure to rescue (Clarke & Aiken, 2003). A novice nurse tends to practice reactively, not anticipating potential problems, and reacting to them after they have already developed (Levett-Jones et al., 2010). Once a life-threatening complication begins to develop, it is the responsibility of the nurse not only to identify the problem early, but also to take control by implementing appropriate interventions (Clarke & Aiken, 2003). The primary reasons for complications to progress include failure to anticipate the problem after it develops, failure to initiate appropriate nursing interventions, and inappropriate management of the complication once it is present.

del Bueno's (2005) research also identified the importance of a nurse's ability to recognize a problem before rescue can take place. It is only when a problem is recognized that the nurse will intervene and do something about it. I have seen clinical situations that foreshadowed a patient's death as a result of the primary nurse's "failure to rescue" and clinically reason when there was a change of status that went unrecognized until it was too late.

Consider This If a nurse is able to clinically reason, patient outcomes will be improved when "rescue" is facilitated.

A Personal Story

I share this story to put a personal face on the current crisis in critical thinking in nursing education (del Bueno, 2005) that results in failure to rescue. Jenny was a new nurse on surgical unit who was responsible for an elderly male patient named Ken (some details changed to ensure confidentiality). He had a perforated appendix, but it had been removed successfully 2 days earlier, and he was clinically stable. Around midnight, he became restless. His blood pressure (BP) was slightly elevated at 158/90, and his heart rate (HR) was in the 100s. He had a history of mild dementia and was unable to readily communicate his needs, so Jenny gave him one tablet of Percocet, assuming he was restless because he was in pain. Two hours later, nothing changed. She noted that he was now more tachypneic with a respiratory rate of 28 per minute. He did have a history of chronic obstructive pulmonary disease and had an albuterol nebulizer prn ordered, so that was given assuming that was the reason for his persistent restlessness.

Two hours later, Jenny called me as the rapid response nurse to come and take a look at her patient. She was concerned, but was unable to recognize what the problem could be and wanted a second opinion. After Jenny explained the course of events that transpired to this point, I took one look at Ken and realized that he was in trouble. He was pale, diaphoretic, and his respirations had increased to 40 per minute despite the nebulizer 2 hours ago. He was not responsive to loud verbal commands. The last BP was still on the screen and read 158/90. I asked, *"When was the last BP checked?"* Jenny stated it was 4 hours earlier. While obtaining another BP,

I touched Ken's forehead. It was notably cold, as were his hands. The BP now read 68/30.

Recognizing that Ken was in septic shock, and that IV fluids and vasopressors would be needed emergently, I looked for an IV and found only one, a 24-gauge catheter in the left hand. This is the smallest-size IV catheter and is typically used with infants and small children.

Realizing that Ken needed a central line and that there was little that could be done to initiate even the most basic life-saving treatments to rescue Ken on the floor, he was emergently transferred to intensive care unit. Within 30 minutes, Ken was intubated, a central line was placed, and three vasopressors—norepinephrine (Levophed), phenylephrine (Neosynephrine), and vasopressin—were required to get his systolic BP greater than 90 mm Hg. Although early signs of sepsis were present at midnight, they were not recognized by Jenny until it was too late for Ken, because he died the next day.

Discussion Point

How do you feel about the responsibility that comes with being a professional nurse? Have you considered that you literally hold the life of another in your hands?

WHY CLINICAL REASONING IS IMPORTANT

To make a correct clinical judgment, clinical reasoning is used to select from all alternatives, understand the rationale for each alternative, collect and recognize the significance of clinical data, process this information to understand the current problem, and identify the current care priority and plan of care (Levett-Jones et al., 2010). Critical Thinking + Clinical Reasoning = Correct Clinical Judgment is the equation of nurse thinking that is required for clinical practice (Alfaro-LeFevre, 2013) (Box 15.3).

Clinical judgments are made on a continual and ongoing basis in practice, and may be influenced by what the nurse brings to the situation based on the length of clinical experience. Knowledge acquired from past experience will lead an experienced nurse to respond intuitively, while a novice nurse will rely on textbook knowledge (Tanner, 2006). Thinking in action by making clinical judgments is an ongoing process for the nurse in practice. One study found that on a typical med/surg floor, over an 8-hour shift, the nurse engaged in an average of 50 significant clinical reasoning concerns that required a clinical judgment (Thompson, Cullum, McCaughan, Sheldon, & Raynor, 2004).

Because clinical judgment is the end result and hallmark of professional practice, nurse educators must ensure that students develop clinical judgment before they graduate (Bussard, 2015). Therefore, it must be properly defined and understood. Tanner (2006) defines clinical judgment as an interpretation or conclusion about what a patient needs and/or the decision as to whether to take action or not. Good clinical judgment requires the nurse to be flexible, recognize what is most important, interpret the meaning of these clinical data, and respond appropriately. Tanner (2006) has developed a model that breaks down clinical judgment using principles of both critical thinking and clinical reasoning. This understanding is essential to practice because it also integrates components of clinical reasoning that include the ability to notice and then interpret the significance of relevant clinical data. This is the essence of the thinking that is required for practice (Box 15.4).

To clinically reason by interpreting the significance of clinical data that have been collected, the significance of any ambiguity of clinical data must also be determined by the nurse. Tanner's model is relevant to the nurse in the clinical setting because it can help develop clinical reasoning in students by integrating the first two steps of Tanner's model in the following questions:

1. *What did you observe?* (noticing) From the nursing assessment and vital signs.
2. *What do you make of what you saw?* (interpreting) Data that have been collected need to be interpreted to identify if it is expected or unexpected,

BOX 15.3 Equation of Nurse Thinking Required for Clinical Practice

Critical Thinking + Clinical Reasoning = Correct Clinical Judgment

Source: Alfaro-LeFevre, R. (2013). *Critical thinking, clinical reasoning, and clinical judgment: A practical approach* (5th ed.). St. Louis, MO: Elsevier.

BOX 15.4 Essence of Thinking Required for Practice

1. **Noticing:** Although this can be part of nursing assessment, it emphasizes the nurse's expectations of the current clinical situation. If the patient is presenting in a way that is expected or unexpected, a decision can be made on the basis of his or her knowledge that is used and applied from the textbook as well as from prior clinical experience.
2. **Interpreting:** Once the essence of the current clinical situation is grasped and relevant clinical data identified, this data must now be interpreted. What do this data mean and what is their significance? Unless a nurse has a deep understanding of the applied sciences, especially pathophysiology, the ability to correctly interpret will be impacted.
3. **Responding:** Based on the correct interpretation, does the nurse need to act or rescue, or is further monitoring warranted?
4. **Reflecting:** Two aspects of reflection are needed by the nurse. Reflection-in-action is the ability of the nurse to "read" the patient and how he or she is responding to current nursing interventions, and to adjust what is done on the basis of the patient's response. Reflection-on-action is done afterward. This completes the four-step cycle by determining what can be learned from what was just experienced and how that experience will contribute to ongoing clinical knowledge development. This is especially important if an error in judgment occurred so that needed learning can take place.

Source: Adapted from Tanner, C. A. (2006). Thinking like a nurse: A research-based model of clinical judgment in nursing. *The Journal of Nursing Education, 45*(6), 204–211.

and what data are relevant or clinically significant. Because novice students are concrete learners who see textbook ranges as the definition of "normal," they have difficulty identifying what is acceptable versus unacceptable ambiguity or deviations from normal. The ability to determine acceptable ambiguity can be developed by having students reflect on the clinical data collected and then research the patient's weight, past medical history, current problem, medications, and other clinical data such as laboratory values and radiology findings that would explain any variations from expected norms (Koharchik et al., 2015).

STRATEGIES TO DEVELOP CLINICAL REASONING

Although the nursing literature defines the constructs of clinical reasoning, nurse educators require tools to develop clinical reasoning in students (Russell et al., 2013). This author used a methodical, sequential approach of applied clinical reasoning based on 30 years of clinical experience to grasp the essence and establish care priorities for each patient cared for. From this lens of clinical practice and drawing from the clinical reasoning work of Patricia Benner, Linda Caputi, and Lisa Day, a clinical reasoning tool was developed that is a template of 12 sequential questions that deconstruct clinical reasoning by identifying the sequential steps a nurse in practice uses to clinically reason from the time they prepare to assume care when reviewing the chart to when the patient is seen for the first time, and then throughout the shift (Box 15.5).

This template of 12 clinical reasoning questions is divided into two parts. First, there is a series of eight questions that represent the sequential thinking that is required before a patient is seen by the nurse. As the nurse reviews the chart and obtains a nurse-to-nurse-report, these eight questions capture the essence of how a nurse in practice prepares to safely assume care. The first segment emphasizes the following aspects of clinical reasoning:

- Relevant data collection
- Care planning priorities/interventions
- Nurse vigilance by identifying the worst possible or most likely complication and what to do if it is realized.

The second part of this template has four clinical reasoning questions to guide nurse thinking after the patient has been seen for the first time and the nurse has collected clinical assessment data firsthand. These four questions emphasize the following aspects of clinical reasoning:

- Relevance of vital signs, assessment data personally collected
- Nursing priority…has it changed?
- Priority educational needs
- Rationale of primary care provider's plan of care.

BOX 15.5 Template of Clinical Reasoning Questions

Formulate and Reflect on the Following BEFORE Providing Care

1. *What is the primary problem, and what is the underlying cause/pathophysiology of this problem?*
2. What clinical data from the chart are RELEVANT and needs to be trended because they are clinically significant?
3. List all relevant nursing priorities. What nursing priority captures the "essence" of your patient's current status and will guide your plan of care?
4. What nursing interventions will you initiate on the basis of this priority, and what are the desired outcomes?
5. What body system(s), key assessments, and psychosocial needs will you focus on based on your patient's primary problem or nursing care priority?
6. What is the worst possible/most likely complication(s) to anticipate based on the primary problem?
7. What nursing assessments will identify this complication EARLY if it develops?
8. What nursing interventions will you initiate if this complication develops?

Formulate and Reflect on the Following WHILE Providing Care

9. *What clinical assessment data did you just collect that are RELEVANT and need to be TRENDED because it is clinically significant to detect a change in status?*
10. Does your nursing priority or plan of care need to be modified in any way after assessing your patient?
11. After reviewing the primary care provider's note, what is the rationale for any new orders or changes made?
12. *What educational priorities have you identified, and how will you address* them?

This template of clinical reasoning questions can also be used to replace the traditional care plan (recommend advanced level) in the clinical setting because it combines care planning, nursing process, and clinical reasoning in one construct that closely mirrors how a nurse thinks in practice.

To correlate this template of clinical reasoning questions with the key constructs of clinical reasoning from the literature, the following explanations will clarify this relationship.

Part 1: Reflect on the Following BEFORE Providing Care

1. *What is the primary problem, and what is its underlying cause or pathophysiology?*

   This is the admission medical problem or diagnosis. The most important aspect of this question is the importance of the nurse to deeply understand the pathophysiology of the illness or problem. This knowledge will lay the foundation for critical thinking by recognizing the clinical relationship between the primary problem and physiologic symptoms and establishing correct nursing care priorities.

2. *What clinical data from the chart are RELEVANT that need to be trended because they are clinically significant?*

   One observation I have made as a nurse educator is that students will take as much time as you give them in the clinical setting to collect data on their patient from the medical record. As novice nurses, students do not have an experiential base to recognize what clinical data are relevant (Benner, 1984). The ability to filter clinical data and focus on what is relevant is something that can be strengthened and developed with clinical experience. This question is also one of the 5 "rights" of clinical reasoning, the importance of the nurse to recognize the right cues of clinical data, when a complication begins to become evident (Levett-Jones et al., 2010).

3. *What nursing priority captures the "essence" of your patient's current status and will guide your plan of care?*

   Capturing the essence of each patient's clinical scenario is an essential component of clinical reasoning (Benner et al., 2010). Students struggle at times with capturing nursing care priorities that capture the essence in the clinical setting when NANDA-I is the primary taxonomy to establish care priorities (del Bueno, 2005). Although there are NANDA-I nursing diagnostic statements that can capture the essence of the care priority such as "acute/chronic pain" or "fluid volume excess/deficit," there are numerous clinical scenarios that I have experienced where NANDA-I diagnostic statements do not "fit" or even come close to describing the care priority with an acute change of status.

   For example, when a patient is found unresponsive without a pulse and agonal respiration, a nurse in practice uses clinical reasoning to grasp the essence of this scenario and simply states the nursing care priority as "No pulse, no respirations," and life-saving interventions such as calling a code and beginning CPR logically follow. The NANDA-I nursing diagnostic statement that would fit this scenario is "Impaired tissue perfusion; cardiac, renal, and neurological." Although technically correct, this statement is vague and does not capture the essence and the gravity of the current clinical scenario.

4. *What nursing interventions will you initiate based on this priority, and what are the desired outcomes?*

Questions 2 to 4 integrate the essence of nursing process by emphasizing the importance of:

- Identifying relevant assessment data (assessment)
- Identifying correct nursing priority (nursing diagnosis/priority)
- Initiating nursing interventions (implementation)
- Identifying desired or expected outcomes.

This is the essence of a nursing care plan, but it is positioned within the framework of applied clinical reasoning. Another aspect of clinical reasoning that is inferred but not clearly specified is to identify the rationale for each nursing intervention. Correctly stating the rationale ensures safe practice.

5. *What body system(s) and key assessments will you focus on based on your patient's primary problem or nursing care priority?*

Although students are taught to perform a systematic head-to-toe assessment for every patient they care for, they must also be able to identify the priority body system that must be focused on and more thoroughly assessed on the basis of the patient's primary problem or nursing care priority.

6. *What is the worst possible/most likely complication(s) to anticipate on the basis of the primary problem?*

Nurse vigilance and early recognition of a complication will prevent failure to rescue by the bedside nurse (Clarke & Aiken, 2003). A practical clinical reasoning skill that situates nurse vigilance is identifying the most likely or worst possible complication before patient care is assumed. When a problem is anticipated and recognized early, it will lead to better patient outcomes because a complication is not allowed to needlessly progress. If a worst possible or most likely complication is recognized later and allowed to needlessly progress, it will likely be more serious and even life threatening. Sepsis that progresses to septic shock is a common example of this clinical reality.

7. *What nursing assessments will identify this complication EARLY if it develops?*

Once the worst possible or most likely complication is identified, the specific assessments to recognize it correctly must be determined. Early recognition of any complication is essential for better patient outcomes. For example, if sepsis/septic shock is the most likely complication, the early assessments that the nurse would need to cluster to confirm its presence and then initiate "rescue" if they develop include the following:

- Temperature: fever >100.8 or <96.8
- HR: >90
- BP: downward trend with mean arterial pressure <65
- WBC: <4,000 or >12,000.

This question is also one of the 5 "rights" of clinical reasoning, the importance of the nurse to initiate needed interventions in the right time, when a complication becomes evident (Levett-Jones et al., 2010).

8. *What nursing interventions will you initiate if this complication develops?*

If you look at the last three questions (6 to 8), they follow the pattern of situating nursing process and care planning in the context of identifying the most likely or worst possible complication. This is another way that nurses in practice develop a care priority. Once the potential priority complication is identified, assessments to recognize it are listed so that this problem does not remain hidden, and then nursing interventions to initiate "rescue" can be implemented if needed (Clarke & Aiken, 2003). This question is also one of the 5 "rights" of clinical reasoning, the importance of the nurse to initiate the right action, when a complication is present (Levett-Jones et al., 2010).

Discussion Point

Do you currently incorporate these clinical reasoning questions as you assume care in the clinical setting? Which questions could you utilize to help you prepare for patient care?

Part 2: Reflect on the Following WHILE Providing Care

9. *What clinical assessment data did you just collect that are RELEVANT and need to be TRENDED because they are clinically significant to detect a change in status?*

   This question is also one of the 5 "rights" of clinical reasoning, the importance of the nurse to recognize the right cues of clinical data, when a complication begins to become evident (Levett-Jones et al., 2010). In addition to recognizing what clinical data are relevant, clinical reasoning requires the nurse to trend data that were collected and put them side by side with data received in report or last recorded in the chart to identify the trajectory of what have been collected. What direction is the data trend suggesting? Has anything changed? Were any of the findings unexpected? Is further assessment or an update to the primary care provider required? Because patients rarely stay static, but can change quickly, trending all clinical data will identify a potential problem early, encourage nurse vigilance, and implement the "right" action to "rescue" if needed.

10. *Does your nursing priority or plan of care need to be modified in any way after assessing your patient?*

    Because clinical reasoning is fluid and not rigid, the nurse must continually reevaluate the nursing priority and plan of care based on the data that were just collected not only during the first encounter but throughout the entire shift of care. This question situates the importance of continually thinking in action (Benner et al., 2010), so that a correct clinical judgment is made (Alfaro-LeFevre, 2013).

11. *After reviewing the primary care provider's note, what is the rationale for any new orders or changes made?*

    This question is also one of the 5 "rights" of clinical reasoning, the importance of the nurse to recognize the right reasons for all that is done in practice (Levett-Jones et al., 2010). When the nurse understands the primary care provider's plan of care and the rationale for any changes that have been made, as well as the current nursing priority and plan of care, medicine and nursing can be recognized as complementary and not in separate "silos." The daily progress note or most recent documentation by the primary care provider is a "must read" by the nurse to clearly understand these priorities and benefit from the primary care provider's current perspective on the patient. When the primary care provider note is understood and this knowledge is "dovetailed" with the data the nurse has collected, the "big picture" of patient care is apparent, and this knowledge will help ensure that proper nursing judgments are made as the nurse clinically reasons.

12. *What educational priorities have you identified, and how will you address them?*

    Identifying patient priorities is a key component of clinical reasoning. It is also a weakness and a work in progress for students and new nurses (Benner, 1982). The nurse is also an educator. When education is done in a way that promotes patient learning and understanding, it can improve patient outcomes and even prevent hospital readmissions. Every patient has a need for education. Therefore, this priority is always relevant and must be identified.

Discussion Point

Do you currently incorporate these clinical reasoning questions as you care for patients in the clinical setting? Which questions could you utilize to help identify care priorities?

TOOLS TO TEACH CLINICAL REASONING

To become proficient with any clinical skill, it must be practiced over and over again. When nursing students are taught technical skills such as medication administration or procedural sterile technique, practice is expected and required to demonstrate needed competence. Thinking like a nurse is also a skill that needs to be practiced in order for students to acquire the knowledge, skills, and experience required for practice (Alfaro-LeFevre, 2013). Developing clinical reasoning is a higher-level cognitive skill that is the crux of nursing education (Koharchik et al., 2015) and that also needs to be practiced in the safety of the classroom because in this context, students can safely make mistakes (Benner et al., 2010).

Case studies provide practice to apply knowledge and acquire experience with complex scenarios in the safety of the classroom (Shoulders et al., 2014). By providing contextualization to practice, case studies develop decision-making skills and connect theory to practice

(Brooks, Harris, & Clayton, 2010). To be effective, case studies must engage students with scenarios that mirror clinical practice and challenge students to build on and apply prior knowledge (Popil, 2011). In a summary of the literature on the efficacy of case studies, Popil (2011) found that case studies are an effective active learning strategy to develop critical-reasoning, analytical, problem–solving, and identification skills but that it is not being implemented enough in nursing education.

The author has developed a classroom tool of a clinical reasoning case study that mirrors clinical practice and emphasizes experiential active learning, problem solving/identification, and practice of clinical reasoning. Each theory topic I taught was contextualized with a clinical scenario of the most salient themes derived from my current lens of clinical practice. The scenario integrated the essence of the 12 clinical reasoning questions I developed that were discussed previously. The case study mirrored clinical practice by unfolding step by step with open-ended questions that assessed the ability of the student to identify what clinical data were relevant and their clinical significance. As a result, students were able to practice the essence of clinical reasoning in the safety of my classroom. At the end of the semester I conducted a written survey of my class to obtain their feedback on this new approach to learning in the classroom. Not one student favored returning to a traditional content lecture, but preferred to continue to utilize clinical reasoning case studies to contextualize student learning to the bedside.

Strengths of Clinical Reasoning Case Studies

There are numerous benefits to student learning that can be facilitated if this active learning tool is used to develop clinical reasoning, some of which are listed here:

1. *Implementation of educational best practice from educating nurses.* Clinical reasoning case studies integrate the three essential shifts from *Educating Nurses* that are needed to transform nursing education:
   - Contextualize content
   - Integrate classroom and clinical learning
   - Emphasize clinical reasoning
2. *Practice thinking like a nurse.* Salient clinical experiences are often random, and not all students get the same degree of learning from the clinical setting. By utilizing clinical reasoning case studies in the classroom, every student has the opportunity to develop and practice the thinking that will directly translate to the bedside regardless of the clinical experience they have had.
3. *Emphasize knowledge usage and application of content.* For students to recognize the relevance of content that is taught, it must be placed into clinical context and applied to the bedside. Knowledge usage is emphasized, and how to apply this knowledge for the good of the patient is practiced.
4. *Rehearse for most common changes of patient status.* It is not likely that a student will care for a patient who will have a change in status that will require the nurse to "rescue" in the clinical setting. But this needed practice can take place in the context of simulation or with a clinical reasoning case study.
5. *Active learning strategy.* The classroom needs to become an active learning environment where students are required to participate in their learning. Students participate and are engaged in the learning process.
6. *NCLEX principles reinforced.* The essence of the NCLEX is that it is an examination that assesses the ability of every graduate nurse to clinically reason. By integrating clinical reasoning, students will be prepared for the NCLEX, as well as professional practice.
7. *Open-ended versus multiple choice.* Once in practice, students do not have the luxury of multiple choices to determine the nursing priority or the most important clinical data. You either situate your knowledge to the bedside or you do not. If a student is unable to determine the relevance of clinical data or recognize the need to "rescue," they will be unsafe in clinical practice. By requiring students to identify relevant data and establish nursing priorities through open-ended questions, clinical reasoning case studies most closely mirror real-world clinical practice and identify knowledge deficits that can be remedied.

HOW REFLECTION CAN DEVELOP CLINICAL REASONING AND JUDGMENT

Clinical reasoning is required by the nurse to make a clinical judgment (Levett-Jones et al., 2010). Reflective practice is a crucial component to develop clinical judgment (Tanner, 2006). Reflective thought is an active process that if done purposefully, can form knowledge and influence future actions (Bussard, 2015). This involves both reflection-in-action as well as reflection-on-action. Reflection-in-action is the ability of the nurse to "read"

Research Study Fuels the Controversy 15.1

SAFETY: An Integrated Clinical Reasoning and Reflection Framework for Undergraduate Nursing Students

Faculty in a pediatric course designed a reflective clinical reasoning activity based on the SAFETY template, which is derived from the National Council of State Boards of Nursing RN practice analysis. SAFETY is an acronym for: S: system-specific assessment, A: assignments and accuracy of orders, F: first/priority, E: evaluate interventions, T: teach and test infection control, Y: cYa/cover your assets.

Source: Russell, B. H., Geist, M. J., & Maffett, J. H. (2013). SAFETY: An integrated clinical reasoning and reflection framework for undergraduate nursing students. *The Journal of Nursing Education, 52*, 59–62.

Study Findings

The SAFETY template is a tool that facilitates students' learning by providing a framework to analyze patient data, individualize interventions, and identify the most important aspects of providing safe, competent, and comprehensive care. SAFETY has proven to be a useful tool for integration of content knowledge, clinical reasoning, and reflection on essential professional practice issues for baccalaureate nursing students.

the patient and how they are responding to current nursing interventions, and adjust what is done based on the patient's response as well as providing students the opportunity to reflect on the interaction to determine what can be learned so they can use this knowledge in the future (Koharchik et al., 2015). A reflective clinical reasoning framework is shown in Research Study Fuels the Controversy 15.1.

Reflection-on-action promotes student knowledge and clinical judgment by thoroughly dissecting and reflecting upon a clinical situation that may have been significant, such as a patient change in status or error in practice. A recent review of the literature on clinical judgment and reasoning summarized a finding in the following words: "Clinical judgment is a process that develops over a time in the nurse who consistently reflects in action and on action and responds accordingly" (Cappelletti et al., 2014, p. 458).

Reflective journaling can help develop reflection-on-action (Bussard, 2015). When students were exposed to structured reflection practice that allowed them to share their reflections in class, by the end of the semester they reported a "perceived improvement related to the development of clinical judgment and clinical confidence" (Glynn, 2012, p. 137). The qualitative clinical judgment themes that Glynn noted included increased student ability to apply acquired knowledge, perceived increased patient care experiences from other students' shared reflections, and improved priority setting and development of a sense of salience. By structuring clinical reflection in the classroom, Glynn (2012) observed that students had the opportunity to develop clinical knowledge that could be applied to future patient care experiences. This strategy was also effective in integrating clinical and classroom learning and helped develop clinical reasoning. (see Box 15.6).

Discussion Point

How do you currently use reflection to learn from your clinical experience, especially when something did not go as expected?

BARRIERS TO INTEGRATING CLINICAL REASONING

Although the need for transformational change in nursing education is evident, there continue to be barriers that limit or oppose needed change in nursing education that includes an emphasis of clinical reasoning to develop clinical judgment. To realize transformational change, it is imperative to directly address each of the following barriers:

1. *Change.* Nursing education has historically been resistant to change. It is imperative that nurse educators recognize the importance of emphasizing clinical reasoning and simplify and decrease the amount of content in nursing education. Any barriers that inhibit or impact student learning need to be addressed. Although change takes time and

BOX 15.6 Structured Reflection in Classroom Guide

- Brief summary of patient problem:
  - Current chief complaint
  - Past medical history
  - Lab/diagnostic results
  - Recent vital signs/nursing assessment
- Clinical learning
  - Summarize and present pathophysiology of patient problem
  - Discuss nursing plan of care including specific interventions and outcomes
- Reflection-on-action
  - Identify nursing interventions you may/would have performed differently
  - Identify any emotional and/or ethical issues that were present

Source: Glynn, D. M. (2012). Clinical judgment development using structured classroom reflective practice: A qualitative study. *The Journal of Nursing Education, 51*, 134–139.

can be painful, when students have deep learning of what is most important and are able to clinically reason, patient outcomes will be improved and needed rescue will be facilitated with a change of status. Everything that is done in nursing education impacts patient care and patient outcomes. Nurse educators must not lose sight of this reality.

2. *Time.* Nurse educators have numerous pressing demands and a struggle to juggle the competing demands of clinical, classroom, and simulation skills lab learning as full-time faculty. To create strategies and tools that incorporate and integrate clinical reasoning requires significant time, work, and effort. Although educators are committed to promoting the learning of students, the challenge to do things differently can at times feel overwhelming.
3. *Student buy-in.* The benefits of an active learning classroom that emphasize collaboration must be explained to students so that the benefit to their learning becomes apparent (Handwerker, 2012). Therefore, any change needs to be explained so that the rationale for an emphasis on active learning strategies that involve clinical reasoning is understood. Students must recognize that an emphasis on clinical reasoning is educational best practice. Just as nursing practice must change when evidence-based practice suggests that it should be done differently, the same is true in academia. Passive learning that requires the student to absorb information and take notes is quickly forgotten. Although active learning requires work and engagement by the student, when the student is a participant and engaged in the learning experience, knowledge is constructed and learning is retained.

Using active learning strategies that incorporate clinical reasoning provides necessary practice of the thinking that is required, which is the highest priority of nursing education. This practice can be done in the safety of the classroom, which will then translate to the bedside in the clinical setting. Adult learners value relevance. Clinical reasoning is a relevant emphasis that will promote and develop the thinking that is required for practice. When this relevance is recognized by students, the value of an emphasis on clinical reasoning and active learning strategies will be evident.

Discussion Point

Do you find active learning strategies relevant to your learning, or do you prefer a traditional lecture-oriented classroom?

Conclusions

To prepare students for the current demands of clinical practice, nursing education needs to be radically transformed by contextualizing classroom content to the clinical setting, integrating and bringing clinical realities to the classroom, and integrating rich experiential learning in both the classroom and clinical settings by emphasizing clinical reasoning. Clinical reasoning is an essential thinking skill that makes it possible for the nurse to make a correct clinical judgment. This will translate to improved patient outcomes and decrease the prevalence of failure to rescue when a complication is allowed to needlessly progress. Although clinical reasoning requires time and clinical experience to develop, it can be taught as well as practiced in the safety of an active learning classroom as well as in the clinical setting. It is the responsibility of nurse educators to ensure that each student is proficient with clinical reasoning before graduating to ensure safe clinical practice.

For Additional Discussion

1. What factors do you think contribute to the ongoing disconnect between nursing education and clinical practice?
2. What content would you decrease or eliminate in nursing education to decrease content overload?
3. As a novice nursing student, describe a clinical situation when you struggled with identifying relevant clinical data or nursing priorities.
4. Reflect on a clinical experience when the care priority of the patient had quickly changed. What aspects of clinical reasoning did you utilize to "think in action?"
5. To state the rationale for everything a nurse does in clinical practice, what theory content must be mastered?
6. What data in clinical practice must be trended in order to recognize a change in status or determine whether care priorities have changed?
7. Reflect on a clinical situation when things did not go as expected. How can you use reflection to learn from this experience and apply this knowledge to strengthen your clinical judgment abilities?

References

Alfaro-LeFevre, R. (2013). *Critical thinking, clinical reasoning, and clinical judgment: A practical approach* (5th ed.). St. Louis, MO: Elsevier.

Benner, P. (1982). From novice to expert. *The American Journal of Nursing, 82*(3), 402–407.

Benner, P. (1984). *From novice to expert: Excellence and power in clinical nursing practice*. Upper Saddle River, NJ: Prentice Hall.

Benner, P., Hooper-Kyriakidis, P., & Stannard, D. (2011). *Clinical wisdom and interventions in acute and critical care: A thinking-in-action approach* (2nd ed.). New York, NY: Springer.

Benner, P., Sutphen, M., Leonard, V., & Day, L. (2010). *Educating nurses: A call for radical transformation.* San Francisco, CA: Jossey-Bass.

Brooks, E., Harris, C. R., & Clayton, P. H. (2010). Deepening applied learning: An enhanced case study approach using critical reflection. *Journal of Applied Learning in Higher Education, 2*, 55–76.

Bussard, M. E. (2015). Clinical judgment in reflective journals of prelicensure nursing students. *The Journal of Nursing Education, 54*, 36–40.

Cappelletti, A., Engel, J. K., & Prentice, D. (2014). Systematic review of clinical judgment and reasoning in nursing. *The Journal of Nursing Education, 53*, 453–458.

Clarke, S. P., & Aiken, L. H. (2003). Failure to rescue. *The American Journal of Nursing, 103*, 42–47.

del Bueno, D. (2005). A crisis in critical thinking. *Nursing Education Perspectives, 26*(5), 278–282.

Felton, M. (2012). Recognizing signs and symptoms of patient deterioration. *Emergency Nurse, 20*, 23–27.

Glynn, D. M. (2012). Clinical judgment development using structured classroom reflective practice: A qualitative study. *The Journal of Nursing Education, 51*, 134–139.

Gonzol, K., & Newby, C. (2013). Facilitating clinical reasoning in the skills laboratory: Reasoning model versus nursing process-based skills checklist. *Nursing Education Perspectives, 34*, 265–267.

Handwerker, S. M. (2012). Transforming nursing education: A review of current curricular practices in relation to Benner's latest work. *International Journal of Nursing Education Scholarship, 9*, 1–16.

Jensen, R. (2013). Clinical reasoning during simulation: Comparison of student and faculty ratings. *Nurse Education in Practice, 13*, 23–28.

Koharchik, L., Caputi, L., Robb, M., & Culleiton, A. L. (2015). Fostering clinical reasoning in nursing students. *The American Journal of Nursing, 115*, 58–61.

Lasater, K., Johnson, E. A., Ravert, P., & Rink, D. (2014). Role modeling clinical judgment for an unfolding older adult simulation. *The Journal of Nursing Education, 53*, 257–264.

Levett-Jones, T., Hoffman, K., Dempsey, J., Yeun-Sim Jeong, S., Noble, D., Norton, C., & Hickey, N. (2010). The 'five rights' of clinical reasoning: An educational model to enhance nursing students' ability to identify and manage clinically 'at risk' patients. *Nurse Education Today, 30*, 515–520.

Olson, I. (2000). *The arts and critical thinking in American education*. Stamford, CT: Bergin & Garvey.

Popil, I. (2011). Promotion of critical thinking by using case studies as a teaching method. *Nurse Education Today, 31*, 204–207.

Potter, P. A., & Perry, A. G. (2009). *Fundamentals of nursing* (7th ed.). St. Louis, MO: Mosby Elsevier.

Russell, B. H., Geist, M. J., & Maffett, J. H. (2013). SAFETY: An integrated clinical reasoning and reflection framework for undergraduate nursing students. *The Journal of Nursing Education, 52*, 59–62.

Shoulders, B., Follett, C., & Eason, J. (2014). Enhancing critical thinking in clinical practice. *Dimensions of Critical Care Nursing, 33*, 207–214.

Tanner, C. A. (2004). The meaning of curriculum: Content to be covered or stories to be heard? *The Journal of Nursing Education, 43*(1), 3–4.

Tanner, C. A. (2006). Thinking like a nurse: A research-based model of clinical judgment in nursing. *The Journal of Nursing Education, 45*(6), 204–211.

Thompson, C., Cullum, N., McCaughan, D., Sheldon, T., & Raynor, P. (2004). Nurses, information use, and clinical decision making: The real potential for evidence-based decisions in nursing. *Evidence-Based Nursing, 7*(3), 69–72.

Bibliography

Andersson, N., Klang, B., & Peterson, G. (2012). Differences in clinical reasoning among nurses working in highly specialized pediatric care. *Journal of Clinical Nursing, 21*, 870–879.

Clarke, C. (2014). Promoting the 6C's of nursing in patient assessment. *Nursing Standard, 44*, 52–59.

Corlett, J. (2012). The perceptions of nurse teachers, student nurses, and perceptions of the theory-practice gap in nurse education. *Nursing Education Today, 20*, 499–505.

Huang, Y. C., Chen, H. H., Yeh, M. L., & Chung, Y. C. (2012). Case studies combined with or without concept maps improve critical thinking in hospital-based nurses: A randomized-controlled trial. *International Journal of Nursing Studies, 49*, 747–754.

Johnson, E. A., Lasater, K., Hodson-Carlton, K., Siktberg, L., Sideras, S., & Dillard, N. (2012). Geriatrics in simulation: Role modeling and clinical judgment effect. *Nursing Education Perspectives, 33*, 176–180.

Kalkbrenner, A., & Brandt, P. A. (2012). Coaching strategies for clinical learning: A strengths-based approach to student development. *Nurse Educator, 37*, 185–186.

Lang, G. M., Beach, N. L., Patrician, P. A., & Martin, C. A. (2013). A cross-sectional study examining factors related to critical thinking in nursing. *Journal for Nurses in Professional Development, 29*, 8–15.

Lewis, R., Strachan, A., & Smith, M. M. (2012). Is high fidelity simulation the most effective method for the development of non-technical skills in nursing? A review of the current evidence. *The Open Nursing Journal, 6*, 82–89.

McCallum, J., Duffy, K., Hastie, E., Ness, V., & Price, L. (2013). Developing nursing students' decision making skills: Are early warning scoring systems helpful? *Nurse Education in Practice, 13*, 1–3.

Munroe, B., Curtis, K., Considine, J., & Buckley, T. (2013). The impact structured patient assessment frameworks have on patient care: An integrative review. *Journal of Clinical Nursing, 22*, 21–22.

16

New Graduate RN Transition to Practice Programs

Deloras Jones and Nikki West

ADDITIONAL RESOURCES

Visit thePoint for additional helpful resources

- eBook
- Journal Articles
- WebLinks

CHAPTER OUTLINE

LEARNING OBJECTIVES

The learner will be able to:

1. Understand the historical gap between academia and practice, and the role that transition to practice programs play in bridging that gap.
2. Identify at least three models of transition to practice programs.
3. Understand the role of transition to practice programs within the larger national initiative to advance nursing through the Institute of Medicine Report on the Future of Nursing.
4. Explain the factors creating the current, pressing need for transition to practice programs to retain new graduate nurses and prepare them for employment.
5. Explain the unique characteristics of academic–practice-based transition to practice programs that make them attractive and applicable for use in preparing nurses for smaller, nonhospital settings that are nontraditional places for first employment.
6. Describe challenges with sustaining transition to practice programs.

INTRODUCTION

This chapter explores the gap between completion of academic programs and entry into employment (also referred to as service or practice) as a registered nurse (RN) and strategies for closing that gap with transition to practice programs (TPPs). The chapter suggests that such programs report fewer patient (medication) errors and better patient safety practices, higher competency levels, less stress and increased job satisfaction as well as lower turnover rates for new graduates. Organizations leading a national call for TPPs or residencies as an expectation of nursing education are presented, as are the challenges to realizing this expectation. The hiring difficulties new graduates began experiencing in 2009 and the impact that has had on TPPs is also discussed. A demonstration project that strives to increase the skills, competencies, and confidence of new graduates in community-based TPPs, housed in schools of nursing, is highlighted. This chapter then summarizes the important evidence regarding the need for TPPs as an expectation of the nursing education process.

TRANSITION TO PRACTICE PROGRAMS: CLOSING THE GAP

What Are Transition to Practice Programs?

TPPs are designed to support newly licensed RNs' progression from education to practice as they move into their first professional nursing role. The National Council for State Boards of Nursing (NCSBN) and the American Association of Colleges of Nursing (AACN) have defined TPPs as a formal program of active learning that includes a series of educational sessions and work experiences for newly licensed RNs (AACN n.d.-b; NCSBN, 2011). Transition to practice is also designated as the period between being a student nurse and an independent professional nurse. TPPs have been given various names including "residencies," "externships," and "internships."

Although multiple types of TPPs exist, all are focused on helping new nurses bridge the transition from school into employment. There are programs that begin in the final year of nursing school and continue through licensure. Others are structured as employer-based "new graduate classes," typically within a hospital. Some of these programs take up to a year to complete, whereas others are only 12 to 16 weeks in length. Still other programs are for new graduates who have yet to be hired, so they may gain skills in order to become more employable.

Also, interest is growing in TPPs for ambulatory care settings, for experienced nurses moving into new roles, and for advance practice RNs. The need for nurse practitioners to have residencies to prepare them as primary care providers in federally qualified health clinics is becoming a priority as these nurses are being called upon to fill the shortfall of primary care providers, traditionally a role held by physicians, who have completed internships and residencies (Flinter, 2011).

Why Have Transition to Practice Programs?

Although the NCSBN reports that there has been a call for TPPs for more than 80 years (Spector et al., 2015), arguments have grown over the last decade regarding the need for these programs for newly licensed nurses. The ever-changing health care delivery system, with its increasing complexity of patient care as people live longer with multiple chronic conditions, rapidly evolving technology, and focus on patient safety, has created expectations from nursing educational systems that are not being met. The practice setting or environment where nurses are working requires highly developed critical thinking and problem-solving skills, the ability to exercise clinical judgment with the know-how to practice from an evidence-based and outcome-driven perspective, and the ability to develop effectively from a novice to an expert in competency.

Acute care hospitals, which are the traditional employers of new graduates, often report an incongruence between the expectations of education and those of employers. This gap is described in a practice brief from the Nursing Executive Center, The Advisory Board Company (Nursing Executive Center, The Advisory Board Company, 2006) following interviews with nurse executives from member hospitals. The brief states,

> *Many arrive at the hospital unprepared to perform even basic clinical tasks and lacking critical thinking skills to apply their classroom learning to real-life clinical practice. New graduates may also be unprepared for the emotional demands of first-year nursing. The stresses of navigating a new environment, working overnight shifts, and caring for acutely ill patients can take a significant toll …* (p. viii)

In addition, del Bueno (2005) reported that 10 years of performance-based competency testing she completed suggested that 65% to 75% of new graduates did not meet expectations for entry-level clinical judgment and that most had difficulty translating knowledge and theory into practice; 50% would miss life-threatening situations. The NCSBN stated in their report for a Regulatory Model for Transition to Practice that "new nurses often engage in concrete thinking and focus on technology, thus miss the bigger picture… and are weak in detecting subtle changes in patient conditions" (Spector & Echternacht, 2009). Furthermore, a survey conducted for the Advisory Board Company of both hospital nurse executives and leaders of nursing education programs found that only 10% of nurse executives felt that new graduates were fully prepared to provide safe and effective care in hospitals, compared with 90% of nurse educators (Berkow, Virkstis, Stewart, & Conway, 2010; Pete Simkinson, personal communication, August 31, 2011).

This academic–practice gap places patient safety and the quality of care at risk if a new graduate does not have the critical thinking skills or competencies needed to apply critical judgments to patient situations. TPPs bridge the gap by providing the new graduate opportunities to take the learnings from nursing school and apply them in an expanded, intensive, and integrated clinical learning situation while providing direct patient care under the guidance of a preceptor. TPPs would assist new nurses to identify subtle changes in patients and avoid practice errors (Spector & Echternacht, 2009).

Consider This Other health care professions, including medicine, pharmacy, clinical laboratory scientists, physical therapists, psychologists, pastoral care, public health, and optometry, require residencies or internships to complete their professional training. During their residencies or internships, academic learning is applied to actual care of patients as the new health professional transitions into the professional role. This is a missing step in nursing education.

Discussion Point

No one expects a fully qualified physician to step forward after the completion of medical school and begin practice without an internship or residency in his/her area of specialty. The same is not expected of nurses. What are the best arguments for changing the perception of nursing education to include TPPs?

Why an Academic–Practice Gap?

New graduates often begin working as RNs with little more than a few weeks of orientation, in contrast to most other health professions, which require formal and, often standardized, internships or residencies. This is largely a residual outcome of the traditional nursing educational system that was grounded in apprenticeship and hospital-based training programs that led to the student receiving a diploma in nursing. A large portion of the education of the diploma-prepared nurse included clinical training by providing direct care to patients in the hospital that sponsored the program. Following graduation, only a few weeks of orientation specific to the hospital or the unit they were assigned to was required, as many were first employed at their training hospital.

New standards were applied to nursing education in 1965, when the American Nurses Association called for a college-based nursing education system (Gallagher & Sullivan, n.d.). With this change in the standards, the primary focus of nursing education changed from the hospital-based program to the college or university setting. At that time, hospital-based programs were preparing 78% of all nurses.

The growth of associate degree programs in community colleges that also took place during this time further exacerbated this change, with these community college programs effectively taking the place of hospital-based diploma programs in most cities. As these academic-based programs did not have the clinical focus found in diploma programs, a gap between academia/education and the practice setting came to exist that the profession and employers of nurses continue to grapple with today. The gap became more problematic when in 1994 the NCLEX examination for licensure provided results electronically that were available in a few days, enabling the newly licensed nurse to be eligible for hire as an RN (NCSBN, n.d.). Prior to this, new graduates were frequently hired after they took the licensing exam and worked as nonlicensed graduates under the supervision of a licensed nurse, at times for several months, before exam results were available and the new nurse could then take accountability as an RN.

CONSEQUENCES OF THE ACADEMIC–PRACTICE GAP

Turnover

Without TPPs or residencies, stresses associated with the first year of employment, concerns about patient care, and feeling unsupported in their new roles often lead to high turnover rates in new graduates who are more likely than experienced nurses to resign within their first year of employment (Nursing Executive Center, The Advisory Board Company, 2006). Studies have reported that turnover rates for new graduates range from 22.6% to 60% (vanWyngeeren & Stuart, n.d.).

High turnover rates result in the "churning of staff," including increased use of temporary staff to fill vacancies. In addition to negatively impacting patient care and continuity of care, this "churning of staff" impacts the stability, and hence the quality, of the work environment. It also places additional stress on senior nursing staff who are called upon to precept and orient new hires, increases management and supervisory time, and decreases staff productivity (Ulrich et al., 2010).

The cost of turnover is high. Estimates of turnover cost per nurse range from US$82,000 to US$88,000 (Jones, 2008). During a typical new nurse training period, which may last anywhere from 2 weeks to 6 months, hospitals essentially pay two nurses (a trainer and a trainee) for the product of one. A survey of hospital CEOs indicates that the average time to onboard a new graduate is 233 hours, or almost 6 work weeks (National Association of Travel Healthcare Organizations, 2011). The investment made in the high cost of onboarding a new graduate is lost by the hospital (employer) when premature turnover occurs. Leaving within 2 years of employment does not allow an effective return on investment (ROI).

However, residency programs provided by hospitals to new graduates they employ have resulted in a significant drop in turnover. For example, one large highly respected metropolitan hospital in Western United States reported that 36% of new graduates were leaving within their first year and that 56% left within 2 years (Ulrich et al., 2010). The hospital implemented a standardized approach for TPPs as a means of increasing retention of new graduates. The 12-month turnover dropped to just over 5%. Versant, the standardized residency program that dramatically decreased the hospital's turnover rate, has continued to produce results in more than 85 hospitals since 1999, providing excellent evidence for the ROI for residencies (Ulrich et al., 2010; Versant.org, 2015).

Expertise Gap and Health Care Reform

A growing concern among nurse leaders is the prediction of an expertise gap in nursing as experienced nurses retire and the ratio of new graduates to experience nurses increases (Orsolini-Hain & Malone, 2007). Considering that in 2013, 53% of the nation's working nursing workforce was 50 years or older, the impact of the expertise gap will be significant, as these nurses retire and are replaced by new graduates (Budden, Zhong, Moulton, & Cimiotti, 2013). Retirements have been delayed because of the economic recession, which began in 2008, but an outward flow of experienced nurses is expected across the country as the economy continues to improve and older nurses retire.

Consider This The argument for ensuring that new graduates have the skills and competencies to transition into the practice environment and provide the safe, quality care that is demanded of them also means that planning for providing TPPs is needed now more than ever—while there are still experienced nurses available to precept new graduates.

Ten years ago, it was reported that a 50% turnover in the nursing profession will be evident within a decade (Dracup & Morris, 2007). A full 18% of California's working nurses are 60 years or older (California Board of Registered Nursing [CBRN], 2013–2014).

Furthermore, there are factors at work in addition to succession planning that need to be considered. Based on economic, demographic, and regulatory factors, nurses are being asked to work in different and more efficient ways. The nation is challenged with a population that is diverse, aging, and mobile. As life expectancy extends, those with chronic conditions will need support to manage their conditions more effectively. The 2008 Affordable Care Act is driving increased demand for health care services for a higher volume of insured individuals, and necessitating the creative rethinking of delivery settings and approaches. New models for delivery care are emerging with emphasis placed on team-based interprofessional care. New roles for nurses are being defined. These changes and evolving roles call for utilizing TPPs as a means for preparing nurses for future and new roles driven by demands of health care reform (HealthImpact, 2013).

NATIONAL CALL FOR TRANSITION TO PRACTICE PROGRAMS

Who Is Calling for Transition to Practice Programs?

In response to the need to provide a bridge for newly graduated nurses from education to practice, fueled by a growing national focus on patient safety, the increasing complexity of patient needs and health care delivery systems, and the need to improve retention in the workplace, the momentum to provide TPPs is increasing. This is occurring with the full recognition that academia alone cannot fully prepare new graduates for the work environment and honing the necessary skills for professional practice. It requires that employers of nurses share in creating sustainable solutions. National and professional organizations are calling for a response to the need for TPPs (Box 16.1)—some are in the national leadership spotlight.

The National Council of State Boards of Nursing (NCSBN)

The NCSBN hosted a convention of national nurse leaders and organizations in 2007 to examine the need for TPPs and the role regulation should have. The participants strongly supported the need for a national, standardized model (for transition into practice) that was implemented through regulation (NCSBN, 2008). Subsequently, the NCSBN has been investigating a regulatory model for transition from education to practice, and believes these transition programs are essential and should be provided postlicensure, not lengthening the time of a nursing program. In 2010, the NCSBN launched a major national study on the impact of residencies on patient outcomes. Outcomes of this study provide the critical evidence of the need for TPPs for patient safety and successful transitioning into the professional role of a nurse (Spector & Li, 2007).

Patricia Benner and colleagues, in their work for the **Carnegie Foundation**, called for radical transformation of the nation's education of nurses, and identified the development of clinical residencies for all new graduates in their key recommendations. They further recommended that all graduates be required to complete a 1-year residency so that they have the opportunity to develop in-depth knowledge in one clinical area of specialization (Benner, Sutphen, Leonard, & Day, 2009).

The University HealthSystem Consortium and the American Association of Colleges of Nursing (UHC/AACN)

The UHC/AACN launched a joint venture on sponsoring residencies for baccalaureate-prepared nurses in academic medical centers. Their position is that new graduates should not be expected to transition into their first jobs without a formal TPP to facilitate bridging the gap between education and practice, and that this should be a nationally accredited program. This curriculum is now the largest in the county with over 92 practice sites in 30 states (Goode, Lynn, Krsek, & Bednash, 2009).

The Institute of Medicine (IOM)

The IOM Report on *The Future of Nursing*, released in October 2010, identified TPPs/residencies as one of the eight key recommendations to actualize nursing contributions to the demands of health care reform. This report provides a framework for a national call for action

BOX 16.1 Additional Organizations Calling for Transition to Practice Programs

American Association of Ambulatory Care Nursing: White Paper on the need for ambulatory nurse residencies programs for nurses transitioning into ambulatory care (2014).

American Nurses Credentialing Center: Practice Transition Accreditation has been added to its credentialing of programs along with Magnet Hospital (2014).

American Organization of Nurse Executives: Guiding Principles for creating a learning and supportive professional environment that will position the new graduate for success (2010).

The Joint Commission: Call for structured postgraduate programs for nurses that would provide the opportunity for skill-building in real clinical settings as do residencies for physicians (2002).

Nurse Executive Center, The Advisory Board: Represents 2,900 chief nursing officers as an important voice of employers on the value of residencies to transition new graduates into practice and increase retention.

States' Nursing Workforce Centers and Action Coalitions: Implementing the IOM Report on the Future of Nursing Recommendation 3.

Veterans Health Administration: Standardized curriculum launched nationally to transition new nurses from entry level to competent professional (2011).

Versant—Leader in standardized residencies with over 85 hospitals utilizing their approach (2015).

in that it states that "State boards of nursing, accrediting bodies, the federal government, and health care organizations should take action to support nurses' completion of a TPP (nurse residency) after they have completed a pre-licensure or advanced practice degree program or when they are transitioning into new clinical practice areas" (IOM, 2010, p. 280).

The report goes on to make specific recommendations to support these programs, including redirecting all graduate medical education funding from diploma nursing programs to support the implementation of residencies. They are also calling for programs to be developed outside of the acute care setting, with the expected shift of care from hospitals to community-based settings with health care reform.

The effort to carry out the IOM recommendations continues as part of a national campaign through the Center to Champion Nursing in America, a partnership between the Robert Wood Johnson Foundation (RWJF) and AARP. Fifty-one Action Coalitions have been established for each state and Washington DC. Other organizations encouraging the establishment of TPPs are shown in Box 16.1.

Consider This Other countries have or are in the process of implementing a national approach to transitioning newly licensed nurses into practice. These countries include Portugal, Ireland, Scotland, and Australia.

HealthImpact

HealthImpact (formerly the California Institute for Nursing and Health Care [CINHC]), the state's nursing workforce center, has led the dialogue among educators, hospital and nonacute care employers, regulators, professional associations, and foundations in California about TPPs as an expectation of nursing education in California, through the development of a *White Paper for Nursing Education Redesign*. This important document, developed in 2008 by thought leaders representing all major stakeholders, serves as a framework for how nursing education needs to be designed to meet the evolving needs of the health care delivery system (HealthImpact, 2008b; Fig. 16.1). In 2015, this work began a process to be updated to reflect the impact and requirements set by the Affordable Care Act and changes in the health care environment that will influence shifts in optimal nursing education.

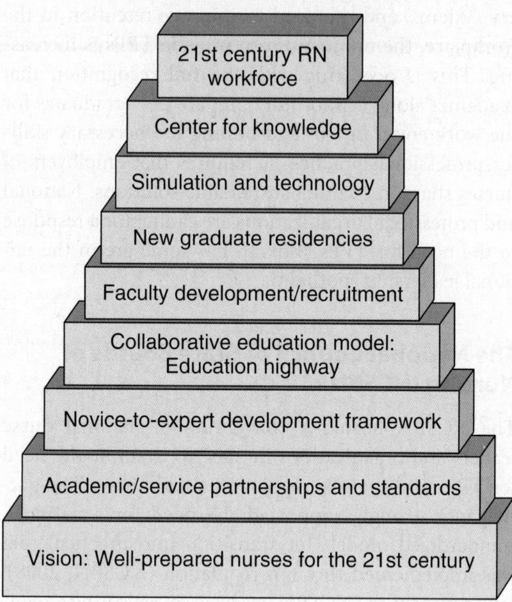

Figure 16.1 Building blocks from White Paper for Education Redesign.
(*Source:* HealthImpact. (2010). *Education redesign building blocks illustration.* Retrieved from http://healthimpact.org/resources/publications/)

In 2008, the California Hospital Association (CHA) and HealthImpact established a statewide workgroup to raise awareness around the importance of residencies for all new graduates within California hospitals. This statewide workgroup continues its efforts and has been identified to carry out the goals of the IOM's recommendation on implementing nurse TPPs and residency programs through the California Action Coalition, which is housed at HealthImpact.

Recommendation 3 of the IOM Report specifically states: "Implement nurse residency programs." This California statewide work group meets regularly to determine goals and action steps for actualizing and defining how to achieve this recommendation. This workgroup has agreed to work toward the goal of strongly recommending that all new graduates have the opportunity to participate in a residency program. The group has developed tools and definitions, which include definitions for "new graduate nurse," "nursing orientation," and "nurse residency/transition to practice programs."

MODELS OF TRANSITION TO PRACTICE PROGRAMS

Characteristics of Quality Transition to Practice Programs

TPPs focus on areas where new graduates need additional skills and competencies and do not repeat a prelicensure academic program. According to the Nursing Executive Center, The Advisory Board Company (2006), areas of focus should include organizing work and priority setting; communicating effectively with physicians, team members, families, and patients; clinical leadership skills to include delegating and overseeing the work of others; emergency response; end-of-life care; and technical skills for specific patient care environments.

Krozek (2008), developer of Versant, describes TPPs as integrated, interconnected programs hardwired throughout the organization that provide a systematic approach to onboarding. He goes on to indicate that characteristics of such programs include standardization leading to core training; practical application of knowledge through clinical immersion to hone patient care skills; support systems that include seasoned nurses prepared for roles as preceptors, coaches, and mentors; rigorous evaluation to ensure that expected outcomes are being met; and continuous improvement based on learning and evolving needs.

Major characteristics of employer-based nurse residency programs designed as a transition from nursing school to professional practice are shown in Box 16.2, and goals of exemplary nurse residency programs are displayed in Box 16.3.

To meet the needs of a variety of practice setting requirements, budgets, and experience with RN preparation, there are several models of TPPs and residencies to prepare nurses for practice.

Examples of program types include:

1. The UHC/AACN Residency Program was formed out of the desire of chief nursing officers for a better educated workforce in their clinical settings. UHC/AACN offers a residency for BSN graduates

BOX 16.2 Major Characteristics of Employer-Based Nurse Residency Programs

- Designed primarily as a transition from nursing school to professional practice, not primarily to teach specialty-specific skills
- Open only to new graduates or nurses with limited work experience following schooling (eg, not to nurses returning to practice after years out of the workforce)
- Involve majority of (and preferably all) new graduates hired into the institution
- Focus on building critical thinking and professional practice skills

Source: Nursing Executive Center, The Advisory Board Company. (2006). *Transitioning new graduates to hospital practice: Profiles of nurse residency program exemplars*. Retrieved from www.advisary.com

BOX 16.3 Nine Goals of Exemplary Nurse Residency Programs

- Bridge gaps in residents' clinical skill set
- Connect "book knowledge" to real-life clinical challenges
- Ensure ongoing support from leadership and peers
- Foster esprit de corps among resident class
- Broaden residents' understanding of health care delivery
- Empower residents to contribute to practice improvement
- Spark continuous professional growth and development
- Demonstrate residency program value
- Facilitate partnerships with area nursing schools

Source: Nursing Executive Center, The Advisory Board Company. (2006). *Transitioning new graduates to hospital practice: Profiles of nurse residency program exemplars*. Retrieved from www.advisary.com

targeted to academic medical centers and is built on an evidence-based curriculum that meets national residency standards. A one-year program designed for direct care roles in the hospital acute care setting, the focus is on in-depth development of the resident's leadership skills, analysis of evidence through reviews of the literature, application of outcome data to patient care improvements, and professional development. The year culminates with the completion of an evidence-based project by the nurse residents (AACN, n.d.-c).

2. Versant is an intense 18-week program, expanding to a year of less intense clinical oversight and mentoring work. The program was created at Children's Hospital in Los Angeles and is employer-based. Versant has evidence from a 10-year longitudinal study that demonstrates both new graduate nurses and their organizations benefit significantly from the implementation of a structured, evidence-based, clinical immersion RN residency (Versant.org, 2015).
3. The National Council of State Boards of Nursing (NCSBN), in collaboration with more than 35 nursing organizations, developed a year-long, employer-based standardized model. The NCSBN conducted a large-scale research effort to assess the value of TPPs in a controlled, blinded, evidence-based manner. Over 3 years, the model was tested and results collected. The evaluation of the NCSBN model that was carried out by Spector and colleagues (2015) is a major contribution to the profession, providing the evidence that supports the arguments for TPPs. The multisite study included 105 hospitals in 3 states in rural and urban settings, and enrolled 1,088 new graduates. The study examined safety, stress, competence, job satisfaction, and retention. The study provided substantial evidence that a standardized TPP does improve patient safety and quality outcome, with fewer reported errors, fewer negative safety practices, high overall competence, less stress, more job satisfaction, and new graduates less likely to leave their positions. The study also demonstrated that the control hospitals with an established transition to practice/residency program had similar results to the NCSBN standardized model.

Furthermore, the study demonstrated that "new nurses who do not have the support of an evidence-based, structured institutional program are at a disadvantage during their first year of practice" (Spector et al., 2015).

4. Hospital-based programs that hire new graduate RNs and prepare them for practice at their specific site exist across the country. These programs are developed by the individual hospital or health care system, with various degrees of rigor and structure. Most hospital-based programs are created as an alternative to a named program, such as Versant or the UHC/AACN model, due to cost constraints or staff/resource requirements needed to implement larger-scale programs.
5. In California, HealthImpact has developed an academic–practice-based RN transition program. Programs are structured as collaborative partnerships offered through a school of nursing, which partners with one or multiple clinical facilities to provide the experience. The program participants are graduated, newly licensed RNs, but not yet employed. The program is versatile enough to prepare RNs for employment both within the hospital and in nonhospital settings. This is compelling as ways are sought to match the supply of nurses for the various community-based, ambulatory settings where care is being delivered (Jones & West, 2011; West et al., 2014) (see following: Academic–Practice-Based Transition to Practice—A Demonstration Project).

Consider This A well-designed TPP strengthens new graduates' skills and competencies and prepares the new nurse for the demands of caring for patients. Furthermore, a systematic approach to transiting not only facilitates "onboarding" (integration into staffing on the nursing unit to provide direct patient care) but also reduces turnover by decreasing the toll associated with insufficient preparation for the work environment. This toll results in stress in new nurses, which in turn increases the risk of patient care errors.

Discussion Point

What are your thoughts to ensure your stress levels do not take a toll on you during your first year as a working new nurse?

THE CALIFORNIA STORY—A CASE STUDY

The Nursing Shortage and an Unanticipated Outcome

The nursing shortage that has long plagued the nation's health care system persists and is likely to worsen in years to come. The 21st century began with the nation preparing for a looming shortage that threatened to result in a public health crisis, driven by 76 million aging baby boomers reaching eligibility for Medicare (sign of the aging of the United States), retirements of an older nursing workforce, and an insufficient number of new nurses to replace those retiring. Analyzing population growth, income, and technology statistics, Buerhaus, Staiger, and Auerbach (2009) estimated the demand for health care would grow 3% every year in the United States. The nursing shortage crisis was brewing and was expected to begin around 2010 (when the first of the baby boomers became eligible for Medicare), reaching a forecasted shortage of 500,000 FTEs by 2025.

Across the country, states responded to this forecasted crisis by building educational capacity to increase the nursing workforce, and a national campaign led by Johnson & Johnson focused on the desirability of nursing as a career. Largely, as a result of these efforts and helped by an influx of foreign-educated nurses and older nurses returning to the workforce, Buerhaus, Auerbach, and Staiger (2009) revised the predicted 2025 shortfall of RNs to 260,000 FTEs.

California's response to the nursing shortage, which was among the worst in the nation, included measures that built educational capacity. In 2004, California ranked 50th out of 50 states for ratio of RNs to population, at 580 RNs per 100,000 population, compared with the nation's average of 825 per 100,000 (Bivano, Fritz, & Spencer, 2004). The state was also forecast to have a shortfall of 116,000 RN FTE by 2020 if the trajectory the state was on at that time continued, meeting only 55% of the state's demand for nurses.

These sobering predictions resulted in a focused and systematic effort, led by the Governor's Task Force for Nursing Education and facilitated by the development of a master plan for building educational capacity under the leadership of HealthImpact, to increase the state's capacity to educate nurses (HealthImpact, 2008a). As a result of these efforts, between 2004 and 2010, educational capacity increased 69%, and the state rose in RN per capita to 644 per 100,000 (compared with a national average of 860 per 100,000 [CBRN, 2009, 2010]).

However, while these statistics were encouraging, the sudden, severe economic downturn in 2008 created an unexpected "perfect storm" for new RN graduates that resulted in unprecedented difficulty securing employment. In spite of preparing for a looming shortage, several factors changed the employment picture for nurses.

First of all, in late 2008, as the nation's economy began to plummet, fewer patients opted for elective surgeries and other treatments as unemployment resulted in the loss of health plan benefits and uncertainty of income; this led to a decrease in hospital days and revenue and decreased demand for nurses.

Second, as a response to the economic recession, experienced nurses worked more. The majority (68%) of nurses in California were married, and to compensate for a spouse's loss or anticipated loss of employment during the recession, many nurses worked extra hours or took on a second job, part-time nurses transitioned to full-time, and others who were not working returned to the workforce. In addition, older nurses who were eligible for retirement delayed leaving the workforce as the value of their investment accounts dropped.

Hospitals, which were also facing financial hardships during this time, found it easier and less expensive to hire experienced nurses than to bring on new graduates, who were costly to hire since hospitals needed to provide extensive orientation or residencies (TPP) to prepare them for employment. Thus, experienced nurses retained and took the jobs that new graduates had expected to fill and competed with the new graduates for the fewer jobs that were available in hospitals—the traditional first places of employment.

In 2010, California hospital RN vacancy rates dropped to an unprecedented low rate of 3.4%, and turnover dropped to 8.2%, compared with 10.2% vacancy rates in 2005 (Hospital Association of Southern California [HASC], 2010). In 2014, low turnover rates have persisted (2.5%) as have hospital RN vacancy rates of 4.7% (HASC, 2014). The California New Graduate Hiring Survey released in January 2015 shows that 35% of new graduates were not yet working in an RN role within 6 months of graduation. These results, however, do provide evidence that a greater percentage of newly licensed nurses obtained jobs within the first year of licensure and are working as RNs compared with each of the four prior years, with 59.3% reported to be working in 2013, 54% in 2012, and 57% in both 2011 and 2010 (HealthImpact, 2015).

The economic climate in the years 2008 to 2012 temporarily concealed the chronic nurse shortage. These conditions are expected to pass, and once they do, the nation's health care system will again see the consequences of an increasing demand for nurses and a grossly inadequate supply. This demand will be exacerbated by the demands of health care reform, which calls for a health care delivery system capable of providing care to 32 million more Americans through health plans and the increasing numbers of the aging population requiring more in the way of health care and chronic disease management. Given this prognosis, California cannot afford to lose its invaluable new RNs.

Consider This The nursing workforce is elastic. Nurses work less when the economy is good and work more when the economy is bad. Nurses find mixed information about career prospects, hearing that "Nursing is a recession-proof profession," yet many struggle to find positions.

Hiring Difficulties of New Graduates

To quantify the extent of new graduate RNs' inability to secure jobs in California, a survey of nurse employers, led by HealthImpact, indicated that approximately 40% of new graduates in 2010 would not be hired in hospitals. Follow-up surveys of new graduate RNs, conducted in 2010 and 2011, confirmed that 43% had not found jobs in nursing after 6 or more months following graduation (HealthImpact, 2009, 2010, & 2012). California's new nurses had fewer opportunities to gain experience and transition successfully into practice.

To address this statewide issue, regional forums were held across the state to report the survey findings and determine solutions to this hiring dilemma. Participants at these forums included health care employers, schools of nursing, state agencies, nursing and health care organizations, workforce investment boards (WIBs), and foundations. After considerable discussion, the solution that resonated was to develop *academic–practice-based transition programs for* newly *graduated RNs, housed in schools of nursing,* to maintain and improve their skills and competencies, and to increase their chances of employability. Santa Rosa Junior College in Santa Rosa, California, led the way in developing this concept with a similar approach, through a partnership with the local WIB and community hospitals to address the increased numbers of their new graduates unable to find jobs.

The concept is that the programs would be designed in collaboration with service and academic partners to address perceived gaps between nursing school and preparation for practice as a professional nurse. The programs would have schools involved in providing didactic (classroom) instruction, and clinical partners would provide intense clinical instruction with preceptorships in various types of settings. Hospitals would be active partners, yet they would not need to first hire the new nurse in order to provide the experience. This important distinction alleviated the issue of limited job openings, which had been preventing service partners from providing new graduates with traditional TPP experiences.

The academic–practice-based TPPs can be customized by each school–clinical partnership providing the education; however, all programs have standard components. Consistently, leaders involved in designing the community-based TPPs agreed the standard basis for the curriculum should be the Quality and Safety Education for Nurses (QSEN) competencies for professional practice.

QSEN Competencies

The national, multiphase QSEN project was developed to address the challenge of preparing future nurses with the knowledge, skills, and attitudes (KSAs) necessary to continuously improve the quality and safety of the health care systems in which they work. QSEN faculty have defined prelicensure and graduate quality and safety competencies for nursing and proposed targets for the KSA to be developed in nursing prelicensure programs for each competency. The agency that accredits baccalaureate nursing programs incorporated QSEN competencies into their Essentials for Baccalaureate Education (AACN, n.d.-b). These competencies are shown in Box 16.4 (QSEN, 2011).

BOX 16.4 Quality & Safety Education for Nurses (QSEN) Competencies

- Patient-centered care
- Teamwork and collaboration
- Evidence-based practice
- Quality improvement
- Safety
- Informatics

Source: Quality and Safety Education for Nurses. (2011). *Quality and safety competencies*. Retrieved from http://www.qsen.org/competencies.php

QSEN pursues strategies to build and develop effective teaching approaches to ensure that future graduates develop competencies in these areas. In terms of new graduate RNs preparing for the workforce, the KSAs in these six competency areas are seen as a solid basis for assessing and creating development plans for nurses as they bridge from student to licensed nurse clinicians serving patients.

Discussion Point

Can you identify what aspects of your nursing school curriculum address QSEN competencies?

Academic–Practice-Based Transition to Practice Programs: A Demonstration Project

In 2009, HealthImpact partnered with several leading statewide organizations, including the CHA, the Association of California Nurse Leaders, and philanthropic organizations invested in advancing nursing—the Gordon and Betty Moore Foundation in Palo Alto, California, and the Kaiser Permanente Fund for Health Education at the East Bay Community Foundation, in Oakland, California—to launch demonstration programs to help new graduates gain skills and experience to become more employable (Jones & West, 2011).

As a first step, the group identified common components for all community-based TPPs. All participants were newly graduated nurses who had passed the NCLEX and were licensed to practice. Programs should be structured to:

- Be offered through local schools of nursing, which provide liability coverage and workers' compensation, with service partners providing the clinical experience, without the requirement to hire.
- Award academic credit or continuing education to participants upon completion.
- Award a common industry-recognized certificate of completion.
- Incorporate clinical, didactic, simulation, skills lab, and e-learning components.
- Run 12 to 18 weeks in length, with a 24-hour-per-week participant commitment.
- Follow QSEN competencies for professional practice as an indicator of improved preparation for clinical practice.
- Use common, QSEN-based evaluation tools to assess participant competence and progress, as well as a common evaluation tool for first employers of program participants, in order to determine the impact of the program.
- Provide extended experiential learning opportunities in generalist, acute, specialty, or community health care settings to advance skills.
- Provide training to program preceptors.
- Recruit and enroll new graduates in (generally) non-salaried positions in programs.

In 2009, four pilot or demonstration TPPs were launched with funding from grants for 250 new graduate RNs. The four programs developed their own curricula based on the core requirements identified above; secured clinical partners including hospitals, clinics, skilled nursing facilities, rehabilitation facilities, and even public schools for school nursing; recruited and enrolled new graduate RN participants; and launched their individual programs. Programs admitted a combination of ADN- and BSN-educated nurses from local nursing schools.

Consider This It is expected that more health care will be provided outside of acute care settings as health care reform is implemented. Academic–practice-based TPPs focused on nonacute settings, such as primary care clinics, behavior health clinics, long-term care, home health, corrections, school nursing, and public health, provide exposure to career paths that new graduates may not have previously considered. These settings also provide an opportunity for nonacute care employers to consider hiring new graduate nurses.

Discussion Point

What are your thoughts about working in a non-acute setting as your first job as an RN? What are some advantages? Some disadvantages?

Outcomes of the Demonstration Project

The academic–practice-based TPPs present a new model for preparing new RNs for the practice setting, as compared with hospital- (employer-) based residencies. These programs do not require clinical sites to hire participants in advance of the program, but do require academia and service to work in a partnership for program design and implementation.

The programs are designed with consistent guidelines and result in an industry-recognized certificate of completion. This certificate has been created to build common understanding and industry recognition around these programs. A statewide database of these TPPs has been created. This model of TPP is being used in a variety of new settings and specialties, including home health, long-term care, school health centers, infection control, and primary care clinics (Jones-Bell et al., 2014).

Interest in the academic–practice-based TPPs is growing. By 2015, over 20 programs were offered throughout California using the same model and evaluation tools. In view of their unique characteristics, these programs are receiving attention as an important new model for providing TPPs. The value of the demonstration programs is of interest not only to funders of the pilots but also to others across the country seeking ways to implement Recommendation 3 of the IOM Report.

Grant funding provided resources to HealthImpact for evaluation and replication of these academic–practice-based TPPs. The evaluation includes working with a university-based research team from the University of San Francisco. The evaluation included an analysis of the new graduate RN program participant's ability to increase the following:

- Perceived self-confidence
- Competence
- Ability to transition to the workforce—ease of transition and decreased time to independent functioning
- Impact on new graduate employability.

Several survey tools have been created to examine the success of the programs, including a competency tool based on QSEN. This analysis builds the body of knowledge supporting the importance of TPPs as a sustainable means to assist new graduate nurses, and supports TPP as an expectation of the nursing education process.

Consider This An initial evaluation of the data from the academic–practice-based TPPs over 2010 to 2012 shows an increase in RN competence and confidence from program start to completion. The programs are meeting the goal of employment for new graduates. Eighty-four percent were employed 3 months after program completion. In addition to these benefits, clinical partners share that they appreciate taking part in the experience and working collaboratively with the schools to watch participants grow in competence and confidence (Berman, Johnson, & West, 2014; Wallace et al., 2014). For organizations that don't have traditional residencies, this model provides a meaningful opportunity for new graduate RN development and a potential pool for recruitment and hiring.

Additionally, HealthImpact led a national webinar hosted by the Center to Champion Nursing in America with a specific focus on the RN Transition Program. Presentations have also been given at statewide conferences of the California Nursing Students' Association, the Association for California Nurse Leaders, and the California Action Coalition.

CHALLENGES TO THE FUTURE OF TRANSITION TO PRACTICE PROGRAMS

Across the country, schools of nursing and nurse employers support TPP. The response is encouraging and reinforced by the important IOM Report on the Future of Nursing. But challenges exist, which need to be overcome to effectively expand and sustain TPPs in all practice settings where newly licensed nurses are employed, and even where experienced nurses seek new clinical opportunities.

Outdated Perspectives of Nurse Training

One of the most important challenges to overcome is an industry-wide expectation that nursing schools provide all the preparation needed for practice as an RN. This is an outcome of the historical hospital-based nursing education, as described earlier. Even though nurse leaders recognize this is not possible, in 2010, 90% of nurse educators were reported to have thought that new graduates were fully prepared to provide safe and effective care in hospitals (Berkow et al., 2010).

Consider This Educators that participated in the HealthImpact academic–practice-based TPP felt that further study of the gaps (between education and practice) could inform prelicensure curriculum and the design of TPP (Berman et al., 2014).

Nurse educators are providing graduates with a foundation upon which to build the skills needed to transition into professional practice. Educators need to recognize the gap between academia and practice and seek opportunities to work with service to build bridges to close the gap. TPP, as part of the nursing education process, is the bridge and is a more contemporary way to view the nursing education trajectory.

Need for Standardization

Standardization of TPP results in consistency in bridging the gap so that employers, new graduates, the nursing profession, health care industry, and the public have confidence in the quality of education provided in the TPP. Without standardization, the quality and expected outcomes of a program may be called into question. Also, programs that are not TPP or residencies, but are actually new hire orientations, may call themselves TPP, thus misguiding or misrepresenting themselves to a new hire.

Common elements have been identified for successful TPP. Furthermore, the Commission on Collegiate Nursing Education, the accrediting body for baccalaureate and graduate education, has already established criteria for accrediting TTP/residencies (AACN [n.d.-a] —Standards for Accreditation of Post-Baccalaureate Nurse Residency Programs). This is a tremendous step not only in standardization, but also in the national call for TPP, which is also a call for standardization.

The residency movement of the UHC/AACN was an early voice for standardization. They also called for federal funds through Medicare to help fund programs that meet standardized criteria (Goode et al., 2009). They have been joined by the Joint Commission, the Kellogg Foundation, the IOM, and the recent work from the NCSBN. Programs such as Versant, the UHC/AACN, and the NCSBN model all provide standardized approaches. An important aspect of the academic–practice-based model of TPP presented by HealthImpact is meeting consistent criteria for implementation and receiving a certificate of completion so that employers have confidence in the expectations and outcomes of new graduates who completed the program—another aspect of standardization (West et al., 2014).

Who Pays?

The greatest obstacle to TPP is "Who pays?" There is widespread agreement that TPPs/residencies are a good idea and a highly desirable approach to providing the bridge from academia to practice for the new graduate, but who is going to foot the bill? Practice has been the payer all these years, but many argue that hospitals (largest employer of new graduates) don't have the dollars any longer as a result of decreasing reimbursement for services from Medicare and insurance companies, and increasingly RNs are being hired in non-acute settings. As long as employers are able to hire experienced nurses, many are doing this rather than hiring new graduates who need TPP. But one can argue that employers, as the benefactor from low turnover rates and improved patient safety indicators, can justify the ROI in hiring newly licensed nurses and should bear the cost of TPP.

There are other approaches to consider. Employers (acute and nonacute clinical sites) investing in academic–practice-based TPPs will find there is value added with shorter onboarding time with a new graduate who has begun the process of closing the gap when hired—even when followed with a traditional employer-based residency. At least one large hospital system with access to graduates of these academic–practice-based programs is accepting applications for RN positions and their new graduate residency program only from newly licensed nurses who have successfully completed one of these TPPs.

An untapped funding source for TPPs/residencies for nurses is the federal government. Currently, Medicare dollars are passed onto a few hospitals that still have diploma programs, in the same manner that Medicare (CMS) passes funding onto hospitals to pay for physician internships and residencies. The national call for TPP needs to include shifting these federal funds to nurse residencies. The IOM Recommendation 3 calls for this shifting of funds. Using these Medicare dollars in medically underserved communities and rural hospitals would go further toward increasing a qualified nursing workforce than perpetuating diploma education.

Consider This The costs of medical residencies are largely underwritten by the federal government through Medicare Graduate Medical Education pass-through dollars to hospitals providing training of physicians. Funding comes from the Centers for Medicare and Medicaid Services (CMS), which also supports the residencies of pharmacy and pastoral care (Spector & Echternacht, 2011). Nursing does not have residencies as a requirement nor federal dollars to fund programs.

However, a pilot has been initiated, with the federal government funding residencies for advanced practice nurses (nurse practitioners) through a CMS Innovation Grant as a response to the Affordable Care Act.

Consider This The Federal Register rules and regulations state that a program is considered to be provider-operated when the hospital directly incurs the training costs, directly controls the curriculum and the administration of the program, controls both the classroom instruction and the clinical training, and employs the teaching staff (CMS, n.d.). In addition, the residency must be accredited by a national accrediting body. When these conditions are met, a residency should qualify for Medicare reasonable cost pass-through payment (Goode et al., 2009).

However, CMS considers nurse residency programs to be continuing education, because it is not a requirement for employment (CMS n.d.). Unless the new graduate is required to have a residency experience in order to be eligible for employment, CMS will not reimburse for these programs.

Discussion Point

Arguments seem to be in favor of requiring residencies or TPPs for nurses. AACN is calling for the profession to come together and seek CMS or other federal funding for TPP for new graduates. What are your thoughts on how this could actually occur?

Consider This A potential financial model for shared funding of an academic–practice-based TPP:

- Schools of nursing have faculty for classes and overseeing preceptorships and the structure for supporting the TPP, including receiving funds that underwrite the costs of the program, providing insurance, and developing curriculum. Simulation labs are also available in most schools of nursing to help hone skills and clinical decision making.
- Practice partners have the clinical sites needed and the preceptors for overseeing and guiding the new graduate's clinical practice. They are also the potential employers for graduates of the TPP. Practice partners contribute preceptors cost. They may also provide a stipend to TPP participants, especially with consideration of hiring. A forgivable loan may also be provided with the intent to hire those who successfully complete the program.
- New graduates pay a fee to the school of nursing to participate in the TPP that would cover the cost incurred by the school and infrastructure funding to support the process. This fee could be considered part of the cost of nursing education. As the new graduate is now licensed, clinical experiences will be more inclusive than those under the restrictions often found with student nurses.
- Private foundations or workforce investment boards may also be considered to help underwrite the costs of TPP or provide stipends to participants.

Discussion Point

- Would you be willing to pay to participate in an academic–practice-based TPP if you thought it would improve your skills and competencies as a new nurse? Would you see this as part of the cost of your nursing education?
- How much would you be willing to pay?

Critical Mass and Call to Action

A critical mass needs to be built to accept TPP as an expectation of nursing education and to initiate a "Call to Action." This critical mass is growing, as evident by all the organizations—including several key national organizations—that are calling for TPP for new graduates. These collective voices should be sufficient one day to reach the tipping point that will result in TTP as an expectation for all newly licensed nurses. But it will be up to the profession of nursing—which includes nurse leaders in academia and in service and practicing nurses in all areas of health care delivery—along with stakeholders to come together to initiate the "Call to Action"—to actualize TPP as an expectation of nursing education.

The NCSBN began the "Call to Action" when they convened a panel of nurse leaders in 2007 to grapple with this compelling issue. The UHC/AACN added their voice, calling the profession to come together with a requirement of residencies for employment and requesting the federal funds through CMS be made available for nurse residency. The work of Benner and colleagues for the Kellogg Foundation and the IOM Report strengthens this "Call to Action." This important work has begun to transform nursing education—preparing new nurses for their professional role in a way that effectively links academic preparation with the practice of nursing. TTP/residencies utilize a much needed contemporary and professional approach to nursing education.

Discussion Point

We talk about a critical mass needed to reach a tipping point when sustaining change occurs. According to Malcolm Gladwell, the *tipping point* is that magic moment when an idea, trend, or social behavior crosses a threshold and subsequently spreads with incredible speed through society. How does this apply to nursing education and the expectation of having TPP as an expectation of nursing education? What more is needed to build the critical mass? What will happen when the tipping point for TPP is reached? (Gladwell, 2002).

Conclusions

TPPs have been designed to provide additional clinical experience under the guidance of a preceptor (experienced RN who has been trained for this mentoring/teaching role) for new RNs and to meet the needs of health care employers by developing a nursing workforce that is better prepared to bridge the gap between education and practice. These programs have demonstrated fewer patient care–related errors and improved safety, more confidence, and lower turnover rates with new nurses—an important retention strategy of employers. In addition, in the case of the public school–based, home care/hospice, and community clinic programs, the experience provides access to employment for health care facilities that lack the resources to fund training programs.

TPPs integrate prior academic learning into guided intensive clinical practice in order to transition new graduates to the professional role of the RN. The professional role includes having the critical thinking skills to make the decisions that positively impact patient care, and having the insight to discern and appropriately act on subtle changes in the patient. The evidence is now available that supports the value of these programs from a patient safety perspective, justifies the ROI, and demonstrates effective bridging of the gap from education to practice.

National support is growing for TPPs for all new nurses as well as experienced nurses transitioning to new roles. But in order to have the call for action that is necessary for TPPs to be an expectation of nursing education, challenges led by "who pays?" must be overcome. It is hoped that in the near future, growing evidence of the difference that TPPs make in safe patient care will provide the momentum to mount the call for action. The foundation laid by the IOM Report on the Future of Nursing will facilitate and justify this critical need.

For Additional Discussion

1. Should TPPs be a standard component of nursing education? Why or why not?
2. What are the pros and cons of new graduates paying to participate in a TPP? Would you be willing to pay?
3. Some labor groups suggest that school-based TPPs are free labor. Most organizations see the programs as an important extension of education that prepares RNs for their first role. What do you think? Can you envision a cost-effective approach that would appeal to new graduates, clinical sites, and labor groups?
4. Do you believe you will be fully prepared for your first RN position upon graduation? If not, which skills or competencies would you need to learn or practice following licensure to feel confident, safe, and ready for direct work with patients?
5. What type of setting do you think you'll be in for your first RN position? Does this setting typically have a TPP in place? Do you believe your prelicensure program adequately prepared you for work in this setting?
6. Do you think TPPs should be available to experienced RNs? Are there certain roles that constitute additional preparation where more RNs will be needed? Which ones?

References

American Association of Colleges of Nursing. (n.d.-a). *Standards for Accreditation of Post-Baccalaureate Nurse Residency Programs.* Retrieved from http://www.aacn.nche.edu/ccne-accreditation/resstandards08.pdf

American Association of Colleges of Nursing. (n.d.-b). *CCNE accreditation.* Retrieved from http://www.aacn.nche.edu/education-resources/baccessentials08.pdf

American Association of Colleges of Nursing. (n.d.-c). *Nurse residency program.* Retrieved from http://www.aacn.nche.edu/education-resources/nurse-residency-program

Benner, P., Sutphen, M., Leonard, V., & Day, L. (2009). *Educating nurses: A call for radical transformation* [Higher and adult education series]. San Francisco, CA: Jossey-Bass.

Berkow, P. C., Virkstis, K., Stewart, J., & Conway, L. (2010). Assessing new graduate nurse performance. *Journal of Nursing Administration, 38*(11), 468–474.

Berman, A., Beazley, B., Karshmer, J., Prion, S., Van, P., Wallace, J., & West, N. (2014). Competency gaps among unemployed new nursing graduates entering a community-based transition-to-practice program. *Nurse Educator, 39*(2), 56–61.

Berman, A., Johnson, T., & West, N. (2014). New license, no job: Nurse leaders' experience with transition-to-practice programs for unemployed new RN graduates. *Nurse Leader, 12*(5), 29–32.

Biviano, M., Fritz, M., & Spencer, W. (2004). *What is behind HRSA's projected supply, demand, and shortage of registered nurses?* Rockville, MD: National Center for Health Workforce Analysis, Bureau of Health Professions, Health Resources and Service Administration, U.S. Department of Health and Human Services.

Budden, J. S., Zhong, E. H., Moulton, P., & Cimiotti, J. P. (2013). Highlights of the National Workforce Survey of Registered Nurses. *Journal of Nursing Regulation, 4*(2), 5–14.

Buerhaus, P. I., Auerbach, D. I., & Staiger, D. O. (2009). The recent surge in nurse employment: Causes and implication [Abstract]. *Health Affairs, 28*(4), 658.

Buerhaus, P. I., Staiger, D. O., & Auerbach, D. I. (2009). *The future of the nursing workforce in the United States*. Sudbury, MA: Jones & Bartlett.

California Board of Registered Nursing. (2013–2014). *Survey of registered nurses in California 2014* (Annual school survey). Retrieved from http://rn.ca.gov/pdfs/forms/survey2012.pdf

Centers for Medicare and Medicaid Services. (n.d.). *Graduate nurse education demonstration*. Retrieved from http://innovation.cms.gov/initiatives/gne/

del Bueno, D. J. (2005). A crisis in critical thinking. *Nursing Education Perspectives, 26*(5), 278–282.

Dracup, K., & Morris, P. E. (2007). Nursing residency programs: Preparing for the next shift. *American Journal of Critical Care, 16*(4), 328–330.

Flinter, M. (2011, November 28). From new nurse practitioner to primary care provider: Bridging the transition through FQHC-based residency training. *The Online Journal of Issues in Nursing, 17*(1), 6.

Gallagher, R. M., & Sullivan, K. (n.d.). *Compendium of ANA education positions, position statements, and documents*, p. 4. Retrieved from http://nursingworld.org/MainMenuCategories/Policy-Advocacy/State/Legislative-Agenda-Reports/NursingEducation/NursingEducationCompendium.pdf

Gladwell, M. (2002). *The tipping point: How little things can make a big difference*. Boston, MA: Little, Brown and Company.

Goode, C. J., Lynn, M. R., Krsek, C., & Bednash, G. D. (2009). Nurse residency programs: An essential requirement for nursing. *Nursing Economic$, 27*(3), 142–147.

HealthImpact. (2008a). *Building educational capacity in California schools of nursing*. Retrieved from http://healthimpact.org/wp-content/uploads/2015/09/Master-Plan-for-building-educational-capacity-2008.pdf

HealthImpact. (2008b). *White Paper: Nursing education redesign for California*. Retrieved from http://healthimpact.org/wp-content/uploads/2015/09/White-paper-on-nursing-education-redesign.-2008.pdf

HealthImpact. (2009). *New RN graduate workforce regional planning meetings: Statewide summary of RN hiring survey*. Retrieved from http://healthimpact.org/wp-content/uploads/2015/09/RN-Job-pres-All-Regions-ed-0809.pdf

HealthImpact. (2010). *Education redesign building blocks illustration*. Retrieved from http://healthimpact.org/resources/publications/

HealthImpact. (2012). *2010–2011 California new graduate hiring survey*. Retrieved from http://healthimpact.org/wp-content/uploads/2015/09/2010-2011-CA-new-graduate-hiring-survey.pdf

HealthImpact. (2013). *Nurse role exploration project: The Affordable Care Act and new nursing roles*. Retrieved from http://healthimpact.org/wp-content/uploads/2015/08/NurseRoles-1009201311.pdf

HealthImpact. (2015). *2013–2014 California new graduate hiring survey*. Retrieved from http://healthimpact.org/wp-content/uploads/2015/09/NewGrad-SurveyReportofFindings2015.pdf

Hospital Association of Southern California. (2010). *Allied for health quarterly turnover and vacancy report (4th quarter)*. Los Angeles, CA: Author.

Hospital Association of Southern California. (2014). *Allied for health quarterly turnover and vacancy report (3rd quarter)*. Los Angeles, CA: Author.

Institute of Medicine. (2010). *The future of nursing: Leading change, advancing health*. Washington, DC: The National Academies Press.

Joint Commission on Accreditation of Healthcare Organizations. (2002). *Health care at the crossroads: Strategies for addressing the evolving nursing crisis*. Retrieved from http://www.jointcommission.org/assets/1/18/health_care_at_the_crossroads.pdf

Jones, C. B. (2008). Revisiting nurse turnover cost. *Nursing Administration, 38*(1), 11–18.

Jones, D., & West, N. (2011). Community-based transition programs: California's answer to the new-graduate hiring crisis. *Journal of Nursing Regulation, 1*(2), 14–17.

Jones-Bell, J., Karshmer, J., Berman, A., Prion, S., Van, P., Wallace, J., & West, N. (2014). Collaborative academic-practice transition program for new graduate RNs in community settings: Lessons learned. *The Journal of Continuing Education, 45*(6), 259–264.

Krozek, C. (2008). The new graduate RN residency: Win/win/win for nurses, hospitals, and patients. *Nurse Leader, 6*(5), 41–44.

National Association of Travel Healthcare Organizations. (2011). *KPMG Releases 2011 U.S. hospital nursing labor costs study*. Retrieved from http://natho.org/kpmgStudy.php

National Council of State Boards of Nursing. (2008, August). *Regulatory mode for transition to practice report*. Retrieved from www.ncsbn.org/Final_08_reg_model.pdf

National Council of State Boards of Nursing. (2011). *Goals of NCSBN's transition to practice model*. Retrieved from www.ncsbn.org/Final_08_reg_model.pdf

National Council of State Boards of Nursing. (n.d.) *History*. Retrieved from https://www.ncsbn.org/history

Nursing Executive Center, The Advisory Board Company. (2006). *Transitioning new graduates to hospital practice: Profiles of nurse residency program exemplars*. Retrieved from https://www.advisory.com

Orsolini-Hain, L., & Malone, R. E. (2007). Examining the impending gap in clinical nursing expertise. *Policy, Politics, & Nursing Practices, 8*(3), 158–169.

Quality and Safety Education for Nurses. (2011). *Quality and safety competencies*. Retrieved from www.qsen.org/competencies/pre-licensure-ksas/

Spector, N., Blegen, M. A., Silvestre, J., Barnsteiner, J., Lynn, M. R., Ulrich, B., . . . Alexander, M. (2015). Transition to practice study in hospital settings. *Journal of Nursing Regulations, 5*(4), 24–38.

Spector, N., & Echternacht, M. (2009). A regulatory model for transitioning newly licensed nurses to practice. *Journal of Nursing Regulation, 1*(2), 18–25.

Spector, N., & Li, S. (2007). A regulatory model on transitioning nurses from education to practice. *JONA's Healthcare Law, Ethics, and Regulation, 9*(1), 19–22.

Ulrich, B., Krozek, C., Early, S., Ashlock, C. H., Africa, L. M., & Carman, M. L. (2010). Improving retention, confidence, and competence of new graduate nurses: Results from a 10-year longitudinal database. *Nursing Economic$, 28*(6), 363–375.

vanWyngeeren, K., & Stuart, T. (n.d.). Increasing new graduate nurse retention from the student nurse perspective. *RN Journal*. Retrieved from http://www.rnjournal.com/journal_of_nursing/increasing_new_graduate_nurse_retention.htm

Versant.org. (2015). *Outcomes*. Retrieved from www.versant.org/about/125-outcomes.html

Wallace, J., Berman, A., Karshmer, J., Prion, S., Van, P., & West, N. (2014). Economic aspects of community-based academic-practice transition to practice programs for unemployed new nursing graduates. *Journal for Nurses in Professional Development, 45*(6), 237–264.

West, N., Berman, A., Karshmer, J., Prion, S., Van, P., & Wallace, J. (2014). Preparing new nurse graduates for practice in multiple settings: A community-based academic-practice partnership model. *The Journal of Continuing Education in Nursing, 45*(6), 252–256.

17

MOOCS and Virtual Learning Spaces

A Withering of the Traditional Classroom

Pamela R. Jeffries, Khadijah A. Mitchell, April M. Clayton, Emily L. Jones, and Cynthia Foronda

ADDITIONAL RESOURCES

Visit thePoint for additional helpful resources
- eBook
- Journal Articles
- WebLinks

CHAPTER OUTLINE

Introduction
Higher Education—State of Evolution and Alternative Learning Environments
Massive Open Online Courses (MOOCs)
Open Source Materials
Virtual Learning Spaces
- *Online Pedagogy*
- *Standards for Distance Education*
- *Virtual Simulation*

Challenges and Barriers to Traditional Learning Environments
- *Faculty and Learner Expectations: Challenges and Impact*
- *Models of Instruction: Barriers to Passive and Active Learning*
- *Environmental Barriers: Time, Setting, and Physical Space*
- *Lack of Flexibility*

Faculty Development Needed for Digital Education and MOOC Teaching
- *Faculty Expectations*
- *Benefits to Faculty*
- *Challenges and Barriers*

Classroom Learning Environments of the Future
Conclusions

LEARNING OBJECTIVES

The learner will be able to:

1. Identify trends in distance education.
2. Define MOOCs and their current purpose in higher education.
3. Discuss the use and purpose of open courseware.
4. Compare/contrast faculty benefits and challenges when incorporating emerging technologies into their teaching/learning environments.
5. Identify various interpretations of the term “virtual classroom.”
6. Discuss multiple methods of instruction for teaching online.
7. Discuss benefits and challenges of using emerging technologies in teaching.
8. Describe uses for virtual simulation in nursing education.
9. Discuss the future classroom and teaching environments in this changing, dynamic higher education landscape.

INTRODUCTION

Technology will continue to influence how we educate learners with advanced new tools and environments that create new strategies for learning. Curriculum for the 21st century is restructured, redesigned, and disruptive in many cases to meet the needs of our learners today and in the future. University education and changes therein will affect nursing education as we see it today. This chapter will describe alternative learning environments, including the massive open online courses (MOOCS), open source materials, and learning spaces, in addition to virtual learning environments that include virtual classrooms, simulations, and other learning spaces. The role and expectations of the educator in these alternative-type learning environments and how educators need to be developed for these new spaces will be described with, finally, the classroom and other learning spaces of the future being thoughtfully discussed.

HIGHER EDUCATION—STATE OF EVOLUTION AND ALTERNATIVE LEARNING ENVIRONMENTS

Higher education is dynamic, with many changes occurring and being seen as disruptive due to the new pedagogies and the infusion of technologies in the teaching–learning environments. Traditional face-to-face learning spaces and pedagogy are being challenged by many educators as they explore new ways to teach and provide quality education to today's diverse learners. A major part of the disruption in higher education is coming from the development and use of emerging technologies into the learning space. The advent of the MOOCS, the notion of open courseware, and the creation of virtual environments are now transforming the way students achieve their educational goals.

New on the horizon, according to EdTech designers ("What's Hot," 2013), are eight new trends or growth areas being seen to "unleash the promise of learner revolution" (p. 7). These changes and potential trends focus on individual learner success. Table 17.1 highlights the eight trends being seen in higher education today that not only influence what we know today as higher education norms but also impact the way we may view and implement nursing education.

Discussion Point

In reviewing the eight growth areas in higher education, what do you see affecting nursing education and the changes in pedagogy and the teaching/learning environments based on these trends?

TABLE 17.1 Eight Growth Areas in Higher Education

Growth Area/Trend in Higher Education	Description
Credit portability	System is being developed that will ensure seamless and transparent agreement where credits earned at one institution are the equivalent of another
21st century skill assessment	An individual's resume/CV will include not only academic credits and certificates, but also credentials demonstrating other skills and attributes that a person possesses and intentionally develops
Competency-based credit	Transparent competency-based credit system—giving students credit for what they know
Personal learner coaching	A personal trainer will provide career advice to set strategies for the learner to acquire the right skills to get a job, promotion, or to change careers
Facilitated peer learning	Online learning has created opportunities for anyone who wants to learn a subject to be able to do so—innovations are developing that will bring students together, online and in person, so one can learn from another
Real-world learning labs	Vendors are looking to create and credential opportunities for the "living learning experience" on a scale broader than internships or study abroad programs
Skills-specific academies	Specific-skill academies or boot camps where professions or skills can be disrupted by third-party skills academy that bypasses the traditional higher education system
Adaptive learning and feedback	Creating new approaches to accommodate different learning styles

Source: What's hot; What's not for 2014. (2013, December). *The JOURNAL: Transforming Education through Technology, 40*(12). Retrieved from http://online.qmags.com/TJL1213/default.aspx?fs=2&pg=1&mode=1#pg1&mode1 and NMC Horizon Report. 2015 Higher Education Edition. (2015). Retrieved October 16, 2015 from http://cdn.nmc.org/media/2015-nmc-horizon-report-HE-EN.pdf

MASSIVE OPEN ONLINE COURSES

MOOCs have shaped the online learning scene, fostered "disruptive" innovations in higher education and lifelong learning, and quickly gained immense popularity over such a short period of time (Miller, 2012; Skiba, 2013). MOOCs are online courses on a wide range of topics open to anyone in the world who has Internet access and computer and language proficiencies. Unlike the standard traditional classroom, registration is open to everyone (and registration usually remains open after the course's start date), without limits on the number of student participants and without the need for prerequisites (Liyanagunawardena & Williams, 2014; McAuley, Stewart, Siemens, & Cormier, 2010). Additionally, MOOCs are free; however, some courses will provide verified certificates (as means for provision of credit) for a fee.

George Siemens and Stephen Downes at the University of Manitoba taught the first MOOC, "Connectivism and Connective Knowledge," in 2008. With around 2,000 students taking the course for free and no credit and 25 paid, enrolled (for credit) students, this inaugural MOOC was pivotal in shaping online education (Downes, 2008; Liyanagunawardena, Adams, & Williams, 2013). Now, many universities offer MOOCs via various platforms. The American edX, Udacity, and Coursera platforms are major players in the MOOC arena (Times, 2012). As of 2014, Coursera has partnered with over 100 institutions from around the world to generate MOOCs covering a multitude of subjects.

Based on pedagogy, two types of MOOCs have prevailed in the online learning world: cMOOCs and xMOOCs (Liyanagunawardena & Williams, 2014). cMOOCs or connectivist MOOCs thrive on the strength of peer networks and learning rather than learning from instructors or course designers. The first MOOC, by Siemens and Downes, was based on this principle of connectivism, in which "knowledge is not a destination but an ongoing activity, fueled by the relationships people build and the deep discussion catalyzed within the MOOC" (Johnson et al., 2013; Liyanagunawardena & Williams, 2014). xMOOCs, or MOOCs "as an eXtension of something else," are much more individualistic, in which learning and understanding content provided by instructors and course designers is assigned more importance. The majority of MOOCs provided by most platforms are of this flavor (Downes, 2013; Liyanagunawardena & Williams, 2014; Mackness, 2013; Rodriguez, 2012; Siemens, 2005).

As with other facets of higher education, there are many benefits and challenges to MOOCs for faculty, course designers, and students. Perhaps an obvious benefit is the globalization of higher education. One MOOC can have as many as thousands of students enrolled from around the world. This open access to a free (or at a minimal cost if one wants a verified certificate) education taught by university experts is also a shining glory of MOOCs. The large networks of communication and discussion fostered by MOOCs are quite impressive. Yet a recent report highlights the structural limitations of these forms of large-scale learning and massive diffusion of information (Gillani, Yasseri, Eynon, & Hjorth, 2014). MOOCs also serve as an alternative (and supplement for many) to the traditional university classroom, and may allow learners to acquire new skills at their own pace. Verified certificates may also enhance employability as per the hopes of major MOOC platforms; however, research into the viability of this claim is slim to none, and recently, edX dropped its plans to implement a job placement service for high-performing MOOC students (Kolowich, 2013).

Consider This How would you want to use the MOOC-type pedagogy in nursing education?

There are other challenges and concerns of MOOCs. A major criticism is the student completion rate of MOOC courses, with a range of 2% to 10% of students completing a MOOC course. This statistic is calculated as the number of participants receiving a certificate of completion divided by the total number of students who registered to take the class. However, some scholars are assessing whether this metric is appropriate to use since it is not taking into account the intent of students signing up for MOOCs in the first place (Koller, Ng, Do, & Chen, 2013).

A recent study from Harvard aimed to dissect student intention and persistence in the landscape of MOOCs on the platform HarvardX for the 2013 to 2014 academic year (Reich, 2014). Study findings highlighted that students who intended to take a course for a certificate were almost five times more likely to do so than students who intended to only browse the course. The study also noted that learner intentions may change over the time of the course and such "intentional flips" may be a better indicator of course success than the standard metric used. Another key finding was that attrition happens early in a MOOC course (Reich, 2014). While this study investigated only MOOCs offered by the HarvardX platform, it may provide a useful reference point for MOOC course designers and instructors and assist them in designing MOOCs aimed to maintain student engagement. This study may also influence how MOOCs are critiqued, charging critics and educational researchers to keep in mind the dynamics of student intention, persistence, and attrition when measuring MOOC success.

Another concern of MOOCs is that the majority of MOOCs are conducted in English. In a recent review of MOOCs on health and medicine, it was determined that over 90% of MOOCs were offered in English (Liyanagunawardena & Williams, 2014). Hence, a barrier is imposed if the learner, albeit interested in a MOOC course, is not proficient in English. To mitigate this, a number of MOOCS are now being offered in other languages such as Spanish, Arabic, Portuguese, and Chinese. Founded in 2012, the MOOC platform Miriada X provides Spanish courses; and Rawq is a MOOC platform that provides courses in Arabic. The Chinese platform XuetangX, Japanese platform Schoo, German platform iversity, and Brazilian MOOC platform Veduca have been formed in recent years to cater to the diverse array of international learners (Grossman, 2013; Liyanagunawardena & Williams, 2014). Additional English-language MOOC platforms are FutureLearn and Open2Study, founded in the UK and Australia, respectively (Liyanagunawardena & Williams, 2014).

Also of concern, MOOCs are not accessible to underprivileged communities, especially to learners of low socioeconomic status and/or learners living in developing countries who may not have access to computers let alone the Internet. A recent study in 2013 from the University of Pennsylvania (Penn) highlighted that in a survey of almost 35,000 students worldwide who took courses on Coursera taught by Penn instructors, the majority of learners were already educated (Christensen et al., 2013). Eighty percent of students surveyed had either a 2- or 4-year degree, and 44% of students had some level of graduate education, further emphasizing the fact that MOOCs are mainly reaching those already educated. Additionally, this study highlighted that more male participants attended MOOCs than their female counterparts (Christensen et al., 2013). Despite it being a charge to provide low-cost, accessible high-quality education to those who need it most, major MOOC platforms have yet to successfully overcome hurdles to provide higher education to underprivileged sets of learners.

The American platform edX has recently partnered with Facebook, Nokia, and Internet service provider Airtel to develop a pilot program called SocialEDU for Rwandan students. Together, these groups will create a teaching app suitable for use at a low bandwidth on affordable smartphones. Students participating in the pilot program will receive free education data for 1 year (Biemiller, 2014). Additionally, the MOOC Research Initiative (https://openlearningandrecognition.wordpress.com/2013/06/14/the-gates-foundation-funds-mooc-research-initiative/), funded by the Bill and Melinda Gates Foundation, has invested funds and efforts to investigate whether MOOCs can successfully engage and prepare underprivileged learners (https://openlearningandrecognition.wordpress.com/2013/06/14/the-gates-foundation-funds-mooc-research-initiative/; Kolowich, 2014). Better access to technology and equitable access to basic education are pivotal in enlarging MOOC's embrace around the world, transcending racial, gender, and class barriers.

Nursing education programs have implemented aspects of online learning in their curricula, and such programs have been embraced as a flexible and cost-effective alternative while maintaining full-time employment (Smith, Passmore, & Faught, 2009). According to the American Association of Colleges of Nursing (AACN), 400 of the 646 RN-to-BSN programs were conducted partially or completely via an online interface (AACN, 2012). This set of nontraditional students is more likely to go to school part-time and less likely to attend face-to-face courses.

However, attrition rates in the online environment are higher than rates in the traditional, physical classroom environment (Cornelius & Glasgow, 2007; Patterson & McFadden, 2009). Suggestions for such high attrition rates may be due to lack of computer competency. A mini MOOC initiative and incentive program, Gateway to Online Learning, at Drexel's College of Nursing and Health Professions (CNHP) was created to curb technological burdens by providing a strong online foundation and encouraging RNs to go back to achieve their BSNs after the completion of the MOOC (Goldschmidt & Greene-Ryan, 2014). This free MOOC initiative proved to be successful in the increase of RN-to-BSN enrollment and online course competency in their initial cohort of 49 students for the 2012 to 2013 academic year. However, enrollment and payment for further classes decreased. This study begins to address how MOOCs can be better implemented at nursing schools to overcome financial and computer literacy burdens in order to encourage continuing education. Since nursing is a critical thinking as well as a hands-on practice, a recent paper highlights the technical utility of merging the MOOC platform OpenEdx and the virtual patient system Open Labyrinth for later use in researching the pedagogical benefits of virtual patients in the MOOC setting (Stathakarou, Zary, & Kononowicz, 2014).

A commentary by Skiba (2013) discussed how MOOCs may be used to achieve key goals outlined in 2011 by the Institute of Medicine (IOM), some of which were to increase the number of nurses with baccalaureate degrees to 80% by 2020, to diversify the nursing workforce to meet the demands of a diverse world, and to increase the use of technology in nursing instruction (IOM, 2011). Skiba suggested that MOOCs can be utilized for nursing prerequisites and introductory courses, to accelerate the completion of nursing baccalaureate programs by offering credit for MOOC courses taken, or be used toward graduate-level degrees in nursing. Skiba ends with suggesting a meeting of the minds in order to critically assess how MOOCs can be ingrained in the nursing education curriculum in order to achieve the IOM goals. The newness of MOOCs warrants much thoughtful discussion on how best to merge technology and pedagogy to ensure nursing student success (Caplan, Myrick, Smitten, & Kelly, 2014).

The overarching success and popularity of MOOCs indicates that the MOOC is the classroom of the present and the future. While careful and continued research is needed to fully understand how MOOCs contribute to higher education (Reich, 2015), the implications of MOOCs in the e-learning landscape as massive villages for which knowledge from the world's best is obtained openly and freely, lifelong learning is made amenable, and students and instructors can engage in virtual discussions is quite astounding. MOOCs have truly turned the axis of higher education.

OPEN SOURCE MATERIALS

Open and free source educational materials provide global access to learning and promote sharing of knowledge. Resting on the shoulders of the philosophy and framework of open source software, open education resources (OER) were originally defined in 2002 by UNESCO (United Nations Educational, Scientific, and Cultural Organization) as "the open provision of educational resources, enabled by information and communication technologies, for consultation, use and adaptation by a community of users for noncommercial purposes" (Parisky & Boulay, 2013).

A forerunner in OER and the original inspiration of UNESCO's definition is the Massachusetts Institute of Technology's (MIT's) OpenCourseWare (OCW) site (http://ocw.mit.edu/index.htm). Launched officially in 2002, MIT's OCW site now has over 2,000 open and free courses. Other universities have followed in MIT's footsteps and played critical parts in the OER revolution. The William and Flora Hewlett Foundation majorly funds this movement, which has been manifested as the Open Education Consortium (http://www.oeconsortium.org/). The William and Flora Hewlett Foundation defines OER as "teaching, learning, and research resources that reside in the public domain or have been released under an intellectual property license that permits their free use and re-purposing by others" (Parisky & Boulay, 2013). While the global access to education is immensely beneficial, there is an obvious concern about the verity of materials presented as it undergoes iterative changes and modifications (Ellaway & Martin, 2008).

As the OER movement progresses and develops, care to maintain valid, expert resources must be a priority. This is particularly important in the field of health care, where the use of electronic resources as a means of education provision has increased over the years.

There is much concern and conflicting data over the use of open source Web sites such as Wikipedia, the editable and collaborative online encyclopedia, in the field of nursing and medical education. A study by Carol A. Haigh involved sampling health-related Wikipedia entries to assess for the quality and reputation of sources cited. She suggested that Wikipedia was an appropriate medium to be used by nursing students (Haigh, 2011). However, a survey among surgical residents and medical students showed that commonly used electronic resources such as UpToDate, Google, Medscape, and Wikipedia had a high rate of answering clinical questions incorrectly and a high rate of misinformation (Egle, Smeenge, Kassem, & Mittal, 2014). In light of such shortcomings, scholars in the health care fields should be better trained in discerning the accuracy of information presented in electronic resources that are not peer reviewed.

While much deserved caution is garnered around open electronic resources being accessed by those in the health care profession, some scholars suggest that health care professionals need to become more active in maintaining the verity and accuracy of such sites as most patients and their relatives use the Internet to investigate health concerns (Heilman et al., 2011; Metcalfe & Powell, 2011). Not only does improving Wikipedia and other sites patients use provide the opportunity to globally educate, but some consider it a professional responsibility of those in health care (Callis et al., 2009). To wield the power of Web-based "collaborationware"—such as Wiki pages, blogs, and podcasts—that have expanded exponentially over the years, health professionals should carefully and accurately implement such tools to foster the dissemination and sharing of accurate knowledge for students and patients (Boulos, Maramba, & Wheeler, 2006).

Consider This Are there nursing courses or content that are consistently provided across nursing curricula that should be developed and used as open courseware for all students to take providing a standardization to these required courses?

VIRTUAL LEARNING SPACES

According to the landmark report *2013—Grade Change: Tracking Online Education in the United States*, 7.1 million higher education students were taking at least one online course in the United States (Allen & Seaman, 2014). The number of college students taking online courses has been on a steady increase for the past decade with 32% of higher education students taking at least one online course (Allen & Seaman, 2013). The majority of academic leaders are predicting that online courses will continue to impact an increasing number of students (Allen & Seaman, 2014). The Alliance for Nursing Accreditation Statement on Distance Education Policies (2007) forecast an increase in distance education courses and programs for delivery of education specific to nursing (AACN, 2015). This explosion of distance learning has forced a paradigm shift in nursing education regarding methods and evaluation of teaching and learning.

The interpretation of the terms *online*, *distance*, or *virtual* education varies depending on one's experience. Ironically, the true meaning of "virtual" is *pseudo* rather than *actual*, although the common connotation has morphed to mean "Internet-based" (Simonson, Smaldino, Albright, & Zvacek, 2012). The term "virtual" is often used when referring to distance education. *Virtual classrooms* have encompassed video-based distance education using satellites, telephones, videostreaming, MOOCs, asynchronous learning through learning management systems, videoconferencing, virtual simulation, and other modalities; thus, the term may be broadly or ambiguously understood.

Online Pedagogy

Online courses are considered as "those in which at least 80% of the course content is delivered online" (Allen & Seaman, 2013, p. 7). Many online courses were originally offered in an asynchronous format, consisting of organized modules, vast amounts of reading, and typed discussion boards, and they involved working independently at a time of one's convenience. However, the online classroom has evolved with advances in technology. Web-conferencing tools such as Adobe Connect, Blackboard's Collaborate, Cisco's Webex, and Citrix's GoToMeeting have enabled nurse faculty to push beyond the asynchronous world to foster synchronous communication in real time. It is now commonplace for online courses to include sophisticated videoconferencing platforms allowing for more traditional pedagogy including demonstration of presentations, case studies, debates, polling, storytelling and more (Foronda, 2014). In fact, Foronda and Lippincott (2014) found that the use of videoconferencing in nursing education resulted in comparable or better student learning outcomes than face-to-face methods. Similarly, Mee (2014) compared the effectiveness of distance education with campus-based learning among nursing students and found no significant differences in learning outcomes.

In addition to the use of refined learning management systems (such as Blackboard, Angel, Canvas, and Moodle) as well as Web-conferencing tools, the conventional ideas behind student learning activities and assessment have changed too. Nurse faculty members are embracing more creative ways of teaching and evaluating. Faculty members are encouraging students to use technology by assigning projects such as developing e-portfolios or Web pages, or guiding students to create online modules through free applications. Faculty members are attending to various learning styles and reaching the affective domain virtually by providing meaningful learning activities such as having students create video-clips, construct a mini-movie, give a virtual presentation, or build an infographic (Foronda, 2014).

When teaching online, critical means of fostering a successful course are to create a learning community and encourage frequent communication. Accessories such as VoiceThread allow faculty to record messages using video and audio for viewing and listening at a time of convenience.

Discussion Point

Through introductory discussion boards and by encouraging use of pictures, is it possible to network and foster a community of scholars comparable to in the classroom?

The importance of communication cannot be overemphasized. Communication is critical. A plethora of research has identified communication as a key factor in making or breaking online courses. The faculty member must provide frequent communication with students and encourage them to communicate as well. Faculty members must demonstrate presence and make it explicit to the student that he or she is available by email or phone call.

In this age of information, faculty members are shifting from teaching *what* to know to teaching one *how* to find out. Instead of having students memorize information, nurse faculty are leaning toward enabling students to use their resources, find information, differentiate reputable sources from poor sources, and apply evidence-based practice. Emphasis is shifting from teaching students specific information to improving one's critical thinking and ability to make connections as well as develop proficiency with technology. Teaching students with technology through online means is especially congruent with these student learning objectives as students become more comfortable using the Internet with exposure and practice in their online courses.

Many faculty members who teach online choose to use a variety of assessment measures such as discussion boards, papers, and projects. Debate continues about the security of objective online testing and whether or not this is an appropriate form of assessment given the possibilities for cheating. To avoid concerns about security, some faculty have decided to offer timed, open-book exams. Meeting the needs of faculty members who prefer to offer formal online proctoring for objective testing in the convenience of the student's home, several products have emerged from the market including ProctorU and Respondus Monitor. With some of these virtual proctoring solutions, students are monitored via Web-camera with browsers locked down to prevent searching for answers. Further, certain products will monitor and report Internet protocol addresses to ensure that students are taking the tests independently rather than with each other in the same location. While a fail-proof method has not clearly emerged—outside of paying for and attending formal proctoring at an official testing center—administrators are receiving direction from federal regulation bodies and accreditation organizations to ensure that the students who register and participate in the online courses are the ones who receive the credit. This security and compliance issue will likely receive more scrutiny in days to come.

Standards for Distance Education

A number of regulatory issues arose when the landscape of nursing education shifted to include more distance delivery. There was a need to ensure quality and that online standards were comparable to face-to-face methods. Quality Matters was an agency that set a national benchmark for online course design and standards from primary education to postsecondary education (Quality Matters, 2014). Many schools of nursing continue to follow the guidance of Quality Matters' standards for developing and administering online courses.

The Alliance for Nursing Accreditation Statement on Distance Education Policies (2007) emphasized nursing education programs must meet the same academic program and learning support standards and accreditation criteria as programs provided in face-to-face formats (AACN, 2015). Faculty members were directed to use accreditation criteria to guide online course development and evaluate student learning outcomes. The Online Learning Consortium (2015), formerly the Sloan Consortium, developed five pillars to measure quality in online courses: Learning Effectiveness, Scale, Access, Faculty Satisfaction, and Student Satisfaction. More recently, the National Council of State Boards of Nursing's Board of Directors convened to develop a white paper regarding nursing regulation recommendations for distance education in prelicensure nursing programs (National Council of State Boards of Nursing, 2014). This white paper synthesizes the hallmarks for quality distance education in nursing and serves as a valuable reference for faculty and administrators in nursing education.

Since Boards of Nursing vary by state and have different regulations, a number of challenges have arisen for educational institutions offering programs in nursing as well as students who would like to study nursing from a distance. One major challenge relates to state authorization for students from an outside state who would like to attend an online program. Each state has different requirements and restrictions. Educational institutions must individually apply and pay a fee to obtain authorization to offer distance education. Additionally, Boards of Nursing have different requirements for clinical practicum as well as licensure of faculty who are qualified to teach within each state. Hence, the faculty member who supervises a clinical practicum should be knowledgeable about the Nurse Practice Act in the state where the education is occurring; however, this legislative requirement has led to difficulties in obtaining clinical learning experiences for distance students. While there still remains room for improvement, quality in online courses has improved greatly because of these leading organizations and high standards.

Virtual Simulation

A highly promising breakthrough in online education in nursing, the emergence of virtual simulation has received much attention. Virtual simulation has been used in multiple contexts. Interpretations of the term *virtual simulation* have included simply being offered on a computer, Web-based, two-dimensional (2D) computerized case studies, CD-ROMs, videos, games, or study programs (Foronda, Godsall, & Trybulski, 2012). Linden Lab was a pioneer in simulation offering Second Life, a Web-based platform, where students could create avatars and interact virtually like never before. Since then, vendors including Elsevier (creators of Virtual Clinical Excursions), Shadow Health (creators of TINA), and Wolters Kluwer (creators of vSim) have developed interactive virtual simulations that place students in an active role in a virtual clinical environment. Innovation in Learning, Inc., developed CliniSpace, a high-fidelity, multiplayer, Web-based gaming software that allows real-time voice-over-Internet communication through headsets and enables faculty members to manipulate the patient's hemodynamics and responses, depending on the students' interventions. This sophisticated software has been used with students internationally, and research has suggested it is effective to teach various skills in nursing education including leadership, communication, and education (Foronda, Budhathoki, & Salani, 2014; Foronda, Gattamorta, Snowden, & Bauman, 2014; Foronda, Lippincott, & Gattamorta, 2014).

As virtual simulation is based on tenets of social and experiential learning theory, it is a promising pedagogy of the future (Foronda, Gattamorta, et al., 2014). The high-level thinking that occurs in virtual simulation, such as considering pathophysiology, pharmacology, and prioritization, is comparable to the thinking that takes place in the clinical setting. Virtual simulation has a place in nursing education, not only to complement theory, but also to provide opportunities for students that are not practically completed in the clinical setting such as high-risk, low-occurring events. For example, virtual simulation may be used to teach disaster management or how to manage a cardiac arrest. Further, virtual simulation may be used to enhance lectures or as a clinical makeup opportunity. The opportunities for uses of virtual simulation are limitless.

Consider This Some predict that virtual simulations will transform the future of online education in nursing. Do you agree or disagree?

CHALLENGES AND BARRIERS TO TRADITIONAL LEARNING ENVIRONMENTS

Faculty and Learner Expectations: Challenges and Impact

Colleges and universities are faced with new challenges such as decreased financial resources, increased accountability to stakeholders, demands for curriculum reform that meets the changing needs of the nursing workforce, and a growing faculty shortage. Additionally, faculty must accommodate Millennial student (1982 to present) learning expectations, which may vary greatly between generations. Millennial learners have unique characteristics that challenge traditional learning environments. This population is assertive, self-reliant, curious, fascinated with new technology, has a need for group activities, and is focused on grades (Skiba & Barton, 2006). Most faculty are from previous generations that focused on text, emphasized rote memorization based on repetition, lacked personalized instruction, and saw the instructor as the authority.

Millennial learners require a student-centered model of instruction with digital literacy, interactivity and collaboration, immediacy and connectivity, and experiential and engaging learning (Skiba & Barton, 2006). In nursing education, inaccessibility to a wireless network in the traditional learning environment poses challenges to learner expectations. As a demographic that frequently uses the Internet, it is important for students to access the appropriate discipline-specific databases such as CINAHL and Medline instead of using Internet search engines. The design of a course Web page that contains class materials, multimedia, and additional links for independent learning or podcasting lectures would help meet student digital literacy needs (Skiba & Barton, 2006). Interaction can be fostered by the use of an interactive response system in a traditional lecture hall environment as well as provide formative assessment information (Skiba & Barton, 2006). To meet the immediacy and connectivity needs of Millennial learners, nursing faculty can utilize different forms of communication during traditional office hours, such as instant messaging (one-on-one) or a group chat room (one-to-many) (Skiba & Barton, 2006). Experiential and engaging learning expectations are satisfied through active learning activities. Blogging is one way for nursing students to reflect on course learning or through the use of the National League of Nursing Chapters interactive book chapters (Skiba & Barton, 2006). Active learning is arguably one of the most impactful models of instruction in nursing education today, but has many barriers to its implementation.

Models of Instruction: Barriers to Passive and Active Learning

The primary model of instruction in higher education is the traditional lecture (Lujan & DiCarlo, 2006). This educational approach features instructor-centered didactic lectures and fosters passive learning of information (Sinclair & Ferguson, 2009). There are several advantages to passive learning. In a traditional learning environment, a large amount of course material can be presented over a short duration of time, lecture content and concepts can be organized in a cohesive manner, and primary and supplementary lecture materials can be prepared in advance. Some students prefer, and may benefit from, the well-structured, instructor-centered approaches. Although it can be beneficial, passive learning also has numerous disadvantages that can greatly hinder learning, such as limited student interactions and a focus on predetermined curricula (Miller & Metz, 2014). This can result in few opportunities for formal assessment to check student comprehension and nominal time to clarify student questions or facilitate class discussions that lead to deeper learning. In nursing education, the passive learning of clinical skills can result in professional barriers such as the inability to translate important clinical information and critical reasoning skills to patient care (Sinclair & Ferguson, 2009).

Although many agree professional students are adept at being successful upon receiving traditional lectures, evidence suggests active learning can increase critical thinking skills, enhance performance, and improve student experiences (Lujan & DiCarlo, 2006). By definition, active learning is any model of instruction that engages students in the learning process. This model of instruction enables students to be responsible for their own learning through various exercises, activities, and discussion. Active learning also encourages higher cognitive thinking on Bloom's taxonomy, such as analysis, synthesis, and evaluation. Student-centered instruction builds upon their knowledge base, skill set, and preferences (Lujan & DiCarlo, 2006). A recent study suggested that the use of simulation, an active learning tool gaining traction in nursing education, increased student self-confidence for nursing practice, course satisfaction, and consistency with their learning style (Ferguson & Day, 2004; Sinclair & Ferguson, 2009). Despite evidence of efficacy, traditional learning environments are slow to adopt active learning models of instruction in higher education. Major barriers reported by instructors are a lack of required class time to deliver active learning lessons, more comfort with traditional lectures, and insufficient time to develop appropriate materials (Miller & Metz, 2014).

Consider This Some believe interactive lectures with elements of both passive and active learning are the best of both worlds. Do you agree or disagree?

Environmental Barriers: Time, Setting, and Physical Space

Many environmental barriers can be impediments to teaching and learning in a traditional environment. Traditional nursing education requires a considerable time commitment from both the instructor and the student. Clinical and research faculty must balance primary responsibilities with teaching commitments and faculty development, which may or may not provide adequate institutional support (DaRosa et al., 2011). Consequently, increasing clinical demands can be challenges to effective teaching. Students that attend a traditional classroom have to balance their own competing employment, familial, and financial priorities. Traditional teaching hospitals are bustling, complex environments and are not ideal to teach every competency a nursing student needs to master. Curriculum in traditional settings may not take into account practice in other health care settings, changing demographics, or future delivery systems (DaRosa et al., 2011). Nursing faculty must take the initiative to bring about the process of curriculum reform, which can be both labor- and time-intensive. Often overlooked, but an insufficient or inappropriately designed physical space can disrupt education delivery by a lack of integration in the facilities planning process (DaRosa et al., 2011). Technology tools and simulation models do not generate revenue, and can sometimes become a lower-priority purchase in the midst of competing priorities.

Lack of Flexibility

Colleges and universities provide various learning environments to accommodate student needs. In traditional learning environments, both faculty and students lack flexibility. Faculty members in traditional settings have geographic restrictions, must teach at appointed times, and to a limited number of students. Students lack control over content and depth, information sequence, pace of learning, and supplementary materials that may include multimedia platforms. Online learning provides more flexibility than traditional learning environments (Ruiz, Mintzer, & Leipzig, 2006). In diverse education settings, blended-learning strategies may be the key for increasing flexibility in traditional learning spaces through instructor-led training along with complementary adaptive, collaborative, and self-directed student learning online.

FACULTY DEVELOPMENT NEEDED FOR DIGITAL EDUCATION AND MOOC TEACHING

Faculty Expectations

Faculty who have had the opportunity to teach MOOCs are surprisingly finding they are paying more attention to their teaching styles and pedagogy when thousands of participants/learners are embarking on their open digital platform in their MOOC courses. It appears teaching in MOOCs may be prompting some faculty to be more vigilant about their teaching styles and communication strategies than ever before. The new focus on teaching methods is coming from potentially two driving forces: (1) faculty wanting to ensure their teaching is high quality for the broad audience they are reaching in the MOOCs and (2) the technologies available in the MOOC platforms that allow different levels of interaction with students worldwide. Faculty members have more of an opportunity to actually understand the students' strengths, weaknesses, and collaborative spirit when teaching in these MOOCS. When teaching in a MOOC, the work, effort, and instruction move to an entirely new level than in the traditional classroom setting or a small online course within a specific university program (Rivard, 2015).

According to Hollands and Tirthali (2014), as shown in Table 17.2, 38% of the institutions participating in their study that were offering or teaching MOOCs and 20% of their interviewees, overall, expected MOOCs to improve overall learning outcomes, some directly within the MOOC format and others indirectly transferring new pedagogical strategies and tactics to traditional-type teaching. A few strategies highlighted in their study include (1) faculty rethinking pedagogy; (2) redesigning courses; (3) creating chunked or small modules of materials with integration of interactive-type questions and assessment points for the learner; (4) ensuring there is prompt feedback from the instructor to the learners; and (5) outreach to various participants to encourage persistence and engagement, to name a few. Overall, however, the researchers declare, for the most part, that the actual impact on learning outcomes in the MOOCs still need to be explored and documented in a rigorous fashion.

Benefits to Faculty

When faculty embark on teaching a MOOC or decide to develop an online course or module within their program, there are challenges and benefits to using this new type of pedagogy, as shown in Table 17.3. When faculty pursue this type of new pedagogy, typically, new knowledge and skills abound regarding the new tools for creating online content. Typically, faculty may work with an instructional designer or other type of technologist to learn the tools and application of using them in their online course development, or at times, faculty may be self-taught.

Teaching in a MOOC where thousands of students participate in the open-enrollment massive open course, faculty need to develop their distinct online voice and presence. No longer is the presence of the faculty member only within the university or within a certain division, but after teaching in a MOOC, the presence becomes global due to the exposure to thousands of students worldwide.

TABLE 17.2 Reasons MOOCS May Be Improving Learning Outcomes (Hollands & Tirthali, 2014)

Faculty rethinking pedagogy, trying new, innovative methods
Faculty redesigning courses to engage students
Opportunity to create small learning "chunks" or small modules with integration questions and comments
Opportunities for prompt feedback, promoting student–faculty interactions
Increased outreach to learners to facilitate engagement and persistence in meeting learning outcomes

TABLE 17.3 Benefits and Challenges to Educators When Teaching MOOCs and Online Courses

Benefits	Challenges
• New knowledge and skills develop • Faculty can develop their own "voice and presence" online • Global presence when teaching a MOOC	• New model of pedagogy to be learned and experienced • Shift from teacher-centered to a student-centered approach • With an MOOC, teachers have the challenges of teaching to thousands of learners—adding a layer of complexity to teacher–student relationships
• Online teaching is also providing methods to improve overall teaching, including face-to-face courses • Potential for using different teaching strategies, for example, "flipping the classroom" if a MOOC or online modules have been created	• Faculty lack knowledge and skills to teach in the online environment when using this type of platform • Teaching in MOOCs and/or providing open course materials, faculty are concerned about "giving content free"
• MOOCs and online teaching provide a greater platform and visibility to speak about their passion, work, and content across the globe	• Faculty sometimes miss the face-to-face interaction with students in an online format
• Teaming opportunities with instructional designers, Web programmers, and others when developing course content	• Preparation ahead of time before the online course or MOOC opens—courses need to be ready for learners to embrace at different times—learning for many occurs at different paces

When teaching a MOOC, the faculty members find ways to improve quality of online presentations and communication to thousands of participants to provide clarity and articulation of specific messages, directions, and overall summaries. When teaching a MOOC and the directions are not clear, confusion reigns, causing many participants to blog, post in the discussion forums, and emotions can erupt. Therefore, when teaching in a massive online course, faculty quickly learn how to improve presentations and their presence within the course. As an example, Dr. Peter Norvig, a Stanford instructor and author of one of the first MOOCs, was inspired to develop short videos by the success of Khan Academy. Norvig challenged himself and his teaching partner to produce videos ranging from 2 to 6 minutes in length, often incorporating a review question at the end to mimic one-on-one tutoring delivered to a course with over 160,000 students (Norvig, 2012).

Another benefit to faculty who teach MOOCs may be the opportunity for the educator to consider flipping their traditional courses if they find the format to be effective by using the MOOC for students to preview content prior to class then using class time more effectively to apply and synthesize the material provided in the MOOC. Once the MOOC has been created and is available, the content and format can be used in many ways, whether it be assigned as part of a "flipped classroom" or the MOOC content integrated into a course as a hybrid and/or as supplementary material for learners needing perhaps more material and review of specific content.

Faculty teaching MOOCs also have greater visibility and a platform to speak about their passion, their work, and content needed across the globe. Teaching a MOOC provides the opportunity to inform large numbers of students and potential students about research or passion. Traditionally, faculty members have been challenged to engage students who may be enrolled in a class simply to check it off as a requirement to graduate. MOOC students represent a different model, however, with many seeking professional growth and development for work or career. Without the traditional forcing function of higher education degrees, every student enrolled in a MOOC is choosing to be there. In most cases, MOOC participants are choosing to engage in a learning opportunity where the potential for reward, course credit, or acknowledgement of their accomplishments in the course is very limited or nonexistent. This lifelong learning model may seem strange to traditional university-based faculty, but it is the long sought-after ideal of higher education.

Faculty's benefits in teaching MOOCs also includes experience teaming with course developers to repurpose or reuse course content as MOOC licensing allows (Brandenburger, 2015). According to Brandenburger

(2015), MOOCs can help to reframe or reorganize curriculum development at home universities. Faculty have the opportunity to gain an appreciation for the project management role of IT and instructional design staff if these professional staff are hired within the institution. For faculty who have never worked with a creative instructional design team, using this resource in the MOOC development phase may be reason for faculty to want to integrate these roles and positions within the university ecosystem.

Challenges and Barriers

Developing and teaching a MOOC provides an opportunity for faculty to reframe their model of teaching. For several hundred years, teaching has been a hands-on, experiential activity. In traditional education, one believes the teacher must be in the same room as the student to make the direct transfer of knowledge. Teaching in an online environment can be challenging to faculty who have not done so before since the model of teaching shifts from a teacher-centered one to a student-centered model, where students are accountable for their own learning. Teaching an online MOOC with thousands of students adds an additional layer of complexity and distance to the teacher–student relationship.

Another challenge in the MOOC online environment is that faculty may lack knowledge and skills in using technologies. Faculty can become overwhelmed with technology and new pedagogies, and course redesign using technology. In addition, there is the challenge and fear of "giving away content for free."

CLASSROOM LEARNING ENVIRONMENTS OF THE FUTURE

What will nursing education look like in the future? This question is somewhat elusive, but some recent innovations and trends may shed some light. There is movement toward interprofessional education to better simulate reality as opposed to educating students in silos. For this reason, schools in health sciences are developing simulation hospitals. One may anticipate that nurses, physicians, pharmacists, and other providers will be educated in a collective, collaborative manner through simulation centers.

As technology advances, some prognosticate expansion of virtual reality for purposes of health education. For example, Microsoft has engineered the HoloLens, a 3D headset that allows users to interact in a virtual environment (Kedmey, 2015). The current sophistication of

Research Study Fuels the Controversy 17.1

Effect of Telemedicine on Patient Outcomes

This quasi-experimental study examined the differences in cost, caring, and family-centered care in relation to pediatric specialty services utilizing telemedicine technology ($n = 112$) compared with traditional face-to-face care ($n = 110$).

Source: Hooshmand, M. A. (2010). *Comparison of telemedicine to traditional face-to-face care for children with special health care needs: analysis of cost, caring, and family-centered care, family cost survey, caring professional scale, measure of processes of care 20-item scale.* Open Access Dissertations. Paper 408. http://scholarlyrepository.miami.edu/oa_dissertations/408

Study Findings

Results indicated that there were no significant differences in family costs when telemedicine was available locally compared with traditional face-to-face care in the local community. Family costs were anticipated to be significantly higher if telemedicine was not available in their communities. There were no differences in the families' perceptions of care as caring for the telemedicine and traditional groups. Results indicated significant differences between the groups in regard to family-centered care, with telemedicine group parents/guardians reporting more positive perceptions of the system of care as family-centered compared with families receiving traditional face-to-face pediatric specialty care.

This well-executed study supported the use of telemedicine. The results underscore the importance of assuring and facilitating access to pediatric specialty care for children with special healthcare needs (CSHCN) and their families by further reducing their burdens and costs (Hooshmand, 2010). The use of innovative systems of care such as telemedicine has promise to promote caring, family-centered systems of care in their home communities (Hooshmand, 2010). Of note, as health care technology has advanced, legislative policy has not always been able to keep up. The complexities of technology, resources, privacy, litigation, and legislation will likely combine for a challenging yet exciting future in nursing education.

children's video games provides hope that similar high-tech opportunities lie ahead for serious gaming in health education. As the use of tablets and applications proliferate, increased opportunities for individualized, interactive learning are expected. Thus, immersive, clinical experiences through simulation appear to be central in the future of nursing education.

To anticipate the future of nurse education, one must envision what health care delivery will look like in years to come. With the growth of personalized electronic health records, tracking applications, and personalized medicine, nursing education will have to adapt and prepare nurses appropriately. Therefore, the need to educate nurses to be technologically savvy appears critical. It is plausible to foresee an increased role in nursing related to telehealth. Telehealth has been expanding, and research has suggested that its use improves access to health care. Telehealth has proven useful for those in rural or urban areas and has allowed an international outreach. From providing mental health counseling virtually to diagnosing skin cancer of individuals at sea, there lies a high potential for growth of telehealth in nursing.

Hooshmand (2010), a nurse executive, educator, and researcher, found that telemedicine resulted in better outcomes than traditional face-to-face care (Research Study Fuels the Controversy 17.1).

Conclusions

The deployment and integration of digital technologies and changes in pedagogy provide unparalleled opportunities for educators to spread knowledge and ideas to students around the world through different avenues including online courses for credit, MOOCS, open course ware, virtual learning environments, and the traditional face-to-face classrooms. To shift the paradigm from traditional lectures and classroom engagement, faculty members need to develop and have access to the technological tools and ways to use them. Promoting faculty development in the area of digital education and initiatives must include facilitating and rewarding of quality education in both digital and traditional educational formats. A coordinated effort in academic institutions and other organizations can focus on elevating the importance of quality education and innovative teaching/learning environments, showcasing the faculty who are innovators and experimenters in and out of the classrooms, and promoting the scholarship of new, educational innovations that are changing the landscape of higher and nursing education. Although higher education is in a disruptive state, it provides many opportunities and possibilities to better educate our health care professionals and other learners today. Rigorous, robust research is needed in these new areas of pedagogy along with identification and evidence of best practices so quality and excellence of these educational changes can be promoted. Nursing education is changing and will continue to evolve as new technologies, learning environments, and innovative faculty pursue new strategies to "connect" with the learners to ultimately promote high-quality education and practice.

For Additional Discussion

1. How will the forecasted trends in higher education impact nursing education as we know it today?
2. Do technological advances always help to facilitate teaching and learning in traditional environments? Can they ever hinder the learning process in this setting?
3. In what nursing education environments is passive learning better than active learning?
4. Is online education in nursing education counterproductive for a hands-on profession?
5. In what context is online education most suitable and least suitable for nursing education?
6. What are the biggest challenges to prepare faculty for changes in nursing and higher education?
7. Will online education continue to expand in nursing education?
8. What are the advantages and disadvantages of an online course?

(continued)

9. Will MOOCs and open courseware become a standard type of pedagogy for required nursing courses?
10. Is virtual simulation an effective way of teaching select skills in nursing? What are the advantages and disadvantages of this pedagogy?
11. In the new world of using and integrating technologies into the teaching–learning environment, what are nurse educators' new challenges and reward systems?

References

Allen, I. E., & Seaman, J. (2013). *Changing course: Ten years of tracking online education in the United States.* Oakland, CA: Babson Survey Research Group. Retrieved from http://www.onlinelearningsurvey.com/reports/changingcourse.pdf

Allen, I. E., & Seaman, J. (2014). *Grade change: Tracking online education in the United States.* Oakland, CA: Babson Survey Research Group. Retrieved from http://onlinelearningconsortium.org/survey_report/2013-survey-online-learning-report/

American Association of Colleges of Nursing. (2012). *White paper: Expectations for practice experiences in the RN to baccalaureate curriculum* (pp. 1–9). Retrieved from http://www.aacn.nche.edu/aacn-publications/white-papers/RN-BSN-White-Paper.pdf

American Association of Colleges of Nursing. (2015). *Alliance for nursing accreditation statement on distance education policies.* Retrieved from http://www.aacn.nche.edu/education-resources/distance-education-policies

Biemiller, L. (2014, February 24). Quickwire: edX and Facebook team up to offer free education in Rwanda. *The Chronicle of Higher Education.* Retrieved from http://chronicle.com/blogs/wiredcampus/quickwire-edx-partners-with-facebook-to-offer-courses-in-rwanda/50693

Boulos, M. N., Maramba, I., & Wheeler, S. (2006). Wikis, blogs and podcasts: A new generation of Web-based tools for virtual collaborative clinical practice and education. *BMC Medical Education, 6*, 41. doi:10.1186/1472-6920-6-41

Brandenburger, E. (2015). Course development and MOOCs—II. *Inside Higher Ed.* Retrieved from https://www.insidehighered.com/blogs/higher-ed-beta/course-development-and-moocs-ii

Callis, K. L., Christ, L. R., Resasco, J., Armitage, D. W., Ash, J. D., Caughlin, T. T., . . . Bruna, E. M. (2009). Improving Wikipedia: educational opportunity and professional responsibility. *Trends in Ecology & Evolution, 24*(4), 177–179. doi:10.1016/j.tree.2009.01.003

Caplan, W., Myrick, F., Smitten, J., & Kelly, W. (2014). What a tangled web we weave: How technology is reshaping pedagogy. *Nurse Education Today, 34*(8), 1172–1174. doi:10.1016/j.nedt.2014.04.005

Christensen, G., Steinmetz, A., Alcorn, B., Bennett, A., Woods, D., & Ezekiel, E. J. (2013). The MOOC phenomenon who takes massive open online courses and why? [Abstract]. *Social Science Research Network.* Retreived from http://ssrn.com/abstract=2350964

Cornelius, F., & Glasgow, M. E. S. (2007). The development and infrastructure needs required for success—One college's model: Online nursing education at Drexel University. *TechTrends, 51*(6), 32–35.

DaRosa, D. A., Skeff, K., Friedland, J. A., Coburn, M., Cox, S., Pollart, S., . . . Smith, S. (2011). Barriers to effective teaching [Research support, non-U.S. gov't]. *Academic Medicine, 86*(4), 453–459. doi:10.1097/ACM.0b013e31820defbe

Downes, S. (2008). Places to go: Connectivism & connective knowledge. *Innovate: Journal of Online Education, 5*(1), 6. Retrieved from http://bsili.3csn.org/files/2010/06/Places_to_Go-__Connectivism__Connective_Knowledge.pdf

Downes, S. (2013). *What the 'x' in 'xMOOC' stands for* [Web log post]. Retrieved from https://plus.google.com/109526159908242471749/posts/LEwaKxL2MaM

Egle, J. P., Smeenge, D. M., Kassem, K. M., & Mittal, V. K. (2014). The Internet School of Medicine: Use of electronic resources by medical trainees and the reliability of those resources. *Journal of Surgical Education, 72*(2), 316–320. doi:10.1016/j.jsurg.2014.08.005

Ellaway, R., & Martin, R. D. (2008). What's mine is yours—Open source as a new paradigm for sustainable healthcare education. *Medical Teacher, 30*(2), 175–179. doi:10.1080/01421590701874058

Ferguson, L. M., & Day, R. A. (2004). Supporting new nurses in evidence-based practice. *The Journal of Nursing Administration, 34*(11), 490–492.

Foronda, C. (2014). Spice up teaching online! *Nurse Educator, 39*(6), 265–266. doi:10.1097/NNE.0000000000000081

Foronda, C., Budhathoki, C., & Salani, D. (2014). Use of multiuser, high-fidelity virtual simulation to teach leadership styles to nursing students. *Nurse Educator, 39*(5), 209–211. doi:10.1097/NNE.0000000000000073.

Foronda, C., Gattamorta, K., Snowden, K., & Bauman, E. (2014). Use of virtual clinical simulation to improve communication skills of baccalaureate nursing students: A pilot study. *Nurse Education Today, 34*(6), e53–e57. doi:10.1016/j.nedt.2013.10.007

Foronda, C., Godsall, L., & Trybulski, J. (2012). Virtual clinical simulation in nursing: A state of the science. *Clinical Simulation in Nursing, 9*(8), e279–e286. doi.org/10.1016/j.ecns.2012.05.005

Foronda, C., & Lippincott, C. (2014). Graduate nursing students' experience with synchronous, interactive videoconferencing within online courses. *Quarterly Review of Distance Education, 15*(2), 1–8.

Foronda, C., Lippincott, C., & Gattamorta, K. (2014). Evaluation of virtual simulation in a master's level nurse education certificate program. *Computers, Informatics, Nursing: CIN, 32*(11), 516–522. doi:10.1097/CIN.0000000000000102

Gillani, N., Yasseri, T., Eynon, R., & Hjorth, I. (2014). Structural limitations of learning in a crowd: Communication vulnerability and information diffusion in MOOCs. *Scientific Reports, 4*, 6447. doi:10.1038/srep06447

Goldschmidt, K., & Greene-Ryan, J. (2014). Massive open online courses in nursing education. *Journal of Pediatric Nursing, 29*(2), 184–186. doi:10.1016/j.pedn.2013.12.001

Grossman, S. (2013, July 5). American MOOC providers face international competition. *The Chronicle of Higher Education.* Retrieved from http://chronicle.com/blogs/wiredcampus/american-mooc-providers-face-international-competition/44637

Haigh, C. A. (2011). Wikipedia as an evidence source for nursing and healthcare students. *Nurse Education Today, 31*(2), 135–139. doi:10.1016/j.nedt.2010.05.004

Heilman, J. M., Kemmann, E., Bonert, M., Chatterjee, A., Ragar, B., Beards, G. M., . . . Laurent, M. R. (2011). Wikipedia: A key tool for global public health promotion. *Journal of Medical Internet Research, 13*(1), e14. doi:10.2196/jmir.1589

Hollands, F. M., & Tirthali, D. (2014). *MOOCs: Expectations and reality: Full report.* New York, USA: Center for Benefit-Cost Studies of Education, Teachers College, Columbia University.

Hooshmand, M. A. (2010). *Comparison of telemedicine to traditional face-to-face care for children with special health care needs: Analysis of cost, caring, and family-centered care, family cost survey, caring professional scale, measure of processes of care 20-item scale.* Open Access Dissertations. Paper 408. Retrieved from http://scholarlyrepository.miami.edu/oa_dissertations/408

Institute of Medicine. (2011). *The future of nursing: Leading change, advancing health.* Washington, DC: The National Academies Press.

Johnson, L., Becker, A. S., Cummins, M., Estrada, V., Freeman, A., & Ludgate, H. (2013). *NMC horizon report: 2013 higher education edition.* Retrieved from http://www.nmc.org/pdf/2013-horizon-report-HE.pdf

Kedmey, D. (2015, February 9). Virtually real Microsoft joins the crowd betting on 3-D headsets. *Time, 185*(4), 12.

Koller, D., Ng, A., Do, C., & Chen, Z. (2013, June 3). Retention and intention in massive open online courses: In depth. *EDUCAUSE Review.* Retrieved from http://www.educause.edu/ero/article/retention-and-intention-massive-open-online-courses-depth-0

Kolowich, S. (2013, December 16). edX drops plans to connect MOOC students with employers. *The Chronicle of Higher Education.* Retrieved from http://chronicle.com/blogs/wiredcampus/edx-drops-plans-to-connect-mooc-students-with-employers/48987

Kolowich, S. (2014, June 27). 5 things researchers have discovered about MOOCs. *The Chronicle of Higher Education.* Retrieved from http://chronicle.com/blogs/wiredcampus/5-things-researchers-have-discovered-about-moocs/53585

Liyanagunawardena, T. R., Adams, A. A., & Williams, S. A. (2013). MOOCs: A systematic study of the published literature 2008–2012. *The International Review of Research in Open and Distributed Learning, 14*(3).

Liyanagunawardena, T. R., & Williams, S. A. (2014). Massive open online courses on health and medicine: Review. *Journal of Medical Internet Research, 16*(8), e191. doi:10.2196/jmir.3439

Lujan, H. L., & DiCarlo, S. E. (2006). Too much teaching, not enough learning: What is the solution? *Advances in Physiology Education, 30*(1), 17–22. doi:10.1152/advan.00061.2005

Mackness, J. (2013, October 22). *cMOOCs and xMOOCs—Key differences* [Web log post]. Retrieved from http://jennymackness.wordpress.com/2013/10/22/cmoocs-and-xmoocs-key-differences/

McAuley, A., Stewart, B., Siemens, G., & Cormier, D. (2010). *The MOOC model for digital practice.* Retrieved form http://www.elearnspace.org/Articles/MOOC_Final.pdf

Mee, S. (2014). Is distance education the answer to the nursing shortage? *Open Journal of Nursing, 4*, 158–162.

Metcalfe, D., & Powell, J. (2011). Should doctors spurn Wikipedia? *Journal of the Royal Society of Medicine, 104*(12), 488–489. doi:10.1258/jrsm.2011.110227

Miller, C. J., & Metz, M. J. (2014). A comparison of professional-level faculty and student perceptions of active learning: Its current use, effectiveness, and barriers. *Advances in Physiology Education, 38*(3), 246–252. doi:10.1152/advan.00014.2014

Miller, T. (2012, December 12). MOOCs break down barriers to knowledge. *The Australian.* Retrieved from http://www.theaustralian.com.au/higher-education/opinion/moocs-break-down-barriers-to-knowledge/story-e6frgcko-1226534770043

National Council of State Boards of Nursing. (2014). *White paper: Nursing regulation recommendations.* Retrieved from https://www.ncsbn.org/6662.htm

Norvig, P. (2012). *"Peter Norvig: The 100,000-student classroom."* Retrieved February 34, 2015, from http://www.ted.com/talks/peter_norvig_the_100_000_student_classroom.html

Online Learning Consortium. (2015). *The 5 pillars.* Retrieved from http://olc.onlinelearningconsortium.org/5-pillars

Parisky, A., & Boulay, R. (2013). Designing and developing open education resources in higher education: A molecular biology project. *International Journal of Technology, Knowledge and Society, 9*(2), 145–155.

Patterson, B., & McFadden, C. (2009). Attrition in online and campus degree programs. *Online Journal of Distance Learning Administration, 12*(2).

Quality Matters. (2014). *A national benchmark for online course design.* Retrieved from https://www.qualitymatters.org/

Reich, J. (2014, December 8). MOOC completion and retention in the context of student intent. EDUCASE Review. Retrieved from http://www.educause.edu/ero/article/mooc-completion-and-retention-context-student-intent

Reich, J. (2015). Rebooting MOOC research. *Science, 347*(6217), 34–35. doi:10.1126/science.1261627

Rivard, Ry (2015). Learning how to teach. *Inside Higher Ed.* Retrieved from https://www.insidehighered.com/news/2013/03/05/moocs-prompt-some-faculty-members-refresh-teaching-styles

Rodriguez, C. O. (2012). MOOCs and the AI-Stanford like courses: Two successful and distinct course formats for massive open online courses. *European Journal of Open, Distance and E-Learning.* Retrieved from http://www.eurodl.org/?p=current&article&article=516

Ruiz, J. G., Mintzer, M. J., & Leipzig, R. M. (2006). The impact of E-learning in medical education [Research support, non-U.S. gov't review]. *Academic Medicine, 81*(3), 207–212.

Siemens, G. (2005). Connectivism—A learning theory for the digital age. *International Journal of Instructional Technology and Distance Learning, 2*(1), 3–10.

Simonson, M., Smaldino, S., Albright, M., & Zvacek, S. (2012). *Teaching and learning at a distance: Foundations of distance education* (5th ed.). Boston, MA: Allyn & Bacon.

Sinclair, B., & Ferguson, K. (2009). Integrating simulated teaching/learning strategies in undergraduate nursing education [Controlled clinical trial multicenter study]. *International Journal of Nursing Education Scholarship, 6*(7). doi:10.2202/1548-923X.1676

Skiba, D. J. (2013). MOOCs and the future of nursing. *Nursing Education Perspectives, 34*(3), 202–204. doi:10.5480/1536-5026-34.3.202

Skiba, D. J., & Barton, A. J. (2006). Adapting your teaching to accommodate the net generation of learners. *Online Journal of Issues in Nursing, 11*(2), 5.

Smith, G. G., Passmore, D., & Faught, T. (2009). The challenges of online nursing education. *The Internet and Higher Education, 12*(2), 98–103.

Stathakarou, N., Zary, N., & Kononowicz, A. A. (2014). Beyond xMOOCs in healthcare education: Study of the feasibility in integrating virtual patient systems and MOOC platforms. *PeerJ, 2*, e672. doi:10.7717/peerj.672

Times, T. N. Y. (2012, November 2). The big three, at a glance. *The New York Times.* Retrieved from http://www.nytimes.com/2012/11/04/education/edlife/the-big-three-mooc-providers.html?_r=0

What's hot; What's not for 2014. (2013, December). *The JOURNAL: Transforming Education through Technology, 40*(12). Retrieved from http://online.qmags.com/TJL1213/default.aspx?fs=2&pg=1&mode=1#pg1&mode1

18

Academic Integrity in Nursing Education

Is It Declining?

George C. Pittman

ADDITIONAL RESOURCES

Visit thePoint for additional helpful resources

- eBook
- Journal Articles
- WebLinks

CHAPTER OUTLINE

LEARNING OBJECTIVES

The learner will be able to:

1. Identify types of cheating common in nursing programs.
2. Identify variables that contribute to integrity failures.
3. Discuss possible reasons for academic dishonesty.
4. Discuss consequences of a lack of academic integrity in nursing programs.
5. Identify methods/strategies to ensure academic integrity and decrease cheating.
6. Analyze conditions that promote academic integrity or that promote cheating.
7. Discuss barriers to self-reporting cheating or reporting others for cheating.
8. Reflect on his or her individual willingness to report other students for cheating.

INTRODUCTION

Loschiavo (2015) suggests that cheating in college has been with us since the inception of higher education and that much of this cheating appears to take shape in high school, with 64% of 24,000 students at 70 high schools admitting to cheating on a test, 58% admitting to plagiarism, and 95% saying they participated in some form of cheating, whether it was on a test, plagiarism, or copying homework.

The cell phone appears to be a cheating vector for many of these teenagers, with one out of three students in grades 7 through 12 admitting they used their cell phones to cheat on tests and 65% saying other kids in their schools are using their cell phones to cheat (The Latest Ways That Kids Cheat on Exams, 2009). In addition, more than half the cheaters said they texted or used their cell phones to call friends to warn them of pop quizzes, and only half of students believed that using their cell phones to cheat during tests was a serious offense.

Equally disconcerting, Buchmann (2014) suggests that about 75% of college students admit to cheating, and that probably even more than three quarters of college students have done something against the rules to improve their grades. "With an increasingly competitive atmosphere and a culture that some say is more accepting of cheating than it was in past generations, cheating has sadly become a somewhat expected phenomenon at universities across the country" (Buchmann, 2014, para. 2).

Indeed, in recent months, cases of cheating, including large-scale cheating at elite colleges, have become front-page headlines. For example, Buchmann (2014) notes that in May 2012, a teaching fellow for a government class at Harvard started noticing similarities between students' final exams that shouldn't have been there. The professor brought the case forward, and it was discovered that approximately 125 students—nearly half the entire lecture class—had been cheating. Buchmann (2014) concluded "that if students at Harvard—the most prestigious school in the world—can be caught cheating in large numbers, it's safe to assume that cheating happens on every campus much more often than we would like to think" (para. 1).

Consider This "It's no secret that students cheat" (Examiner.com, 2012). Indeed, research increasingly suggests that cheating from middle school through college is epidemic.

Discussion Point

Does a legacy of cheating exist in academe today? Are cheating cultures accepted or even condoned in contemporary secondary and collegiate settings?

CHEATING IN NURSING EDUCATION

Nurses are viewed as among the most trustworthy, ethical, and honest professionals in American society. From 1999 to 2014, Gallup polls found between 73% and 85% of respondents viewed the honesty and ethical standards of nurses as high to very high (GALLUP, 2014). It would seem to follow, then, that nursing students would exhibit high or very high ethical standards. The comment of a student who participated in a longitudinal study on academic dishonesty illustrated this view: "I think that…the type of people who choose to go into nursing… results in less cheating than in other disciplines" (McCabe, 2009). Unfortunately, the data don't seem to support this view of nursing students.

Cheating is a concern in any academic discipline. It is of particular concern to nursing educators because nurses hold the well-being and health of their patients in their hands. Lapses of integrity can have grave consequences for patients. It follows, then, that nursing educators and leaders must inculcate the highest standards of honesty and integrity in students to create a culture of trustworthiness in the nurses who graduate from their programs. While there isn't a great deal of data that defines the link between academic integrity and professional integrity, there is some evidence, beyond the intuitive, that there is a correlation.

Lapses in academic integrity can take many forms. Cheating in the classroom can include copying answers from another's exam, offering answers to exam questions to another student, soliciting answers to exam questions from students who have already taken the exam, collaborating with other students on assignments when collaboration is not allowed, quoting without appropriate attribution, using disallowed materials to get answers on exams or quizzes, or any of a myriad of practices that pass another's work as one's own. It can also include downloading papers from the Internet, taking photos of tests and posting them online, hiring someone to take their online tests, purchasing an instructor's version of a book to get copies of tests and answers, and faking test scores or letters of recommendation for employers or academic pursuits.

In the clinical setting, dishonest practices include recording vital signs that weren't actually taken or recorded accurately, reporting medications as given that were not administered, reporting patient/client responses to treatment that weren't observed, attempting procedures without adequate knowledge or asking for guidance from the instructor, breaking sterile technique without reporting it or replacing contaminated items, and discussing protected client information in public places or with nonmedical personnel (McCrink, 2010).

Discussion Point

Do you believe that students who lack academic integrity are more likely to demonstrate the same behaviors in clinical practice?

OVERVIEW OF THE LITERATURE

Numerous studies of nursing students' academic misconduct have been published in the last 30 years. Two of the earliest studies were by Hilbert in 1985, with a follow-up study in 1987. Other studies that documented academic dishonesty among nursing students were conducted by Bailey in 2001, Gaberson in 1997, Sheer in 1989, McCrink in 2010, McCabe in 2009, Krueger in 2014, Beasley in 2014, Stonecypher and Willson in 2014, and Woith, Jenkins, and Kerber in 2012. These studies, and others, indicate that nursing students engage in a wide variety of dishonest academic practices in both the classroom and clinical settings. More than just documenting the size of the problem, these studies examined the attitudes among nursing students that caused them to engage in these behaviors as well as the strategies that may be employed to deter such behavior. These studies also suggest that students engage in a variety of rationalizations to explain their misconduct such as time constraints, unfair course assignments, and the unrealistic expectations of nursing faculty, among others (McCrink, 2010).

Prevalence of the Problem in Nursing

The question of whether academic dishonesty is rising among nursing students may not be answerable. However, there is considerable evidence that such behavior is common. McCrink (2010) studied nursing students in two associate degree nursing programs in the northeastern United States (193 respondents), and found a mean score of 21.58 (range 19 to 95, SD 3.46) for frequency of self-reported misconduct. Krueger (2014) found that 216 of 334 (64.7%) participants admitted to engaging in some form of academic dishonesty in the classroom setting and that 181 of 335 (54%) engaged in academic dishonesty in the clinical setting.

Similarly disconcerting data were noted in a 2007 study by McCabe (2009) that involved nursing students from 12 schools. A request to participate was sent to 6,290 students, and 1,057 responses were received (a return of 16.8%). He found that more than half of undergraduate students and almost half of the graduate students self-reported engaging in one or more of 16 behaviors identified as classroom cheating.

Clearly, there is cause for concern. Moreover, since all these studies involved self-reporting of academic dishonesty, there is likely considerable underreporting. As one of McCabe's (2009) participants put it, "I think that you may have difficulty generating accurate statistics. I don't think that people who cheat are willing to give out that information."

There also seems to be a correlation between self-reported cheating in the classroom and self-reported cheating in the clinical setting. Krueger (2014) found a statistically significant correlation between the two behaviors ($r = 0.42$, $p < 0.01$). This correlation suggests that students who cheat in the classroom are likely to cheat in the clinical setting as well.

McCrink's data recorded the most common self-reported behaviors of academic dishonesty as discussing clients in public or with nonmedical personnel (35.3%), paraphrasing material without appropriate attribution (35.2%), working collaboratively when it was not allowed (24.3%), obtaining test questions from other students (21.8%), and recording vital signs that were not taken or recorded accurately (13%) (Box 18.1). Moreover, 8.8% of McCrink's respondents reported recording client treatments that were neither performed nor observed, 6.7% reported they'd recorded client responses to treatment they hadn't observed, and 2.1% reported they'd recorded administration of medications that had not been administered.

Discussion Point

What do you believe is driving these significant numbers of self-reported academic dishonesty? Is it a quest for a higher grade? For recognition of success? Is it driven by more intrinsic or extrinsic factors?

BOX 18.1 Commonly Self-Reported Types of Academic Dishonesty by Nursing Students

- Discussing clients in public places or with nonmedical personnel
- Paraphrasing material without appropriate attribution
- Working collaboratively on assignments or tests when it was not allowed
- Obtaining test questions from other students
- Recording vital signs that were not taken or recorded accurately
- Recording client treatments that were neither performed nor observed
- Recording administration of medications that had not been administered
- Reporting patient/client responses to treatment that weren't observed
- Attempting procedures without adequate knowledge or asking the instructor for guidance
- Breaking sterile technique without reporting it or replacing contaminated items

Another finding by Krueger (2014) was also disturbing. In her study of 335 participants in two associate degree nursing programs in the Midwest, 329 participants (98.2%) believed that plagiarism occurs at their college, and 97 participants (28.9%) reported witnessing another student cheating. Further, 291 of 329 participants (88.4%) said they'd never reported an incident of cheating, and 74 of 332 (22.3%) believed that the typical student would never report an incident of cheating they observed. In a recent student survey of graduating students in the author's nursing program, graduating students rated the academic integrity of their classmates at a mean of 3.58, the lowest score of the questions related to how these students viewed their classmates. Students who had reported cheating to the faculty were extremely reluctant to name the students they'd observed cheating. This, of course, makes taking action against the perpetrators even more difficult.

WHY DO STUDENTS CHEAT?

Many researchers have explored the question of why students cheat, and the responses are varied. Running out of the time needed to complete an assignment correctly or to study for an exam adequately is the most common reason students give for resorting to cheating (Colorado State University [CSU], 1993–2015). A second reason students give for cheating is not having fully understood the material or assignment at hand. In addition, sloppy note-taking leads to unintentional plagiarism, which is often treated just as seriously as intentional plagiarism (CSU, 1993–2015).

Woith et al. (2012) found that student participants identified competition among students for grades as fostering an environment conducive to cheating. Buchmann (2014) suggests that competitive pressures placed on children at a very young age carry on with them through high school and college. With so much pressure to stand out as the smartest in a class, some students may give in to the opportunity to succeed at the price of integrity.

Another reason cited by participants as pressures that led to cheating were the time constraints related to acquiring a vast amount of knowledge in the short period offered by nursing programs (typically, approximately 2 years). Krueger (2014) found that participants in her study who worked more than 40 hours per week rated academic dishonesty as more ethical than participants who worked 1 to 10 hours per week.

Institutional apathy has also been identified as a reason why students cheat (Buchmann, 2014). Students may cheat when they do not see the academic environment as one that deserves their honesty. "Just like cheating at Monopoly is easier to justify than tax evasion, if students don't believe their university deserves high standards then they may see no reason to follow all the rules about grading. Lack of respect for the collegiate institution may also prevent students from reporting instances of dishonesty they see around them" (Buchmann, 2014, para. 8).

Buchmann (2014) suggests that self-interest is also a factor in why people cheat and that this factor appears to encompass all cheating. Students who cheat hope to see a return on their investment of time and resources in college, and watching someone else make a better grade can be painful. "With only his or herself in mind, cheating is hard not to justify when someone can get away with it" (Buchmann, 2014, para. 10).

Reasons that students identify as compelling them to cheat are shown in Box 18.2.

Learning theory also offers insight into the development of a culture of cheating. As Krueger (2014) found

BOX 18.2 Why Students May Feel Compelled to Cheat

- Procrastination on assignments and studying
- Time constraints
- Not fully understanding the material or assignment at hand
- Sloppy note-taking, leading to unintentional plagiarism
- Competition for grades or success
- Ambiguous attitudes among students about what qualifies as cheating
- Institutional apathy
- Self-interest

Source: Buchmann, B. (2014, February 20). Cheating in college: Where it happens, why students do it and how to stop it. *The Huffington Post.* Retrieved May 28, 2015, from http://www.huffingtonpost.com/uloop/cheating-in-college-where_b_4826136.html; Colorado State University. (1993–2015). *Why do students cheat?* Retrieved May 28, 2015, from Learning@CSU Website: http://learning.colostate.edu/integrity/faqs/why_do_students.cfm

in her study, students who witness other students engaging in academically dishonest behavior, or who believe their peers are cheating are, themselves, more likely to cheat. The study of Woith et al. (2012) had this same observation. This was one of the situational conditions related to cheating that Krueger (2014) identified for her study. The other two were consequences and enforcement of academic dishonesty policies, and the students' personal beliefs and values related to cheating and academic honesty. Krueger's study found that students generally perceived that the risk of being caught was high and the consequences severe. Krueger also found a significant negative correlation between a commitment to integrity and the occurrence of dishonest behaviors. In other words, students who valued integrity highly cheated less. These findings suggest some possible approaches to deterring cheating.

STUDENT ATTITUDES REGARDING ACADEMIC DISHONESTY

There seems to be some disagreement among nursing students as to what constitutes academic dishonesty, and even more disagreement as to the seriousness of the conduct described. Most students in McCrink's study agreed that reporting vital signs that aren't taken is highly or severely unethical. Similarly, falsely reporting medication administration, recording responses to treatment that weren't observed, failure to report an error or incident that involved a client/patient, and coming to the clinical setting under the influence of alcohol or drugs were all viewed as highly unethical or severely unethical by these same students. However, 21.6% of the participants felt that working with another student when it wasn't allowed wasn't unethical or only slightly unethical. Sixteen percent of students felt the same way about getting answers from another student.

McCabe also noted that students tended to engage more readily in behaviors they viewed as less serious (McCabe, 2009). Such a result might be expected, but the question remains as to why students who rate behaviors as very unethical still engage in those behaviors. Similarly, how are we to reconcile the observation that most nursing students in the various studies felt the likelihood of, and penalties for, getting caught cheating were very high with the large number of students who self-report engaging in these behaviors? (McCabe, 2009; McCrink, 2010; Woith et al., 2012). In some cases, students reported that they didn't know that their actions constituted unethical conduct or cheating (Beasley, 2014; Bezek, 2014; McCrink, 2010).

Consider This Loschiavo (2015) notes that cheating "can be an intentional, calculated decision in order to get ahead. Often, it is motivated by the path to success that they see around them—people cheating without incurring any real consequences. Students then come to believe that dishonest behavior is rewarded and often do not hesitate to engage in it" (para. 8).

FERTILE GROUND FOR CHEATING?

Nursing school may be a breeding ground for academic dishonesty, despite nursing students' generally wide acceptance that trust, honesty, and fairness are essential to the formation of the therapeutic relationships that are

Research Study Fuels the Controversy 18.1

What Can Stop Student Academic Dishonesty?

This study explored the responses of 298 students who had been caught cheating and were assigned to a remediation class to answer the question "What, if anything, would have stopped you from committing your act of academic dishonesty?"

Source: Beasley, E. M. (2014). Students reported for cheating explain what they think would have stopped them. *Ethics & Behavior, 24*(3), 229–252. doi:10.1080/10508422.2013.845533

Study Findings

The researcher analyzed the responses and found several themes. Students said they were ignorant of what constituted academic dishonesty and ignorant of the consequences and/or seriousness of those violations; students deflected blame, usually by saying the instructor could have done something differently; students felt they didn't have sufficient time, resources, and/or skills to get the desired result, but didn't take responsibility for this lack of time, resources, or skills.

Students also felt they did not manage their time appropriately, and did take responsibility for the poor time management; some said a bad grade was not an option; and some cited peer behavior as a contributing factor. Beasley concluded that many of the students in his study believed that having better information about what constituted academic dishonesty and the penalties for such behavior would have inhibited them. In addition, students cited ideas consistent with neutralization and strain theories and felt that lack of time was a major factor in ultimately leading them to cheat (Beasley, 2014).

foundational to practice. While nursing educators and leaders, and even nursing students, may disagree as to whether the factors that promote cheating are actually causes, or rationalizations for bad behavior, or just excuses for moral laxity, if we are to deter academic dishonesty we must understand and acknowledge the context within which it occurs. Without question, many of the reasons, cited by students, for cheating exist in nursing programs in abundance: time constraints, large body of knowledge to assimilate in a short time, significant culture challenge for many students, great pressure for grades, and so on.

Since the first studies of cheating by nursing students in the mid-1980s, the use of Internet-based research and sources, electronic media, electronic submission of papers and exams, online management of courses, complete with quizzes, exams, and various assignments completed online, has made the burden of detecting and deterring academic dishonesty even more difficult.

As McCabe (2009) observed, nursing students are exposed to the same influences as students in other disciplines. Opportunities for cheating have certainly increased with the increased use of electronic technologies, but there is little evidence that the actual number of students cheating has increased as a result (McCabe, 2009). The ease with which students can access material is certainly a time saver, a valuable incentive in nursing programs (McCabe, 2009). In McCabe's (2009) study, more than a third of nursing students reported "copying a few sentences from a Web source without citing it." Among the questions raised by this finding is whether students are ignorant of appropriate citation of sources, seduced by the ease of such plagiarism, or whether there is some other explanation for such widespread cheating (Research Study Fuels the Controversy 18.1).

Interestingly, participants in two of the studies (McCrink, 2010; Woith et al., 2012) rejected the neutralization statements (rationales) for academic dishonesty and recognized the correlation between public/patient safety and academic integrity. This finding may offer insight into ways that both faculty and students may cooperate to decrease the incidence of cheating in both the classroom and clinical settings.

WHAT SHOULD THE CONSEQUENCES BE FOR CHEATING?

Both Krueger (2014) and McCabe (2009) report that students who observe their classmates engaging in academic dishonesty are more prone to engage in such activity themselves. Bezek (2014) noted that 71% of students performed acts of academic dishonesty because their peers did so and "got away with it." Clearly then, academic dishonesty must be immediately confronted and addressed so that a culture of cheating is not allowed to exist, much less condoned.

Consider This According to the Boston Globe, cheating is no more prevalent today than it was 50 years ago (Buchmann, 2014).

Given that the number of students who admit to cheating has remained constant since it was first measured in 1963, whatever is being done to stop cheating today clearly isn't working (Buchmann, 2014). What, then, should the consequences be for cheating? Clearly, consequences can range from no action to disciplinary expulsion (Box 18.3). Finding an appropriate balance between an excessively punitive culture that allows for no exceptions and an apathetic attitude that actually encourages cheating may be more difficult than one would expect. Expulsion and formal disciplinary actions clearly affect a student's future as well as career choice. Perhaps even more importantly, and not often addressed, is the fact that students who cheat their way through their education may be missing critical information they need to safely perform in their chosen career path. Certainly, this is the case in nursing, and allowing students who cheat to earn professional degrees clearly places patients at risk.

Consider This Some students cheat because they believe that grades and test scores are the only thing that really matter, not mastery of the content.

Discussion Point

If the consequences for cheating were more severe, would students be less inclined to cheat?

HOW CAN ACADEMIC INTEGRITY BE FOSTERED?

Nursing students and faculty, alike, recognize the importance of academic integrity as fostering the kind of ethical behavior essential to nursing care (McCrink, 2010; Woith et al., 2012). Given the positive correlation between academic misconduct in the classroom and unethical behavior in the clinical setting, classroom and clinical faculty as well as nursing leaders must be alert to instances of cheating in both arenas.

The approach to fostering academic integrity, however, must not be just reactive (negative sanctions when punishment is discovered). It must be proactive and include establishing an ethical culture, using

BOX 18.3 Common Consequences of Academic Misconduct

- No action
- Warning or written reprimand
- General disciplinary probation
- Disciplinary probation with loss of good standing
- Discretionary sanctions such as:
  - Educational programs
  - Restorative justice assignments
- Grading penalties such as:
  - An "F" on the assignment or exam
  - Failure in the class
  - Reduced grade
  - Academic Misconduct "AM" noted on transcript
- Loss of Repeat/Delete privilege
- Disciplinary suspension
- Disciplinary expulsion
- Revocation of admission or degree
- Withholding of degree

Source: Colorado State University. (1993–2015). *Why do students cheat?* Retrieved May 28, 2015, from Learning@CSU Website: http://learning.colostate.edu/integrity/faqs/why_do_students.cfm

professional standards as a guide for ethical behavior, establishing clear guidelines and expectations, increasing faculty supervision, fostering self-discipline, implementing honor codes, teaching students about research and appropriate citation, and providing mentoring and support.

Establishing an Ethical Culture

Ethical conduct and its role in establishing trustworthiness and a caring, therapeutic relationship among nursing students, nurses, and clients must be a central focus of students, faculty, and professional nurses. The establishment of a culture of ethical behavior and trustworthiness in nursing programs, however, must be a joint endeavor between faculty and students. Without significant participation, "buy in" by students, faculty efforts to stop cheating are likely to fail. As Krueger (2014) and other researchers point out, if the perceptions among students that they are likely to get caught cheating and the consequences for cheating are quite severe don't deter cheating, a punitive approach alone seems unlikely to solve the problem. Nevertheless, faculty, students, and the institution must be resolute that academic dishonesty will not be tolerated.

If the development of a culture of cheating is a result of socialization as Krueger (2014) and Woith et al. (2012) suggest, then one avenue toward reversing that course would be to socialize student nurses into a culture of caring, trustworthiness, and accountability. An emphasis on the importance of these attributes to the professional nurse should come early and be repeated often during the course of a student's progression through a nursing program. This socialization would involve teaching and role modeling ethical behavior and integrity. Educators also need to establish the relevance of the work they assign, and endeavor to help students manage their time better in order to deal with the increasing complexity and amount of knowledge required of the professional nurse (Woith et al., 2012).

Using Professional Standards as a Guide for Ethical Behavior

McCrink (2010), Krueger (2014), and Woith et al. (2012) agree that faculty play a central role in helping students incorporate such exemplars as the American Nurses Association (ANA) Code of Ethics (2001) into their interactions with students. Faculty must also provide clear guidelines and expectations for ethical behavior, and model such behavior. In addition, they must help students identify and discuss lapses of ethical conduct they encounter in the clinical setting by both students and professional nurses. Student peer leaders can be helpful in modeling and promoting accountability and trustworthiness (Beasley, 2014; Woith et al., 2012).

Indeed, Buchmann (2014) suggests that since cultural ideas may influence the prevalence of cheating, the best long-term solution may be to take a societal approach. Instead of seeing cheating as something that can't be done, students must come to recognize that it should not be done. Faculty have a clear responsibility to model ethical behavior. Not only should clinical standards and expectations regarding original work, allowed collaboration and so on be crystal clear, but faculty must also be sure to credit sources in lectures, assignments, and so on.

Establishing Clear Guidelines and Expectations

Buchmann (2014) suggests that many students lack understanding of what constitutes cheating since they may not have fully read or comprehended their student rules. This lack of understanding may lead students to cheat by accident or in a way that isn't known to be called cheating. In addition, "ambiguous attitudes among students about what qualifies as cheating may cause more academic dishonesty than intended by students. While most students will call plagiarism cheating, many of them will define plagiarism in a way that allows them to indirectly copy the work of others" (Buchmann, 2014, para. 6).

In addition, faculty should revisit the parameters and expectations of ethical conduct frequently, rather than only at the beginning of the program. Clear delineation of the types of activities that are approved for collaborative work and of those that require individual work would eliminate the rationalization that students didn't realize they weren't to work together. Faculty and students should work together to establish the policies that govern behavior in the academic and clinical settings (Stonecypher & Willson, 2014).

Faculty should also encourage discussions regarding ethical dilemmas associated with academic integrity. This is particularly important in the clinical setting when students may be exposed to unethical conduct by the staff nurses they are working with. Clinical instructors should be very clear about their expectations for ethical conduct and the consequences for failing to report errors in an appropriate manner.

Increasing Faculty Supervision

The quality of faculty supervision in test taking can be either a deterrent or a promoter of academic dishonesty. Indeed, Buchmann (2014) suggests that tightening the rules on classroom behavior during exams seems like the most obvious and readily available solution to reducing academic dishonesty. He goes on to detail extensive efforts made by universities to record everything suspicious, efforts made to prevent students from photographing a test, and not allowing students to chew gum since it provides a way to hide that they're talking into a hidden microphone.

Similarly, more faculty are requiring online students to take exams under the supervision of a proctor. Indeed, research demonstrates that students taking online unproctored exams perform better than when they sit for exams before a proctor enforcing the closed-book exam rules (Winneg, n.d.). In other words, more students cheat when taking exams unproctored, online at home.

Unfortunately, the Internet is filled with strategies students can use to individually or collaboratively cheat, including "the long-sleeved shirt method" (students write important information on their arms for an exam and then roll up their sleeves when instructor is not looking); the "buddy system" (students sit near a student they believe will do well on the test, and that student holds up their exam as if reflecting on their answers so that the other person can copy); "the telephone scam" (students are allowed to use the calculator on their phone for exams, but actually use the telephone to text answers to other students or search online); "the distraction method" (one student distracts the instructor so that other students can exchange answers); using crib notes written on band aids, Kleenex, gum wrappers, and other commonly used innocuous items; and "sign language" (using a series of coughs, morse code, hand or foot tapping, or other nonverbal cues to let another student know which answer is the correct one), to name just a few.

An attentive instructor may be able to detect some of these strategies, but it is equally clear that the sophistication and skill of academic cheaters is continuing to increase. Using multiple test proctors may be a useful strategy in increasing the degree of faculty supervision.

But new technology is unfolding that includes smartwatches, smart pens, and Google glasses to help students cheat (Vandoorne, 2014). Some new devices are almost impossible to see—such as "invisible" Bluetooth earpieces. They work with a tiny microphone, which is synced to a Bluetooth cell phone and enable questions, whispered from exam rooms, to be answered from someone outside the room. Such wearable technology will only make it more difficult for instructors to spot cheating when it is occurring.

Discussion Point

Can observant teachers detect academic dishonesty, or are cheating strategies so sophisticated or well practiced that being caught is unlikely?

Discussion Point

Is collaborative cheating typically instigated by a few people and others simply follow, or do you believe academic dishonesty is simply more common than most people would like to admit?

Using Test Security or Plagiarism Assessment Tools

Some instructors have begun Computerized Adaptive Testing (CAT) to address cheating concerns. CAT uses an algorithm to choose test items based on the students' strengths and weaknesses (Bleiberg & West, 2013). Every student takes a different test when using CAT, which decreases the number of items tests have in common. Students take the test online, eliminating inappropriately administered testing accommodations and making it difficult for students to share answers.

In addition, plagiarism assessment tools such as Turnitin.com and SafeAssign have become commonplace. These sites have millions of catalogued articles, papers, and webpages to determine what percentage of student papers are original work and what percentage is the work of others.

Instructors are also using webcams to monitor students taking tests offsite and increasingly requiring some type of biometric sign-in to make sure that the student taking the test is the same student taking the course. (The 2008 Higher Education Opportunity Act contains a requirement that schools offering distance learning programs have a system in place to authenticate the identity of their online students). More computers are being recessed into desktops so that students who attempt to photograph screens are more obvious.

In addition, some schools have begun using jamming devices to block the use of cellphones during testing.

Fostering Self-Discipline

A focus on quality improvement rather than a punitive approach to each mistake may encourage students to report errors rather than hiding them. Frank discussion between clinical faculty and students about the problems students observe can help inculcate an attitude of vigilance regarding their own personal practice.

Faculty should also emphasize the findings of the Institute of Medicine's (2004) report linking errors with outcomes in discussions with students regarding academic integrity. While the evidence that students who cheat become nurses who cheat in the workplace is sketchy, it seems intuitively true, and student respondents in several of the studies cited noted the link (McCabe, 2009; McCrink, 2010; Woith et al., 2012). Instructors should continually discuss with students the importance of the data they're collecting, the procedures they perform, and the dependence of patients' well-being on their honesty and ethical behavior (Krueger, 2014).

Implementing Honor Codes

An academic honor code is a set of rules or expectations that govern an academic community, and is based on ideals that define honorable behavior within that community. An honor code's utility depends on the notion that members of the community can be trusted to act with honor. Infractions of the honor code are enforced with various sanctions, including expulsion from the program or institution (Wikipedia, the Free Encyclopedia, 2015). Honor codes may be quite complex, listing various types of infractions, or they may be quite brief: a statement that the student who has signed the honor code pledges that all work is his or her own and that he or she has received no disallowed assistance.

Woith et al. (2012) and Krueger (2014) both noted that earlier researchers had found that schools that had formal honor codes reported fewer instances of student cheating. It may be that the formalization and discussion of these codes not only lay clear guidelines for student behavior, but also cause students to actively consider their behavior in the context of the fundamental principles of the nursing profession. Stonecypher and Willson (2014) notes that honor codes are effective if students understand the expectations of the code. Honor codes place the responsibility for academic integrity on the student, and must be written with clear, easy-to-understand expectations and steps that guide both students, faculty, and administrators (Stonecypher & Willson, 2014).

A common feature of honor codes is a "no tolerance" policy that obligates students to report infractions of academic honesty. Others may opt for a policy that allows a student to first confront another student about violations and encourage the accused to self-report before the formal reporting obligation is in force (Wikipedia, 2015). Failure to report a violation is generally considered a violation.

Discussion point

Would you report one of your classmates for academic dishonesty? What factors would influence your decision? How does tolerance of academic dishonesty affect the culture of integrity in the nursing program?

Teaching Students About Research and Appropriate Citation

Loschiavo (2015) suggests that one reason students cheat is that they are unprepared for college-level work. He suggests that the reason many students plagiarize is that they were never taught how to write a research paper. He also suggests that students are not being taught how to paraphrase and instead are just expected to cut and paste from the articles they read on the Internet.

In addition, Loschiavo suggests that some students don't have any confidence in their own ideas, so when given the chance to write a paper in which they must share their own thoughts, they simply go to the Internet and use others' words or ideas, thinking they are worth more than their own. Or students think that the author's words were so eloquent that they are afraid of their ability to interpret what has been read and to translate it into their own words.

Educators might help students with these deficiencies by requiring submission of intermediate steps (summaries, rough drafts, etc.) before deadline for finished papers and assignments. Students might also benefit from a course on research and writing during nursing school. Such a course could also help students learn how to evaluate other research papers and articles in their quest for evidence-based practice.

Providing Mentoring and Support

Loschiavo (2015) suggests that some students cheat because they don't know how to manage their time and thus underestimate how long assignments or studying will take them. They then panic and take shortcuts. In addition, he suggests that some students cheat as a cry for help, subconsciously wishing to be caught so they can share what is going on in their lives with someone they believe may be able to help. He suggests then that faculty should always ask questions about why students made the choices they did.

Conclusions

Unethical conduct and cheating in both the classroom and the clinical setting are a serious concern for nursing faculty, nursing leaders, and students. Recognition and amelioration of some of the factors in nursing programs that may encourage student dishonesty is critical. Since integrity and trustworthiness are foundations of good nursing practice, faculty must be prepared to help students develop and incorporate these values. As McCabe (2009) put it, "Nursing schools, as the gateway to a profession whose members are assumed to have a strong professional identity that is built on integrity and a desire to serve should assume some responsibility for developing these standards among future members of its profession" (p. 622).

Creating a culture of honesty and accountability is crucial to this end, and has been shown to deter cheating. Both Stonecypher and Willson (2014) and McCrink (2010) noted that student attitudes toward ethical standards of behavior made the strongest contribution to an ethic of caring and honesty. As one of McCabe's faculty respondents put it, "We have to help students learn that being a student with integrity is a critical part of their socialization into the role of professional health care provider with responsibility for life and death decisions" (McCabe, 2009, p. 620).

For Additional Discussion

1. Which is more important to you—building a culture of integrity in the nursing program and the profession, or loyalty to your classmates or coworkers? How do you handle conflicts between these two values?
2. Do you support the development and use of honor codes in nursing programs? What should an honor code for nursing school look like?
3. Do you believe there is a culture of cheating in your nursing program? What do you do personally to promote academic integrity?
4. What do you think is the relationship between academic integrity and professional integrity? Is a student who cheats in nursing school more likely to cheat in the professional realm? Would you want a nurse who cheated in nursing school caring for someone you cared about?
5. What steps would you recommend to build a culture of strict academic integrity in your nursing program?

References

American Nurses Association: Code of ethics for nurses. (2001). Retrieved May 27, 2015, from Indiananurses .org Website: http://indiananurses.org/isnapsite/articles/code_of_ethics.pdf

Bailey, P.A. (2001). Academic misconduct: responses from deans and nurse educators. *Journal of Nursing Education*, 40 (3), 124-131.

Beasley, E. M. (2014). Students reported for cheating explain what they think would have stopped them. *Ethics & Behavior, 24*(3), 229–252. doi:10.1080/10508422.2013.845533

Bezek, S. M. (2014). Who is taking care of you? A study of the correlation of academic and professional dishonesty. *Dissertation Abstracts International: Section A. Humanities and Social Sciences,* 114. (Publication No. 3630808)

Bleiberg, J., & West, D. (2013, August 20). How technology can stop cheating. *The Huffington Post.*

Retrieved June 2, 2015, from http://www.huffingtonpost.com/darrell-west/how-technology-can-stop-c_b_3784392.html

Buchmann, B. (2014, February 20). Cheating in college: Where it happens, why students do it and how to stop it. *The Huffington Post.* Retrieved May 28, 2015, from http://www.huffingtonpost.com/uloop/cheating-in-college-where_b_4826136.html

Colorado State University. (1993–2015). *Why do students cheat?* Retrieved May 28, 2015, from Learning@CSU Website: http://learning.colostate.edu/integrity/faqs/why_do_students.cfm

Examiner.com. (n.d.). *7 common ways students cheat.* Retrieved June 2, 2015, from http://www.examiner.com/article/7-common-ways-students-cheat

Gaberson, K.B. (1997, Jul-Sep). Academic dishonesty among nursing students. Nursing Forum, 32 (3), 14-20.

GALLUP. *Honesty/ethics in professions.* (2014, December). Retrieved May 17, 2015, from http://www.gallup.com/poll/1654/honesty-ethics-professions.aspx

Hilbert, G.A. (1985, July-August). Involvement of nursing students in unethical classroom and clinical behaviors. Journal of Professional Nursing, 1 (4), 230-4.

Institute of Medicine. (2004). *Keeping patients safe: Transforming the work environment of nurses.* Washington, DC: National Academic Press.

Krueger, L. (2014, February). Academic dishonesty among nursing students. *Journal of Nursing Education, 53*(2), 77–87.

The latest ways that kids cheat on exams. (2009). Retrieved June 2, 2015, from http://www.cbsnews.com/news/the-latest-ways-that-kids-cheat-on-exams/

Loschiavo, C. (2015, May 19). Why do students cheat? Listen to this dean's words. *The Conversation.* Retrieved May 28, 2015, from http://theconversation.com/why-do-students-cheat-listen-to-this-deans-words-40295

McCabe, D. L. (2009, November). Academic dishonesty in nursing schools: An empirical investigation. *Journal of Nursing Education, 48*(11), 614–623.

McCrink, A. (2010). Academic misconduct in nursing students: Behaviors attitudes rationalizations and cultural identity. *Journal of Nursing Education, 49*(11), 653–659.

Sheer, B.L. (1989). *The relationships among socialization, empathy, autonomy and unethical student behaviors in baccalaureate nursing students.* (Unpublished doctoral dissertation) Widener University School of Nursing, Chester, Pa.

Stonecypher, K., & Willson, P. (2014, May). Academic policies and practices to deter cheating in nursing education. *Nursing Education Perspectives, 35*(3), 167–179.

Vandoorne, S. (2014, June 19). From smartwatch and smartpen... to smartcheat? *CNN.* Retrieved June 2, 2015, from http://www.cnn.com/2014/06/19/business/high-tech-cheating/index.html

Wikipedia, the Free Encyclopedia. (2015, May 28). *Academic Honor Code.* Retrieved June 1, 2015, from http://en.wikipedia.org/w/index.php?title=Academic_honor_code&oldid=664372276

Winneg, D. (n.d.). Students will cheat—So, deal with it! [Web log post]. *Software Secure.* Retrieved June 2, 2015, from http://www.softwaresecure.com/students-will-cheat-so-deal-with-it/

Woith, W., Jenkins, S. D., & Kerber, C. (2012, October). Perceptions of academic integrity among nursing students. *Nursing Forum, 47*(4), 253–259.

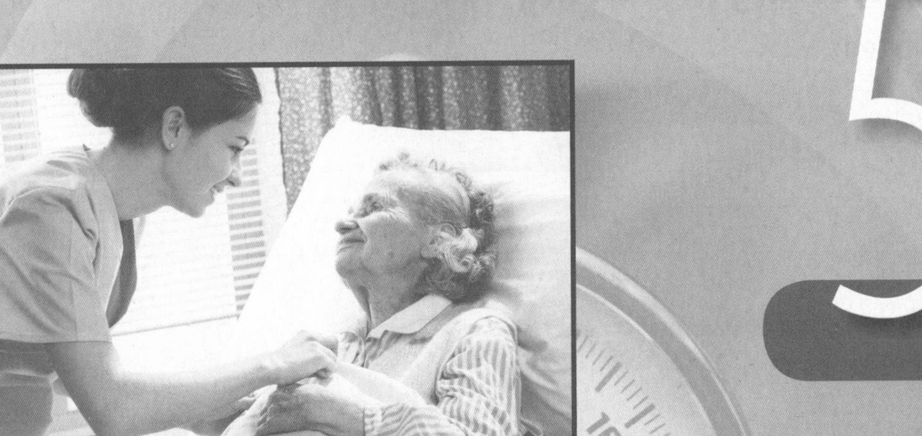

5

Legal and Ethical Issues

19

Whistle-Blowing in Nursing

Carol J. Huston

ADDITIONAL RESOURCES

Visit thePoint for additional helpful resources
- eBook
- Journal Articles
- WebLinks

CHAPTER OUTLINE

LEARNING OBJECTIVES

The learner will be able to:

1. Define whistle-blowing and differentiate between internal and external whistle-blowing.
2. Identify conditions that should be met before whistle-blowing occurs, as well as situations in which whistle-blowing is clearly indicated.
3. Examine how cultural background may affect a nurse's willingness to blow the whistle on unsafe practices.
4. Identify risks and retaliatory consequences frequently experienced by whistle-blowers as a result of their actions.
5. Explore why reactions to whistle-blowers are often mixed and why the courage to speak out is something we honor more often in theory than in fact.
6. Differentiate among the consequentialist, deontological, and utilitarian viewpoints regarding the purposes of whistle-blowing.
7. Analyze how whistle-blowing could be considered a failure of organizational ethics.
8. Delineate strategies to create an organizational climate that both discourages the need for whistle-blowing and supports the whistle-blower when it is necessary for him or her to come forward.
9. Identify strategies that whistle-blowers should use to reduce the likelihood of retaliation and to reduce their legal liability.
10. Analyze existing and proposed federal and state legal protections for whistle-blowers.
11. Identify the process used by a whistle-blower to file a *qui tam* or whistle-blower lawsuit under the False Claims Act and the potential benefits of doing so.
12. Reflect on his or her willingness to assume the personal risks associated with whistle-blowing, should the need arise.

INTRODUCTION

Watergate break-in ... Enron and the artificial manipulation of energy prices ... Martha Stewart and insider trading ... WorldCom and accounting fraud ...Bridgestone and Firestone tires ... Dow Corning and silicone breast implants ... Morgan Stanley and overcharging customers ... fraudulent bank loans and artificial home price inflation. All of these high-profile cases, involving some degree of ethical malfeasance, have led the US public to an increased sense of moral awareness about what is right and what is wrong. In addition, these cases have all come to the attention of the public as the result of *whistle-blowing*.

Dictionary.com ("Whistleblowing," 2015) suggests whistle-blowing occurs when a person informs on another or makes public disclosure of corruption or wrongdoing. Similarly, the Free Online Dictionary ("Whistleblower," 2003–2015) defines a whistle-blower as "an informant who exposes wrongdoing within an organization in the hope of stopping it" (para. 3).

Consider This Virtually all definitions of whistle-blowing suggest the importance of advocating for others who may be harmed.

It is generally accepted that there are two types of whistle-blowing: internal and external. *Internal whistle-blowing* typically involves reporting concerns up the chain of command within an organization in the hope that whatever the problem is, it will be resolved. *External whistle-blowing* involves reporting concerns outside the organization and, in particular, to the media. In many cases, whistle-blowing becomes external only if inadequate action is taken at the organizational level to address the concerns of the whistle-blower. In some cases, however, whistle-blowing becomes external in an effort to embarrass an organization publicly or to seek financial redress.

Discussion Point

Is it ever appropriate to whistle-blow externally before attempting to resolve the problem internally?

In an era of transparency in quality reporting, declining reimbursements, and the ongoing pressure to remain fiscally solvent, the risk of fraud, misrepresentation, and ethical malfeasance in health care organizations has never been higher. As a result, the need for whistle-blowing has also likely never been greater.

This chapter explores the effect of "groupthink" on the likelihood that whistle-blowers will come forward. In addition, it presents select cases of whistle-blowing. Personal risks associated with whistle-blowing are described, as are the mixed feelings many individuals hold about whistle-blowing. Whistle-blowing is also explored as a failure of organizational ethics, and strategies are identified to create an organizational climate that both discourages the need for whistle-blowing and supports the whistle-blower when it is necessary for him or her to come forward. Finally, legal protections (or the lack thereof) for whistle-blowing are discussed.

Consider This "To see what is right, and not do it, is want of courage, or of principles."

—Confucius

GROUPTHINK AND WHISTLE-BLOWING

Being a whistle-blower takes great courage and self-conviction because it requires the whistle-blower to avoid *groupthink*—an inappropriate conformity to group norms. Going outside group norms often carries significant personal and professional risks. Unfortunately, these risks are more common than not, as whistle-blowers may be viewed as disloyal rather than as courageous. For example, Colvin (2002) recounted how Sherron Watkins, an accountant, first blew the whistle on Enron's complex "special-purpose entities." She detailed them in a memo to Chief Executive Officer Ken Lay, her boss's boss's boss. She understood that something wrong was going on—something everyone else seemed to think was perfectly okay—and that public revelation would be disastrous.

What Colvin argued was most important in this scandal was that Watkins had access to the same facts as many other people inside Enron, yet somehow she was able to escape the groupthink that ensnared her colleagues. Soon after writing the memo, she identified herself as its author and met with Mr. Lay. When her memo eventually became public, the wrongness of what happened was apparent even internally (Colvin, 2002).

Colvin recounts a similar story at WorldCom, where Cynthia Cooper, another internal auditor, saw something that did not look right and took matters into her own hands. In this case, Cooper began investigating some of the company's capital expenditures and discovered bookkeeping entries that would eventually uncover what is likely the largest accounting fraud in US history.

Faced with disturbing facts, Cooper discussed her findings with the company's controller and with Scott Sullivan, the chief financial officer. Sullivan tried to explain to her why costs that had previously been expensed were suddenly being capitalized. Then he asked her to stop the audit, which was being conducted early, and to put it off until the third quarter. She did not. Instead, she continued—and immediately went over her boss's head and called the chairman of the board's audit committee. He arranged to meet with her and the company's new auditor, KPMG. Two weeks later, WorldCom announced that it would restate earnings by US$3.9 billion—the largest restatement ever.

Again, Colvin (2002) suggested that the importance of Cooper's refusal to postpone her audit, as Sullivan had asked, is even greater than it may appear. Facts uncovered about the company, combined with the memo Sullivan wrote to the board in a last-ditch attempt to defend himself, show that if Cooper had "been a good soldier," the whole problem might have been concealed forever.

A similarly unsettling case was reported by Smith (2008), who profiled corporate whistle-blower Dana de Windt, a stockbroker at the financial services firm of Morgan Stanley. de Windt complained to government regulators that the company was cheating brokerage clients, having overcharged brokerage customers on 2,800 purchases of US$59 million of bonds. de Windt repeatedly confronted his bosses with "questions tucked inside a thick, three-ring binder" for more than 4 years, and management's response was simply for "him to get over it" (para. 5). Finally, de Windt reported the situation to regulators, and in August 2007, Morgan Stanley settled the resulting complaint brought by the US Securities and Exchange Commission (SEC) by paying a US$ 6.1 million fine.

Finally, Schulman (2007) presented the story of Leroy Smith, a safety manager at a federal prison in California, who exposed "hazardous conditions in a prison computer recycling program where inmates were smashing monitors with hammers, unleashing clouds of toxic metals" (para. 1), despite being threatened with termination and other types of retaliation. Although Smith eventually went on to be named "Public Servant of the Year" by the U.S. Office of Special Counsel (the federal agency charged with protecting government employees who expose waste, fraud, and abuse), his recognition ceremony was canceled at the last minute due to what Schulman called "ludicrous" reasons. In addition, things did not change at the prison as a result of the whistle-blowing. Smith concluded that his experience "was a beacon of false hope for public servants who are trying to correct wrongdoing," and Schulman (2007) agreed, noting that "given the current climate for whistle-blowers, false hope might be all the hope there is" (para. 3).

> **Consider This** Although the US public wants corruption and unethical behavior to be unveiled, the individual reporting such behavior is often looked on with distrust and considered to be disloyal.

Indeed, Schulman (2007) alleged that "a series of court rulings, legal changes, and new security and secrecy policies have made it easier than at any time since the Nixon era to punish whistle-blowers" (para. 3). William Weaver, a professor of political science at the University of Texas-El Paso and a senior adviser to the National Security Whistle-blowers Coalition, agreed and stated that he now counsels federal employees against coming forward in any situation (Schulman, 2007). He said that he warns them that it will destroy their lives, cost them their families and friends, and squander their life savings on attorneys.

More recently, whistle-blower Jeffrey Sterling, an ex-CIA officer, was convicted of exposing a dubious covert operation without presenting clear-cut evidence that he did, something Solomon (2015) calls "a chilling message to others" (para. 1). Solomon alleges that prosecutors were trying to vindicate *Operation Merlin*, 9 years after a book by James Risen reported that it "may have been one of the most reckless operations in the modern history of the CIA." "That bestselling book, *State of War*, seemed to leave an indelible stain on Operation Merlin while soiling the CIA's image as a reasonably competent outfit" (Solomon, 2015, para. 2).

Interestingly, journalist Risen was beyond the reach of the law, but Sterling, as a CIA employee, was not. Sterling had gone through channels in 2003 to warn Senate Intelligence Committee about Operation Merlin, and he was later indicted for allegedly giving Risen classified information about it. "For CIA officials, the prosecution wasn't only to punish Sterling and frighten potential whistle-blowers; it was also about payback, rewriting history and assisting with a PR comeback for the operation as well as the agency" (Solomon, 2015, para. 1).

Perhaps the most frightening aspect of all these cases is that the responses to the whistle-blower are not unique. Many organizations are aware of problem situations but choose to ignore them until a crisis occurs or the problem becomes public.

Some nurses take comfort in thinking that nursing is different and that any moral professional would report substandard care. The reality, however, is often very different, and many professionals are torn between what they believe they should do and what they actually do. "When surveyed, over 99% of all nurses understood that reporting unethical practices was part of their obligations as nurses. However, less than 45% of surveyed nurses strongly believed they would have the courage to do so" (IV Infusion Home, 2015). This is particularly disconcerting, since those who bear witness are required to overcome groupthink despite their moral distress. This is a primary reason why so many whistle-blowers delay reporting their concerns outside the organization.

Discussion Point

Why is speaking out often honored more in theory than in fact?

Discussion Point

In the United States, there is some evidence that the events of September 11, 2001, have made people more public spirited and more inclined to blow the whistle. Do you think this inclination is driven more by fear or by a desire to promote public good?

EXAMPLES OF WHISTLE-BLOWING IN NURSING

Complaints about unsafe staffing and unlicensed assistive personnel performing nursing tasks outside their scope of practice are fairly common. In addition, some nurses claim that they have been told to participate in illegal or unethical activities such as fraudulently altering medical records, falsifying insurance claims, and covering up the failure to meet mandated staffing ratios. A review of the literature reveals multiple case studies of whistle-blowing by nurses.

Mason (2011) shared the story of two nurses, Anne Mitchell and Vicki Galle, who blew the whistle on a physician for a variety of charges including unprofessional conduct, via what they thought was a confidential report to the state board for medicine. Instead of the physician being investigated, the nurses found themselves the target of unprofessional conduct charges brought by the local sheriff and county attorney, who were friends and business associates of the reported physician. In the end, the nurses who had a combined 47 years of experience at the hospital were fired. The charges for Galle and Mitchell were eventually dropped, and the sheriff, county attorney, and hospital administrator were indicted for retaliating against the whistle-blowers. Each faces six counts, including misuse of official information and retaliation, which are third-degree felonies (Sack, 2011). The nurses sued the county and settled for a shared US$750,000 (Sack, 2011).

Rohner (2015) wrote about a recent case in Cape Dorset, Nunavut, Canada, following the "preventable" death of a 3-month-old baby in 2012. The Government of Nunavut's policies and procedures for nurses state that nurses must examine sick children less than 1 year old when a parent contacts them after normal working hours. Gwen Slade, the whistle-blower nurse, alleges that another nurse told the mother not to bring the baby into the health center (to bathe the infant instead), and that the accused nurse faced numerous complaints that coworkers and members of the public had filed against her. The territory's health minister ordered an immediate independent review, but this had not begun nearly 3 months later. In the meantime, the accused nurse was promoted to acting nurse-in-charge despite restrictions being placed on her license by the Registered Nurses Association of the Northwest Territories and Nunavut.

In addition, Slade said she was suspended for speaking out against what she believed to be misdiagnoses and irresponsible behavior by a coworker. An investigation ensued, and Slade was eventually cleared of any wrongdoing. Slade suggests, however, that she continues to suffer the consequences of speaking out and that she has not been able to find work in Nunavut as a nurse since the alleged incidents. Slade also suggests that the investigation into her own conduct prevented her from getting two teaching jobs in Ontario and that she is only months away from losing her farm, her dream. Slade suggests that she is the victim of an extraordinary abuse of power, that has brought pain, devastation, and destruction to someone who did nothing wrong.

Clearly, patient advocacy has a central role in nursing. So too does professional advocacy, through which nurses are committed to improving the practice of nursing and maintaining the integrity of the health care profession. Both advocacy roles suggest that the nurse is accountable for ensuring that at least minimum standards are met. Both of these cases depict nurses who believed that they were acting honorably in the role of patient advocate. Yet all suffered negative consequences, including job loss. Unfortunately, this is more common than not.

Consider This Advocacy is the foundation and essence of nursing, and nurses have a responsibility to promote human advocacy (Marquis & Huston, 2015).

It is important, however, to remember that whistle-blowing should never be considered the first solution to ethically troubling behavior. Indeed, it should be considered only after other prescribed avenues of solving problems have been attempted. This is true, however, only if patients' lives are not at stake. In those cases, immediate action must be taken.

In addition, the employee should typically go up the chain of command in reporting his or her concerns. This process, however, must be modified when the immediate supervisor is the source of the problem. In such a case, the employee might need to skip that level to see that the problem is addressed. Indeed, Foose, Penman, and Petry (2015) noted that most would rather raise the issue internally to their manager than take it outside. Thus, companies generally get the opportunity to resolve issues internally—the question is whether they will take this opportunity or miss it.

There are other general guidelines for blowing the whistle that should also be followed, including carefully documenting all attempts to address the problem and being sure to report facts and not personal interpretations. These guidelines, as well as others, are presented in Box 19.1.

CULTURAL BACKGROUND AND WHISTLE-BLOWING

For some minority nurses, cultural issues further complicate whether a decision is made to blow the whistle

BOX 19.1 Guidelines for Blowing the Whistle

- Stay calm and think about the risks and outcomes before you act.
- Know your legal rights, because laws protecting whistle-blowers vary by state.
- First, make sure that there really is a problem. Check resources such as the medical library, the Internet, and institutional policy manuals to be sure.
- Seek validation from colleagues that there is a problem, but do not get swayed by groupthink into not doing anything if you should.
- Follow the chain of command in reporting your concerns, whenever possible.
- Confront those accused of the wrongdoing as a group whenever possible.
- Present just the evidence; leave the interpretation of facts to others. Remember that there may be an innocent or good explanation for what is occurring.
- Use internal mechanisms within your organization.
- If internal mechanisms do not work, use external mechanisms.
- Private groups, such as The Joint Commission or the National Committee for Quality Assurance, do not confer protection. You must report to a state or national regulator.
- Although it is not required by every regulatory agency, it is a good rule of thumb to put your complaint in writing.
- Document carefully the problem that you have seen and the steps that you have taken to see that it is addressed.
- Do not lose your temper, even if those who learn of your actions attempt to provoke you.
- Do not expect thanks for your efforts.

Source: American Nurses Association. (2015). *Things to know about whistle blowing.* Retrieved March 20, 2015, from http://nursingworld.org/MainMenuCategories/ThePracticeofProfessionalNursing/workforce/Workforce-Advocacy/Whistle-Blowing.html; Blecher, B. M. (2001–2010). *What color is your whistle?* Retrieved May 20, 2011, from http://www.minoritynurse.com/?q=workplace-issues/what-color-your-whistle

and, if so, how it should be done. For example, "nurses with certain cultural backgrounds—for example, some Asians, Filipinos, and Africans—may be more reluctant to blow the whistle because they've been raised to respect a clear chain of command and hierarchy" (Blecher, 2001–2015, para. 12). The same goes for nurses whose first language is not English. According to Winifred Carson, nurse practice counsel for the ANA, "They fear problems related to communication—whether they accurately communicate the magnitude of the problem and whether not speaking English as a first language would be used against them if they continue to challenge authority" (Blecher, 2001–2015, para. 14).

Bitoun Blecher (2001–2015) suggested that "reporting incidents of wrongdoing in the workplace is always a risky business—but for minority nurses who blow the whistle, the stakes are even higher" (para. 1). Carson stated that minority nurses are more apt to be retaliated against, especially if they are working in nonminority settings (Blecher, 2001–2015, para. 7).

THE PERSONAL RISKS OF WHISTLE-BLOWING

Being a whistle-blower is not without risks. Indeed, it is filled with risks. Unfortunately, most whistle-blowers set out believing that their actions will be welcomed, only to discover that the problems raised go much deeper than they imagined and the personal consequences can be overwhelming. Such consequences include negative reactions from coworkers, losing one's job, and, in the extreme, legal retaliation. In many cases, whistle-blowers are fired from their jobs, especially those who are termed *at-will* employees.

Bitoun Blecher (2001–2015) concurs, noting an Australian survey of 95 nurses that suggested that there were severe repercussions for the 70 nurses who reported incidents of misconduct but few professional consequences for the 25 nurses who remained silent: "Fourteen percent of the whistle-blowers reported being treated as traitors, 16% received professional reprisals in the form of threats, 14% were rejected by peers, 11% were reprimanded, 9% were referred to a psychiatrist and 7% were pressured to resign" (para. 6).

Consider This Our culture still often labels whistle-blowers as "snitches," "moots," and "tattletales" (Hill, 2010, p. 8).

Peters et al.'s (2011) interviews with Australian nurses whose actions had been affirmed by whistle-blowers or who were whistle-blowers themselves also suggested that whistle-blowing brought about negative effects in virtually every aspect of their lives. The nurses shared such problems as tremendous and chronic distress, acute anxiety, flashbacks, nightmares, and disturbing thoughts. Peters et al. concluded that many nurse whistle-blowers were not prepared for the impact on their personal, emotional, physical, and professional welfare.

In addition, Wilkes, Peters, Weaver, and Jackson (2011) noted that many whistle-blowers report negative impacts on their family life, including strained relationships with family members, dislocation of family life, and exposing family to public scrutiny. Wilkes et al. note that the harm caused to the nurses who blow the whistle is not restricted to one party, but is echoed in family life as well.

Consider This There isn't an employee in your organization who doesn't gauge the potential for retaliation when considering raising an issue (Foose et al., 2015).

Not all whistle-blowing, however, results in repercussions from employers. For example, in late 2014, Anderson Cooper featured the story of Nurse Briana Aguirre who spoke out about the treatment of Ebola patient Thomas Duncan and others at Texas Presbyterian Hospital, where she worked (Cable News Network [CNN], 2014). Ms. Aguirre described chaos, a lack of training, confusing protocols from the CDC, and unnecessary risks that she says nurses were exposed to on the job. She also claimed that 2 weeks into the hospital's Ebola crisis, nurses like her did not have the same level of protection as sanitation workers at the hospital. Although Ms. Aguirre expressed concerns about recrimination for openly sharing her concerns, the hospital responded that "Her employment status is the same today as it was yesterday. We would welcome the opportunity to learn more about her observations when she is willing" (CNN, 2014, para. 4).

It is imperative then that nurses working on the frontline be encouraged to speak up and that they be supported in their actions to do so. For example, nursing departments within hospitals should provide their nurses with an ethics committee chaired by a nurse with experience in bioethical issues (not one who has a vested interest in promoting administrative or hierarchical constraints). Nurse managers should promote the values inherent in patient advocacy, and the organization should openly support individuals who are willing to take the risk of being a whistle-blower. The reality is that if an employee is willing to go to the trouble and risk the repercussions of blowing the whistle, those concerns should be taken seriously and investigated.

Consider This The motive of most whistle-blowers is advocacy, not troublemaking.

More research, however, is being conducted on the motivation behind whistle-blowing. Recent research conducted by Guthrie and Taylor at North Carolina State University and Bucknell University suggests that strong, reliable antiretaliation policies can encourage employees to notify internal authorities of possible wrongdoing, but that offering monetary incentives does not necessarily influence whistle-blowing behavior—or at least not right away (North Carolina State University, 2015). However, when monetary incentives increase, so too does the incidence of whistle-blowing (Research Study Fuels the Controversy 19.1).

The bottom line, though, is that whistle-blowers should never assume that doing the right thing will result in a financial incentive or protect them from retaliation. Instead, potential whistle-blowers should determine their legal duty for reporting and carefully research the specifics of their protection under the law. In addition, they should try to report anonymously when possible. Moreover, they must be prepared to defend their claims. In addition, prospective whistle-blowers should always at least try to solve problems internally before going public. When that is impossible and there is a clear indication of serious harm, they must document their actions and go public. They should also seek support and counsel before taking any steps.

Clearly, whistle-blowers often face both social and work-related retaliation, and that at times this retaliation can be severe and life altering. Yet it must be noted that at least some self-satisfaction and pride must come with the recognition that unethical behavior has been exposed and that at least the potential for correction is possible because of the whistle-blower's actions. Box 19.2 summarizes some of the pros and cons of whistle-blowing.

ETHICAL DIMENSIONS OF WHISTLE-BLOWING

Ethical organizations practice in such a way that patients and workers are protected from harm. Sometimes,

Research Study Fuels the Controversy 19.1

Protections, Not Money, Boost Whistle-blowing

The researchers surveyed 283 adults who were asked to respond as though they were employees of a company that appeared to be committing fraud. The participants were split into three groups: one in which there was no payment for reporting fraud; one in which employees received a percentage of their salary as payment for reporting fraud; and one in which employees received a percentage of the fraud reported as payment. Each of these three groups was then split in half: half of each group received no promise of protection from retaliation, while the other half were told they'd be protected from retaliation.

Source: North Carolina State University. (2015, March 2). Protections, not money, can boost internal corporate whistleblowing. *Science Daily.* Retrieved March 21, 2015, from http://www.sciencedaily.com/releases/2015/03/150302091701.htm

Study Findings

Protection from retaliation made people significantly more likely to report possible wrongdoing; however, this was contingent largely on whether the employee trusted the company. Money, on the other hand, was not a significant factor in determining whether someone would report a problem. However, there was an interesting secondary effect regarding money. After the first set of questions, all study participants were offered a much larger amount of money for reporting the fraud internally. Participants who were not offered money in the first place were no more likely to report. But both groups that had been offered money in the first set of questions (based on salary or the size of the fraud) were more likely to report the fraud when the amount of monetary compensation increased. This suggests that the initial offer of money for reporting framed reporting as an economic decision, rather than as an altruism decision—so when the money went up, they were more likely to report.

BOX 19.2 Pros and Cons of Whistle-Blowing

Pros

- Protects patients
- Improves quality of care
- Meets professional expectations and standards
- Satisfies ethical duty
- Brings problems out into the open
- Provides validation of concerns and moral rightness

Cons

- Poses personal and professional risks
- Casts doubt on motives
- Leads to possible job loss or employer retaliation
- Is typically a tiring, anxiety-producing, and often frustrating experience

however, health care organizations fail to provide accountability for the safety and welfare of their patients and workers. Nurses or other employees then feel compelled to take action against the wrongdoing in an effort to fulfill their professional obligations.

Whistle-blowing, however, can create considerable moral distress for nurses as they weigh the consequences of their actions against the duties of their profession. Clearly, nurses are bound to the role of patient advocacy by ethical codes of conduct. The problem is that nurses also have professional commitments to their employer and to other health care professionals, and this loyalty to the employer can be misplaced when it leads to patient harm. The end result all too often, then, is a conflict between principles and duty. This tension between loyalty to employer and the need to protect patients is a major reason so many nurses delay in blowing the whistle.

Matthewson (2012) agrees, suggesting that the question of whether whistle-blowing is ethical can be addressed by a broad scope of dizzying philosophies, but when kept simple, one must remember that whistle-blowing does cause a conflict of interest between the personal, organizational, and societal spheres. Much of this conflict stems from the context in which a whistle-blower is viewed: whether as someone sharing knowledge of misconduct for the benefit of others or as someone who is acting "disloyal" to their organization. Matthewson argues that the whistle-blower is ultimately torn between loyalty to their employer (or the subject of their revelation) and their moral commitment to the law and society at large. Many feel they have the most to lose, at least in the first instance.

Lachman (2008) suggested that the ethics of this divided loyalty can be viewed in relation to its moral purpose, whether that is to maximize the benefit and minimize the harm (a consequentialist view) or to fulfill a duty (a deontological Kantian view). If whistle-blowing is aimed at changing a situation for the better, the consequentialist moral framework becomes paramount. If whistle-blowing is viewed as the fulfillment of a duty to keep promises or protect patients, then the deontological framework becomes paramount.

A strong argument can be made, however, for the precedence of the nurse's duty to the patient over his or her duty to the employer. Indeed, nurses must always remember that their primary professional responsibility is to their patients, not to their employers. As such, the need to uphold the rights of others, to promote fairness, and to provide for the greater good becomes paramount.

Discussion Point

Can you think of a situation in which you have been involved in which utilitarianism (the greater good) would support not blowing the whistle on unethical behavior?

Consider This A whistle-blower must blow the whistle for the right reason for it to be a moral action.

McKee (2013) suggests that justice and fidelity are other ethical principles that must be examined when considering the ethics of whistle-blowing. McKee argues that society could not function if individuals routinely broke their agreements. Employees of all types owe fidelity to their employers, if not to a professional code of conduct. At times, however, claims of justice may supersede the claims of fidelity, and one's professional duty sometimes includes a legal and moral duty to report violations, especially if they are being covered up.

The ANA *Code of Ethics for Nurses with Interpretive Statements* may also provide guidance for nurses who are considering becoming a whistle-blower. Provision 3 of the *Code of Ethics* states that the nurse "promotes, advocates for, and strives to protect the health, safety, and rights of the patient" (ANA, 2015, p. 9). In addition, Section 3.5 states:

> *When incompetent, unethical, illegal, or impaired practice is not corrected and continues to jeopardize patient well-being and safety, nurses must report the problem to appropriate external authorizes such as practice committees or professional organizations, licensing boards, and regulatory or quality assurance agencies. Some situations are sufficiently egregious as to warrant the notification and involvement of all groups and/or law enforcement.* (ANA, 2015, p. 12)

Ethical codes of conduct from Canada, the United Kingdom, Australia, and Japan mandate similar action. Such ethical codes bind nurses to the role of patient advocacy and compel them to take action when the rights or safety of patients is jeopardized. The bottom line is that although whistle-blowing can result in negative consequences for both the employing institution and the whistle-blower, nurses must uphold a professional standard and protect their patients.

LEGAL PROTECTION FOR WHISTLE-BLOWERS

There is no universal legal protection for whistle-blowers; however, under the 1st and 14th Amendments to the US Constitution, state and local government officials are prohibited from retaliating against whistle-blowers. In addition,

> *Although they do not fall under the category of "whistle-blower" protections, the laws protecting individual employees from mistreatment in the workplace, such as Title VII of the Civil Rights Act or the Fair Labor Standards Act, also protect employees from retaliation for asserting their rights under those laws. For example, it is illegal to terminate an employee for reporting sexual harassment, or for challenging an employer's failure to pay overtime.* (Joseph & Kirschenbaum, LLP, 2015)

In addition, there is some whistle-blower protection at the state level. As of 2014, 32 states (Box 19.3) had passed some type of whistle-blower legislation, although a number of other states are considering the introduction of such legislation. The problem is that although some of these state laws prohibit retaliation, the standards for proving retaliation vary.

Employees in most states, however, increase their likelihood of whistle-blower protection under general statutes or common law if they meet criteria similar to those established at the federal level: (1) They must be acting in good faith that the employer or its employees are breaking the law in some way, (2) they must complain about that violation either to the employer or to an outside agency, (3) they must refuse to be a party to the violation, and (4) they should be willing to assist in any official investigations of the violation.

BOX 19.3 States With False Claims Acts/Qui Tam Laws as of 2014

California	Minnesota
Chicago	Montana
Colorado	Nevada
Connecticut	New Hampshire
Delaware	New Jersey
District of Columbia	New Mexico
Florida	New York City
Georgia	New York
Hawaii	North Carolina
Illinois	Oklahoma
Indiana	Rhode Island
Iowa	Tennessee
Louisiana	Texas
Maryland	Virginia
Massachusetts	Wisconsin
Michigan	Washington

Source: WhistleblowerLaws. (2014). *What is a qui tam?* Retrieved March 9, 2015 from http://www.whistleblowerlaws.com/what-is-qui-tam/

Discussion Point

What whistle-blowing protections, if any, exist in the state where you live? Is any legislation pending?

The False Claims Act

Some whistle-blower legislation has been enacted at the federal level, however, to encourage people to report wrongdoings. One such piece of legislation is the False Claims Act (FCA), originally a Civil War statute, which encourages whistle-blowers to come forward regarding fraud committed against the federal government and to file a lawsuit seeking lost monies in the government's name.

The individual would file a *qui tam* or whistle-blower lawsuit and provide knowledge that a person defrauded the government. Qui tam law suits are brought by a citizen, known as a "relator" or whistle-blower, against a company, person, or entity that he or she believes is cheating the federal or state government in some way (WhistleblowerLaws, 2014). Since the qui tam suit is brought in the name of the whistle-blower on behalf of the government, the government may actually join the case and litigate alongside the whistle-blower's lawyers. These FCAs or "*qui tam* laws" exist at the federal level and have been adopted by 29 states, the District of Columbia, the city of New York, and the city of Chicago (WhistleblowerLaws, 2014). An individual who successfully pursues a *qui tam* action is entitled to a bounty that ranges from between 15% and 30% of the government's recovery.

For example, a whistle-blower may have knowledge of a colleague inappropriately billing Medicare or Medicaid. The FCA provides protection for government whistle-blowers, thereby prohibiting employers from punishing employees who report the fraud or assist in the investigation of the fraud. If the whistle-blower is dismissed or discriminated against in any way as a result of the lawsuit, the whistle-blower can file a claim against that employer for unlawful retaliation.

To have a case brought to trial under federal law, the whistle-blower must first exhaust his or her internal chain of command and then file a complaint with the Department of Health and Human Services (DHHS). If the DHHS decides that the complaint is valid, the government proceeds with litigation against the employer, and the whistle-blower receives a percentage of the damages awarded. The case discussed earlier in this chapter involving the two nurses in Missouri who alleged nursing home abuse and fraud was a FCA *qui tam* lawsuit.

One recent case involving the FCA occurred with Good Shepherd Hospice (a for-profit hospice headquartered in Oklahoma City that provides hospice services in Oklahoma, Missouri, Kansas, and Texas), which agreed to pay $4 million to settle allegations that it submitted false claims for hospice patients who were not terminally ill (Schwarz, 2015). "Medicare's hospice benefit is available to patients with terminal illnesses and a life expectancy of six months or less. When a Medicare patient receives hospice services, that patient is no longer entitled to Medicare coverage for care designed to cure their illness. Here, the government alleged that Good Shepherd knowingly submitted or caused the submission of false claims for hospice care for patients who were not terminally ill" (Schwarz, 2015, para. 1).

Schmitt (2014) details the story of a strip mall with two dozen or so health care businesses listed on the building's directory. Yet, when visited by the US DHHS, the offices were empty, despite one of the businesses billing Medicare for $2.2 million in 3 months in 2007. Schmitt also details the story of a Los Angeles doctor charged with conspiracy in connection with a $33 million scheme in which he allegedly signed prescriptions and other documents for medically unnecessary home health services, hospice service, and durable medical equipment. The prescriptions were then allegedly used by supply companies and other firms to bilk Medicare.

Similarly, Schwarz (2014) noted that in a nationwide takedown by Medicare Fraud Strike Force operations, 90 people, including 27 doctors, nurses, and other medical professionals, were charged for their alleged participation in fraud schemes involving approximately $260 million in false billings to Medicare. The defendants were charged with various health care fraud-related crimes including submitting claims to Medicare for treatments that were either not provided or not necessary, recruiters paying kickbacks to get Medicare billing numbers of patients so that providers could submit fraudulent bills to Medicare, supplying motorized wheelchairs that were not needed, and conspiring to bill Medicare for medically unnecessary home health services.

Another case in which a *qui tam* lawsuit was filed occurred when a former employee at a nursing home in Tennessee filed a lawsuit after he was fired for pointing out instances of Medicare and Medicaid fraud at the nursing home (Rosenfeld, 2011). The employee alleged that the nursing home was double-billing for some patient services as well as billing Medicare and Medicaid for the care of unqualified patients. Vanguard denied any wrongdoing, but did pay back US$2 million as compensation for the amount it allegedly overbilled the federal health care systems (Rosenfeld, 2011).

Because the FCA has been fairly effective in detecting fraud at the federal level, state versions of the FCA have also passed. Under these state laws, whistle-blowers can file lawsuits seeking lost monies in the state or local government's name and share in the proceeds.

Other Federal Legislation Related to Whistle-Blowing

Another piece of legislation, the *Whistleblower Protection Act of 1989*, protects federal employees who disclose government fraud, abuse, and waste. The *Whistleblower Protection Enhancement Act of 2007* extended the *Whistleblower Protection Act of 1989* to federal employees who specialize in national security issues. In addition, the *Paul Revere Freedom to Warn Act* protects federal employee whistle-blowers who speak out about abuse, harassment, and unethical behavior in the workplace.

The National Labor Relations Act might protect employees in the private sector from retaliation when employees act as a group to modify working conditions or ask for better wages. The best protection for employees who work for publicly traded companies or companies that are required to file certain reports with the SEC in the United States at this time, however, is likely the *Sarbanes-Oxley Act of 2002* (further amended by the *Dodd-Frank Wall Street Reform and Consumer Protection Act* in 2010). This act dramatically redesigned federal regulation of public company corporate governance and reporting obligations and provided some protection for whistle-blowers who report fraud in publicly traded companies to the proper authorities (Joseph & Kirschenbaum, LLP, 2015).

Employees in these companies who experience retaliation for whistle-blowing have 180 days to file a written complaint with OSHA. If the evidence supports an employee's claim of retaliation and a settlement cannot be reached, OSHA will issue an order requiring the employer to reinstate the employee, pay back wages, and restore benefits (Occupational Safety and Health Administration [OSHA], 2011, para. 11). After OSHA issues its final ruling, either party may request a full hearing before an administrative law judge of the Department of Labor. That decision can then be appealed to the Department's Administrative Review Board for final review.

WHISTLE-BLOWING AS AN INTERNATIONAL ISSUE

Whistle-blowing cases involving nurses are not limited to the United States. In November 2014, the U.S. SEC issued its Annual Report to Congress on the Dodd-Frank Whistleblower Program. The report notes that during 2014, the Commission received submissions from individuals in all 50 states, as well as from individuals in 60 countries (Foose et al., 2015). The highest numbers of international reports came from the UK, Canada, Australia, China, and India, with the most coming from the UK (70 reports). After a lengthy study by a commission formed by the Bank of England and the U.K. Financial Conduct Authority (FCA), the commission rejected US-style "bounties" for individuals who report financial crimes to government authorities (Foose et al., 2015).

The lack of protection for whistle-blowers, then, is a global problem. Boumil, Nariani, Boumil, & Berman (2010) suggest that international adoption of legislation such as the FCA or qui tam laws would do much to expose fraud and increase the protection for whistle-blowers from retaliation globally.

Discussion Point

Would international adoption of legislation similar to the FCA increase the likelihood that whistle-blowers will both come forward and be protected from recrimination globally?

Conclusions

Nurses as health care professionals have a responsibility to uncover, openly discuss, and condemn shortcuts that threaten the clients they serve. Clearly, however, there has been a collective silence in many such cases. The reality is that whistle-blowing offers no guarantee that the situation will change or the problem will improve, and the literature is replete with horror stories regarding negative consequences endured by whistle-blowers. The whistle-blower cannot even trust that other health care professionals with similar belief systems about advocacy will value their efforts because the public's feelings about whistle-blowers are so mixed. In addition, state laws vary, and protections for the nongovernment employee whistle-blower are often limited.

For all these reasons, it takes tremendous courage to come forward as a whistle-blower. It also takes a tremendous sense of what is right and what is wrong, as well as a commitment to follow a problem through until an acceptable level of resolution is reached. Whistle-blowers are heroes and should be treated as such; their courage is nothing short of exceptional. How unfortunate that we frequently do not treat them that way.

For Additional Discussion

1. Why do Americans have a "love–hate" relationship with whistle-blowers? Is this dichotomy prevalent in other countries as well?
2. Which is greater for you personally—your duty to your patients, your duty to your employer, or your duty to yourself? How do you sort out what you should do when these duties are in conflict?
3. Do you believe that most whistle-blowing must be external before appropriate action is taken?
4. Should whistle-blowers receive compensation under the FCA?
5. Would you be willing to bear the risks of becoming a whistle-blower?
6. Do you believe that there is more, less, or the same amount of whistle-blowing in health care as in other types of industries?
7. Can you identify a whistle-blowing situation in which it might be appropriate to go outside the chain of command in reporting concerns about organizational practice?

References

American Nurses Association. (2015). *Code of ethics for nurses with interpretive statements.* Silver Spring, MD: Author.

Blecher, B. M. (2001–2015). *What color is your whistle?* Minority Nurse Magazine (Archived). Retrieved February 20, 2015, from http://minoritynurse.com/?s=what+color+is+your+whistle%3F

Boumil, S., Nariani, A., Boumil, M., & Berman, H. (2010). Whistleblowing in the pharmaceutical industry in the United States, England, Canada, and Australia. *Journal of Public Health Policy, 31*(1), 17–29.

Cable News Network. (2014, October 16). Whistle-blower nurse: I would do anything and everything not to be a patient there. *Anderson Cooper 360˚.* Retrieved March 8, 2015, from http://ac360.blogs.cnn.com/2014/10/16/whistleblower-nurse-i-would-do-anything-and-everything-not-to-be-a-patient-there/

Colvin, G. (2002). Wonder women of whistleblowing. *Fortune, 146*(3). Retrieved February 20, 2015, from http://money.cnn.com/magazines/fortune/fortune_archive/2002/08/12/327047/index.htm

Foose, A., Penman, C., & Petry, E. (2015). *2015 trends: #8 top whistleblowing priorities for compliance professionals.* Sausalito, CA: JD Supra. Retrieved March 20, 2015, from http://www.jdsupra.com/legalnews/2015-trends-8-top-whistleblowing-prior-00132/

Hill, T. (2010). Whistleblowing: The patient or the paycheck? *Kansas Nurse, 85*(2), 4–8.

IV Infusion Home. (2015, February 22). Whistleblowing and nursing practice [Web log post]. Retrieved March 19, 2015, from https://ivinfusion.wordpress.com/2015/02/22/whistleblowing-and-nursing-practice/

Joseph & Kirschenbaum, LLP. (2015). *Whistleblower and Sarbanes-Oxley claims.* New York, NY: Author. Retrieved March 20, 2015, from http://www.jhllp.com/lawyer-attorney-1324989.html

Lachman, V. D. (2008). Whistleblowers: Troublemakers or virtuous nurses? *Medsurg Nursing, 17*(2), 126–128, 134.

Marquis, B., & Huston, C. (2015). *Leadership roles and management functions in nursing* (8th ed.). Philadelphia, PA: Lippincott Williams & Wilkins.

Mason, D. J. (2011, January 14). Public officials indicted in RN whistleblowing case [Web log post]. Retrieved November 6, 2011, from http://centerforhealthmediapolicy.com/2011/01/14/public-officials-indicted-in-rn-whistleblowing-case/

Matthewson, K. (2012, January 22). What's ethical about whistleblowing? *The Corporate Social Responsibility Newswire*. Retrieved March 20, 2015, from http://www.csrwire.com/blog/posts/280-what-s-ethical-about-whistleblowing

McKee, C. (2013, September 23). Whistleblower ethics. *America Press*. Retrieved March 19, 2015, from http://www.americamagazine.org/issue/whistleblower-ethics

North Carolina State University. (2015, March 2). Protections, not money, can boost internal corporate whistleblowing. *Science Daily*. Retrieved March 21, 2015, from http://www.sciencedaily.com/releases/2015/03/150302091701.htm

Occupational Safety and Health Administration. (2011). *OSHA fact sheet: Filing whistleblower complaints under the Sarbanes-Oxley Act*. Retrieved March 19, 2015, from http://www.osha.gov/Publications/osha-factsheet-sox-act.pdf

Peters, K., Luck, L., Hutchinson, M., Wilkes, L., Andrew, S., & Jackson, D. (2011). The emotional sequelae of whistleblowing: Findings from a qualitative study. *Journal of Clinical Nursing, 20*(19/20), 2907–2914.

Rohner, T. (2015, February 6). Whistle-blowing nurse wants action on Nunavut nursing scandal. *Nunatsiaq Online*. Retrieved February 18, 2015, from http://www.nunatsiaqonline.ca/stories/article/65674whistle-blowing_nurse_wants_action_on_nunavut_nursing_scandal/

Rosenfeld, J. (2011, November 22). *Nursing home operator to reimburse government for double billing*. Retrieved May 20, 2012, from http://www.nursinghomesabuseblog.com/whistleblower-qui-tam-claims/nursing-home-operator-to-reimburse-government-for-double-billing/

Sack, K. (2011, January 14). Sheriff charged in Texas whistle-blowing case. *The New York Times*. Retrieved November 7, 2011, from http://www.nytimes.com/2011/01/15/us/15nurses.html?_r=1

Schmitt, R. (2014, November). Medicare Special Report: Inside the Medicare strike force. *AARP Bulletin, 55*(9), 10–12.

Schulman, D. (2007). Office of special counsel's war on whistleblowers. *Mother Jones*. Retrieved August 17, 2008, from http://www.motherjones.com/news/feature/2007/05/dont_whistle_while_you_work.html

Schwarz, K. (2014, May 23). Case of the week: 90 people charged with submitting more than $260 million in false claims to Medicare. *WhistleblowerLaws*. Retrieved March 8, 2015, from http://www.whistleblowerlaws.com/submitting-million-medicare/

Schwarz, K. (2015, February 26). Case of the week: Good Shepherd Hospice to pay $4 million to resolve allegations of fraudulent billing in violation of the false claims act. *WhistleblowerLaws*. Retrieved March 8, 2015, from http://www.whistleblowerlaws.com/allegations-fraudulent-violation/

Smith, R. (2008, May 24). A Morgan Stanley crusader: Bond-pricing issues prompt one broker's inside investigation. *The Wall Street Journal* (Eastern edition, p. B1). Retrieved May 20, 2012, from http://online.wsj.com/article/SB121158398445518845.html

Solomon, N. (2015, February 4). Convicting sterling to chill whistleblowing. *Consoritumnews.com*. Retrieved February 18, 2015, from https://consortiumnews.com/2015/02/04/convicting-sterling-to-chill-whistleblowing/

Whistleblower [Definition]. (2003–2015). In *The Free Online Dictionary*. Retrieved February 21, 2015, from http://www.thefreedictionary.com/whistleblower

Whistleblowing [Definition]. (2015). In *Dictionary.com*. Retrieved February. 20, 2015, from http://dictionary.reference.com/browse/whistleblowing?s=t

WhistleblowerLaws. (2014). *What is a qui tam?* Retrieved March 9, 2015 from http://www.whistleblowerlaws.com/what-is-qui-tam/

Wilkes, L. M., Peters, K., Weaver, R., & Jackson, D. (2011). Nurses involved in whistleblowing incidents: Sequelae for their families. *Collegian, 18*(3), 101–106.

20

Impaired Nursing Practice
Is Progress Being Made?

Jennifer Lillibridge

ADDITIONAL RESOURCES

Visit thePoint for additional helpful resources

- eBook
- Journal Articles
- WebLinks

CHAPTER OUTLINE

LEARNING OBJECTIVES

The learner will be able to:

1. Examine the prevalence of substance abuse in the nursing profession.
2. Describe early risk factors that result in an increased risk of chemical addiction in the nursing profession.
3. Identify links between national nursing policies about impaired practice and local implementation of strategies to address the problem.
4. Describe some of the challenges and barriers nurses face when confronting and/or helping an impaired colleague.
5. Explore the concept of drug diversion and how nurses and managers can prevent or detect drug diversion in the workplace.
6. Examine the role of nursing education in the prevention of impaired nursing practice.
7. Examine the role of nurse leaders in the workplace in the prevention of impaired nursing practice.
8. Explore reasons why nurses with substance abuse problems often fail to receive the same caring attitude or approach from their peers that is extended to other individuals who misuse drugs and alcohol.
9. Identify State Board of Nursing reporting requirements for nurses suspected of chemical dependency or of diverting drugs for personal use.
10. Describe typical components of a state diversion program, as well as a "return to work" agreement, for a chemically impaired nurse.

(continues on page 294)

11. Identify the driving forces that compelled most State Boards of Nursing in the United States to move from mandatory disciplinary action for impaired nurses to diversion program treatment.

12. Reflect on personal feelings regarding the extent to which a State Board of Nursing has the right and/or responsibility to invade the impaired nurse's privacy to ensure recovery is ongoing.

INTRODUCTION

"Helping the impaired nurse is difficult but not impossible. The choices for action are varied. The only choice that is clearly wrong is to do nothing" (National Council of State Boards of Nursing [NCSBN], 2001, p. iv). Definitions of impaired practice vary, but most include that professional judgment is impaired due to the use of drugs or alcohol (or mental illness) and that this compromises patient safety.

The problem of impaired nursing practice has plagued nursing for decades; however, it continues to remain both underresearched and underreported. Monroe and Kenaga (2010) suggest that some of the reasons rest with the taboo nature of the topic among many health care providers and nursing school faculty and staff. In addition, the NCSBN (Darbro, 2011) suggests that stigma and negative stereotyping also leads to underreporting as well as "the tendency to protect or ignore workplace indicators of problem behaviors" (p. 42).

A discussion about impaired nursing practice often raises more questions than it answers. Two key issues surround impaired nursing practice. The first is concern for patient safety. The second is concern for the health of the impaired nurse. With denial being common, the problem can go undetected or untreated for years. Typically, patient harm from drug diversion by nurses can occur in several ways, such as being denied pain medication, receiving an unsafe substitution or reduced dose of medication, and receiving injections from contaminated needles, syringes, or vials (Kunyk & Austin, 2011; New, 2014). Supervisory actions to protect patients are shown in Box 20.1.

Without wanting to discount the individual nurse with a substance abuse problem, patient safety has been at the forefront of national considerations about professional nursing practice and the future of nursing since the seminal publication by the Institute of Medicine, *To Error Is Human* (1999), and has been reinforced repeatedly in the literature (Cook, 2013; Kunyk, 2015). Given this agenda, it seems critical that preventing impaired practice and dealing with it when it does happen should be inclusive in all discussions about patient safety. Kunyk (2015) states, "If active and hidden, SUD [substance use disorder] presents threats to patient safety, the health of nurses with these disorders and to the professional image of nursing" (p. 54).

BOX 20.1 Three Supervisory Actions to Protect Patients

Check in Early	Correct Early	Contain the Risk
Follow routine procedures	Investigate further	Escort nurse from practice setting immediately
Conduct check-in meetings	Document the facts	Follow policy for fitness evaluation
Observe and assess nurse performance	Request on-demand meeting when indicated	Request alcohol and drug screen
Document safe practice	Follow disciplinary procedures if warranted	Document the facts
Submit routine written reports	Report a compliance issue immediately	Submit incident report

Source: O'Neill, C., & Cadiz, D. (2014). Worksite monitors protect patients from unsafe nursing practices. *Journal of Nursing Regulation, 5*(2), 22.

PREVALENCE OF THE PROBLEM

Estimates on the prevalence of chemical dependency in the nursing profession are varied; efforts to quantify the prevalence are fraught with problems. It has been suggested that the difficulty may be due in part to the fact that self-disclosure is reduced due to the stigma, shame, and denial associated with substance abuse (Kunyk, 2015). Estimates often state that prevalence mirrors statistics from the general population. The American Nurses Association (ANA) estimate of 6% to 8% is dated; NCSBN (2011a) reports other estimates of between 10% and 15%. Another estimate suggests "between 10 and 20 percent of nurses will have a substance abuse problem at some point in their lives" ("I Think," 2011, p. 24). Kunyk's (2015) recent study in Canada supports the suggestion that the prevalence of substance use disorder in nursing is similar to that in the general population.

Previously, it has been suggested that prevalence is not as important as patterns of abuse among health professionals, such as physicians and nurses. Although patterns of abuse may still be important, the critical consideration must be the behavior of the nurse and whether the nurse is making safe, appropriate decisions in the provision of quality patient care.

Consider This Given current estimates of impaired nursing practice, it is likely that 1 out of every 10 nurses you work with will struggle with a substance use problem.

OVERVIEW OF THE LITERATURE

While gaps about many issues related to impaired practice continue to exist, research on this persistent problem is beginning to emerge. Kunyk (2015) investigated the prevalence of substance use disorder in nurses and impaired nursing practice, including nurse health, in a disciplinary jurisdiction in Canada. Underreporting, which has been identified as a significant problem with impaired practice, was also found in Kunyk's study. Over 95% of self-identified impaired nurses were currently employed and unknown to their employers as having a substance use problem. This finding highlights the critical nature of substance use disorder as impaired nurses continue to put patients and themselves at risk. Cook (2013) conducted a study to examine whether nurses could trust their recovering (from substance use) colleagues in direct care. Cook discovered that nurses were willing to trust recovering nurses and found strong agreement that they should be able to return to work in health care. Although a small study, this finding might suggest a change in perceptions of nurses generally that previously were thought to not take care of their own.

Bettinardi-Angres and Bologeorges (2011) focused on the challenges of confronting/reporting impaired work colleagues, and found that most nurses were not comfortable confronting or reporting a suspected impaired colleague. Several consistent reasons were cited, such as lack of knowledge of chemical dependence in the workplace and lack of clear protocols or policies about intervention. Burman and Dunphy (2011) explored the barriers that exist with advanced practice nurses confronting a colleague in which they believed practice misconduct had occurred due to substance abuse. These authors recommended standardizing practices, discussing ethical obligations, and addressing institutional policies and procedures.

Boulton and Nosek (2014) investigated the perceptions of nursing students and substance abusing nurses. They found that students generally had positive perceptions of nurses with a substance use problem and that these perceptions were reinforced with education. A nonstatistically significant finding supported previous research that nursing education falls short of effectively preparing nurses to identify and respond supportively to an impaired colleague. Participants also believed that even after exposure to an educational program on the topic, they would not be able to recognize or support an impaired nurse. The authors suggest this might be indicative of the reluctance of the profession to deal with the problem.

While there is no consistent theme in recent literature on substance use disorder among nurses, nursing students, and health care professionals generally, it is encouraging to note that research is being conducted and that the topic remains active. However, without comprehensive empirically based research, there is limited help for the profession to move closer toward prevention, recognition, management, and resolution of the problem, if indeed resolution is even possible.

Discussion Point

Why hasn't more nursing research been conducted that explores the experiences and perspectives of nurses with a substance use disorder?

Identifying Early Risk Factors for Substance Abuse

The very nature of the work of nurses seems to be challenged when risk factors are considered. Nurses have constant access to narcotics, and fatigue seems to come with the job, no matter what shift is worked. It is difficult to avoid job strain in the current health care environment, which is in the middle of the worst nursing shortage ever reported. Despite the difficulties inherent in the practice setting today, many nurses do work hard to get experience and increase knowledge so they can become specialists, only to find this, too, can put them at higher risk of turning to drugs or alcohol when coping is difficult. These issues highlight the complexity of the problem for the profession, requiring that all nurses become more aware of how to prevent it from occurring.

Discussion Point

Workplace risk factors for nurses are access, stress, lack of education, and attitude. Whose responsibility is it to address these issues?

Darbro and Malliarakis (2012) analyzed specific risk factors that affect nurses. They identified them as specialty, gender, and workplace, as well as the more general risk factors that apply to everyone. Unique to the article is the discussion of what is termed "protective factors," which would assist nurses to avoid destructive coping that leads to a substance use disorder as well as to recover from an existing problem. Identification of risk factors has been presented in previous literature; the more interesting component of the article is discussion of the protective factors. Workplace protective factors include work satisfaction, workplace social support, and workplace constraints regarding use. Identifying these areas highlights the importance of the role of the workplace and employers in the prevention and support for nurses with a substance use problem and those nurses who might be at risk.

National: Impaired Practice Position and Policies

For policies to be in place at the local level, it is imperative that there be support from leading national nursing organizations about impaired practice. The ANA's position about impaired practice can be found on its website. The ANA (2015) supports treatment as opposed to discipline and a process that facilitates reentry of the recovered nurse back into practice.

The American Association of Colleges of Nursing (AACN, 1998) focuses on policy development in nursing education. Their policy was written in 1994 and updated in 1998. The AACN's policy can be found on its website. The policy has guidelines for prevention and management of substance abuse in the nursing education community. There are specific features that address the issue for students, faculty, and staff. Critical to successful policy development is attention to confidentiality and legal perspectives. From the perspective of process and content, the necessary areas are identification, intervention, evaluation, treatment, and reentry into practice. The AACN is in agreement with the ANA regarding the importance of treatment over a reasonable time frame and a process for successful reentry into practice.

The NCSBN published *Substance Use Disorder in Nursing* in 2011a, and the manual can be found on their website. The purpose of the *Substance Use Disorder in Nursing* manual "is to provide practical and evidence-based guidelines for evaluating, treating and managing nurses with a substance use disorder" (NCSBN, 2011b, p. 16). As with the AACN and the ANA, the NCSBN also supports early detection and treatment of the impaired nurse with the goal of returning a recovered nurse to work. National nursing organizations support alternative to discipline programs in the treatment of substance use disorder in nursing.

Local: Impaired Practice Policies in the Workplace

In keeping with the position at the national level, it is imperative that health care organizations and educational institutions have a policy in place about impaired practice that clearly identifies the process to be followed if a substance use problem is suspected. A commitment to a drug- and alcohol-free educational setting or workplace environment is critical to policy development. Some state boards of nursing have detailed documents about return to work processes, such as those outlined by the Massachusetts Nurses Association (2011). Their guidebook of interventions and resources about impaired nursing practice provides detailed information about topics such as how to assist a nurse with a substance use problem, an algorithm, available resources, legal considerations, and a sample return to work agreement.

Nurses Reporting an Impaired Colleague—Issues and Ethics

It is a difficult and often traumatic experience for a nurse to report an impaired peer. The important considerations are that patients are not harmed, the nurse is helped, and the provider is protected. It is the responsibility of every nurse to be aware of reporting requirements when a colleague is suspected of substance abuse or of diverting drugs for personal use. No uniform agreement exists among the states as to what those reporting requirements are. Information regarding reporting requirements can be found from each State Board of Nursing, which can often be easily accessed via its website. Before a nurse can be reported or referred to a treatment program, there must be recognition that the nurse needs help. Recognizing that a nurse is impaired might not be easy and has been addressed in the literature as an area in which nurses lack knowledge and skills, making them uncomfortable to act.

Consider This Considering your nursing education, practice experience, and workplace support, how comfortable do you feel in recognizing and reporting an impaired colleague?

In theory, reporting an impaired nurse seems like a decision that would be easy to make. The position of the ANA and other nursing organizations is clear: It is the ethical and legal duty of a nurse to advocate for public safety, their colleagues, and the profession (Burman & Dunphy, 2011). This means simply that it is a nurse's job to protect the patient from harm; if that means reporting an impaired colleague, that is what one must do. In practice, however, the situation is anything but clear.

Research conducted with both nurses and physicians suggests that although both groups of professionals understand the need for reporting an impaired colleague, most do not report (Bettinardi-Angres & Bologeorges, 2011; DesRoches et al., 2011). Previous literature suggests that there is a "code of silence" about impaired practice. However, these newer studies suggest that other reasons are responsible for a lack of peer reporting.

In the DesRoches et al. (2011) study, the main reason physicians did not report seemed to be that they thought someone else was dealing with the problem. However, Bettinardi-Angres and Bologeorges (2011) found the reasons were more complex. These authors identified some barriers as lack of general knowledge of substance abuse in the workplace, lack of a clear protocol or process for reporting or intervening, and lack of compassion in the workplace for peers. They also found that the word *confrontation* itself was a barrier to reporting and that perhaps more compassionate terminology would help, such as assisting a nurse, addressing a problem, and so forth. While the removal of all barriers might not be realistic, Cook's (2013) findings that nurses were willing to report an impaired colleague suggest that some barriers might be lessening (Research Study Fuels the Controversy 20.1).

Drug Diversion

Identifying and investigating drug diversion is a current topic in health care literature and is critical to consider when examining impaired nursing practice. New (2014) discusses the harm that drug diversion can cause to patients, staff members, the community, and diverting nurses. New stresses the importance of all health care facilities having in place comprehensive preemployment screening, drug security, diversion-risk rounds, and a clear policy in place for investigation of drug diversion if it is suspected. The importance of programs to detect and prevent drug diversion is supported by recent publications from the Mayo Clinic (Berge, Dillion, Sikkink, Taylor, & Lanier, 2012; Lien, 2012) that has instituted policies in an effort to improve patient safety. These authors also focus on the harm that is extended beyond the patient to other health care workers, and to employers. Also highlighted is the significance of education for all health care workers, as many may not be aware of the serious nature of the problem.

Dittman (2012) investigated male nurses' perspectives on impaired professionals. Findings of this phenomenological study included that "lack of awareness, poor adherence to drug control procedures, and apathy of reporting impaired practitioners provided a culture where their diversion thrived" (p. 39). Findings from this study suggest that drug diversion may persist due to the lack of automated processes required to discourage self-medication administration and/or diversion. Automated systems and appropriate management oversights may identify medication diversion early so that nurses could be removed from practice, evaluated, and offered a recovery program so that they could be returned to the profession. This would help ensure a safe environment for the nurse and the patient.

Wright (2013) examines factors that contribute to drug diversion that have been identified elsewhere, such as increases in workload, mandatory overtime, floating to unfamiliar units, fatigue, and medical issues requiring the need for prescription pain medication.

Research Study Fuels the Controversy 20.1

The Issue of Trust: Can Nurses Trust Nurses in Recovery Reentering the Workplace?

While much research has highlighted the reluctance of nurses to report an impaired colleague or determine the causes that nurses divert drugs for personal use, this researcher-designed quantitative study examined direct care nurses' ability to trust nurses in recovery from substance use disorders reentering the workplace. Trust is critical in a caring profession such as nursing, yet there is a paucity of research into the important consideration as to whether nurses returning to work will be trusted and accepted by their colleagues, which potentially affects the success of the reentry program.

Source: Cook, L. (2013, March). Can nurses trust nurses in recovery reentering the workplace? *Nursing, 43*(3), 21–24.

Study Findings

The study found that most nurses would report a nurse colleague that was impaired in a variety of circumstances including alcohol, illegal drugs, prescription medication and drug diversion. Nearly 75% of nurses had worked with an impaired colleague in their career. While nurses were willing to work with nurses recovering from alcohol (96%) or drug addiction (90%), they were less likely to trust a nurse who had diverted medication from patients (61%). The majority of nurses thought their recovering colleagues should be allowed to return to work in health care.

An important implication of this study is that most nurses wanted to help nurses in recovery but were not knowledgeable about substance use disorder generally, how to help a colleague, or find support about treatment programs. Other studies about the specific concept of trust could not be found, but further investigation in this area might improve understanding about how to better educate nurses about substance use disorder in the profession as well as providing support for nurses in recovery when they return to work.

A common factor identified in the literature is the easy access nurses have to controlled substances. Other issues identified that contribute to the problem are the reluctance of nurses to believe that a trusted colleague is diverting drugs. Wright highlights the importance of professional awareness in recognizing and combating drug diversion, and presents eight strategies to identify and detect drug diversion. While identification and detection are critical, only one of the eight strategies focuses on education programs about stress management and coping techniques that might prevent drug diversion before it occurs.

Investigated by a medical center were three dimensions related to workplace access that influenced diverting behaviors. These included "perceived availability of controlled substances, frequency of administration, and the degree of workplace control" (Rohman, 2012, p. 29). Following a lengthy process of trial and error, the facility adopted a drug diversion surveillance program that included a public safety officer, the director of public safety, director of pharmacy, and appropriate nurse leaders. This process identified nurses who were diverting drugs. An unexpected outcome of this process was an increased awareness of direct care nurses about appropriate policies and procedures for medication administration that were not being followed.

While having policies about drug diversion in place is important for patient safety and for the health and safety of the diverting nurse, another issue receiving limited discussion in the literature is how to prevent drug diversion and possibly addiction initially. This involves consideration of education and the environment in which nurses work. Contributing workplace factors are mentioned, but a thorough dialogue of the impact these factors have on leading to impaired practice was not found.

Boulton and Nosek (2014) suggest that nursing students are not taught how to recognize an impaired colleague or what to do about it if they did. For nurse educators, are students being taught how to keep themselves healthy as they deal with the often traumatic nature of nursing? If not, this means the new generation of nursing graduates may not have the necessary tools to help address this serious problem. If schools of nursing do not consider this content a critical component of the curriculum, how is the problem ever going to be satisfactorily addressed? What are health care facilities doing to prevent or discourage drug diversion prior to it occurring? For nurse leaders, are nurses working in a toxic environment that is fraught with short staffing, trauma, and stress that all can contribute to a nurse turning to drug diversion as a way to cope? The challenge then becomes not only putting in place surveillance programs to detect and investigate drug diversion, but also mechanisms to support a population of nurses that are increasingly being taxed to their limit so that they remain healthy and their patients remain safe. Box 20.2 lists some of the common methods of drug diversion.

Discussion Point

You suspect that a coworker/friend is diverting drugs for personal use. You find yourself covering up for her because you know that she is depressed, exhausted, and having family problems. Your supervisor makes a casual comment with similar suspicions. Your first instinct is to make excuses for your friend; what would you do?

Consider This Most addiction specialists and the American Medical Association view addiction as a chronic medical illness and argue that it should be approached in an analogous way to, say, diabetes or asthma.

Alternative to Discipline Programs

Although most states now offer treatment options, the types of programs vary. The first treatment program offered was the Intervention Project for Nurses (IPN, 2015) in Florida in 1983. The IPN has a comprehensive website offering information about the history of the program, including frequently asked questions and available services.

California also offers a diversion program; information is available from the California Board of Registered Nursing (CBRN). Established in 1985, its goal is to "protect the public by early identification of impaired registered nurses and by providing these nurses access to appropriate intervention programs and treatment services" (CBRN, 2011, para. 2). Impaired nurses can be self-referred or can be referred by family, coworkers, or the board. All licensed registered nurses residing in California are eligible to enter the program, but they must agree to enter the program voluntarily. Since 1985, more than 1,900 nurses have successfully completed the diversion program in California. Requirements for completion include "a change in lifestyle that supports continuing recovery and [having] a minimum of 24 consecutive months of clean, random, body-fluid tests" (CBRN, 2011, para. 14). Law protects the confidentiality of participants, and nurses who successfully complete the program have their records regarding chemical impairment destroyed.

A different approach is followed in the Texas Peer Assistance Program (TPNAP) for Nurses. This program offers services to nurses suffering from chemical dependency, as well as from anxiety and other mental health disorders. It requires abstinence, maintains confidentiality, is strictly voluntary, and is independent of the state licensing board (TPNAP, n.d.). Information from the TPNAP website includes how and when to make

BOX 20.2 Common Methods of Diversion

- Removal of medication when a patient does not need it
- Removal of medication for a discharged patient
- Removal of a duplicate dose
- Removal of fentanyl patches
- Removal of medication without an order
- Removal under a colleague's sign-on
- Substitution of a noncontrolled substance for a controlled substance
- Theft of patient medications brought from home
- Failure to waste when indicated
- Frequent wasting of entire doses

Source: New, K. (2014). Preventing, detecting, and investigating drug diversion in health care facilities. *Journal of Nursing Regulation, 5*(1), 18–23.

referrals, how the program works, and important links to services and organizations.

> **Consider This** Although most states lean toward treatment rather than discipline for substance use problems, many nurses still attach a stigma and think that impaired nurses should be punished and not allowed to return to work.

The Recovered Nurse: Reentry Into Practice

When a nurse has completed a treatment or rehabilitation program and is ready to return to work, he or she typically encounters a number of issues. These issues include whether the nurse's practice is limited or restricted in some way, how long the nursing board has a right to invade the nurse's privacy to ensure that recovery is ongoing, where organizational responsibility ends, who bears the cost if the nurse does not return to work at full capacity, and ensuring that confidentiality is maintained (Box 20.3).

Although many anecdotal or discussion articles were found on the topic of what constitutes a disciplinary or treatment approach to impaired practice, limited information was found that addressed the concerns of reentry of the impaired nurse to the practice setting.

O'Neill and Cadiz (2014) propose that the monitoring of a recovered nurse requires two agreements, one between the nurse and the external body, such as a disciplinary board or alternative to discipline program. The second agreement is with the employer and may be in the form of an individualized contract with the nurse. This document would outline the terms and conditions in which the nurse can return to direct care.

Despite a lack of standardized guidelines, there are some general considerations that should be taken into account when a recovered nurse returns to work. To protect patient safety, practice restrictions may be in place for a varying time, depending on the length of the program and whether it was treatment based or disciplinary action occurred. It is important that staff nurses realize the commitment of the recovering nurse to reestablish his or her career and continue in the profession.

Most Board of Registered Nursing websites offer little information about the reentry process. Instead, they focus primarily on what should be done if someone suspects an impaired colleague, how to report it, the treatment or disciplinary action once impairment is identified, and the specific aspects of each program. A question that is left unanswered is how long the board follows a recovered nurse in terms of random drug testing. Some hospitals or health care agencies already do random drug testing, so the question of invasion of privacy has in some instances already been dealt with.

> **Discussion Point**
>
> You just came from a staff meeting at which the nurse-manager informed everyone that a substance abuse recovered nurse would begin working on the unit in a few weeks. Some nurses had the attitude that the nurse not be allowed back to work because he or she could not be trusted. How would you respond to your colleagues?

Research Dissemination—Is It Happening?

While there are some new research findings to disseminate, the question still needs to be asked: Are the profession and education community applying/using what findings are available? Issues have been raised about

BOX 20.3 Issues to Consider When the Recovered Nurse Returns to Work

- Should the nurse returning to work following rehabilitation have his or her practice limited or restricted in some way, such as no exposure to the drug of choice or no access to controlled substances for a period of time?
- How long does the Board of Nursing have a right to invade the privacy of a recovered nurse?
- Where does the organizational responsibility end?
- Who bears the cost if the recovered nurse is not able to return to work at full capacity?
- Can confidentiality be maintained?
- Should the nurse be allowed to work in stressful practice areas?
- Should the nurse initially be allowed to work full time?

student substance abuse. If you work in an educational setting or interact with students in your workplace, do you know what policies are in place if a student is suspected of impaired practice? More important, what is being done in the educational community to address the issue of alcohol and substance use by students that might be affecting their performance in the clinical setting? Is impaired nursing practice part of the nursing curricula, and if not, why not? As suggested by the AACN (1998), it is critical that policies regarding impaired practice be clear and in place in the educational community and that all faculty and students be aware of the content of the policy.

The literature clearly supports that impaired practice policies should be in place in every health care setting. However, anecdotal evidence suggests that many nurses in clinical practice have no knowledge of such policies and would not know what to do if they suspected a colleague was impaired. Impaired practice policies should be introduced during hospital orientation for new employees and during annual renewal of hospital safety procedures. This would highlight the issue for everyone and put the problem clearly in the spotlight, especially if issues such as barriers to reporting an impaired colleague and prevalence of the problem were discussed. Nurses should be allowed to ask questions so that they are clear about the process of reporting and so that a nurse who is using substances irresponsibly knows where to go for help.

HOW CAN WE STOP LOSING NURSES TO SUBSTANCE ABUSE?

Preventative health care is finally receiving much needed attention in the media and in practice. Insurance companies are increasingly paying for prevention and screening procedures, yet many areas of health care still lag behind what would be ideal for preventative practices. The issue of preventing substance abuse is no exception to this situation. How can nurses individually and as a profession help to prevent the cycle of nurse addiction from starting?

Some of the risk factors for substance abuse that have been identified are difficult to modify. Nurses will always have easy access to narcotics, do shift work, and suffer from fatigue. The ongoing stress that has worked its way into clinical settings due to the nursing shortage seems a long way from dissipating. What, then, can be done to diminish the effects of these factors so that nurses do not turn to substances as an inappropriate coping mechanism?

Perhaps one avenue is to more fully explore the experiences of nurses who do not turn to substances. Do nurses who use self-care strategies to cope with a stressful work environment and to prevent burnout also use those same strategies to avoid harmful substance use? Perhaps this information about how nurses cope with difficulties of the workplace when they do not turn to drugs or alcohol will contribute to prevention.

Most research focuses on the nurse who abuses drugs, when a great deal could be learned about positive coping behaviors from nurses who manage stress without abusing drugs. Does the professional generally take a closer look at the protective factors outlined by Darbro and Malliarakis (2012) as a means to prevent a path to substance abuse?

Where does the education about substance abuse begin? Student nurses need to be made not only aware of the risks of substance abuse but also self-aware about their attitudes and beliefs regarding those who do abuse substances, whether those people are patients or colleagues. Nursing school is an incredibly stressful time for students. Appropriate education in nursing school could not only help to prevent the onset of substance abuse, but might also allow students to explore their feelings and beliefs about impaired practice. This increased self-awareness might help students to have empathy toward impaired nurses and encourage them to take the appropriate steps to assist a nurse or fellow student in getting help.

Nursing is going through a very tumultuous time. The nursing shortage is never far from the minds of most nurses as they struggle on a daily basis with low staffing levels and a stressed work setting. How this stress is channelled can lead a nurse to have positive or negative coping strategies. What are hospitals doing to acknowledge and diffuse this stress? Are nurses too stressed to seek counsel from each other when they have a particularly bad day? Are nurses debriefing with each other or at home so they can let go of the often traumatic nature of work and move forward? Nurses and nurse-managers need to answer these questions for their particular work settings to know whether they are doing enough for themselves, their colleagues, and their staff.

Conclusions

Losing one nurse to substance abuse is losing one nurse too many. We are a profession known for its caring nature toward others, yet we often fail to care for ourselves. The harmful coping strategies that lead to substance abuse can begin even before nursing school. Educating our students may help us to increase awareness about this ever-present problem. If new graduates can bring current information to their nursing practice and be self-aware about their attitudes, beliefs, and coping strategies, then perhaps they can come armed with more positive strategies to help them when times get tough.

Do we teach our students, new graduates, and seasoned nurses to ask for help when they need it, or do we expect them to "do it all?" All nurses who suspect an impaired colleague need to take action as they have an ethical, regulatory, and legal obligation in the interest of patient safety (Tanga, 2011). If all nurses are aware of the problem of substance use disorder and take the initiative to confront or intervene when they suspect a colleague of impaired practice, we are one step closer to decreasing the incidence of substance abuse in the nursing profession.

Finally, responsibility rests not just with individual nurses. Educators must accept the challenge to teach students about impaired practice and how to recognize it when they see it and, in addition, to assist them to develop positive coping strategies so they don't turn to substances to deal with stress. Employers must also accept the challenge to create a work environment that supports nurses to deal with stress successfully, to know employees so that confrontation can occur early, to increase awareness about substance abuse so that nurses are not afraid to ask for help, to support nurses if they do suspect drug diversion or an impaired colleague, to ensure that an impaired practice policy is in place, and lastly to provide a process that facilitates reentry into practice following recovery.

For Additional Discussion

1. Explore your attitudes and beliefs about impaired nursing practice. How would you treat a colleague suspected of diverting drugs for personal use? Would you trust a recovered nurse returning to work?
2. What kind of peer support exists in your work setting? How do staff debrief from stressful situations?
3. Should recovered nurses who return to work have a limited practice? If so, for how long, and with what types of limitations? How does this affect the workload of other nurses?
4. What practices are in place in your work setting that could deter a nurse from diverting drugs for personal use?
5. Have you known a colleague who was caught diverting drugs for personal use? If so, how was it handled? Did the nurse seek treatment and return to work? Could it have been managed better?
6. You are a nurse-manager for an intensive care unit and have been asked to talk to student nurses about impaired practice. What key points would you make?
7. Does your workplace have an impaired practice policy in place? If so, have you read it, and was it discussed during your initial hospital orientation? Is it discussed annually? If not, what might you do to ensure that one is in place?

References

American Association of Colleges of Nursing. (1998). *Substance abuse statement: Policy and guidelines for prevention and management of substance abuse in the nursing education community*. Retrieved from http://www.aacn.nche.edu/publications/position/substance-abuse-policy-and-guidelines

American Nurses Association. (2015). *Impaired nurse resource center*. Retrieved from http://nursingworld.org/MainMenuCategories/WorkplaceSafety/Healthy-Work-Environment/Work-Environment/ImpairedNurse

Berge, K. H., Dillion, K. R., Sikkink, K. M., Taylor, T. K., & Lanier, W. L. (2012). Diversion of drugs within health care facilities, a multiple-victim crime: Patterns of diversion, scope, consequences, detection, and prevention. *Mayo Clinic Proceedings, 87*(7), 674–682.

Bettinardi-Angres, K., & Bologeorges, S. (2011). Addressing chemically dependent colleagues. *Journal of Nursing Regulation, 2*(2), 10–15.

Boulton, M. A., & Nosek, L. J. (2014). How do nursing students perceive substance abusing nurses? *Archives of Psychiatric Nursing, 28*, 29–34.

Burman, M. E., & Dunphy, L. M. (2011). Reporting colleague misconduct in advanced practice nursing. *Journal of Nursing Regulation, 1*(4), 26–31.

California Board of Registered Nursing. (2011). *What is the diversion program?* Retrieved from http://www.rn.ca.gov/diversion/whatisdiv.shtml

Cook, L. M. (2013, March). Can nurses trust nurses in recovery reentering the workplace? *Nursing, 43*(3), 21–24.

Darbro, N. (2011). Model guidelines for alternative programs and discipline monitoring programs. *Journal of Nursing Regulation, 2*(1), 42–49.

Darbro, N., & Malliarakis, K. D. (2012). Substance abuse: Risk factors and protective factors. *Journal of Nursing Regulation, 3*(1), 44–48.

DesRoches, C. M., Rao, S. R., Fromson, R. J., Iezzoni, L., Vogeli, C., & Campbell, E. G. (2011). Physicians' perceptions, preparedness for reporting, and experiences related to impaired and incompetent colleagues. *Journal of the American Medical Association, 304*(2), 187–193.

Dittman, P. W. (2012). Mountains to climb: Male nurses and their perspective on professional impairment. *International Journal of Human Caring, 16*(1), 34–41.

"I think my colleague has a problem …" (2011). *The Canadian Nurse, 107*(3), 24–28.

Institute of Medicine. (1999). *To error is human: Building a safer health system.* Retrieved from http://www.nap.edu/catalog/9728/to-err-is-human-building-a-safer-health-system

Intervention Project for Nurses. (2015). *Intervention project for nurses: IPN History*. Retrieved from http://www.ipnfl.org/ipnhistory.html

Kunyk, D. (2015). Substance use disorders among registered nurses: Prevalence, risks and perceptions in a disciplinary jurisdiction. *Journal of Nursing Management, 23*, 54–64. doi:10.1111/jonm.12081

Kunyk, D., & Austin, W. (2011). Nursing under the influence: A relational ethics perspective. *Nursing Ethics, 19*(3), 380–389.

Lien, C. A. (2012). A need to establish programs to detect and prevent drug diversion. *Mayo Clinic Proceedings, 87*(7), 607–609.

Massachusetts Nurses Association. (2011). *Impaired practice in nursing: A guidebook for interventions and resources.* Canton, MA: Author. Retrieved from http://www.massnurses.org/files/file/Nursing-Resources/Nursing-Practice/Impaired_Practice.pdf

Monroe, T., & Kenaga, H. (2010). Don't ask don't tell: Substance abuse and addiction among nurses. *Journal of Clinical Nursing, 20*, 504–509. doi:10.1111/j.1365-2702.2010.03518.x

National Council of State Boards of Nursing. (2001). *Chemical dependency handbook for nurse managers.* Retrieved from https://www.ncsbn.org/chem_dep_handbook_intro_ch1.pdf

National Council of State Boards of Nursing. (2011a). *Substance use disorder in nursing.* Retrieved from https://www.ncsbn.org/SUDN_10.pdf

National Council of State Boards of Nursing. (2011b). *Substance use disorder in nursing: A resource manual and guidelines for alternative and disciplinary monitoring programs.* Retrieved from https://www.ncsbn.org/2038.htm

New, K. (2014). Preventing, detecting, and investigating drug diversion in health care facilities. *Journal of Nursing Regulation, 5*(1), 18–25.

O'Neill, C., & Cadiz, D. (2014). Worksite monitors protect patients from unsafe nursing practices. *Journal of Nursing Regulation, 5*(2), 22.

Rohman, C. (2012). Roads to recovery: Drug diversion surveillance programs. *Nursing Management, 43*(3), 28–31.

Tanga, H. Y. (2011). Nurse drug diversion and nursing leader's responsibilities: Legal, regulatory, ethical, humanistic, and practical considerations. *JONA'S Healthcare Law, Ethics and Regulation, 13*(1), 13–1

Texas Nurses Association. (n.d.). *Texas peer assistance program for nurses.* Retrieved from http://www.texasnurses.org/?page=TPAPN

Wright, R. L. (2013). Drug diversion in nursing practice: A call for professional accountability to recognize and respond. *Journal of the Association of Occupational Health Professionals in Healthcare, 33*(1), 27–30.

21

Collective Bargaining and the Professional Nurse

Carol J. Huston

ADDITIONAL RESOURCES

Visit thePoint for additional helpful resources

- eBook
- Journal Articles
- WebLinks

CHAPTER OUTLINE

LEARNING OBJECTIVES

The learner will be able to:

1. Explore possible motivations behind nurses' decisions to join or not join unions.
2. Identify major US legislation that has affected the ability of nurses to unionize over time.
3. Describe the shifting balance of power between unions and management in the United States over the last century and analyze the power balance that currently exists between the two entities.
4. Identify the largest unions representing health care employees, and nurses in particular.
5. Investigate the current status of rulings by the National Labor Relations Board and the courts regarding the definition of "supervisor" in nursing and the effect those rulings have on the eligibility of nurses for protection under the National Labor Relations Act.
6. Delineate common union organizing strategies as well as specific steps for starting a union.
7. Debate the potential conflicts inherent in having the American Nurses Association serve as both a professional association for all nurses and as a collective bargaining agent.
8. Explore the impact management has on creating a work environment that eliminates or reduces the need for unionization.

(continues on page 305)

This chapter is reproduced, in part, with permission from Marquis, B., & Huston, C. (2015). Understanding collective bargaining, unionization, and employment laws. In *Leadership roles and management functions in nursing* (8th ed., pp. 514–539). Philadelphia, PA: Lippincott Williams & Wilkins.

9. Reflect on whether going on strike can be viewed as an ethically appropriate action for professional nurses.
10. Explore his or her beliefs about whether belonging to unions, a practice historically reserved for blue-collar workers, undermines nursing's quest for increased recognition as a profession.

INTRODUCTION

There is likely no greater dichotomy than stereotypical images of gentle nurse angels of mercy and images of angry nurses in picket lines waving strike placards at passersby. Although both the images are stereotypical, they are at the heart of the debate about whether nursing, long recognized as a caring and altruistic profession, should be a part of collective bargaining efforts to improve working conditions.

Collective bargaining involves activities occurring between organized labor and management that concern employee relationships. Such activities include negotiation of formal labor agreements and day-to-day interactions between unions and management. A *labor union* (hereafter referred to as a *union*) is an organization of workers, often in a trade or profession, formed to protect their rights and interests and improve their economic status and working conditions through collective bargaining with employers.

Many nurses have strong feelings about unions and collective bargaining activities. Often these feelings have to do with their exposure to unions while growing up. Many nurses from working-class families were raised in a cultural milieu that promoted unionization. Other nurses know little about unions and know only what they have seen portrayed in the media. Some nurses, however, have been actively involved in collective bargaining in their place of employment and have emerged from the experience with either positive or negative impressions or a combination thereof.

Despite this tension, collective bargaining and unions are very much a part of many nurses' experiences. Union activity tends to change in response to workforce excesses and shortages. For decades, employment demand for nurses has increased and decreased periodically. High demand for nurses is tied directly to a healthy national economy, and, historically, this has been correlated with increased union activity. Similarly, when nursing vacancy rates are low, union membership and activity tend to decline.

Moberg (2013) notes that as of 2012, just over 18% of the nation's registered nurses (RNs) belonged to unions, down from almost 20% in 2008. Not only did the proportion of unionized nurses drop in those 4 years, but so did the actual number, despite the total number of nurses increasing by about 70,000. Still, nurses are roughly twice as likely to be in a union as are other workers (Moberg, 2013). Similarly, OR Manager ("Be Constructive," 2015) suggests that approximately 21% of hospitals in the United States in 2012 had a union nursing staff but noted that percentage may increase as an unintended consequence of health care reform.

The issues driving nurses to pursue unionization, however, continue to exist. Increased nursing workloads and a feeling that management does not care are significant factors encouraging increased union activity during the second decade of the 21st century. This chapter explores the historical development of unions in the United States, particularly in nursing. The motivations behind nurses' decisions to join or not join unions are explored, and the unions that represent the majority of nurses are described. Union organizing strategies are presented, as are specific steps for starting a union. Emphasis is given to the importance of management creating a work environment that eliminates or reduces the need for unionization in the first place. The chapter concludes with a discussion of the definition of "supervisor" in nursing, types of labor union–management relationships, and whether striking can be viewed as an ethically appropriate action for professional nurses.

HISTORICAL PERSPECTIVE OF UNIONIZATION IN THE UNITED STATES

Unions have been present in the United States since the 1790s. Skilled craftsmen formed early unions to protect themselves from wage cuts during the highly competitive era of industrialization. Strikes were rare, and when they did occur, they were short and peaceful. This changed in the early 1800s, with strike activity increasing during economic prosperity and declining during less prosperous economic times. By the mid- to late 1800s, the labor movement began to more closely resemble what we see today. Unions started negotiating with employers, addressing not only wages but also work rules, hours, and grievances, thus arbitrating contracts between employees and employers.

By the 1930s, and after 4 years of the Great Depression, repressive management was the norm, and tensions were high between workers and their employers. There were no legal protections for workers, no overtime compensation, no child labor laws, and no health or safety regulations. Workers attempted to form unions to improve working conditions, but business owners responded by blacklisting organizers and using force to prevent strikes (Franklin D. Roosevelt Presidential Library and Museum, 1935).

President Franklin Roosevelt attempted to intervene by promoting the National Industrial Recovery Act, but he was forced to take an even bolder stand alongside labor when the Supreme Court ruled that act unconstitutional. Roosevelt promoted the National Labor Relations Act (NLRA), also known as the Wagner Act after New York Senator Robert Wagner, which was enacted in 1935. This act gave workers the right to form unions and bargain collectively with their employers (Box 21.1). It also provided for the creation of the National Labor Relations Board (NLRB) to oversee union certification, arrange meetings with unions and employers, and investigate violations of the law (Franklin D. Roosevelt Presidential Library and Museum, 1935).

With this rapid shift in power from management to labor, labor–management relationships were turbulent throughout the 1930s and 1940s. History books are filled with battles, strikes, mass-picketing scenes, and brutal treatment by both management and employees. The balance of power, however, fell to labor unions.

Because of this, it was necessary to pass additional federal legislation to restore what was perceived to be a balance of power with management. Passed in 1947, the Taft–Hartley Labor Act, also known as the Labor–Management Relations Act, retained the provisions under the Wagner Act that guaranteed employees the right to collective bargaining but added the provision that employees had the right to refrain from taking part in unions ("closed shops" were illegal) (Box 21.2). In addition, the act permitted the union shop only after a vote of a majority of the employees. It also forbade *jurisdictional strikes* ("an illegal strike about which trade union should have the right to represent a particular group of employees in an organization" ["Jurisdictional Strike," 2015]), secondary boycotts, and unions from contributing to political campaigns.

Discussion Point

The Taft–Hartley Labor Act also required union leaders to affirm they were not supporters of the Communist Party. Why was this requirement a part of the act and how did it mesh with the culture of the time?

BOX 21.1 Unfair Management Practices Identified in the Wagner Act (1935)

1. To interfere with, restrain, or coerce employees in a manner that interferes with their rights as outlined under the act. Examples of these activities are spying on union gatherings, threatening employees with job loss, or threatening to close down a company if the union organizes
2. To interfere with the formation of any labor organization or to give financial assistance to a labor organization
3. To discriminate with regard to hiring, tenure, and so on to discourage union membership
4. To discharge or discriminate against an employee who filed charges or testified before the NLRB
5. To refuse to bargain in good faith

BOX 21.2 Unfair Labor Union Practices Identified in the Taft–Hartley Amendment (1947)

1. Requiring a self-employed person or an employer to join a union
2. Forcing an employer to cease doing business with another person. This placed a ban on secondary boycotts, which were then prevalent
3. Forcing an employer to bargain with one union when another union has already been certified as the bargaining agent
4. Forcing the employer to assign certain work to members of one union rather than another
5. Charging excessive or discriminatory initiation fees
6. Causing or attempting to cause an employer to pay for unnecessary services

Eventually, federal legislation such as the Fair Labor Standards Act (1938), the Occupational Safety and Health Act (1970), and the Equal Employment Opportunity Act (1972) were passed, providing federal protection for workers. These acts were important in the history of unions because unions no longer had to be the primary source of security for workers. As a result, there has been little growth of unions in the private and blue-collar sectors since membership peaked in the 1950s.

To counteract these dwindling numbers, several major unions merged, and new affiliations were formed. In addition, new organizing tactics were developed. Nowhere is this turnaround more apparent than in the health care industry.

HISTORICAL PERSPECTIVE OF UNIONIZATION IN NURSING

Collective bargaining was slow in coming to the health care industry for many reasons. Until labor laws were amended, unionization of health care workers was illegal. In addition, nursing's long history as a service commodity further delayed labor organization in health care settings.

Discussion Point

Is it appropriate for nurses to organize into collective bargaining units, something historically reserved for blue-collar workers?

Initial collective bargaining in nursing took place in government or public organizations as a result of Executive Order 10988 issued by President John Kennedy. This 1962 order lifted restrictions that prevented public employees from organizing. As a result, city, county, and district hospitals and health care agencies joined collective bargaining in the 1960s.

In 1974, Congress amended the Wagner Act, extending national labor laws to private nonprofit hospitals, nursing homes, health clinics, health maintenance organizations, and other health care institutions. These amendments opened the door to much union activity for professions and the public employee sector. Indeed, a review of union membership figures shows that since 1960, most collective bargaining activity in the United States has occurred in the public and professional sectors of industry, most notably among faculty at institutions of higher education, teachers at primary and secondary levels, and physicians.

Discussion Point

Why is white-collar union membership growing when the private and blue-collar sectors are not? Have societal norms altered perceptions regarding the appropriateness of unionization in white-collar industries?

From 1962 through 1989, there were slow but steady increases in the numbers of nurses represented by collective bargaining agents. In 1989, the NLRB ruled that nurses could form separate bargaining units, and union activity increased. However, the American Hospital Association immediately sued the American Nurses Association (ANA), and the ruling was put on hold until 1991 when the Supreme Court upheld the 1989 decision by the NLRB. A summary of the legislation affecting the development of unionization in nursing is shown in Table 21.1.

TABLE 21.1 Labor Legislation

Year	Legislation	Effect
1935	National Labor Relations Act/Wagner Act	Gave unions many rights in organizing; resulted in rapid union growth
1947	Taft–Hartley Amendment	Returned some power to management; resulted in a more equal balance of power between unions and management
1962	Executive Order 10988 (President John Kennedy)	Amended the 1935 Wagner Act to allow public employees to join unions
1974	Amendments to the Wagner Act	Allowed workers in nonprofit organizations to join unions
1989	National Labor Relations Board ruling	Allowed nurses to form separate bargaining units

UNIONS REPRESENTING NURSES

Various unions represent nurses and other health care workers. The *California Nurses Association* (CNA)/*National Nurses Organizing Committee* joined with two other nurses' unions (*United American Nurses* [UAN] and the *Massachusetts Nurses Association*) to create a new 150,000+ member advocacy association known as *National Nurses United* (NNU) in 2009. While all three unions maintained their separate identities, the merger did give these members a greater national voice, with the end result being that NNU won most—if not all—of the organizing efforts it has undertaken since the merger (Commins, 2012).

The *Service Employees International Union* (SEIU) is another large union in the health care industry, representing more than 1.1 million nurses, licensed practical nurses (LPNs), doctors, lab technicians, nursing home workers, and home care workers (SEIU, 2015a). In addition, the National Federation of Nurses (NFN) merged with the American Federation of Teachers (AFT) in February 2013, making AFT the nation's third largest nurses' union, after NNU and SEIU (Moberg, 2013).

Also in 2013, the National Union of Healthcare Workers (NUHW), which formed in 2009 when SEIU took control of California local United Healthcare Workers West, affiliated with CNA. This affiliation unites 10,000 health care workers at NUHW with 85,000 RNs in CNA (Robertson, 2013). Like NNU, this is a strategic alliance, and not a merger. Such alliances are becoming increasingly commonplace as unions recognize that increased negotiating power comes with greater membership.

Some of the other unions that represent nurses include the ANA; the National Union of Hospital and Health Care Employees of the Retail, Wholesale and Department Store Union; the American Federation of Labor–Congress of Industrial Organizations (AFL-CIO); the United Steelworkers of America; the American Federation of Government Employees, AFL-CIO; the American Federation of State, County, and Municipal Employees, AFL-CIO; the International Brotherhood of Teamsters; the American Federation of State, County, and Municipal Employees, which operates mostly in the public sector; the "24/7 Frontline Service Alliance"; and the United Auto Workers.

Union representation also varies by state. The states with the most unions organizing for all industries, including health care, are New York, California, Pennsylvania, Michigan, and Illinois.

Discussion Point

Is it appropriate for RNs to be represented by nonnursing unions? Why would nurses seek out nonnursing unions for representation?

MOTIVATION TO JOIN UNIONS

Knowing that human behavior is goal directed, it is important to examine what personal goals union membership fulfills. Nurse-managers often tell each other that health care institutions differ from other types of industrial organizations. This is really a myth because most nurses work in large and impersonal organizations, just like workers in other industries.

Consider This People are motivated to join or reject unions as a result of many needs and values.

Deciding whether to join a union is a personal and often complex decision because there are typically many influencing factors. Both choices can be justified, however, so both driving and restraining forces for union membership are presented here.

There are six primary motivations for joining a union (Box 21.3). The first is to increase the power of the

BOX 21.3 Reasons Nurses Join Unions

1. To increase the power of the individual
2. To achieve wage advantages
3. To increase their input into organizational decision making
4. To eliminate discrimination and favoritism
5. Because they are required to do so as part of employment (closed shop)
6. To satisfy a social need to be accepted
7. Because they believe it will improve patient outcomes and quality of care

individual. Employees know that singly they are much more dispensable. Because a large group of employees is generally less dispensable, nurses greatly increase their bargaining power and reduce their vulnerability by joining a union.

Consider This The rapid downsizing and restructuring of the 1990s left many nurses feeling that management did not listen to them or care about their needs. This discontentment provides a fertile ground for union organizers because unions thrive in a climate that perceives the organizational philosophy to be insensitive to the worker.

This is a particularly strong motivating force for nurses when jobs are scarce and nurses feel vulnerable. Indeed, during the massive downsizing and restructuring of the 1990s, collective bargaining priorities shifted from wages and benefits to job security. This focus shifted again to worker safety when the first US Ebola patient died in Fall 2014 in Dallas ("Be Constructive," 2015). Union leaders argued that hospitals were not providing nurses with adequate training and protective equipment to care for infected patients. The protests succeeded in focusing public awareness on Ebola readiness and safety.

Indeed, Weinstock and Failey (2014) argue that unions, joined at times by worker advocacy groups (eg, Public Citizen and the American Public Health Association), have played a critical role in strengthening worker safety and health protections. They have sought to improve standards that protect workers by participating in the rulemaking process, through written comments and involvement in hearings; lobbying decision makers; petitioning the Department of Labor; and defending improved standards in court. Their efforts have culminated in more stringent exposure standards, access to information about the presence of potentially hazardous toxic chemicals, and improved access to personal protective equipment, further improving working conditions.

A second reason for joining unions is economics. In some organizations, pay is neither fair nor competitive, and most economists agree that joining a union is typically an effective means of raising one's pay. Indeed, the median weekly earnings of union workers are 28% higher than those of nonunion workers (average yearly difference of US$10,400), and according to a January 2011 Bureau of Labor Statistics report, workers who belong to a union typically earn higher pay than nonunion workers doing the same kind of job (SEIU, 2015b). In addition, 92% of union employees in the United States had access to health care benefits in 2009, as compared with only 68% of nonunion workers, and companies with 30% or more unionized workers were five times as likely to have their entire family health insurance premium paid for, in comparison to companies with no unionized workers (SEIU, 2015b).

Another reason nurses join unions is to communicate their aims, feelings, complaints, and ideas to others. The desire to have input into organizational decision making is a strong motivator for people to join unions. A feeling of powerlessness or the perception that administration does not care about employees is one of the most common reasons for seeking unionization. Indeed, research conducted by Deery, Iverson, Buttigieg, and Zatzick (2014) suggested that union citizenship behavior is a form of voice and that when employees perceive that voice is heard and respected, workplace retention and climate are improved (Research Study Fuels the Controversy 21.1).

Consider This Although historically, unions focused heavily on wage negotiations, current issues that nurses deem just as or more important are nonmonetary, such as guidelines for staffing, float provisions, shared decision making, and scheduling.

In addition, nurses join unions because they want to eliminate discrimination and favoritism. Unions emphasize equality and fairness. This might be an especially strong motivator for members of groups that have experienced discrimination, such as women and minorities.

The fourth primary motivation for joining a union stems from the social need to be accepted. Sometimes, this social need results from family or peer pressure. Because many working-class families have a long history of strong union ties, children are frequently raised in a cultural milieu that promotes unionization.

Another reason nurses join unions is that the union contract dictates that all nurses belong to the union. This has been a big driving force among blue-collar workers. However, the *closed shop*, or requirement that all employees belong to a union, has never prevailed in the health care industry. Most health care unions have *open shops*, allowing nurses to choose whether they want to join the union. Finally, some nurses join unions because they believe that patient outcomes are better in unionized organizations due to better staffing and supervised management practices.

Research Study Fuels the Controversy 21.1

Union Membership as a Form of Voice

The researchers surveyed 1,631 (sample = 1,125) unionized employees from 367 international banking organizations in Australia. Using aggregated attitudinal data and longitudinal retention data, the researchers conducted a confirmatory factor analysis examining union citizenship behavior, union loyalty, union instrumentality, union responsiveness, general prounion attitudes, union socialization, and industrial relations climate.

Source: Deery, S. J., Iverson, R. D., Buttigieg, D. M., & Zatzick, C. D. (2014). Can union voice make a difference? The effect of union citizenship behavior on employee absence. *Human Resource Management, 53*(2), 211–228. doi:10.1002/hrm.21549

Study Findings

Researchers concluded that union citizenship behavior (positive nonspecific behaviors such as attending union meetings, voting in union elections, and supporting coworkers with grievances) results in improved communication between employees and management. This is especially true when bringing forth grievances or concerns that might not be vetted through nonunion channels. Employees who feel their union voice is heard experience lower absenteeism and turnover rates, which results in reduced labor costs and increased organizational performance.

REASONS NOT TO JOIN UNIONS

Just as there are many reasons to join unions, there are also many reasons nurses reject unions, including societal and cultural factors (Box 21.4). Many people distrust unions because they believe that they promote the welfare state and oppose the US system of free enterprise. Other individuals reject unions because they feel a need to demonstrate that they can get ahead on their own merits.

In addition, some professional employees reject unions for reasons that deal with class and education. They argue that unions were appropriate for the blue-collar worker but not for the university professor, physician, or engineer. Nurses rejecting unions on this basis are usually driven by a need to demonstrate their individualism and social status.

Other employees identify with management and thus frequently adopt its viewpoint toward unions. These nurses, therefore, reject unions because their values more closely align with management than with workers.

In addition, although most employees are protected under the NLRA, some nurses reject unions because of fears of employer reprisal. Nurses who reject unions on this basis could be said to be motivated most of all by a need for job security.

Finally, some employees reject unions because they fear losing income associated with a strike or walkout. Strikes and walkouts are a reality of unionization; however, they are heavily regulated by law (striking is discussed later in this chapter).

Once managers understand the needs and driving forces behind nurses' decisions to join or reject unions, they can begin to address them. Organizations with unfair management policies are more likely to become unionized. It is certainly then within managerial power to eliminate some of the needs staff feel for joining unions.

BOX 21.4 Reasons Nurses Do Not Want to Join Unions

1. The belief that unions promote the welfare state and oppose the US system of free enterprise
2. The need to demonstrate individualism
3. The belief that unionization allows for mediocrity and substandard practice
4. The belief that professionals should not unionize
5. Identification with management's viewpoint
6. Fear of employer reprisal
7. Fear of lost income associated with a strike or walkout

Managers can encourage feelings of power by allowing subordinates to have input into decisions that will affect their work. Managers also can listen to ideas, complaints, and feelings and take steps to ensure that favoritism and discrimination are not part of their management style. In addition, managers can strengthen the drives and needs that make nurses reject unions. By building a team effort, sharing ideas and future plans from upper management with the staff, and encouraging individualism in employees, managers can facilitate identification of the worker with management.

When nurses begin showing signs of job dissatisfaction (frustration, stress, perceived powerlessness), they are sending a wake-up call to nursing management. Leaders must be alert to employment practices that are unfair or insensitive to employee needs and intervene appropriately before such issues lead to unionization. However, organizations offering liberal benefit packages and fair management practices may still experience union activity if certain social and cultural factors are present. If union activity does occur, managers must be aware of specific employee and management rights so that the NLRA is not violated by either managers or employees.

ELIGIBILITY FOR UNION MEMBERSHIP

The NLRA defines a supervisor as

> *any individual having authority, in the interest of the employer, to hire, transfer, suspend, lay off, recall, promote, discharge, assign, reward, or discipline other employees, or responsibly to direct them, or to adjust their grievances, or effectively to recommend such action, if in connection with the foregoing the exercise of such authority is not of a merely routine or clerical nature, but requires the use of independent judgment.* (Matthews, 2010, para. 12)

Up until two decades ago, only *supervisors* in nursing were considered managers, and, as such, they were prohibited from joining unions. However, a 2006 NLRB ruling deemed that *charge nurses* might also be considered supervisors since they are responsible for the coordination and provision of patient care throughout a unit (Matthews, 2010). Even part-time charge nurses were so labeled. This finding has been contested legally since that time and several interpretations have occurred. Reinterpretations by the NLRB are expected in the future.

In addition, the definition of supervisor in nursing came into question with several administrative and court rulings in the early 1990s. These rulings came about as a result of a case involving four licensed practical nurses/licensed vocational nurses (LPNs/LVNs) employed at Heartland Nursing Home in Urbana, Ohio. During late 1988 and early 1989, these LPNs complained to management about what they thought were disparate enforcement of the absentee policy; short staffing; low wages for nurses' aides; an unreasonable switching of prescription business from one pharmacy to another, which increased the nurses' paperwork; and management's failure to communicate with employees (National Labor Relations Board [NLRB], n.d.-a). Despite assurances from the vice president for operations that they would not be harassed for bringing their concerns to headquarters' attention, three of the LPNs were terminated as a result of their actions.

In response to what they perceived to be illegal termination, the LPNs filed for protection under the NLRA. The NLRB ruled that because the LPNs had responsibility to ensure adequate staffing, to make daily work assignments, to monitor the aides' work to ensure proper performance, to counsel and discipline aides, to resolve aides' problems and grievances, to evaluate aides' performances, and to report to management, they should be classified as "supervisors," thereby making them ineligible for protection under the NLRA.

On appeal, the administrative law judge (ALJ) disagreed, concluding that the nurses were not supervisors and that the nurses' supervisory work did not equate to responsibly directing the aides *in the interest of the employer*, noting that the nurses' focus is on the well-being of the residents rather than on the employer.

In another turnabout, the U.S. Court of Appeals for the Sixth Circuit then reversed the decision of the ALJ, arguing that the NLRB's test for determining the supervisory status of nurses was inconsistent with the statute and that the interest of the patient and the interest of the employer were not mutually exclusive. The court said that, in fact, the interests of the patient are the employer's business, and argued that the welfare of the patient was no less the object and concern of the employer than it was of the nurses. The court also argued that the statutory dichotomy the NLRB first created was no more justified in the health care field than it would be in any other business in which supervisory duties are necessary to the production of goods or the provision of services ("*NLRB v. Health Care & Retirement Corp.*," 1994).

The court further stated that it was up to Congress to carve out an exception for the health care field, including nurses, should Congress not wish for such nurses to be considered supervisors. The court reminded the NLRB that the courts, and not the board, bear the final responsibility for interpreting the law. After concluding that the board's test was inconsistent with the statute, the court found that the four LPNs involved in this case were indeed supervisors and ineligible for protection under the NLRA ("*NLRB v. Health Care & Retirement Corp.*," 1994).

This same interpretation, at least for full-time charge nurses, was used in another landmark court case in September 2006 to determine whether charge nurses, both permanent and rotating, at Oakwood Healthcare Inc. were "supervisors" within the meaning of the NLRA, and thus could be excluded from a unit of nurses represented by a union (Mayer & Shimabukuro, 2012). Upholding the definition that supervisors "assign," and "responsibly direct" employees as well as exercise "independent judgment," the NLRB concluded that 12 permanent charge nurses employed by Oakwood Healthcare were supervisors. Rotating charge nurses were not if this role was less than 10% to 15% of their work time.

Matthews (2010) notes that the Oakwood case has set precedence and figured in approximately 35 subsequent decisions in both health care and industrial settings, although there have been no further rulings addressing the charge nurse/supervisor status. Hence, the *Oakwood* ruling is still in effect today, specifying that nurses, on average, with less than 10% to 15% (equal to about one shift per pay period) of their time as charge nurse are considered staff nurses, while nurses working more than 15% of their professional time as charge nurses are considered supervisors.

Discussion Point

Would the NLRB's definition of supervisor affect charge nurses' eligibility for union membership at the facility in which you work?

ORGANIZING A UNION AND SEEKING REPRESENTATION

Unions use a variety of tactics when organizing health care workers (Box 21.5). The first step in seeking union representation is determining that adequate levels of desire for unionization exist. The NLRB requires that at least 30% of employees sign an interest card before an election for unionization can be held. Most collective bargaining agents, however, require 60% to 70% of the employees to sign interest cards before they begin an organizing campaign. Union representatives are generally careful to keep a campaign secret until they are ready to file a petition for election. They do this so that they can build momentum without interference from the employer.

After enough interest cards have been signed, the organization must hold an election. At that time, all employees of the same classification, such as RNs, vote on whether they desire unionization. A choice in every such election is *no representation*, which means that the voters do not want a union. During the election, 50% plus one of the petitioned units must vote before the union can be recognized. Unions can also be decertified by a process similar to that of certification. *Decertification* can occur when at least 30% of the eligible employees in the bargaining unit initiate a petition asking to no longer be represented by the union.

There are important differences, however, between organizing in a health care facility and in other types of organizations. Generally, the solicitation and distribution of union literature are banned entirely in immediate patient care areas. Managers should never, however, independently attempt to deal with union organizing activity. They should always seek assistance and guidance from higher-level management and the personnel department. The entire list of rights for management

BOX 21.5 Union Organizing Strategies

1. Meetings (both group and one-on-one)
2. Leaflets and brochures
3. Pressure on the hospital corporation through media and community contacts
4. Political pressure of regional legislators and local lawmakers
5. Corporate campaign strategies
6. Activism of local employees
7. Using lawsuits
8. Bringing pressure from financiers
9. Technology

and labor during the organizing and establishment phases of unionization is beyond the scope of this book.

Throughout the years, Congress has amended various labor acts and laws in the attempt to balance power between management and labor. At times, the balance of power has shifted to management or labor, but Congress eventually enacts laws that attempt to restore what it judges to be the balance. The manager must ensure that the rights of management and employees are protected.

LABOR–MANAGEMENT RELATIONSHIPS

In the last 30 years, employers and unions have substantially improved their relationships. Although evidence is growing that contemporary management has come to accept the reality that unions are here to stay, businesses in the United States are still less comfortable with unions than their counterparts in many other countries. Likewise, unions have come to accept the fact that there are times when organizations are not healthy enough to survive aggressive union demands.

Consider This It is possible to create a climate in which labor and management can work together to accomplish mutual goals.

Once management is faced with dealing with a collective bargaining unit, it has a choice of either accepting or opposing the union. It may actively oppose the union by using various union-busting techniques, or it may more subtly oppose the union by attempting to discredit it and win employee trust. *Acceptance* also may run along a continuum. The company may accept the union with reluctance and suspicion. Although they know that the union has legitimate rights, managers often believe they must continually guard against the union encroaching further into traditional management territory.

There is also the type of union acceptance known as *accommodation*. As is increasingly common, accommodation is characterized by management's full acceptance of the union, with both union and management showing mutual respect. When these conditions exist, labor and management can establish mutual goals, especially in the areas of safety, cost reduction, efficiency, waste elimination, and improvement of working conditions. Such cooperation represents the most mature and advanced type of labor–management relationships.

The bottom line is that the attitudes and the philosophies of the leaders in management and the union determine what type of relationship develops between the two parties in any given organization. When dealing with unions, managers must be flexible. It is critical that they do not ignore issues or try to overwhelm others with power. The rational approach to problem solving must be used.

It is also important to remember that employees have a right to participate in union organizing under the NLRA, and managers must not interfere with this right. Prohibited managerial activities include threatening employees, interrogating employees, promising employees rewards for cessation of union activity, and spying on employees. However, if management picks up early clues of union activity, the organization may be able to take legitimate steps that will discourage unionization of its employees.

Discussion Point

When unions are present in the workplace, what should be the relationship between them and management? What is accomplished by having a competitive or hostile relationship?

AMERICAN NURSES ASSOCIATION AND COLLECTIVE BARGAINING

One difficult union issue faced by nurse-managers is the dual role of their professional organization, the ANA. The NLRB recognizes the ANA, at most state levels, as a collective bargaining agent. The use of state associations as bargaining agents is divisive among US nurses. Some nurse-managers believe that they have been disenfranchised by their professional organization. Other managers recognize the conflicts inherent in attempting to sit on both sides of the bargaining table. Even for members who feel that the issue presents no real dilemma, there appears to be some conflict in loyalty.

This conflict has manifested itself in the recent splitting away of state nurses associations from the parent ANA organization. Since California RNs broke from the ANA in 1995 over dissatisfaction with the control held by nurses in managerial positions in hospitals, other states have also disaffiliated, including Massachusetts, Maine, New York, and Pennsylvania. In addition, many nurses unions, including the just-absorbed NFN, split off from the ANA as a result (Moberg, 2013).

In 1999, the ANA responded by establishing, then spinning off, the UAN as a parallel association of state collective bargaining organizations. NFN consisted of some of the UAN groups that did not want to join with NNU, but then the New York State Nurses Association left NFN. Moberg questions whether new mergers will lead to more cooperation among the sometimes rancorous nursing unions—or to more progress in organizing a field that is growing faster than its union membership.

There are no easy solutions to the dilemma created by the dual role held by the ANA. Clarifying issues begins with the manager examining the motivation of nurses to participate in collective bargaining. The manager must at least try to hear and understand the employees' points of view.

Discussion Point

If you are a student, do you belong to the state student nurses association? If you are an RN, have you joined your state nurses association? Why or why not?

Consider This The ANA acts as both a professional association for RNs and a collective bargaining agent. To some nurses, this dual purpose poses a conflict in loyalty.

Discussion Point

Should the ANA—the recognized professional association for nurses in the United States—also be a collective bargaining agent?

NURSES AND STRIKES

The NLRA states in part that employees shall have the right to engage in "other concerted activities" for the purpose of collective bargaining or other mutual aid or protection (application of the National Labor Relations Board [NLRB], n.d.-b). The phrase "other concerted activities" refers to "the right to effectively communicate with one another regarding self-organization at the jobsite" (para. 8).

The law then gives union members time to work together to determine whether strikes are necessary to achieve desired goals. Such strikes, however, are not allowed without giving the employer and the Federal Mediation and Conciliation Service 10 days' notice of the intent to strike. In doing so, the facility should have a reasonable amount of time to stop admitting patients, transfer existing patients to other facilities, and reduce medical procedures that require nurse-intensive labor. Problems occur when management continues to admit new patients or maintains normal operations.

Discussion Point

Can strikes, walkouts, "blue flu epidemics," and picket lines be considered ethical actions if nurses believe that they are the only ways in which they can improve working conditions or ensure safe patient care?

The controversy over whether nurses should strike is long-standing, and is likely at the heart of why so many individuals fear union activity. Critics of nurses having the ability to strike suggest that it is unethical because it leaves patients without care providers. Unions argue that strikes must be supported because they are used only as a last resort and after careful consideration of every factor. The issue of striking then continues to divide the nursing profession. Ironically, both proponents and opponents of strikes in nursing argue that they aim for the same goal: safe patient care.

Indeed, the ANA has held consistently for 50+ years that nurses not only have a right to strike but also have a professional responsibility and ethical duty to do so if it means maintaining work conditions conducive to providing high-quality care.

In addition to the moral dilemmas related to the decision to strike, nurses must also determine how they feel about crossing the picket line should a strike occur. Nurses do have a choice not to participate in strikes or to cross picket lines when strikes occur. They risk derision by their peers in doing so, however, because strikebreakers, commonly known as "scabs," are viewed as taking management's side on the issue and may never be fully accepted by their peers after the strike action has ended.

Conclusions

The question of whether nurses should participate in collective bargaining has been around since legislation made such organization possible. Advocates on both sides of the issues present earnest, well-reasoned arguments to support their positions. Clearly, nurses working in unionized organizations appear to have some economic advantage, and their individual vulnerability to arbitrary action on the part of their employer is reduced.

Yet nursing's long-standing struggle to be recognized as a profession underscores concerns that the profession's involvement in collective bargaining associations, historically reserved for blue-collar industries, may undermine this goal. In addition, some nurses think that union activities draw attention away from patients and patient-related activities. Union advocates argue the opposite—that improving pay, benefits, and working conditions ultimately leads to improved patient care.

There are also issues related to who can belong to a union, what the definition of "supervisor" is in nursing, and whether strikes and walkouts are ethically justified for nursing professionals. In addition, the dual role of the ANA as both the national organization for nurses and a collective bargaining agent poses ethical dilemmas for many nurses. Even unionized nurses cannot agree on the intensity and direction their unions should take, resulting in state unions breaking off from the ANA.

Finally, the relationships health care organizations have developed with their collective bargaining agents vary from direct opposition to collaboration. The effect of that relationship on working conditions and quality of patient care cannot be overstated. Unionization, then, is likely to continue to be fraught with challenges and will be one of the most passionate issues nurses will debate for some time to come.

For Additional Discussion

1. Does the presence of unions increase the likelihood that management will be fairer and more consistent with employees?
2. Can the need for unionization be eliminated simply by management being more attentive to worker needs and being willing to provide employees with reasonable working conditions and a voice in decision making?
3. Would you be willing to cross a picket line to work during an authorized strike?
4. Are there other ways nurses can increase their group power other than by unions? If so, are they as effective?
5. Some state unions are choosing to break off from the ANA. Does this further fragment nursing's collective power in the political arena by diminishing group size, or does it increase the broad-based support of nursing issues?
6. Do you believe that the current nursing shortage will accelerate the rate of unionization in nursing?
7. How does a nursing shortage affect a union's power in negotiating wages, benefits, and working conditions?

References

Be constructive, not combative, with union staff. (2015). *OR Manager, 31*(1), 24–26.

Commins, J. (2012, January 3). *Why do nurses join unions? Because they can.* Retrieved May 25, 2015, from http://www.strategiesfornursemanagers.com/ce_detail/275275.cfm

Deery, S. J., Iverson, R. D., Buttigieg, D. M., & Zatzick, C. D. (2014). Can union voice make a difference? The effect of union citizenship behavior on employee absence. *Human Resource Management, 53*(2), 211–228. doi:10.1002/hrm.21549

Franklin D. Roosevelt Presidential Library and Museum. (1935). *Our documents: National Labor Relations Act (The Wagner Act).* Retrieved May 26, 2015, from http://docs.fdrlibrary.marist.edu/odnlra.html

Jurisdictional Strike [Definition]. (2015). In *Business Dictionary*. Retrieved May 26, 2015, from http://www.businessdictionary.com/definition/jurisdictional-strike.html

Matthews, J. (2010). When does delegating make you a supervisor? *The Online Journal of Issues in Nursing, 15*(2). Retrieved December 30, 2011, from http://www.nursingworld.org/MainMenuCategories/ANAMarketplace/ANAPeriodicals/OJIN/TableofContents/Vol152010/No2May2010/Delegating-and-Supervisors.aspx

Mayer, G., & Shimabukuro, J. O. (2012, July 5). *The definition of "supervisor" under the National Labor Relations Act*. Washington, DC: Congressional Research Service. Retrieved May 25, 2015, from http://www.fas.org/sgp/crs/misc/RL34350.pdf

Moberg, D. (2013, February 20). Are mergers the answer for fractious nurses unions? *In These Times*. Retrieved May 26, 2015, from http://inthesetimes.com/working/entry/14631/are_mergers_the_answer_for_nurses_unions

National Labor Relations Board. (n.d.-a). *Case 09-CA-026348*. Retrieved May 26, 2015, from http://www.nlrb.gov/search/simple/all/Case%2009-CA-%20026348

National Labor Relations Board. (n.d.-b). *National Labor Relations Act*. Retrieved May 26, 2015, from https://www.nlrb.gov/national-labor-relations-act

NLRB v. Health Care & Retirement Corp., 114 S. Ct. 1778. (1994, May 23). Retrieved May 25, 2015, from http://www.law.cornell.edu/supct/html/92-1964.ZS.html

Robertson, K. (2013, January 4). Unions join forces to fight nursing cutbacks. *Sacramento Business Journal*. Retrieved May 25, 2015, from http://www.bizjournals.com/sacramento/news/2013/01/04/unions-join-forces-to-fight-nursing.html?page=2

Service Employees International Union. (2015a). *About SEIU*. Retrieved May 26, 2015, from http://www.seiu.org/about

Service Employees International Union. (2015b). *The union advantage: Facts and figures*. **SEIU Local 105.** Retrieved May 26, 2015, from http://www.seiu105.org/the-union-advantage/

Weinstock, D., & Failey, T. (2014). The labor movement's role in gaining federal safety and health standards to protect America's workers. *New Solutions: A Journal of Environmental and Occupational Health Policy, 24*(3), 409–434. doi:10.2190/NS.24.3.k

22

Assuring Provider Competence Through Licensure, Continuing Education, and Certification

Carol J. Huston

ADDITIONAL RESOURCES

Visit thePoint for additional helpful resources

- eBook
- Journal Articles
- WebLinks

CHAPTER OUTLINE

LEARNING OBJECTIVES

The learner will be able to:

1. Differentiate between competence and continuing competence in a profession.
2. Identify stakeholders who would be affected by a movement to mandate continuing competence in nursing.
3. Identify driving and restraining forces to implementing mandatory reexamination as a prerequisite for license renewal in nursing.
4. Compare support for mandatory reexamination for license renewal in nursing with that of other health professions such as medicine and pharmacy.
5. Identify arguments for and against mandated continuing education for license renewal.
6. Compare continuing education requirements for nurses with those for other health care professionals.
7. Describe personal and professional benefits of professional certification.
8. Delineate the roles/responsibilities assumed by the American Board of Nursing Specialties as the accrediting body for nursing certification.

(continues on page 318)

9. Identify the strengths and weaknesses of using professional certification as an indicator of entry-level competence in advanced practice nursing.
10. Describe how portfolios and self-assessment, as tools for reflective practice, can further the goal of professional competence.
11. Explore the roles and responsibilities of the individual, employers, the State Board of Nursing, and professional associations in assuring both the initial and the continued competence of health care practitioners.
12. Reflect on his or her beliefs regarding the need for and efficacy of mandating reexamination for licensure, continuing education, and certification for nurses to assure continuing competence.

INTRODUCTION

How can one determine whether a nurse is competent? Does licensure assure competence? Does clinical performance assure competence? Does competence require recency of clinical practice? Is it assured by professional certification? Would nurse residencies increase the competency of the new graduate nurse?

Unfortunately, in many states, a practitioner is determined to be competent when initially licensed and thereafter unless proven otherwise. Yet, clearly, passing a licensing examination and continuing to work as a clinician does not assure competence throughout a career. Competence requires continual updates to knowledge and practice, and this is difficult in a health care environment characterized by rapidly emerging new technologies, chaotic change, and perpetual clinical advancements based on new evidence.

For example, the Institute of Medicine (IOM) (2010) report *The Future of Nursing* suggests that nursing graduates now need competency in a variety of areas including continuous improvement of the quality and safety of health care systems, informatics, evidence-based practice, a knowledge of complex systems, skills and methods for leadership and management of continual improvement, population health- and population-based care management, and health policy knowledge, skills, and attitudes. One must at least question how many nurses currently in practice would be able to demonstrate competency in these areas.

In 1995, the Task Force on Healthcare Workforce Regulations of the Pew Health Professions Commission recommended changing how health care professions, including nursing, were regulated, and suggested that continued competence should be assured as a regulatory board function (North Carolina Board of Nursing [NCBN], 2015). The Citizens Advocacy Center, a public policy organization located in Washington, DC, concurred, as did the 1999 IOM in its report *To Err Is Human*, which included a recommendation for professional licensing bodies to assume the responsibility for determining licensees' competence and knowledge.

There is little disagreement that the knowledge health care professionals' need must be current and appropriate to their area of practice and that their care should be competent at the minimum. The challenge lies, however, in determining how best to assure that competence and in determining who should be responsible for its oversight.

This chapter explores definitions of *competence*, giving particular attention to that of *continuing competence*. Licensure, periodic relicensure, continuing education (CE), and professional certification are examined as potential strategies for assuring provider competence. The chapter also discusses the limitations of each of these strategies for assessing both initial and continuing competence, as well as the difficulties inherent in standardizing continuing competence requirements in a health care system composed of varied stakeholders. Finally, the chapter concludes with an exploration of portfolio development and reflective practice: contemporary strategies that allow health care professionals to carry out a self-assessment of their practice and to develop a personal plan for maintaining competence.

DEFINING COMPETENCE

Competence in nursing can be defined in many ways. Dictionary.com (2015) defines competence as adequacy or the possession of required skill, knowledge, qualification, or capacity. As such, it is tied to experience and context. Hence, professional competence can be defined as the capacity to handle events and challenges effectively.

In 1999, the American Nurses Association (ANA) convened an expert panel that defined three types of competence in nursing: *continuing competence*, *professional nursing competence*, and *continuing professional nursing competence*. Special attention was given, however, to continuing competence because so many assumptions exist regarding the rights and responsibilities of consumers, individual nurses, and employers to see that such competence is present and promulgated. Indeed, it is continuing competence that is a primary focus of this chapter, given that initial licensure suggests that at least minimum competence levels were met at that time.

In 2007, the ANA released a draft position statement on competence and competency for public review and comment. The purpose of this position paper was to define *competence* ("performing successfully at an expected level") and *competency* ("an expected level of performance that results from an integration of knowledge, skills, abilities, and judgment within the context of current and projected professional directions"). Key excerpts from the final document released in 2008 and reaffirmed in 2014 are shown in Box 22.1.

Clearly, although there is some overlap among these definitions, there is still some lack of consensus around what competence is and how it should be measured. There also appears to be difficulty in relating the continuing competence of providers with the roles they are asked to assume in the clinical setting. For example, some nurses develop high levels of competence in specific areas of nursing practice as a result of work experience and specialization at the expense of staying current in other areas of practice. Yet employers, who espouse the support of continuing competence, often ask registered nurses (RNs) to provide care in areas of practice outside their area of expertise because staffing shortages encourage them to do so. In addition, many current competence assessments focus more on skills than they do on knowledge.

Consider This Nurses are often asked to float to or work in areas where their competence may be in question because their license allows them to work in virtually any area of practice.

In addition, new competencies must be integrated into nursing practice as new science emerges. For example, Watson Dillon and Mahoney (2015) note that population health will be a new competency for nurse executives given the movement from individual patient care.

Calzone, Jenkins, Culp, Caskey, and Badzek (2014) argue that genomics is another such emerging competency. In their study of a 1-year genomics competency integration effort, the majority (89%) of nurses felt it was very or somewhat important to become more educated in the genetics of common diseases, but a competency deficit affecting all nurses regardless of academic preparation or role was observed. Thus, despite a recognized need to develop new clinical competencies, the workplace did not support or provide an environment that promoted such learning (Research Study Fuels the Controversy 22.1).

In addition, professional nursing organizations decline to implement continuing competence mandates because they fear membership repercussions. For example, the ANCC continues to offer certification examinations for RNs without baccalaureate degrees, despite the recognition that such certification suggests advanced rather than basic practice.

BOX 22.1 Excerpts from the American Nurses Association (ANA) Draft Statement on Professional Role Competence (Approved March 28, 2008, and reaffirmed November 12, 2014)

The ANA supports the following principles in regard to competence in the nursing profession:

- The public has a right to expect nurses to demonstrate competence throughout their careers.
- Nurses are individually responsible and accountable for maintaining professional competence.
- The nursing profession must shape and guide any process assuring nurse competence.
- Regulatory bodies define minimal standards for regulation of practice to protect the public.
- Employers are responsible and accountable to provide an environment conducive to competent practice.
- Assurance of competence is the shared responsibility of the profession, individual nurses, professional organizations, credentialing and certification entities, regulatory agencies, employers, and other key stakeholders.

Source: American Nurses Association. (2014, November 12). *ANA position statement: Professional role competence*. Retrieved April 6, 2015, from http://gm6.nursingworld.org/MainMenuCategories/Policy-Advocacy/Positions-and-Resolutions/ANAPositionStatements/Position-Statements-Alphabetically/Professional-Role-Competence.html

Research Study Fuels the Controversy 22.1

Integrating Genomics Competencies Into Practice

This longitudinal study provided a cross-sectional analysis of baseline data from 7,798 RNs employed at 23 American Nurses Credentialing Center (ANCC) designated Magnet Recognition Program hospitals. The institutions were in 17 states, representing all regions of the United States, and included 1 rural, 3 children's, 1 Veterans Administration, and 1 psychiatric hospital as well as 1 cancer center. The number of RNs employed per institution ranged from 80 to 3,000 at the time of the baseline survey.

Source: Calzone, K. A., Jenkins, J., Culp, S., Caskey, S., & Badzek, L. (2014). Introducing a new competency into nursing practice. *Journal of Nursing Regulation, 5*(1), 40–47.

Study Findings

Overwhelmingly, nurses in this study felt that genomics was important and expressed intentions to learn more and to do so on their own time. However, gaps that facilitate innovation adoption existed in the practice health care environment. The researchers concluded that introducing new competencies related to clinically relevant science into patient care is challenging. In addition, introducing a complex competency into the nursing scope of practice has ramifications for institutional systems, policies, and workforce preparation. This then requires understanding the nursing workforce's social system, attitudes, confidence, and knowledge in designing and adopting new, effective nursing competencies.

Discussion Point

Should certification be limited to nurses with baccalaureate degrees or even higher education?

The ANA advocates that states defer competence monitoring to the professional association, without governmental involvement in the process, partly because of concern about misconduct charges if state regulators are involved and partly because memberships and revenues are likely to increase if the association monitors competence. Clearly, then, stakeholders and politics continue to influence how continuing competence is defined, used, and promulgated.

The issue is also complicated by the fact that there are no national standards for defining, measuring, or requiring continuing competence in nursing. In addition, specialty nursing organizations, state nurses associations, state boards of nursing, and professional nursing organizations have not reached consensus about what continuing competence is and how to measure it, although there is little debate that it is needed. The reality is that given the multiplicity and variations of the definition of continuing competence and the number of stakeholders affected by its promulgation, identifying and mandating strategies that assure the continuing competence of health care providers will be very difficult.

Consider This There is no consensus about how to define or objectively measure competence in nursing practice.

PROFESSIONAL LICENSURE

Licensure can be defined as

> *the granting of permission by a competent authority (usually a government agency) to an organization or individual to engage in a practice or activity that would otherwise be illegal. Licensure is usually granted on the basis of education and examination rather than performance. It is usually permanent, but a periodic fee, demonstration of competence, or continuing education may be required.* (The Free Dictionary by Farlex, 2003–2015, para. 1)

Most health care professionals must be licensed, and this license is assumed to provide at least some assurance that the practitioner is competent in his or her field at the time of initial licensure.

Licensure Processes in Nursing

One of the most important purposes of the National Council State Boards of Nursing (NCSBN) and its 59 state boards of nursing (1 in each of 50 states, 2 in 3 states, 1 in the District of Columbia, 1 in each of 4 US territories, and 1 with both a Board of Nursing and a board for advanced practice nurses) is to protect the health, safety, and welfare of the public (NCSBN, 2015a; "State Boards of Nursing," 2015). This is done by having a regulatory role in the accreditation of nursing education programs, through licensure, and by implementing and enforcing the Nurse Practice Act. In addition, the NCSBN has created and disseminated numerous nursing practice and regulation resources on nursing practice and education, and maintains a database on nursing disciplinary actions taken across the nation.

It is for the licensing examinations for RNs and licensed practical nurses/vocational nurses (LPNs/LVNs), however, that the NCSBN and its state boards of nursing are probably best known. The NCSBN has developed two licensure examinations to test the entry-level nursing competence of candidates for licensure as RNs and as LPNs/LVNs. These examinations, the National Council Licensure Examinations (NCLEX-RN and NCLEX-PN), are administered with the contractual assistance of a national test service (NCSBN, 2015b) and test integrated nursing content. Passage of the NCLEX suggests that the individual has been deemed by the state to have met minimal competence standards for entry into practice; however, this does reflect or measure the many higher-level competencies achieved in different types of education programs for nurses.

Discussion Point

Does having just one NCLEX for multiple levels of educational levels into practice argue that the associate degree in nursing provides an appropriate knowledge base for competence in all areas of professional nursing practice?

Despite this flaw, licensure by examination continues to be a highly regarded strategy for assuring competence levels of health care professionals such as nurses. Indeed, some professional organizations and regulatory bodies suggest that RNs should be required to repeat the NCLEX periodically or that nurses should be required to take examinations similar in scope to the NCLEX for license renewal.

Efforts to implement mandatory reexamination as a prerequisite for license renewal in nursing, however, have met with minimal success. This is because there is little agreement about what such an examination should look like, how it would be administered, and how often it should be required. Nonetheless, multiple states have introduced legislation with varying approaches from retesting to requiring a provider to demonstrate competence in the workplace, but resistance is high, and there is little hope that periodic reexaminations to assess competence will be a part of nursing's immediate future.

In addition, 25 states (as of 2015) participate in the Nurse Licensure Compact (NLC), which allows a nurse to have a license in one state and to practice in other states, as long as that nurse is subject to each state's practice laws and discipline. Such a compact further reduces the likelihood that a nurse would require NCLEX reexamination during his or her career, despite crossing state lines where the initial nursing license was obtained.

Licensure Processes in Medicine

In contrast to the NCLEX, US medical licensure examinations are developed using a competence-based process that requires examinees to be cognizant of practice changes, the evidence required for practice, and the knowledge necessary to be competent into the future. In addition, to achieve full authority to practice independently, physicians are required to pass three licensure examinations (U.S. Medical Licensing Examination, 1996–2015). Furthermore, a clinical skills examination was implemented in 2004.

In addition, although periodic reexamination was recommended in 1967 by the Bureau of Health Manpower of the U.S. Department of Health for licensure of physicians as of 1971, the decision regarding whether to do so has been left to the discretion of individual states. In most states, this is simply a matter of completing mandatory CE requirements and having no disciplinary actions filed against their license.

Licensure Processes in Pharmacy

Pharmacists have also been reluctant to embrace the IOM's *To Err Is Human* recommendation that periodic reexamination of key providers is critical to resolving health care quality problems, especially medical errors. Pharmacists take a licensing exam on graduation, known as the North American Pharmacist

Licensure Examination (NAPLEX). The NAPLEX is a computer-adaptive examination that consists of 185 multiple-choice test questions. The NAPLEX is just one component of the licensure process and is used by the boards of pharmacy as part of their assessment of a candidate's competence to practice as a pharmacist (National Association of Boards of Pharmacy [NABP], 2015a).

In addition, 48 boards require a Multistate Pharmacy Jurisprudence Examination (MPJE), which combines federal- and state-specific questions to test the pharmacy jurisprudence knowledge of prospective pharmacists both for initial licensure and for license transfer (NABP, 2015b). The MPJE consists of 90 multiple-choice test questions. Reciprocity is then granted between states by an electronic licensure transfer program. At present, pharmacists are not required to retake the NAPLEX at any point for license renewal.

Discussion Point

Why are professional health care organizations reluctant to support reexamination as a means of assuring continuing competence? Who are the stakeholders involved? What are some ramifications of adopting such a mandate?

CONTINUING EDUCATION

Instead of requiring health care providers to periodically repeat their initial licensure examinations, many professional associations and states have mandated CE for license renewal. This has been done in an attempt to promote continued competence and is less controversial than periodic reexamination for licensure.

CE in Nursing

A majority of the states in the United States have some kind of requirements for CE for professional nurse license renewal. These requirements typically vary from a few hours to 30 hours, every 2 years (Box 22.2). There is no requirement for CE for RNs in Arizona, Colorado, Connecticut, Georgia, Hawaii, Idaho, Illinois, Maine, Maryland, Mississippi, Missouri, Montana, New York, Oklahoma, South Dakota, Tennessee, Vermont, Virginia, Washington, and Wisconsin ("Nursing CEU Requirements," 1999–2015). Every other state has some sort of requirement for RNs.

Some states—Colorado, for example—required CE at one time, but removed that requirement because it felt that CE did not guarantee competence. Similarly, Hawaii discontinued CE requirements for many professions, including nursing and physical therapy, because of the high costs of these courses to the individual practitioner,

BOX 22.2 Sample State CE Requirements for Nurses

- *Arkansas:* 15 practice-focused contact hours every 2 years, or certification or recertification during the renewal period by a national certifying body or completion of 1 college credit hour course in nursing with a grade of C or better during licensure period (Arkansas Board of Registered Nursing, 2011).
- *California:* 30 hours every 2 years (California Board of Registered Nursing, 2015).
- *Florida:* One contact hour per calendar month of the renewal period (Florida Board of Registered Nursing, 2015).
- *Iowa:* 36 hours for a 3-year license and 24 hours for licenses less than 3 years (Iowa Board of Nursing, n.d.).
- *Michigan:* Not less than 25 hours of CE, with at least 1 hour in pain and symptom management (Michigan Nurses Association, 2014).
- *New Jersey:* 30 hours every 2 years plus a one-time requirement as part of student curricula or CE: organ, tissue donation, and recovery (Continuing Education Requirements, 2015).
- *New York:* 3 contact hours infection control every 4 years and 2 contact hours child abuse (one time; Continuing Education Requirements, 2015).
- *North Dakota:* 12 contact hours every 2 years (Continuing Education Requirements, 2015).
- *Ohio:* 24 hours every 2 years including a minimum of 1 contact hour related to the law (ORC 4723) and the rules (OAC 4723 1–23) governing nursing practice in Ohio (Continuing Education Requirements, 2015).
- *Oregon:* One-time, 6-hour course on pain management (Continuing Education Requirements, 2015).
- *Texas:* All nurses with an active Texas license are required to demonstrate continuing competency for relicensure. This includes 20 hours of CE every 2 years. In 2010, rules were changed to require contact hours to be in the nurse's area of practice (Texas Board of Nursing, 2015).

considerable costs to the state to administer the legislation, and the inability to demonstrate positive outcomes.

Discussion Point

Is the need for CE greater for one type of health care professional than another? When required, should the minimum number of mandated hours be the same for all health care professionals? If not, how many should be required for each health care specialty?

CE in Medicine

Forty-six states plus Guam, Puerto Rico, and the Virgin Islands require some form of continuing medical education (CME) for relicensure of medical doctors (MDs) and for doctors of osteopathy (DOs), although the requirements frequently differ for the two groups (Medscape Education, 2014).

The number of required hours also varies dramatically by state. For example, Colorado, Indiana, Montana, and South Dakota require no CME hours for either MDs or DOs (Medscape Education, 2014). New York requires only infection control and child abuse content. North Carolina and Illinois require 150 hours every 3 years, whereas Wisconsin requires only 30 hours every 2 years, and Arkansas requires only 20 hours each year (Medscape Education, 2014). It should be noted, however, that some medical specialty societies, specialty boards, hospital medical staffs, the Joint Commission, and insurance groups require physicians to demonstrate CE, even if the state does not require this for relicensure.

In addition, some states have laws that direct the format of the CME. Required topics often include pain management, AIDS, and domestic violence. Other states require that physicians renewing their licenses must receive instruction on ethics and professional responsibility.

Furthermore, unlike nursing CE, which is typically monitored by the state boards of nursing, there is no central repository of CME. Instead, accredited CME providers are required to keep records of *CE credits* awarded to physicians who participate in their activities for 6 years, and physicians are responsible for maintaining a record of their CME credits from all sources.

CE in Other Health Care Professions

Almost all states require CE for pharmacists, and most require the CE be from approved sources such as the American Council on Pharmacy Education. Sometimes carryover of hours or units is allowed, and sometimes the type is proscribed.

In addition, many states require acupuncturists, audiologists, and occupational therapists to have CE for license renewal. Physician assistants (PAs) must log 100 hours of CME every 2 years and sit for a recertification every 6 years to maintain their national certification (American Academy of Physician Assistants, n.d.).

Discussion Point

CE is mandated in most states for certified public accountants, optometrists, real estate brokers, nursing home administrators, and insurance brokers. Why are there fewer states mandating CE for health care professionals? What rationale can be given for why these occupations have a greater need for CE than health care professionals?

Does Requiring CE Ensure Competence?

The CE approach to continuing competence continues to be very controversial because there is limited research demonstrating correlation among CE, continuing competence, and improved patient outcomes. In addition, many professional organizations have expressed concern about the quality of mandated CE courses and the lack of courses for experts and specialists. Likewise, there is no agreement on the optimal number of annual credits needed to ensure competence. Until consensus can be reached regarding how CE should be provided and how much is needed, and until research findings show an empirical link between CE and provider competence, it is difficult to tout CE as a valid and reliable measure of continuing competence. Taft and Sparks (2008) summarized the pros and cons of mandating CE for nurses (Box 22.3).

CERTIFICATION

The Accreditation Board for Specialty Nursing Certification suggests certification "is the formal recognition of the specialized knowledge, skills, and experience demonstrated by the achievement of standards identified by a nursing specialty to promote optimal health outcomes" (American Nurses Credentialing Center [ANCC], 2014a, para. 3). Certification does not, however, include a legal scope of practice. The ANCC

BOX 22.3 Pros and Cons of CE Requirements for Nurses

Pros

- Demonstrates professionalism
- Demonstrates commitment to maintaining competence
- Demonstrates attention to patient safety and a reduction in medical errors
- Motivates employers to support CE needs of RN employees
- Raises the standard for CE for all nurses
- Research supports the conclusion that CE positively affects nursing practice

Cons

- Seat time does not guarantee learning
- Difficult to agree on competence standards
- Administrative and monitoring costs
- Concerns about the cost, access, quality, and relevance of CE offerings
- Research is inconclusive about the benefits of mandatory CE over voluntary CE
- Difficult to measure outcomes of mandatory CE on patient care due to the many variables that influence patient outcomes, including the individual nurse, the choice of the CE program, the CE program itself, learning styles, professionalism, and accountability

Source: Taft, L., & Sparks, R. K. (2008). Mandatory continuing education for nurses. *Nursing Matters, 19*(3), 4.

suggested, however, that it does protect the public by enabling anyone to identify competent people more readily; aids the profession by encouraging and recognizing professional achievement; recognizes specialization, enhances professionalism, and, in some cases, serves as a criterion for financial reimbursement (ANCC, 2014a). Organizations offering specialty certifications for nurses include the ANCC, the American Association of Critical Care Nursing, the American Association of Nurse Anesthetists, The American College of Nurse Midwives, the Board of Certification for Emergency Nursing, and the Rehabilitation Nursing Certification Board.

Becoming Certified

To achieve professional certification, nurses must meet eligibility criteria that may include years and types of work experience, as well as minimum educational levels, active nursing licenses, and successful completion of a nationally administered examination. Certifications normally last 5 years.

The American Board of Nursing Specialties

In addition to the large numbers of certified nurses, there are many different types of nursing certification credentials, and certification programs often have very different standards. This makes it difficult for providers and consumers to determine the value of a particular nursing certification. For this reason, the ABNS was created in 1991 to bring about uniformity in nursing certification, advocate for consumer protection by establishing specialty nursing certification, and increase public awareness of the value of quality certification to health care.

The ABNS is composed of nurse-certifying organizations from around the world. As the only accrediting body specifically for nursing certification, the Accreditation Council provides a peer-review process for accrediting nursing certification programs that demonstrate compliance with ABNS standards.

The American Nurses Credentialing Center

The ANA established the ANA Certification Program in 1973 to provide tangible recognition of professional achievement in a defined functional or clinical area of nursing. The ANCC, a subsidiary of the ANA, became its own corporation in 1991, and since then has certified more than a quarter million nurses and approximately 75,000 advanced practice nurses (ANCC, 2014a). The ANCC, as of 2015, administers 27 specialty certification and 12 advanced practice certification examinations each year at authorized testing agencies across

BOX 22.4 Personal Benefits of Professional Certification

- Provides a sense of accomplishment and achievement
- Validation of specialty knowledge and competence to peers and patients
- Increased credibility
- Increased self-confidence
- Promotes greater autonomy of practice
- Provides for increased career opportunities and greater competitiveness in the job market
- May result in salary incentives

the country. In addition, they administer 12 specialty certification exams for clinical nurse specialists (CNS) (ANCC, 2014b).

Certification and the Advanced Practice Nurse

Advanced practice nurses were the first nurses to use professional certification as a means of documenting advanced knowledge in practice. In 1946, the American Association of Nurse Anesthetists began certifying nurse anesthetists. The American College of Nurse Midwives soon followed. Most states now use certification as an indicator of entry-level competence in advanced practice nursing, which includes CNS and nurse practitioners (NPs).

Even the NCSBN, which originally proposed second licensure for NPs, now recognizes the certification examination as the regulatory mechanism for advanced nursing practice. A master's degree is required to take the certification examinations for advanced practice nurses. Certification, then, in the case of the advanced practice nurse is not really voluntary; it is required to ensure public safety and enhance public health.

Discussion Point

The ANCC currently does not allow educational waivers for the CSN- or NP-certifying examination (all applicants must have at least a master's degree). Do you support this decision to not "grandfather" advanced practice nurses who completed their educations through certifying programs (no master's degree) and who are currently practicing in an advanced role? Why or why not?

The Effect of Professional Certification

A great deal of research has been completed in the last decade regarding the use of certification to ensure competence and its inherent value. Most of these studies suggest that certification does have an effect on both improved patient outcomes and the creation of a positive work environment (Box 22.4). For example, Boyle, Cramer, Potter, Gatua, and Stobinski (2014) examined the impact of specialty nursing certification on patient outcomes in surgical intensive care units and perioperative units, and found lower rates of central line–associated bloodstream infections when nurses held specialty certification. In addition, Fitzpatrick, Campo, and Gacki-Smith (2014) found significant differences in perceived empowerment between emergency department staff nurses who held specialty certification and those who did not.

Creating Work Environments That Value Certification

It is middle- and top-level nurse managers who play the most significant role in creating work environments that value and reward certification. For example, nurse managers can grant tuition reimbursement or salary incentives to workers who seek certification. This is critical because significant barriers to nurses obtaining specialty certification are time and cost. Managers can also show their support for professional certification by giving employees paid time off to take the certification exam and by publicly recognizing employees who have achieved specialty certification.

Managers should also encourage certified nurses to promote their achievements by introducing themselves as certified nurses to patients and wearing their certification pins. In doing so, the certified nurse acts as a role model to other nurses considering specialty certification.

Discussion Point

Do most employers value professional certification? Do nurses value it? Does the general public value it? On what criteria do you base your answer?

REFLECTIVE PRACTICE

Reflective practice is defined by the NCBN (2015) as "a process for the assessment of one's own practice to identify and seek learning opportunities to promote continued competence" (para. 7). Inherent in the process is the evaluation and incorporation of this learning into one's practice. Such self-assessment is gaining popularity as a way to promote professional practice and maintain competence. Often this is done through the use of professional portfolios for competence assessment.

For example, North Carolina now requires RNs to use a reflective practice approach to carry out a self-assessment of her or his practice and develop a plan for maintaining competence (NCBN, 2015). This assessment is individualized to the licensed nurse's area of practice. RNs seeking license renewal or reinstatement must attest to having completed the learning activities required for continuing competence and be prepared to submit evidence of completion if requested by the board on random audit (NCBN, 2015).

Similarly, the Nurses Association of New Brunswick (NANB) developed a mandatory continuing competence program for implementation in 2008 (again revised in 2013) that requires RNs to demonstrate on an annual basis how they have maintained their competence and enhanced their practice (NANB, 2015). The NANB argues that continuing competence is a necessary component of practice and the public interest is best served when nurses enhance their knowledge, skill, and judgment on an ongoing basis; and reflective practice, or the process of continually assessing one's practice to identify learning needs and opportunities for growth, is the key to continuing competence (NANB, 2015).

The three steps of the NANB mandatory Continuing Competence Program (CCP) are as follows:

1. Self-assessment of nursing practice to determine learning needs.
2. Development and implementation of a learning plan to meet the identified learning needs.
3. Evaluation of the effect of learning activities.

The College of Registered Nurses of British Columbia (CRNBC) also has a mandatory CCP in place. This program was created in 2000 in response to the Health Professions Act, which required the establishment and maintenance of a CCP to promote high practice standards among RNs (CRNBC, 2015).

Consider This Competence is continually maintained and acquired through reflective practice, lifelong learning, and integration of learning into nursing practice (NANB, 2015).

Portfolios and Self-Assessment

Portfolio development is another strategy the individual RN can use to be reflective about his or her practice and/or to assess or demonstrate competence. The professional portfolio typically contains a number of core components, such as biographical information; educational background; certifications achieved; employment history; a resume; a competence record or checklist; personal and professional goals; professional development experiences, presentations, consultations, and publications; professional and community activities; honors and awards; and letters of thanks from patients, families, peers, organizations, and others.

Consider This All nurses should maintain a portfolio to reflect their professional growth throughout their career.

WHO IS RESPONSIBLE FOR COMPETENCE ASSESSMENT IN NURSING?

Who, then, has the responsibility for competence assessment in nursing? Should it be the individual, the employer, the regulatory board, or the certifying agency? Is it a shared responsibility? If so, are these entities willing to work together to create an integrated and systematic approach to promoting continuing competence in nursing?

Certainly, an individual responsibility for maintaining competence is suggested by the *ANA Code of Ethics for Nurses with Interpretive Statements* in its assertion that nurses are obligated to provide adequate and competent nursing care (ANA, 2015). State Nurse Practice Acts also hold nurses accountable for being reasonable and prudent in their practice. Both standards require the nurse to have at least some personal responsibility for continually assessing his or her professional competence through reflective practice.

Consider This The individual RN has a professional obligation to maintain competence.

The role of the professional association also lacks clarity. Although professional associations develop and promote standards, there is no oversight function of either initial or continuing competence.

Employers also play a role in assuring competence of employees by performing periodic performance appraisals and by carrying out the requirements of the accrediting bodies to ensure the ongoing competencies of employees. Yet employers are often among the first to argue that "a nurse is a nurse is a nurse" when it comes to meeting mandatory staffing or licensure requirements.

Regulatory boards, such as the state boards of nursing, regulate initial licensure, monitor compliance with requirements for license renewal, and take action when professional standards are breached. Yet, clearly, licensure and relicensure per se do not guarantee competence, particularly in a discipline as broad in scope and practice as nursing.

Finally, certifying organizations do help to identify those individuals who have expertise in a specific area of practice; however, knowledge expertise does not always translate into practice expertise. A lack of professional certification does not necessarily mean that the nurse lacks continuing competence. Recertification does not ensure continued expertise because recertification is usually a product of meeting CE requirements rather than reexamination.

Conclusions

The challenge in assuring competence in nursing is that nursing practice is dynamic, and thus best practice must be continually redefined as a result of new discoveries. Licensure, CE, and professional certification can ensure provider competence only if they reflect the latest thinking, research, and clinical practice needs. In addition, each of these three strategies is limited in its effectiveness as a competence assessment strategy.

Clearly, the NCLEX, as it currently exists, assures only minimum entry-level competence for professional nursing practice. Given that NCLEX content derives from a retrospective model and that technological changes and the rate of knowledge acquisition are increasing exponentially in the 21st century, the knowledge base of the newly licensed nurse has a great likelihood of being dated even before examinations are scored. In addition, as long as a single NCLEX exists and there are multiple levels of educational entry into practice, the examination will continue to have to meet educational content directed at the lowest educational level of entry.

In addition, health care professionals, professional organizations, and regulatory bodies are reluctant to implement mandatory reexamination for licensure. One must at least question whether this is because of the fear that many providers would be unable to demonstrate the continuing competence necessary for relicensure.

CE has similar limitations for assuring provider competence. Some states do not require nurses to complete CE. Those that do demonstrate wide variation in how much CE is required, what content can be included, and how that CE can be provided. In addition, there is no guarantee that completing CE courses results in a change in the provider's knowledge level or practice or even that the content provided in the CE course is current and relevant.

Finally, professional certification does ensure that the nurse has some specialized area of knowledge and practice expertise. The reality, however, is that many nurses perform outside of the area of their certification expertise each and every day in their jobs, particularly if their area of specialty certification expertise is narrow. In addition, there are multiple certifying bodies and numerous types of certification. Determining the exact value of that certification in terms of improving patient care has not completely been ascertained.

How best to ensure provider competence cannot yet be answered. Efforts that address the need to do so are under way, but these efforts have not been coordinated or integrated by the professional associations, regulatory bodies, and stakeholders that are affected. In addition, most professional entities involved in ensuring continuing competence are reluctant to mandate interventions for fear of alienating stakeholders. Individual practitioners also seem reluctant to embrace reflective practice or to put the thought and effort into creating portfolios that identify continuing competence in concrete and measurable ways. Until the focus rests solely on the need to protect patients and improve the quality of health care, mandated interventions for continuing competence are likely never to occur and provider competence will not be assured.

For Additional Discussion

1. Who should be responsible for the cost of ensuring provider competence—the provider, the employer, the clients that are served, or some other entity?
2. How likely is it that states, professional organizations, professional certifying organizations, and employers will be willing to agree on standardized measures for assessing professional competence?
3. Would most RNs support mandatory development of a portfolio? Are most RNs actively engaged in reflective practice in an effort to assess their ongoing competence?
4. Why should the entry-level examination for nursing be broad and general in scope, whereas continuing competence is arguably demonstrated by professional certification in specialty areas?
5. Are cost and access deterrents to professional certification? If so, how can these barriers be overcome?
6. Do most nurses view CE coursework as a reliable and valid tool for increasing provider competence?
7. Should nurses be required to complete mandated CE hours in the area of nursing practice in which they work?
8. Are there core competencies all licensed nurses must achieve regardless of the setting in which they practice?

References

American Academy of Physician Assistants. (n.d.). *Information about PAs and the PA profession.* Retrieved April 6, 2015, from http://www.orthocarolina.com/assets/user/media/Information_About_PAs_and_the_PA_Profession.pdf

American Nurses Association. (2014, November 12). *ANA position statement: Professional role competence.* Retrieved April 6, 2015, from http://gm6.nursingworld.org/MainMenuCategories/Policy-Advocacy/Positions-and-Resolutions/ANAPositionStatements/Position-Statements-Alphabetically/Professional-Role-Competence.html

American Nurses Association. (2015). *Code of ethics for nurses with interpretive statements.* Washington, DC: Author.

American Nurses Credentialing Center. (2014a). *Why ANCC certification?* Retrieved April 26, 2015, from http://www.nursecredentialing.org/Certification/Certified-Nurses-Day/Overview/WhyCertification

American Nurses Credentialing Center. (2014b). *ANCC certification center.* Retrieved April 26, 2015, from http://www.nursecredentialing.org/certification.aspx#specialty

Arkansas Board of Registered Nursing. (2011). *Continuing education.* Retrieved April 26, 2015, from http://www.arsbn.arkansas.gov/education/Pages/continuingEducation.aspx

Boyle, D. K., Cramer, E., Potter, C., Gatua, M. W., & Stobinski, J. X. (2014). The relationship between direct-care RN specialty certification and surgical patient outcomes. *AORN Journal, 100*(5), 511–528. doi:10.1016/j.aorn.2014.04.018

California Board of Registered Nursing. (2015). *Continuing education for license renewal.* Retrieved April 26, 2015, from http://www.rn.ca.gov/licensees/ce-renewal.shtml

Calzone, K. A., Jenkins, J., Culp, S., Caskey, S., & Badzek, L. (2014). Introducing a new competency into nursing practice. *Journal of Nursing Regulation, 5*(1), 40–47.

College of Registered Nurses of British Columbia. (2015). *Quality assurance for RNs and NPs.* Retrieved September 15, 2015, from https://www.crnbc.ca/QA/Pages/Default.aspx

Continuing education requirements by state. (2015). *Advance for Nurses.* Retrieved May 3, 2015, from http://nursing.advanceweb.com/Article/Continuing-Education-Requirements-by-State.aspx?CP=5

Dictionary.com. (2015). Competence [Definition]. Retrieved April 7, 2015, from http://dictionary.reference.com/browse/competence

Fitzpatrick, J. J., Campo, T. M., & Gacki-Smith, J. (2014). Emergency care nurses: Certification, empowerment, and work-related variables. *Journal of Emergency Nursing, 40*(2), e37–e43. doi:10.1016/j.jen.2013.01.021

Florida Board of Registered Nursing. (2015). *Continuing education requirements.* Retrieved April 26, 2015, from http://floridasnursing.gov/renewals/registered-nurse-rn/

The Free Dictionary by Farlex. (2003–2015). Licensure [Definition]. (2009). Retrieved April 7, 2015, from http://medical-dictionary.thefreedictionary.com/licensure

Institute of Medicine. (2010, October). *The future of nursing: Leading change, advancing health.* Retrieved January 31, 2015, from http://thefutureofnursing.org/IOM-Report

Iowa Board of Nursing. (n.d.). *Continuing education.* Retrieved September 15, 2015, from https://nursing.iowa.gov/continuing-education

Medscape Education. (2014, October). *State CME requirements.* Retrieved April 6, 2015, from http://www.medscape.org/public/staterequirements

Medscape. (2015, February 10). *State boards of nursing: How to find them.* Retrieved April 7, 2015, from http://www.medscape.com/viewarticle/482270

Michigan Nurses Association. (2014). *Michigan Board of Nursing continuing education requirements.* Retrieved September 15, 2015, from http://minurses.org/nursing-practice/ce-requirements

National Association of Boards of Pharmacy. (2015a). *North American Pharmacist Licensure Examination (NAPLEX).* Retrieved April 6, 2015, from http://www.nabp.net/programs/examination/naplex/

National Association of Boards of Pharmacy. (2015b). *NAPLEX—North American Pharmacist Licensure Examination/MPJE—Multistate Pharmacy Jurisprudence Examination candidate registration bulletin.* Retrieved April 6, 2015, from http://www.nabp.net/system/rich/rich_files/rich_files/000/000/902/original/naplex-mpje-bulletin-04022015.pdf

National Council State Boards of Nursing. (2015a). *Member boards.* Retrieved April 7, 2015, from https://www.ncsbn.org/member-boards.htm

National Council State Boards of Nursing. (2015b). *NCLEX and other exams.* Retrieved April 7, 2015, from https://www.ncsbn.org/nclex.htm

North Carolina Board of Nursing. (2015). *Continuing competence requirements.* Retrieved April 7, 2015, from http://www.ncbon.com/dcp/i/licensurelisting-renewalreinstatement-continuing-competence-requirements-submission-of-evidence

Nurses Association of New Brunswick. (2015). *Continuing competence program.* Retrieved April 26, 2015, from http://www.nanb.nb.ca/index.php/practice/ccp

Nursing CEU requirements. (1999–2015). Retrieved April 6, 2015, from http://www.ehow.com/facts_4969045_continuing-education-does-nurse-need.html

Taft, L., & Sparks, R. K. (2008). Mandatory continuing education for nurses. *Nursing Matters, 19*(3), 4.

Texas Board of Nursing. (2015). *Education: Continuing nursing education and competency.* Retrieved May 5, 2015, from http://www.bon.texas.gov/education_continuing_education.asp

U.S. Medical Licensing Examination. (1996–2015). *Overview.* Retrieved April 7, 2015, from http://www.usmle.org/bulletin/overview/

Watson Dillon, D. M., & Mahoney, M. A. (2015). Moving from patient care to population health: A new competency for the executive nurse leader. *Nurse Leader, 13*(1), 30–36. doi:10.1016/j.mnl.2014.11.002

6

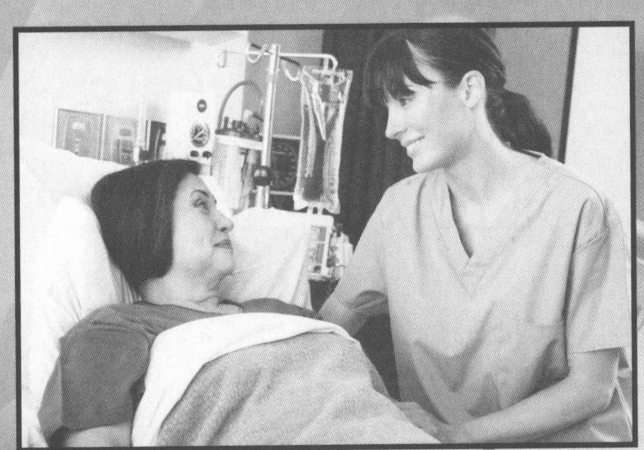

Professional Power

23

The Nursing Profession's Historic Struggle to Increase Its Power Base

Carol J. Huston

ADDITIONAL RESOURCES

Visit thePoint for additional helpful resources

- eBook
- Journal Articles
- WebLinks

CHAPTER OUTLINE

LEARNING OBJECTIVES

The learner will be able to:

1. Explore factors that historically led to nursing's limited power as a profession.
2. Examine characteristics of oppressed groups, and analyze whether the nursing profession displays those characteristics.
3. Examine factors that led to the divergence of the nursing profession and feminism in the 1960s and 1970s and subsequently to their convergence in the mid-1980s as part of second-wave feminism.
4. Analyze the influence of gender on how many nurses view policy and politics, the willingness of nurses to work together collectively to achieve common goals, and the mentoring opportunities available to the profession's future leaders.
5. Identify driving forces in place to increase the nursing profession's power base.
6. Identify potential partners/external stakeholders/alliances that could strengthen the nursing

(continues on page 333)

profession's power in national and global policy arenas.

7. Identify nurses currently holding elected office in Congress and state legislatures, as well as the significant committees they serve on or positions they hold.
8. Identify issues currently being debated in the legislature that affect nursing and health care.
9. Explore individual, organizational, and professional responsibilities for succession planning to ensure that an adequate number of highly qualified nursing leaders exist in the future.
10. Reflect on whether the need to be politically competent should be internalized by nurses as a moral and professional obligation.

INTRODUCTION

Power is an elusive concept. The word *power* is derived from the Latin verb *potere*, meaning "to be able"; thus, power may be appropriately defined as that which enables an individual or a group to accomplish goals. Power can also be defined as the capacity to act or the strength and potency to accomplish something (Marquis & Huston, 2015). Having power then gives an individual or a group the potential to change the attitudes and behaviors of others.

How individuals view power, however, varies greatly. Indeed, power may be feared, worshipped, or mistrusted, and it is frequently misunderstood (Marquis & Huston, 2015). Many women (and thus nurses) have historically demonstrated ambivalence toward the concept of power, and some have even eschewed the pursuit of power.

This likely occurred as a result of how some women have been socialized to view power, believing that women do not inherently possess power (formal or informal) or authority. In addition, rather than feeling capable of achieving and managing power, many women feel that power manages them. These gender-based perceptions are changing, yet women still have much ground to make up in terms of learning to use power as a tool for personal and professional success.

Similarly, the nursing profession has not historically been the powerful force it could be in dealing with issues directly affecting health care and the profession itself. In a 2010 Gallup poll of more than 1,500 thought leaders from insurance, corporate, health services, government, and industry, as well as university faculty, the majority felt that nurses should have more influence in many areas of the health care system, including reducing medical errors, increasing the quality of care, promoting wellness, improving efficiency, and reducing costs (Robert Wood Johnson Foundation [RWJF], 2010). In addition, these thought leaders said that "nurses should have more influence than they do now on health policy, planning, and management. But when asked how much influence various professions and groups are likely to have in health reform, opinion leaders put nurses behind government, insurance, and pharmaceutical executives, and many others—and they see real barriers to nursing leadership" (RWJF, 2010, para. 2).

Indeed, Nault and Kettering Sincox (2014) suggest that the idea of getting involved with legislation and legislators seems far removed from nursing practice and patient care for most nurses. But clearly, nursing can no longer afford to be reactive in the policy arena. Instead, the profession must determine its priorities and then create a plan for action that is strategic and timely relative to the debates taking place at the national and global levels.

Unfortunately, nurses are often thought of as an apolitical group. As a result, nursing has more often than not been reactive (rather than proactive) in the policy arena, addressing proposed legislation after its introduction rather than drafting or sponsoring legislation that reflects nursing's agenda. As a result, external forces (typically, male dominated and medically focused) have often controlled nursing.

All of these factors have contributed to the nursing profession having a relatively small power base in the political arena and some invisibility as a force in health care decision-making. This chapter explores factors that have led to this relative powerlessness as a profession. Driving forces are identified, however, that are in place to increase nursing's professional power. The chapter concludes with an action plan to increase nursing's power base so that the profession is recognized as an increasingly significant force in health care decision-making in the 21st century.

Discussion Point

Why is it that nurses, the largest group of health professionals, with perhaps the greatest firsthand knowledge of the health care problems faced by consumers, have not historically been an integral part of health care policy decision-making?

BOX 23.1 Factors Contributing to Powerlessness in Nursing

1. The oppression of nurses as a group
2. Nursing's failure to fully align with the feminist movement
3. Limited collective action by nurses
4. The socialization of women to view power and politics negatively
5. The inadequate recognition of nursing as an educated profession with evidence-based practice
6. The nursing profession's history of being reactive (rather than proactive) in national policy setting

FACTORS CONTRIBUTING TO POWERLESSNESS IN NURSING

Many factors have contributed to the nursing profession's relative powerlessness in health care policy setting. Six factors are discussed in this chapter (Box 23.1).

Oppression of Nurses as a Group

The attributes of oppression are unjust treatment, the denial of rights, and the dehumanizing of individuals. As such, it has been suggested that nurses and the nursing profession both work with oppressed groups and are themselves an oppressed group. Indeed, nursing has historically been controlled by outside forces with greater prestige, power, and status. Generally, these forces were patriarchal and male dominated, such as medicine and hospital administration. For example, in the early 1900s, physicians attempted to exclude women from knowledge emerging from the basic sciences. Their refusal to let nurses use new instrumentation sustained women's subordination in nursing, although many nurses continually and actively sought greater scientific knowledge and techniques and incorporated these into their education.

Even at the start of this decade, some physicians openly suggested they should be the only health care professionals qualified to directly treat patients, despite the fact that many of the health care professions, including nurses, now hold advanced degrees including doctorates. Indeed, some physicians and their allies are currently pushing legislative efforts to restrict the right to use the title of "doctor," arguing that "nurses who want to be called doctors in a clinical environment should pay their dues and go to medical school" (O'Donnell, 2012, para. 7). One must question whether this elitism is more an effort to control money, power, and prestige than it is a concern about whether patients will be confused. Thus, the battle over the title "doctor" is likely a proxy for a larger struggle related to dominance and status.

In addition, some nurse practitioners work with physicians or within physician groups so that they can receive 100% insurance reimbursement for their services. This is called "incident to" billing and indicates that the physician is somehow involved with the care of the nurse practitioner's patients (Nursing Power, 2015). In many states in the United States, however, nurse practitioners have autonomous practice and do not require physician involvement or presence within their practice. In performing identical services, such as a primary care visit for yearly physical exam, the nurse practitioner typically receives only 75% to 85% compensation from Medicare, Medicaid, and private insurance companies. The Medicare Payment Advisory Commission (MedPAC) examined this payment disparity and determined that there was "no specific analytic foundation" for paying nurse practitioners less than physicians for the same services. This creates nurse practitioner invisibility and decreases nurse practitioner accountability for their own services (Nursing Power, 2015).

When a group is oppressed, it tends to have value confusion and low self-esteem. This occurs because the dominant groups identify their norms and values as the "right ones" and use their initial power to enforce them as the status quo. Oppressed groups accept these norms, at least externally, in an effort to gain some power and control. For example, nursing's oppressors have not always held the same values as nursing (ie, caring, nurturance, and advocacy). This has led to confusion for some nurses and even, at times, contempt for their own profession and what it represents.

Consider This Badmouthing one's own profession may be a sign of oppression and values confusion.

Failure to Align Fully With the Feminist Movement

A second factor contributing to nursing's relative powerlessness is the profession's failure to align fully with the feminist movement. Although both nurses and women have improved their status in the last five decades, nursing has not kept pace with the progress women have made in other areas. This has occurred because, at least in part, nurses have not been fully engaged in the feminist movement.

This occurred for several reasons. One was that many feminists in the 1960s and 1970s were influenced by a more radical feminist perspective and, as a result, spoke out against women becoming nurses because it suggested that female nurses were in subordinate, caregiving roles. In addition, many nurses feared public identification with feminism.

The reality, however, is that nursing continues to be a profession composed of approximately 90% women, and this figure has changed only very slowly over time. This is noteworthy, given that there have been major gender shifts in virtually all of the other traditionally female-dominated professions (such as social workers, librarians, K-to-12 teachers) since the 1970s.

Discussion Point

Many nursing leaders in the early 1900s were political activists, actively involved in social issues such as women's suffrage and public health. At what point did nursing diverge from a sociopolitical agenda and why?

Although having female dominance in the profession may have some benefits, it also poses some liabilities. Indeed, some nursing leaders have suggested that nursing will never attain greater status and power until more men join the ranks (see Chapter 8). Others think that adding men to nursing's ranks is not the answer. Instead, nurses need to accept the responsibility for addressing the problems that have historically plagued the profession, and take whatever steps are necessary to proactively build a power base that does not depend on gender.

Consider This Being a female professional in a male-dominated health care system brings to mind the "Ginger Rogers syndrome." Both Ginger Rogers and her dancing partner, Fred Astaire, were known as wonderful dancers, but Fred Astaire's name always came first, and he always received the greater recognition. In reality, Ginger Rogers danced the same steps as Fred Astaire, but she did them backward and in high heels. So, who deserved the greater recognition?

In addition, recognition that assertive, independent nurses cannot exist if they have been socialized to be dependent women is growing. Similarly, it is improbable, if not impossible, for female nurses to implement expanded roles in advanced practice if they are unaware of or unwilling to recognize the social constraints imposed on them because they are women. Clearly, the battles between the American Medical Association (AMA) and advanced practice nurses about scope of practice, reimbursement, and the need for medical oversight are likely related as much to gender as they are to competition over patients (see Chapter 4).

Nurses need, then, to continue to examine the progress women have made in other professions and work with them inside and outside of nursing to strengthen power for women everywhere. This holds true for the men in nursing as well because the relative powerlessness of the profession transfers to them too, despite gender differences. Both male and female nurses must solve problems, work to advance the science of nursing, network to increase nursing's knowledge base and power, and provide mutual support.

Limited Collective Representation of Nurses

A third factor limiting the development of the nursing profession's power base is the inadequate collective representation of nurses by groups, such as collective bargaining agents and professional nursing organizations. Only about 18% of the 3.1 million nurses in the United States belong to collective bargaining units (Marquis & Huston, 2015). Only about 5% of nurses (approximately 163,011) belong to the American Nurses Association (ANA), the nationally recognized professional organization for all registered nurses (RNs), whose mission is to advance and protect the profession (Union Facts, 2014). These relatively small membership numbers directly reflect the money that is available for lobbyists to represent nursing in the political arena. In contrast, the AMA has one of the most powerful lobbying organizations in the United States.

Consider This Nurses must be represented in mass before they will be able to significantly affect the decisions that directly influence their profession.

There are many reasons for the small representation of nurses in the ANA. The dual and often conflicting role of the ANA as both a professional organization for nurses and a collective bargaining agent is certainly one reason (see Chapter 21). In addition, some nurses think that state nurses associations have been burdened with the task of collective bargaining under the federation model of the ANA and that other programs have suffered as a result of funds being used for collective bargaining. Other nurses have expressed concerns about the cost of membership in the ANA or argued that the ANA is not responsive enough to the needs of the nurse at the bedside. Other nurses look on nursing as a job and not as a career and have little interest in professional issues outside of their immediate work environment.

Discussion Point

Do you belong to a professional nursing organization? Why or why not? Do contemporary nursing leaders espouse this as a value? Is it encouraged in the workplace and in the academic world?

Whether these issues are valid is almost immaterial. The reality is that as long as such a small percentage of nurses belong to the ANA, the economic power of the ANA will be limited, as will its ability to significantly influence policy setting and legislation. Perhaps even more importantly, until nurses are willing to work together collectively in some form, they will be unlikely to increase either their personal or their professional power.

Consider This At times, nurses have lacked pride in their collective groups and have viewed alignment with other nurses as alignment with other powerless persons, something that does little to advance an individual's professional power.

Unfortunately, more often than not, nurses in this country have not acted cohesively, whether at the local level, fighting for wage increases, or at the national level, attempting to influence health policy. Even the various professional nursing organizations to which nurses belong have not historically worked together cooperatively. The reality is that nurses continue to be widely divided on basic issues such as entry into practice, mandatory staffing ratios, and collective bargaining. Strategies to promote greater nurse unity are shown in Box 23.2.

Consider This A metaphor for increasing nursing's power base through collective action would be a snowball. Individual snowflakes are fragile, but when they stick together, they become a powerful force.

Socialization of Women to View Power and Politics Negatively

A fourth factor contributing to powerlessness in the nursing profession has been the socialization of women to view power and politics negatively. Politics is the art of using legitimate power wisely, and it requires clear decision-making, assertiveness, accountability, and the willingness to express one's views (Marquis & Huston, 2015). It also requires being proactive rather than reactive and demands decisiveness.

Unfortunately, there is a persistent belief that political positioning is antithetical to quality nursing care. Perron (2013) suggests that nurses are not faced with choosing between caring for their patients and engaging with politics. Instead, she argues that the ethical merit of nursing care relies instead on positioning nurses squarely at the center-of-care activities, experiences, and functions. Nurses, then, become not a group that needs

BOX 23.2 Strategies for Promoting Unity Within the Nursing Profession

1. Nurses must respect each other's specialties and work toward enriching each other's job and work environments.
2. Nurses must acknowledge the different expertise that will help promote the quality care expected of them.
3. Nurses need to be self-aware regarding their behaviors that lead to disunity.
4. Nurses need to examine and learn from the nursing legacy that has negatively affected their behavior individually and collectively.
5. Accommodation of new vibrant views should be encouraged. This could be done through proper mentoring of the newly graduated nurses.
6. Collaboration among nursing organizations and working collectively, would strengthen nursing.

Source: Thupayagale-Tshweneagae, G., & Dithole, K. (2007). Unity among nurses: An evasive concept. *Nursing Forum, 42*(3), 143–146.

to be controlled and governed, but individuals who must care for their selves before they may care for anyone else.

The International Council of Nurses (ICN) and the World Health Organization agree, suggesting that nurses can and should be involved in policy development since they are uniquely positioned to provide crucial policy information (ICN, 2014). Furthermore, health policy often has a direct effect on nurses, and it is in their best interest to be engaged in its formulation. The ICN (2014) argues that a cultural shift must occur within the nursing profession to emphasize the importance of policy and nurses' role in setting and implementing it. In addition, a clear understanding of how policy affects nurses as well as how their unique knowledge regarding client care is crucial for policy development must be embedded at the institutional level. This cultural shift must also occur in educational institutions where the integration of policy in practice must be emphasized in nursing classrooms and faculty must be given the proper support to develop and carry out policy research so that policy makers and administrators can draw from the evidence base when developing policy.

Consider This Changing nurses' view of both power and politics is perhaps the most significant key to proactive rather than reactive participation in policy setting.

Nurses, then, must perceive a need not only to be more knowledgeable about power, negotiation, and politics but also to be more involved in broad social and political issues. This requires becoming politically astute. Nurses need to understand what politics means, and they need to become experts in using politics to help nursing achieve both its professional goals and the needs of their clients.

Inadequate Recognition of Nursing as an Educated Profession With Evidence-Based Practice

A fifth factor contributing to the nursing profession's relative powerlessness is the inadequate recognition of nursing as a profession driven by research and the pursuit of higher education. Although nurses should value highly the caring, intuitive, nurturing part of nursing practice, the nursing profession has been negligent about equally emphasizing their extensive scientific knowledge base and the high level of critical thinking and analysis professional nurses use every day in their clinical practice.

Both the art and the science of nursing require highly developed skills and a well-developed knowledge base. The nurse of the 21st century has an extensive knowledge base in the sciences as well as in the arts. In addition, nurses must be expert critical thinkers, as they are required to continually look for and analyze subtle clues in their client data, make independent nursing diagnoses, and create plans of care. Constant assessment of and adjustment to the plan of care are almost always necessary, so nurses must be highly organized and know how to set priorities. In addition, nurses must have highly refined communication skills, well-developed psychomotor skills, and sophisticated leadership and management skills. This is the image nurses must promote to the public.

Discussion Point

If the public was asked to list five adjectives to describe nursing, what would they be? Would the art or the science of nursing be recognized more? Would nurses themselves use different adjectives?

The Nursing Profession's History of Being Reactive in National Policy Setting

The last factor discussed here as contributing to a relative lack of professional power in nursing is the profession's history of being reactive rather than proactive in national policy setting regarding nursing practice. *Reactive* means waiting until there is a problem and then trying to fix it. *Proactive* is more anticipatory; it means developing appropriate policy before taking action or a problem occurs.

Unfortunately, the nursing profession has been far from proactive in shaping its own course or that of the health care system. In the 1990s, health care became big business. Managed care proliferated, and gatekeepers, not providers and consumers, began deciding who needed care and how much care was needed. Hospitals lost their place as the center of the health care universe as client care shifted from inpatient hospital stays to outpatient and ambulatory health care settings. Physicians lost much of their autonomy to practice medicine as they saw fit as insurers increasingly placed restrictions not only on which physicians patients could see but also on what services the physician was authorized to prescribe.

Patients found themselves with limited choices of providers, longer wait times for care, more rules to follow, and more confusion about what would and would not be a covered expense. At the same time, RNs in record numbers, for the first time in history, were downsized, restructured, and often replaced by a cheaper counterpart in an effort to reduce costs.

Many nurses felt both overwhelmed and helpless with this degree of change. However, these changes did not happen overnight. Many of them were incremental and insidious, and the health care system changes occurred with little concerted effort by nurses to stop them.

Senge (1990) wrote about a brief parable in *The Fifth Discipline* that nurses should keep front and foremost when they think about the need to be proactive, even with incremental change. It is called "The parable of the boiled frog," and it goes like this:

> *If you place a frog in a pot of boiling water, it will immediately try to scramble out. But if you place the frog in room temperature water, and don't scare him, he'll stay put. Now, if the pot sits on a heat source, and if you gradually turn up the temperature, something very interesting happens. As the temperature rises from 70 to 80 degrees Fahrenheit, the frog will do nothing. In fact, he will show every sign of enjoying himself. As the temperature gradually increases, the frog will become groggier and groggier, until he is unable to crawl out of the pot. Though there is nothing restraining him, the frog will sit there and boil. He will boil to death, oblivious to what is happening to him.*

Consider This Gradual but constant change may be even more dangerous than cataclysmic change because resistance is less organized.

DRIVING FORCES TO INCREASE NURSING'S POWER BASE

So what is the likelihood that the nursing profession will ever be a powerful force in health care decision-making and the political arena? The answer is unclear, although the likelihood of this happening is increasing because of several driving forces in place. This chapter discusses six of these forces (Box 23.3).

Timing Is Right

Timing is everything. The political ferment regarding health care reform continues to escalate, and issues of cost and access are paramount in this country. For 2015, the United States is budgeted to spend US$1.4 trillion on health care, an amount equal to 22% of the gross domestic product (U.S. Government Spending, 2015). In fact, the United States spends more than any other industrialized country in the world (two to three times that of most industrialized countries). Yet its rankings in terms of life span, infant mortality, and teenage pregnancy are much lower than those of many countries that spend significantly less on health care.

The passage and implementation of the Affordable Care Act (ACA) has only escalated public awareness and debate about flaws in publicly funded or subsidized health care in the United States. Gardner (2014) suggests, however, that despite significant negative public opinion regarding the ACA, a return to the status quo wouldn't be tolerated by most Americans. Instead, she argues that nurses have influence, especially if our numbers are leveraged, and that as a profession, we must vigorously oppose legislation that undermines or compromises the goals of the ACA and be a part of the solution in directing policy through political goodwill.

Furthermore, as a result of publications like *To Err Is Human*, consumers, health care providers, and legislators are more aware than ever of the shortcomings of the current health care system, and the clamor for action has never been louder (see Chapter 15). Clearly, the public wants a better health care system, and nurses want to be able to provide high-quality nursing care. Both are powerful elements for change, and new nurses are entering the profession at a time when their energy and expertise will be more valued than ever.

BOX 23.3 Driving Forces to Increase Nursing's Power Base

1. The timing is right
2. The size of the nursing profession and the diversity of our practice
3. Nursing's referent power
4. The increasing knowledge base and education for nurses
5. Nursing's unique perspective
6. The desire for change among consumers and providers

Nault and Kettering Sincox (2014) agree, suggesting that the present health care system is unreasonably costly with a myriad of access and patient safety issues. They argue that the creativity of nurses is needed to provide new solutions to problems and that it is time to individually and collectively determine what can be done to effectively influence the legislative process and policy development.

Size of the Nursing Profession and Diversity of Our Practice

The second driving force for increasing nursing's professional power base is the size of the profession and the diversity of nursing practice. Numbers are the lifeblood of politics. If nurses do not vote as a block, however, their political voice becomes diluted. The nursing profession's size, then, is perhaps its greatest asset, and its potential for a collective voting block should increasingly be recognized as a force to deal with.

Consider This Collective involvement of only a fraction of the nation's 3.1 million RNs in health care policy would produce a significant voting block.

Discussion Point

Have nurses ever made a concerted effort to vote collectively? What positions have professional organizations such as the ANA taken on recent election issues or candidates for office? Have endorsements by professional nursing organizations influenced how you vote?

Nursing's Referent Power

A third driving force for increasing the power of the profession is the referent power nurses hold. *Referent power* is the power one has when others identify with you or what you symbolize; therefore, you have their admiration or respect (Marquis & Huston, 2015). Nurses have a high degree of referent power because of the trust and credibility given to them by the public.

An Increasing Knowledge Base and Education for Nurses

A fourth driving force for increasing the power of the profession is nursing's increasing knowledge base. Indeed, the Institute of Medicine (IOM, 2011) in *The Future of Nursing: Focus on Education* notes that:

> *Transforming the health care system to provide safe, quality, patient-centered, accessible, and affordable care will require a comprehensive rethinking of the roles of many health care professionals, nurses chief among them. To realize this vision, nursing education must be fundamentally improved both before and after nurses receive their licenses.* (para. 1)

Fortunately, more nurses are being prepared at the master's and doctoral levels than ever before. Eileen Breslin, current President of the American Association of Colleges of Nursing, stated she "expects to see the momentum continue to build for advancing nursing education at all levels" since "employers are looking for highly skilled nurses able to translate the latest scientific evidence into practice" (Wood, 2015, para. 19). One of the greatest areas of growth will be in the number of doctor of nursing practice students, with more than 15,000 students now pursuing a practice doctorate. Additionally, during the past decade, enrollment in PhD in nursing programs increased by 49% and is expected to further increase this year (Wood, 2015).

Furthermore, leadership, management, and political theory are increasingly a part of baccalaureate nursing education, although the majority of nurses still do not hold baccalaureate degrees. These are learned skills, and, collectively, the nursing profession's knowledge of leadership, politics, negotiation, and finance is increasing. This can only increase the nursing profession's influence outside the field.

Nursing's Unique Perspective

A fifth driving force for increasing the nursing profession's power base is the unique philosophical perspective nursing brings to the health care arena. Nursing's perspective is unique as a result of its blending of art and science—a blending of "caring" and "curing," so to speak. The caring part of the nursing role is better known and better understood by the public. It is what historically has defined nursing. It is important that nurses not forget or underappreciate the unique values nursing represents because these are the values that make the profession different from all the others. These same values will make nursing irreplaceable in the current health care system.

The "science" part of nursing is less understood by the public. Nursing has an extensive scientific knowledge base, and the high level of critical thinking and

BOX 23.4 Action Plan for Increasing the Power of the Nursing Profession

1. More nurses must be placed in positions of influence.
2. Nurses must stop acting like victims.
3. Nurses must become better informed about all health care policy efforts.
4. Coalition building must occur within and outside of nursing.
5. More research must be done to strengthen evidence-based practice.
6. Nursing leaders must be supported.
7. Attention must be paid to mentoring future nurse leaders and leadership succession.

analysis professional nurses use every day in their clinical practice is enormous. Nursing practice is increasingly becoming *evidence based*, meaning that nursing practice reflects what the literature says is "best practice." That is, the practice of nursing is research based and scientifically driven (see Chapter 2). Unfortunately, consumers, legislators, and sometimes even other health care professionals fail to recognize this. Nursing then must do a better job of explaining and emphasizing both the art and the science of its practice.

Nault and Kettering Sincox (2014) agree, suggesting that since issues that can dramatically affect nursing practice can easily come through the legislative process, nurses must be at that table. Too much can go wrong if legislators, who do not understand these changes, are left to make decisions without the input of those who provide professional care 24 hours a day, 365 days a year.

Consumers and Providers Want Change

Finally, health care restructuring and health care reform are resulting in unrest for health care consumers, as well as providers. Limited consumer choice, hospital restructuring, the downsizing of registered nursing, and the IOM medical error reports were the sparks needed to mobilize nurses, as well as consumers, to take action. Nurses began speaking out about how downsizing and restructuring were affecting the care they were providing, and the public began demanding accountability. The public does care who is caring for them and how that affects the quality of their care. The good news, then, is that the flaws of the health care system are no longer secret and nursing has the opportunity to use its expertise and influence to help create a better health care system for the future.

ACTION PLAN FOR THE FUTURE

Based on these driving forces, an action plan can be created to increase the power of the nursing profession in the 21st century. This chapter identifies seven possible strategies to achieve this goal (Box 23.4).

Place More Nurses in Positions of Influence

The IOM (2011) suggested that for health care reform to work, nurses must be a part of decision-making processes in the health care system. This means placing nurses on advisory committees, commissions, and boards where policy decisions are made to advance health systems to improve patient care (IOM, 2011).

Training will be required, however, since many nurses lack basic skills in health care finance and policy. Indeed, a 2015 study suggested that increased orientation to liabilities and fiduciary duties were needed for nurses to be present and active on boards at all levels (Walton, Lake, Mullinix, Allen, & Mooney, 2015) (Research Study Fuels the Controversy 23.1).

Unfortunately, although nurses typically represent the greatest percentage of the workforce in hospitals, few nurses serve on hospital boards or hold positions of significant power. A survey by the American Hospital Association (AHA) of over 1,000 hospitals in 2010 found that nurses made up only 6% of board members, whereas physicians held more than 20% of board seats (Walton et al., 2015).

For this reason, the Honor Society of Nursing, Sigma Theta Tau International (STTI, 2015) has created a number of resources for nurses interested in gaining the skill set necessary to serve on the boards of health care institutions. One resource is a 2-year *Board Leadership Development* program that focuses on increasing knowledge and skills in the areas of strategic thinking and planning, fiduciary oversight, board and staff partnerships, and generative governance. Online educational resources are also available for nurses interested in learning how to be knowledgeable, contributing leaders on national and international not-for-profit boards.

Research Study Fuels the Controversy 23.1

Preparing Nurses for Boards

The purpose of this study was to examine the orientation experiences of nurses to boards and their preparation to influence health care and health care policy. A Web-based survey about the efficacy of board orientation was sent to members of three local boards made up exclusively of nurses. A convenience sample of 46 board members was eligible and invited to participate in the survey about their board orientation experience.

Source: Walton, A., Lake, D., Mullinix, C., Allen, D., & Mooney, K. (2015). Enabling nurses to lead change: The orientation experiences of nurses to boards. *Nursing Outlook, 63*(2), 110–116. doi:10.1016/j.outlook.2014.12.015

Study Findings

Liabilities and fiduciary duties were least likely to be addressed in board orientation for nurses. Board members requested more training in finance and a more formal/structured orientation process. One respondent in the narrative comments mentioned wanting more information about "teamwork and group process." Two respondents said they wanted more information about "strategic planning." The researchers concluded that orientation elements for nurses serving on boards would best prepare them to serve on interprofessional hospital boards and work in the health policy arena.

In addition, the ANA, the American Academy of Nursing, and the American Nurses Foundation, the charitable and philanthropic arm of ANA, have founded the *Nurses on Boards Coalition*. This coalition is implementing a national strategy to bring nurses' valuable perspective to governing boards, as well as state-level and national commissions, with an interest in health. The goal is to put 10,000 nurses on boards by the year 2020 ("National Coalition Launches," 2015).

In addition, nurses must be placed in national positions that influence public policy. For example, a significant effort began in 2005 to establish an *Office of the National Nurse* in the United States, who would serve as an assistant to the surgeon general. A National Nursing Network Organization was formed, and legislation has repeatedly been introduced in Congress since 2006 to achieve this goal.

Most recently, HR 379, The National Nurse Act of 2015, was introduced. This bill would designate the same individual serving as the Chief Nurse Officer of the Public Health Service as the National Nurse for Public Health (American Nurses Association [ANA], 2015a). This bill elevates this nurse into a full-time leadership position to focus on the critical work needed to address national priorities of health promotion and disease prevention. Major efforts would be directed at improving health literacy and decreasing health disparities in America (The National Nurse for Public Health, 2015). Proponents of the idea suggest that such a position would raise the profile of nursing and assist in a nationwide cultural shift to prevention and health promotion. Opponents suggest that this might not be the best way to effect change both within nursing and in the health care system.

Not all positions that influence public policy, however, occur at the national level. Indeed, few leaders burst on to the national scene directly. Instead, they assume leadership roles in entities such as medical centers, community hospitals, government agencies, and insurance companies.

Running for and holding elected office is, however, the ultimate in political activism and involvement. A total of six nurses were serving in Congress as of 2015 (ANA, 2015b). Many more nurses hold elected office in state legislatures.

In fact, nurses are uniquely qualified to hold public office because they have the greatest firsthand experience of problems faced by patients in the health care system, as well as an ability to translate the health care experience to the general public. As a result, more nurses must seek out this role. In addition, because the public respects and trusts nurses, nurses who choose to run for public office are often elected. The problem, then, is not that nurses are not being elected … the problem is that not enough nurses are running for office.

Stop Acting Like Victims

A second part of the action plan to increase the power of the nursing profession in the 21st century is that nurses must stop acting like victims. This is not to say that some nurses have not been victimized. The reality, however, is that nursing, like any other profession, has positive and negative attributes. Whining and acting like a victim never fixes problems. Nurses unhappy with their career choice either need to fix what is wrong or leave and find a job that fulfills their expectations.

In addition, it is critical that each nurse never lose sight of his or her potential to make a difference. Some legislators and nursing employers have argued that "a nurse is a nurse is a nurse." This is wrong. Nurses can be whatever they want to be in nursing, and they can achieve that goal at whatever level of quality they choose. The bottom line, however, is that the profession will only be as smart, as motivated, and as directed as its weakest link. If the nursing profession is to be the powerful force it can be, it needs to be filled with bright, highly motivated people who want to make a difference in the lives of the clients with whom they work, as well as in the health care system itself.

Consider This Individuals may be born average, but staying average is a choice.

Nurses also must realize that part of the reason nursing has been invisible or portrayed inappropriately in the media is that nurses have not assumed the spokesperson roles they could have or should have for their profession. More nurses need to gain the skills needed to effectively interact with the media about nursing and health care.

Become Better Informed About All Health Care Policy Efforts

The third step of the action plan is that nurses must become better informed about all health care policy efforts—especially those that influence their profession. This is difficult because no one can do this but nurses. This means grassroots knowledge building and involvement. O'Connor (2014) agrees, suggesting that the privileged intimacy the nursing role affords carries with it responsibilities beyond practice and professional responsibilities. It carries political responsibilities as well.

Consider This Nurses who do not understand the legislative process will not be able to influence the policy-making process.

One effort to increase the number of nurses who are well prepared to influence health policy at the local, state, and national levels was the launch of the American Nurses Advocacy Institute (ANAI) in 2009. ANAI fellows attend a 2+ day seminar in Washington, DC to strengthen their competence in the political arena and participate in a year-long formal mentoring program. The institute covers content such as the advocacy process, criteria and methods for conducting political environment scans, effective strategies for creating and sustaining policy change, and coalition building ("RNs Hone Their Advocacy Skills," 2015).

Another program that helps nurses acquire the leadership skills to shape health care locally and nationally is the *Robert Wood Johnson Foundation Executive Nurse Fellows* program (RWJF, 2015). This 3-year program allows fellows to strengthen their leadership capacity and improve their abilities to lead teams and organizations in improving health and health care. The program targets leadership competencies focused on leading oneself, leading others, leading the organization, and leading in health care.

Not all nurses, however, need to or want to be this involved in politics and policy setting. Determining how directly or indirectly one should be involved is a personal decision. Certainly, being an informed voter should be considered a minimum expectation. O'Connor (2014) suggests that voting is an expression of respect for our freedom; conversely, not to vote is to disrespect our freedom, to take it for granted.

Fortunately, nurses are in the enviable position of having great credibility with legislators and the public. Nurses who choose to be directly involved in politics and policy setting can seek public office or become more involved in lobbying legislators about issues pertinent to health care and nursing. Such lobbying can be done either in person or by writing, and there are many good sources on how to do both. The legislator needs to understand why this is an issue that is critical not only to the nursing profession but also to his or her constituents. It is important, then, to create a need for the legislator to listen to what is being said.

Nurses can also give freely of their time and money to support nursing's position in the legislative arena. This can be done indirectly by contributing to professional associations such as the ANA, which have lobbyists in the legislative arena to protect nursing's interests, or by giving money directly to a political campaign. In this case, nurses should try to give early and to make as large a contribution as possible. It is the early and significant contributions that are remembered most.

Nurses interested in a more indirect contribution to policy development may work to influence and educate the public about nursing and the nursing agenda to reform health care. Either role is helpful—at least the nurse will have made a conscious decision to be involved. Other strategies for effecting change through political involvement are noted in Box 23.5.

BOX 23.5 Political Activities to Effect Change

1. Campaigning
   a. Know the issues associated with pending or potential legislation, and formulate a view related to that legislation.
   b. Organize a "call to action" by urging nursing health professionals to contact a legislator and identifying a legislator's position on an issue.
   c. Work for a political candidate.
   d. Attend political meetings.
   e. Make a campaign contribution.
   f. Provide links to a candidate's website.
2. Communicating
   a. Join organizations and assist in the development and wide dissemination of policy statements.
   b. Write letters to the editors of well-known lay newspapers and professional health care journals.
   c. Contact legislators.
   d. Present congressional testimony.
   e. Become a consultant to political candidates, help write their campaign message, and prepare policy briefings.
   f. Use social network media to get the message out to broader audiences.
   g. All television networks are required to provide free advertising space for public service announcements (PSAs). Volunteer to write the script for those PSAs.
3. Voting
   a. Register to vote and take the lead in organizing voter registration activities.
   b. Public universities are mandated to ensure that all college students are made aware of the process for registering to vote. Ensure that nursing students are aware of the process, and engage them in debating the issues.
   c. Promote the appointment of qualified nurses of key governmental positions.
4. Protesting
   a. Participate in a boycott.
   b. Support an action to strike.
   c. Organize a march.
   d. Oppose legislation.

Source: McNeal, G. J. (2011). Politicization: The power of influence. *ABNF Journal, 22*(3), 51–52.

Build Coalitions Inside and Outside of Nursing

The fourth step of the action plan to increase professional power in the 21st century is for the nursing profession to look within itself as well as beyond its organizations for coalition building. For example, in September 2011, National Nurses United (the largest union of and professional association of RNs in the United States with more than 150,000 members) coordinated more than 10,000 RNs across the nation as they "staged 61 actions in 21 states to call for a tax on Wall State in order to raise revenue for healing Main Street America." This protest was likely the biggest series of events ever hosted by nurses in US history ("Nurses Hold Record Number," 2011).

Belonging to professional nursing organizations is another way in which nurses can network for coalition building. Coalitions have been formed within nursing groups as well. The Tri-Council for Nursing is an alliance of four autonomous nursing organizations: the AACN, the ANA, the AONE, and the NLN. The Tri-Council focuses on leadership for education, practice, and research.

The Council for the Advancement of Nursing Science (CANS) is another example of coalition building among nursing groups. The Council is composed of representatives from the four major regional research societies, STTI, the American Academy of Nursing, and the National Institute of Nursing Research (CANS, 2015).

Similarly, the National Federation for Specialty Nursing Organizations and the Nursing Organizations Liaison Forum, an entity of the ANA, merged in 2001 to become the Nursing Organizations Alliance (NOA), also known as The Alliance. The Alliance provides a forum for identification, education, and collaboration building on issues of common interest to advance the nursing profession (The Alliance, 2015).

Consider This More collaboration among nursing organizations would increase the power of the nursing profession.

Discussion Point

All too frequently, the AMA and the ANA stand in opposition to each other in the legislative arena. Are there health care issues on which they could partner? Are there issues on which the ANA and the AHA could partner?

Nurses have not done as well, however, in building political coalitions with other healthcare professionals with similar challenges. Nurses have also not done well in building political coalitions with legislators. Most legislators have a great deal of respect for nurses, but know little about their qualifications to speak with authority about the health care system. Nurses need to become experts at political networking, making tradeoffs, negotiating, and coalition building. They also need to see the bigger picture of health care. This is not to say that nurses should lose sight of client needs but that they must do a better job of seeing the bigger picture and of building and strengthening alliances with others before they will be seen as powerful and capable.

Conduct More Research to Strengthen Evidence-Based Practice

Another critical strategy for increasing nursing's power base is to continue to develop and promote evidence-based practice in nursing. Great strides have been made in researching what it is that nurses do that makes a difference in patient outcomes (research on *nursing sensitive outcomes*), but more needs to be done. Nursing practice must reflect what research has identified as best practices, and a better understanding of the relationship between nursing practice and patient outcomes is still needed.

Consider This Only relatively recently has research been able to prove that patients get better because of nurses and not in spite of them.

Building and sustaining evidence-based practice in nursing will require far greater numbers of master's and doctorally prepared nurse researchers, as well as entry into practice at an educational level similar to that of other professions. Social work, physical therapy, and occupational therapy all now have the master's or doctoral degree as the entry level into practice. Nursing cannot afford to continue debating whether a bachelor's degree is necessary as the minimum entry level into professional practice (see Chapter 1).

Support Nursing Leaders

Another part of the action plan to increase the profession's power is that nurses must support their nursing leaders and recognize the challenges they face as visionary change agents. Nurses have often viewed their leaders as rule breakers, and this has often occurred at a high personal cost to innovators.

In addition, nurses often resist change and new ideas from their leaders, and instead look to leaders in medicine and other health-related disciplines. Some of this occurs as a result of nurse leaders being discounted, at least in part, because of their female majority, and also in part to the low value placed on nursing expertise.

It is important to remember that, typically, it is not outsiders who divide nursing followers from nursing leaders. Instead, the division of nursing's strength often comes from within. Nursing leaders must be perceived as the profession's best advocates. Differing viewpoints should be not only acknowledged but also encouraged. There is a proper arena for conflict and argument, but the outward force presented must be one of unity and direction.

Mentor Future Nurse Leaders, and Plan for Leadership Succession

Finally, and perhaps most important, before nursing can become a powerful profession, nurses must actively plan for leadership succession and care for younger members by providing mentoring opportunities. It is the future leaders who face the task of increasing nursing's power base in the 21st century.

Female-dominated professions have a history of exemplifying what is known as the *queen bee syndrome.* The queen bee is a woman who, after great personal struggle, becomes successful in her career. Her attitude, however, is that because she had to make it on her own with so little help, other novices should have to do the same. Thus, there has been inadequate empowering of young nurse leaders by older, more established nurse leaders. It is the young who hold not only the keys to the present but also the hope for the future. The nursing profession is responsible for ensuring leadership succession and is morally bound to do it with the brightest, most highly qualified individuals.

Discussion Point

Is the nursing profession proactive in planning its leadership succession, or is it a change that occurs by drift?

Conclusions

D'Antonio, Connolly, Wall, Whelan, and Fairman (2010) suggest that while marginalization, invisibility, and gender issues have been and continue to be a part of nursing's history, there is also evidence of strength, purpose, and successful political action. Still, there is little doubt that nursing, as a female-dominated profession, will face more challenges than male-dominated professions in having a strong voice in health care policy. Nursing lobbyists in the nation's capitol are influencing legislation on quality, access to care, patient and health worker safety, health care restructuring, reimbursement for advanced practice nurses, and funding for nursing education. Representatives of professional nursing organizations regularly attend and provide testimony at government agency meetings to be sure that the "nursing perspective" is heard on health policy issues.

Yet, clearly, nurses, as health care professionals, need to have greater input into and control over how the health care system evolves in this country. We need a health care system that will guarantee basic, affordable health care coverage for all citizens and in which all the members of the multidisciplinary health care team work together to create policy and provide care based on what is best for the patient. We also need a health care system that is accountable for its outcomes—that recognizes that individuality, autonomy, quality, and basic human dignity are essential components of health care services and that the bottom line is not always a number.

The nursing profession must be held accountable for being an integral force in shaping such a health care system. Indeed, nursing has a moral and professional obligation to do so. McNeal (2011) perhaps says it best:

> *For too long the discipline of nursing has quietly watched as other disciplines have slowly taken over many duties that were once only within the purview of the nursing profession. Pharmacy chains now conduct blood pressure screening and provide immunizations; retail stores have opened convenience clinics throughout the nation staffed by family nurse practitioners; and, social workers perform case management activities. At no other time in the history of this profession has the Office of the President recognized the value of nursing by creating ample provisions within the Healthcare Reform Act to facilitate nursing's ability to take the lead. This is our time, this is our moment. Let's not permit this time to pass us by.* (p. 52)

For Additional Discussion

1. Should the nursing profession target the recruitment of men into nursing in an effort to increase professional power?
2. What partners/external stakeholders should the nursing profession seek in terms of alliances or coalitions to strengthen its position in the policy arena?
3. What are the priority issues the nursing profession should identify in creating a proactive legislative agenda?
4. Will nursing ever be able to increase its power base if it does not increase its educational entry level to a level similar to that of other health care professions?
5. Do nursing schools provide enough content on politics, policy, and leadership for nurses to develop some degree of political competence? If not, what is missing?
6. Do most nurses internalize the need to be politically competent as a moral and professional obligation?
7. What legislative issues being debated have the greatest potential effect on nursing and health care?

References

The Alliance. (2015). *About us*. Retrieved April 5, 2015, from http://syllabus.nursing-alliance.org/dnn/AboutUs.aspx

American Nurses Association. (2015a). *The National Nurse for Public Health*. Retrieved April 5, 2015, from http://www.nursingworld.org/ONN

American Nurses Association. (2015b). *Nurses currently serving in Congress*. Retrieved April 5, 2015, from http://www.nursingworld.org/MainMenuCategories/Policy-Advocacy/Federal/Nurses-in-Congress

D'Antonio, P., Connolly, C., Wall, B., Whelan, J., & Fairman, J. (2010). Histories of nursing: The power and the possibilities. *Nursing Outlook, 58*(4), 207–213.

Gardner, D. B. (2014). Dismantle or improve ObamaCare? Nurses must take action. *Nursing Economics, 32*(6), 323–326.

Institute of Medicine. (2011). *The future of nursing: Focus on education*. Retrieved December 29, 2011, from http://www.iom.edu/Reports/2010/The-Future-of-Nursing-Leading-Change-Advancing-Health/Report-Brief-Education.aspx

International Council of Nurses. (2014). Moving towards the greater involvement of nurses in policy development. *International Nursing Review, 61*(1), 1–2. doi:10.1111/inr.12092

Marquis, B., & Huston, C. (2015). *Leadership roles and management functions in nursing* (8th ed.). Philadelphia, PA: Lippincott Williams & Wilkins.

McNeal, G. J. (2011). Politicization: The power of influence. *ABNF Journal, 22*(3), 51–52.

National coalition launches effort to place 10,000 nurses on governing boards by 2020. (2015). *The American Nurse*. Retrieved April 3, 2015, from http://www.theamericannurse.org/index.php/2015/01/05/national-coalition-launches-effort-to-place-10000-nurses-on-governing-boards-by-2020/

The National Nurse for Public Health. (2015). *Special interest: HR 3679*. Retrieved April 5, 2015, from http://www.nationalnurse.blogspot.com/

Nault, D. S., & Kettering Sincox, A. (2014). Nursing's voice in politics: The ongoing relationship between nurses and legislators. *Michigan Nurse, 87*(3), 17–21.

Nursing Power. (2015). *Invisibility, just another NP skill?* Posted by Nurse Sally on March 23, 2015. Retrieved April 5, 2015, from http://www.nursingpower.net/nursingpower/invisibility-just-another-np-skill/

Nurses hold record number of actions calling for tax on Wall Street. (2011). *National Nurse, 107*(7), 4–6.

O'Connor, T. (2014). Wanted: Politically aware and involved nurses. *Kai Tiaki Nursing New Zealand, 20*(8), 24–25.

O'Donnell, M. (2012, April 23). Why nurses should not be called doctor. *HealtheCareers Network*. Retrieved April 3, 2015, from http://www.healthecareers.com/article/career/why-nurses-should-not-be-called-doctor

Perron, A. (2013). Nursing as 'disobedient' practice: Care of the nurse's self, parrhesia, and the dismantling of a baseless paradox. *Nursing Philosophy, 14*(3), 154–167. doi:10.1111/nup.12015

Robert Wood Johnson Foundation. (2010, January 20). *Nursing leadership from bedside to boardroom: Opinion leaders' perceptions*. Retrieved April 5, 2015, from http://www.rwjf.org/content/dam/web-assets/2010/01/nursing-leadership-from-bedside-to-boardroom

Robert Wood Johnson Foundation. (2015). *Robert Wood Johnson Foundation executive nurse fellows*. Retrieved April 5, 2015, from http://www.rwjfleaders.org/programs/robert-wood-johnson-foundation-executive-nurse-fellows-program

RNs hone their advocacy skills through leadership program. (2015). *The American Nurse*. Retrieved April 5, 2015, from http://www.theamericannurse.org/index.php/2015/01/05/rns-hone-their-advocacy-skills-through-leadership-program/

Senge, P. (1990). *The fifth discipline*. New York, NY: Doubleday/Currency.

Sigma Theta Tau International Honor Society of Nursing. (2015). *Board leadership institute*. Retrieved April 5, 2015, from http://www.nursingsociety.org/learn-grow/leadership-institute/board-leadership-institute-(bli)

Union Facts. (2014, August 22). *American Nurses Association (ANA)*. Retrieved April 5, 2015, from https://www.unionfacts.com/union/American_Nurses_Association

U.S. Government Spending. (2015). *Total budgeted government spending expenditure GDP—CHARTS—Deficit debt*. Retrieved April 5, 2015, from http://www.usgovernmentspending.com/

Walton, A., Lake, D., Mullinix, C., Allen, D., & Mooney, K. (2015, March–April). Enabling nurses to lead change: The orientation experiences of nurses to boards. *Nursing Outlook, 63*(2), 110–116. doi:10.1016/j.outlook.2014.12.015

Wood, D. (2015, January 12). *Top 10 things nurses can expect in 2015. NurseZone.com*. Retrieved April 4, 2015, from http://www.nursezone.com/Nursing-News-Events/more-news/Top-10-Things-Nurses-Can-Expect-in-2015_42417.aspx

24

Professional Identity and Image

Carol J. Huston

ADDITIONAL RESOURCES

Visit thePoint for additional helpful resources

- eBook
- Journal Articles
- WebLinks

CHAPTER OUTLINE

LEARNING OBJECTIVES

The learner will be able to:

1. Explore the roots and prevalence of historical and contemporary nursing stereotypes, including nurse as angel of mercy, love interest (particularly to physicians), sex bombshell/naughty nurse, handmaiden to the physician, and battle-axe, as well as the stereotype of the male nurse as being gay, effeminate, or sexually predatory.
2. Identify common public portrayals or descriptions of nurses in terms of gender, dress, and role responsibilities.
3. Examine the role that organizations such as the *Center for Nursing Advocacy* and *Truth About Nursing* have assumed in addressing inaccurate or negative portrayals of nursing in the media and the process they use to raise public and professional awareness of the issues surrounding nursing's public image.
4. Analyze the effect of inaccurate nursing stereotypes on the profession's ability to recruit the best and brightest students to nursing, as well as on the collective identity and self-esteem of all nurses.
5. Name well-known fictional nurse characters depicted in contemporary media (television and movies), and identify the nursing stereotypes they best represent.

(continues on page 348)

6. Discuss the challenges inherent in attempting to change deeply ingrained stereotypes about nursing that are likely instilled very early in childhood.
7. Analyze how a lack of uniformity in dress and the way in which nurses introduce themselves to patients may contribute to the public's confusion about who is a nurse.
8. Explore the roles and responsibilities that individual nurses, employers, professional associations, and the media have to ensure that nurses are portrayed accurately and positively to the public.
9. Assess the effect of strategies undertaken by professional coalitions and corporations to improve recruitment and retention in nursing.
10. Reflect on the premise that every nurse controls the image of nursing.
11. Reflect on what image he or she would like the public to have of the nursing profession.

INTRODUCTION

An *image* can be defined as a reproduction or an imitation of something or as a mental picture or impression of something (Image, 2015). In other words, an image is often an unknown reality because it depends on the subjective perception of others. Perhaps that is why the public image of the nursing profession is typically one-dimensional and inaccurate.

If asked to describe a nurse, most of the public would use such terms as *nice*, *hardworking*, or *caring*. They would also use the terms *ethical* and *honest*. There is little question that the public trusts and respects nurses. In fact, since they were added to the list in 1999, nurses have ranked number one on every Gallup poll on honesty and ethics with the exception of 2001 (Nutty, 2015; Riffkin, 2014). Few people, however, would use the terms *highly educated*, *bright*, *powerful*, *professional*, or *independent thinker* to describe a nurse. Even fewer would call the nursing profession *prestigious*.

Discussion Point

If the nursing profession is so well thought of and so highly recommended, why do many of the brightest students look to medicine rather than nursing? Why are there such significant differences in terms of occupational prestige and status between medicine and nursing?

Many people would, however, describe a nurse as a caring young woman, dressed in a white uniform dress, cap, and shoes, altruistically devoted to caring for the ill ("angel of mercy"), under the supervision of a physician. Common job functions would be identified as making beds, passing out pills, emptying bedpans, giving shots, and helping doctors. Some people, however, would allude, at least subtly, to a lustier image of sexy young females dressed in provocative attire and seeking sexual gratification from both patients and physicians. Still others might depict stern, aged "battle-axe" females thrusting hypodermic needles into recalcitrant patients and seemingly enjoying the discomfort they cause and the power that they hold.

What do these portrayals have in common? Almost nothing and yet everything. All are part of the convoluted, often conflicting stereotypical images of nurses. In addition, all of these images demean the true nature and complexity of nursing, and most are based almost entirely in fiction. Yet these stereotypes are pervasive, and efforts to change them have yielded only limited progress. A review of nursing image studies by Ten Hoeve, Jansen, and Roodbol (2014) confirmed that the public image of nursing is diverse and incongruous, noting nursing's public image is obfuscated by the profession's relative invisibility and lack of public discourse about the topic. The researchers expressed concern that this lack of image clarity may negatively impact nurses' self-concept and the development of their professional identity (Research Study Fuels the Controversy 24.1).

Clearly, public perceptions about the nursing profession are mixed and even contradictory at times. The public trusts and admires nurses, but this does not necessarily equate to respect. Nor does the public consider the profession prestigious or understand what nursing is all about.

The result of this public image confusion is that old stereotypes of nurses as overbearing, brainless, sexually promiscuous, and incompetent women are perpetuated, as are images of nurses as caring, hardworking, altruistic, and selfless. This image conflict is an enduring issue

Research Study Fuels the Controversy 24.1

Nursing Image: A Diverse Picture

The researchers completed a literature search of MEDLINE, CINAHL, and PsycINFO databases for the period 1997 to 2010 using the terms nurses, nurse*, perception, public image, professional image, stereotyp*, self-concept, power, public opinion, and social identification, identifying 1,216 relevant studies. Eighteen studies met the final inclusion criteria.

Source: Ten Hoeve, Y., Jansen, G., & Roodbol, P. (2014). The nursing profession: Public image, self-concept and professional identity. A discussion paper. *Journal of Advanced Nursing, 70*(2), 295–309. doi:10.1111/jan.12177

Study Findings

The findings suggested a rather diverse picture of the actual view of the public on the nursing profession. The heterogeneity of setting, sample, and population of the studies made it quite difficult to explain these differences. Furthermore, traditional, cultural, and social values determined the way the public perceived the nursing profession. The researchers noted that the self-concept of nurses and their professional identity are determined by many factors, including public image, work environment, work values, education, and culture. The researchers concluded that to improve their public image and to obtain a stronger position in health care organizations, nurses need to increase their visibility. This could be realized by ongoing education and a challenging work environment that encourages nurses to stand up for themselves. Furthermore, nurses should make better use of strategic positions, such as case manager, nurse educator, or clinical nurse specialist, and use their professionalism to show the public what their work really entails.

for nursing, and the profession's efforts to address the problem have been fragmented and largely unsuccessful. Indeed, many nurses believe nursing's image to be one of the most important and enduring issues they face as a profession.

This chapter explores common historical and contemporary nursing stereotypes. The effect of these inaccurate stereotypes on recruitment into the profession and the collective self-esteem and identity of nurses is examined. In addition, strategies for improving the public image of nursing are presented, as are the challenges inherent in trying to change stereotypes that are ingrained in the profession's history and even in how nurses view themselves.

NURSING STEREOTYPES

Of the many nursing stereotypes, the most common ones are shown in Box 24.1: the nurse as an angel of mercy; the nurse as a love interest (particularly to physicians); the nurse as a sex bombshell or "naughty nurse"; the nurse as a handmaiden to physicians; the nurse as a battle-axe; and the male nurse as gay, effeminate, or sexually predatory. All of these stereotypes are profiled in this chapter. In addition, contemporary nursing images as depicted in movies and on television are profiled in an effort to better identify what images of nursing are before the public, especially the young people who represent the potential future nursing workforce.

BOX 24.1 Common Nursing Stereotypes

1. Angel of mercy
2. Love interest (particularly to physicians)
3. Sex bombshell/naughty nurse
4. Handmaiden to the physician
5. Battle-axe
6. Male nurses as homosexual, effeminate, or sexually predatory

Angel of Mercy

One of the oldest and most common nursing stereotypes is that of the nurse as an angel of mercy. Some individuals suggest that the image of the nurse as an angel with wings actually comes from the capes nurses historically wore as part of their uniforms. When most people think of nurses as angels of mercy, the image of Florence Nightingale bringing comfort to maimed soldiers during the Crimean War comes to mind. Clearly, Florence Nightingale's legacy of caring is beyond remarkable; however, few individuals outside of nursing would recognize Nightingale as a politically astute, assertive change agent who used her knowledge of epidemiology and statistics to document the effectiveness of nursing interventions. Both images should be equally important parts of her legacy.

The nurse "angel of mercy" stereotype continues to persist today, more than 100 years after Florence Nightingale's death. Indeed, a book published by Harlequin in 2008 titled *Single Dad, Nurse Bride* details the fictional life of an orthopedic doctor, Dr. Dane Hendricks, "who is every nurse's dream—handsome and a take charge kind of guy when it comes to medicine but also warm and humorous" (Amazon.com, 1996–2015, para. 2). He is also wealthy. Rikki Johansen, "a conscientious nurse, taking to heart all the lessons she learned in nursing school, … always puts others before herself and as a result, she must drive a car that doesn't always start right away" (Amazon.com, 1996–2015, para. 4). "When Dane's brother is diagnosed with cancer and Rikki turns out to be the only bone marrow match, there is never any doubt what her choice will be" (Amazon.com, 1996–2015, para. 8).

The Center for Nursing Advocacy (2008–2015) has suggested that such images of the nurse as an "angel" or "saint" are generally unhelpful to the profession because they "fail to convey the college-level knowledge base, critical thinking skills, and hard work required to be a nurse. They also suggest that nurses are supernatural beings who do not require decent working conditions, adequate staffing, or a significant role in health care decision-making or policy" (para. 1).

Some individuals argue that the angel of mercy stereotype is unconsciously promoted by nurses even today—in the Nightingale pledge, for instance (Box 24.2). When one looks closely at the pledge, which originated in 1893 but is still cited frequently in nursing graduation ceremonies, it speaks of nurses forgoing their personal wants and needs for the good of others. Being giving and caring in nature is a wonderful thing, but to suggest that it should be done to the extent of self-neglect is likely not the desired message.

It is important to remember, however, that being an angel of mercy is not all bad. It does encompass behaviors that many nurses typify, such as caring and dedication. Unfortunately, the angel of mercy image all too often also carries with it the idea that pay is never an issue and that suffering must be a part of the nurse's life if the role is to have value. This intrapersonal conflict between the values of altruism and pay befitting a professional is still experienced by many nurses.

Love Interest (Particularly to Physicians)

Another historical stereotype of nurses is that of a love interest, particularly to physicians. Doctor–nurse romance novels first appeared in the 1930s and 1940s, when becoming a nurse was one of the few career opportunities available to women. Nurses in these novels were generally cast as intelligent, strong women who felt fulfilled in their careers until they met the physician who would eventually become their husband. Then their career would end, and the nurses would live happily ever after, caring for their spouse and children.

BOX 24.2 The Nightingale Pledge

I solemnly pledge myself before God and in the presence of this assembly, to pass my life in purity and to practice my profession faithfully. I will abstain from whatever is deleterious and mischievous, and will not take or knowingly administer any harmful drug. I will do all in my power to maintain and elevate the standard of my profession, and will hold in confidence all personal matters committed to my keeping and all family affairs coming to my knowledge in the practice of my calling. With loyalty will I endeavor to aid the physician, in his work, and devote myself to the welfare of those committed to my care.

Source: *Florence Nightingale. The "Nightingale Pledge."* (n.d.). Retrieved May 25, 2015, from http://www.countryjoe.com/nightingale/pledge.htm

With the women's rights movement of the 1970s, women's career opportunities expanded, and fewer books were devoted to women as nurses. In addition, readers' interest in medical romances dwindled. This is not to say that there are not still doctor–nurse romance novels. There are, but the characters typically are different from what they were in decades past. The female character is now often a determined but compassionate physician or at least a charge nurse of a critical care unit in a large, urban medical center, who is beautiful. The male character, however, almost always continues to be a physician, coping with a tragedy in his past, who is "brilliant, tall, and muscular" and "with chiseled features, working in emergency medicine" ("Lovesick Doctors," 2007).

Consider This Romantic relationships between nurses and doctors abound on recent television shows as well, such as *Scrubs*, *House*, *Nurse Jackie*, and *Gray's Anatomy*. It could be argued, however, that most of these relationships are not so much love interests as sexual liaisons.

Sex Bombshell/Naughty Nurse

Another common nursing stereotype is that of the nurse as a sex bombshell or "naughty nurse." Use of the word *naughty* probably is not powerful enough, however, given that the depiction of nurses in the sex and pornography industry is even more rampant than the general sexual stereotyping of nurses in the media. In fact, for at least 50 years, nurses have been portrayed as sex objects both on television and in the movies. Indeed, movies in the 1960s, 1970s, and 1980s were filled with images of nurses garbed in miniskirts, sleazy, low-cut tops, and high heels, who spent all of their time fulfilling sexual fantasies and virtually no time providing care to patients.

Nurses are even depicted as sex objects in television commercials. In 2003, Clairol Herbal Essences shampoo launched a commercial that showed a nurse abandoning her patient to wash her hair in his bathroom and then tossing her hair sensually at the patient as she left the room. Many nurses and nursing organizations condemned the unprofessional stereotype perpetuated in the ad and asked sponsor Procter & Gamble to discontinue it (Procter & Gamble Pulls Offending Ad, 2003). Procter & Gamble did issue an apology to nurses and pull the ad, stating that the company "holds the nursing profession in the highest esteem" (p. 35).

Discussion Point

Do you think that the public truly believes that a nurse would abandon patient care duties to wash her hair in a patient's bathroom and then sensually shake her hair at the patient? If not, does the commercial still cause harm?

Another commercial sexualizing nurses was launched in September 2007 by Cadbury Schweppes Canada for Dentyne gum (Truth About Nursing, 2007). The Cadbury Schweppes ads showed female nurses being lured into bed with male patients the instant the male patients popped Dentyne into their mouths. The tag line for the commercial was "Get Fresh," and the message was that when hospitalized patients used Dentyne products, there would be an instant, erotic reaction from the "always available" bedside nurse.

More than 1,000 protest letters were sent from the website of the Registered Nurses Association of Ontario (RNAO) in response to the Cadbury Schweppes commercial (Truth About Nursing, 2007). Another 500 supporters from the Center for Nursing Advocacy wrote letters to top Cadbury Schweppes executives, leaving long messages explaining that such imagery reinforces a stereotype of workplace sexual availability that contributes to the global nursing crisis. Initially, the company responded that its ads were causing no harm. On October 6, 2007, however, the company told the Center and RNAO that it would pull the ads and consult nurses in creating future US and Canadian ads that involved nurses.

Another recent example of the perpetuation of the naughty nurse stereotype became apparent when the Heart Attack Grill, a theme restaurant in Arizona, began dressing their waitresses in naughty nurse uniforms, which included micro miniskirts, fishnet stockings, and high heels. Because nurses are already a highly sexually fantasized profession, the Center for Nursing Advocacy asked the Heart Attack Grill to reconsider their uniform choice when the restaurant opened in 2006. The Grill's owner, Jon Basso, who calls himself "Dr. Jon" and works in a medical lab coat, refused. In November 2011, a peaceful rally was held in front of the restaurant to protest the image of nursing being presented (Truth About Nursing, 2011a). Rally supporters argued that the Heart Attack Grill was reinforcing stereotypes that discouraged practicing and potential nurses (especially men), fostered sexual violence in the workplace, and contributed to a general atmosphere of disrespect that weakened nurses' claims to adequate resources.

In addition, the State Board of Nursing filed a complaint with the Arizona Attorney General's office that Basso was illegally using the term *nurse* in advertising for his restaurant (Arizona Statute A.R.S. 32–1636 states only someone who has a valid nursing license can use the title "nurse"). The Attorney General sent Basso a letter informing him that he was illegally using the word "nurse" at his restaurant and on his website. Basso's response was a refusal to remove the word "nurse" from his website, but he did agree to insert an asterisk next to every nurse reference and to include a disclaimer that none of the women pictured on the website actually had any medical training or provide any real medical services.

Discussion Point

Do you feel that the uniform policy at Heart Attack Grill is simply good fun, or does it truly denigrate the nursing profession and sexualize nursing?

Even more recently, in October 2014, Subway launched a television ad that used a naughty nurse costume, among others, to encourage US customers to dine at the sandwich chain (Truth About Nursing, 2014a). In the ad, a young female office worker urged two colleagues not to eat burgers for lunch, but instead to emulate her Subway choices, because Halloween was coming and they must "stay in shape for all the costumes!" She proceeded to demonstrate, donning a quick series of mostly naughty costumes that she helpfully labeled as "attractive nurse... spicy Red Riding Hood... Viking princess warrior... hot devil... sassy teacher... and foxy fullback!" "The nurse outfit wasn't the naughtiest ever, but it was a ridiculously short, flimsy dress" (Truth About Nursing, 2014a, para. 8).

Handmaiden to the Physician

Perhaps the most pervasive stereotype of nurses is that of handmaiden to physicians. In the handmaiden role, the nurse simply serves as an adoring backdrop to the omnipotent physician, demonstrating little, if any, independent thought or action. Certainly, this image is perhaps the most common image perpetuated on contemporary television and movie screens.

The image, however, is not new. This view of nurses as a handmaiden to physicians was reported in classic research by Philip and Beatrice Kalisch, in the 1970s, a time when nurses generally had no substantial role in television stories and were a part of the hospital background in programs that focused on physician characters. When nurses were the focus of a program, the storyline frequently involved the nurse's personal problems rather than his or her role as a nurse, and attributes such as obedience, permissiveness, conformity, flexibility, and serenity were emphasized.

Sometimes, though, even health care employers perpetuate this image, even if unintentionally. For example, in 2014, the Baylor Health Care System ran a television ad based on the idea that its employees were faithful "servants" (Truth About Nursing, 2014b). The one-minute ad featured many apparent nurses in clinical settings, intending to show them in a positive light. But many nurses objected to being presented as "servants." And the nurse scenes in the ad emphasized what seem to be the most unskilled tasks with which nurses are associated, including hand-holding, mopping brows, wheeling gurneys, changing "hearts" and sheets, and picking things up off the floor. Meanwhile, apparent physicians in the ad acted as servants by doing research and cutting-edge surgeries, changing "minds" and "tomorrow" (Truth About Nursing, 2014b, para. 13). Truth About Nursing suggested that "the servanthood theme may hold some appeal as a matter of spirituality or marketing, but it's dangerous to apply to a traditionally female profession that has struggled to overcome the notion that it simply serves physicians and to get respect for its advanced education and skills" (Truth About Nursing, 2014b, para. 13).

Consider This Nursing care is frequently perceived by the public as simple and unskilled.

Many of the commercial representations of nurses today continue to represent the stereotype of nurse as a handmaiden. For example, in spring 2008, the Angela Moore jewelry catalog featured "Nurse Nancy" bracelets and necklaces. According to Truth About Nursing (2008), the jewelry was composed of four different types of balls; one ball featured a smiling, rosy-cheeked nurse in white uniform and cap giving a balloon to a girl; the second ball had a ladybug next to a stethoscope; the third ball featured a nurse's cap with a thermometer; and the fourth ball had a stuffed bear holding flowers next to a lollipop. The text in the catalog "asked readers to buy the Nurse Nancy jewelry to celebrate the ladies who give lollipops and band aids a whole new meaning" (Truth About Nursing, 2008, para. 1).

In response to letters of concern from nurses, the jewelry maker did agree to modify the description of the jewelry. According to Truth About Nursing (2008), however, what they changed it to was "Here's a special theme to celebrate the wonderful women who promote health and make us feel so much better. Talented, terrific and leaders to love!" (para. 3). Truth About Nursing suggested that "while this was probably an improvement over lollipops and band aids" (Truth About Nursing, 2008, para. 4), it was still problematic in that it suggested that only women are nurses. In addition, they argued that "statements such as 'makes us feel so much better,' 'leaders to love,' and 'wonderful women' sound like adoration for someone's loving mom who makes them feel so much better by making them soup or tea" (Truth About Nursing, 2008, para. 5), not that nurses are highly trained health care professionals who use both science and art to make a difference in their patient's outcomes.

Battle-Axe

Few stereotypes in nursing are as dark or demented, however, as that of the nurse as a battle-axe. The battle-axe stereotype often depicts an overbearing, unhappy, mean, senior nurse who intimidates both patients and staff. The movie *One Flew Over the Cuckoo's Nest* (1975) provides a perfect example of the battle-axe. Nurse Ratched, a nurse in a mental hospital, who fits the description of a battle-axe in almost every way. She craves power and control over others and forces patients to obey her every whim or suffer the repercussions.

Nurse Diesel, in the movie *High Anxiety* (1978), was another stereotypical battle-axe nurse, with the addition of enormous prosthetic breasts. As an overbearing, evil-charge nurse, Nurse Diesel continually displayed a dark sneer and a love of domination. Annie Wilkes from the novel and movie *Misery* gave new meaning to the sociopathic battle-axe nurse as she kidnapped, maimed, and held hostage a writer she admired and wanted to be close to. Similarly, the book *Doctors and Nurses* (Ellman, 2006) depicts Jen, a significantly obese nurse who partners (both sexually and career wise) with her married physician boss, to kill their patients. Jen's appetite for food, sex, and violence is whetted when her physician boyfriend happily scams patients and shrugs off lawsuit-worthy mistakes.

Battle-axe stereotypes of nurses have always existed; however, they seemed to hit their peak in the 1970s and 1980s. There are, however, still multiple images of battle-axe nurses available on the Internet. It is also of interest that the battle-axe counterpart of male physicians in medicine is viewed less negatively. For example, the television show *House* stars a drug-addicted, rule-breaking, rude, and crude male physician whose bad behavior is excused by his brilliance and ability to often cure patients when all hope is lost.

The Male Nurse: Gay, Effeminate, or Sexually Predatory

Female nurses are not the only ones who are stereotyped. Male nurse stereotypes are at least as prevalent as those for females, which only adds to the difficulty of recruiting men to the profession.

For example, male nurses are frequently stereotyped as being homosexual (or at least effeminate). Indeed, a recent study (Goodier, 2013) reviewed one season of each of five American medical television dramas, including *Grey's Anatomy*, *Hawthorne*, *Mercy*, *Nurse Jackie*, and *Private Practice*, evaluating aspects of the episodes such as dialogue, costumes, casting, cinematography, and editing to compile a perspective on the ways that male nurses are characterized. Unfortunately, the shows tended to reinforce a stereotype of male nurses as men who are not traditionally masculine. The shows also reinforced images of the male nurse being mistaken for a doctor and the gay or emasculated male nurse. In addition, male nurses and midwives in the shows tended to suffer condescension from their colleagues and patients and were the object of comedy (Goodier, 2013).

Male nurses may also be stereotyped as being hypersexual and, as a result, the intent of their actions may be questioned as being either sexual in nature or, in some cases, even sexually predatory. This makes it very difficult for male nurses to demonstrate the caring, therapeutic interactions that are such an important part of nursing.

> **Consider This** Many male nurses live in fear of how their caring actions might be interpreted.

Another popular stereotype for male nurses is that they are nonachievers for going into nursing rather than more traditionally male occupations. This was certainly the case in the 2000 movie *Meet the Parents*.

Unfortunately, despite the protestations of Greg Focker, the male registered nurse (RN) in the movie, that he loves nursing and became a nurse by choice, his future in-laws and other relatives constantly questioned his sexual orientation and manliness. They also clearly implied that Greg must have become a nurse because his test scores were not high enough for him to qualify for medical school.

Research by Wallen, Mor, and Devine (2014) suggested that the extent to which male nurses perceive others respect nursing plays an integral role in determining their job satisfaction and affective commitment. Hospitals and other organizations can encourage perceived respect by offering interventions that cultivate feelings of increased occupational status among nurses, and male nurses in particular. Wallen et al. (2014) conclude that an apparent incompatibility exists between the expectations some people have for men, and the communal skills people think are necessary for such jobs. Their research suggests that how men in female-dominated jobs view their gender and professional identities—as compatible and overlapping, or conflicting and divided—affects their ability to navigate these different expectations.

CONTEMPORARY NURSING STEREOTYPES ON TELEVISION

Television medical dramas currently provide the greatest number of visual images of nurses at work. There is little doubt, however, that television medical dramas build on traditional stereotypes of nurses, as well as suggest new ones. One of the best known medical dramas in the past two decades, with strong nurse figures, was *ER* (1994 to 2009). This medical drama focused on the lives and events of the emergency department staff at County General Hospital in Chicago, a level I trauma center.

The character Carol Hathaway was perhaps the best known nurse on *ER*. After surviving the September 1994 pilot episode in which she tried to commit suicide, Hathaway became the charge nurse of the emergency department. She went on to have a sexual relationship with a physician and bore twins out of wedlock. Nurse Hathaway left the show in 1999—to join her physician love interest in another state.

Even with the departure of Nurse Hathaway, *ER* continued to provide probably the most influential portrayals of nurses on television. One of the highest-profile nurses remaining on the show was Abby Lockhart, an alcoholic, former obstetrical nurse from a family afflicted with bipolar disorder. She started on the show as a medical student, dropped out of medical school, worked as a nurse, and then became a doctor. Abby had sexual relationships with several doctors on the show and eventually married one of them.

In addition, Samantha Taggart, a nurse who joined the *ER* cast in 2003, was a tough, free-spirited, single mother of an emotionally troubled child, who almost immediately entered into a sexual relationship with one of the physicians. In her introductory scene, "Sam" (who had come to the hospital inquiring about employment) grabbed a syringe and leaped to sedate an unruly patient through a central vessel in his neck. This behavior earned her not only a job but also the respect of her soon-to-be coworkers.

One newer TV show to stir nurses to action, however, is *Grey's Anatomy* (2005 to present). Physician characters on this show provide all of the direct patient care as well as the emotional support of the patient and family. Nurses hold only trivial roles. Even more distressing is the fact that one of the few visible nurses on the show gave sexually transmitted diseases to the male physicians. Truth About Nursing (2011b) notes that a few episodes in season 7 did feature a handsome male nurse (Eli), who "displayed a little skill and briefly stood up to the physicians, but by season's end, he was mainly a love interest for attending surgeon Miranda Bailey and no longer did any nursing work onscreen" (para. 8).

One of the most alarming contemporary visualizations of a nurse on TV, however, is *Nurse Jackie* (2009 to 2015). The title character Jackie Peyton is a drug-addicted nurse who works in the emergency ward at All Saints' Hospital in New York City. Jackie often makes unethical and illegal decisions for the "good" of her patients, such as forging organ donor authorizations. In addition, although married, she has sex with the pharmacist at the hospital in exchange for drugs. In season 2, her drug addiction led her to falsify an MRI to get a phony prescription and to rip off a local drug dealer who embarked on revenge. Eventually, Jackie's addictions deepened to the point that she stole drugs from the oncology unit. When her theft was discovered, she was placed on probation by her employer, and a sympathetic colleague in the lab perpetuated her employment by discarding her next contaminated urine drug test. In addition, Jackie is a "world class liar," particularly about her addictions, and had alienated almost everyone in her life by the end of the 2014 season (Truth About Nursing, 2015).

Perhaps what is most disturbing about Nurse Jackie is the attention this utterly dislikable nurse character receives solely as a result of her independent and strong-willed thinking. The reality is that this is a drug-addicted nurse who has little regard for any codes of ethics or the patients she is charged to care for. Her primary mission in life and at work is to attain the drugs she needs to fuel an ever-increasing addiction, and this is often at the expense of patients. Unfortunately, *The Truth about Nursing* suggests that "Jackie turned out to be arguably the strongest and the most skilled nurse ever depicted on serial U.S. television" (Campbell, 2013, para. 3).

Even more recently, MTV aired a new reality show, *Scrubbing In*, which follows a group of 20-something travel nurses in Southern California (Campbell, 2013). Based on the trailer, in which these nurses are shown with a heavy focus on looking attractive, partying, and being "hell raisers," many nursing organizations launched campaigns to convince MTV Executives that the show should be cancelled for its unfair portrayal of nurses (most of these petitions occurred before the show had aired even one episode). Despite more than 30,000 letters of protest, the show aired as planned.

THE IMAGE OF NURSING ON THE INTERNET

The Internet is also filled with images of nurses, some accurate and some very stereotypical. A recent review of nurse images on Google found thousands of inappropriate images of nurses. Many were sexually suggestive, as well as demeaning. Some were in caricature, but many were of young women dressed in cleavage-baring uniforms and wearing fishnet stockings, high heels, and garter belts.

Even YouTube includes numerous stereotypical and distorted images. A 2012 study of the most viewed videos for "nurses" and "nursing" on YouTube suggested that nurses were depicted in three main ways—as a skilled knower and doer, as a sexual plaything, and as a witless incompetent (American Association for the Advancement of Science [AAAS], 2015).The 10 most viewed videos reflected a variety of media, including promotional videos, advertising, excerpts from a TV situation comedy, and a cartoon. Some texts dramatized, caricatured, and parodied nurse–patient and interprofessional encounters. Four of the 10 clips, however, were posted by nurses and presented images of them as educated, smart, and technically skilled. They included nurses being interviewed, dancing, and performing a rap song, all of which portrayed nursing as a valuable and rewarding career. The nurses were shown as a distinct professional group working in busy clinical hospitals, where their knowledge and skills counted.

HOW INGRAINED ARE NURSING STEREOTYPES?

Increasingly, researchers are concluding that inaccurate and negative stereotypes of nurses are not only well ingrained but also instilled early in life. Indeed, gender stereotyping about career opportunities begins at a very early age. By 3 years, most children already have firmly rooted gender-based ideas about the roles they can and should hold when they grow up.

The reality, then, is that by the end of middle school, most students report having their minds made up about desirable and undesirable careers. An unpublished study by Huston (Research Study Fuels the Controversy 24.2) suggested that basic beliefs and stereotypes about professions such as nursing may be ingrained at a far younger age, and that waiting until fifth, sixth, or even seventh grade to address inaccurate or negative images of nursing might be too late. Clearly, an early positive image for students is important if this is the population group the profession hopes will solve the current shortage.

THE CENTER FOR NURSING ADVOCACY AND TRUTH ABOUT NURSING

Most nurses are upset about their depiction in contemporary media, but their efforts to respond to and change the situation have been fragmented. A more unified voice became possible with the creation of the Center for Nursing Advocacy in 2001. The center was created when Sandy Summers and seven other graduate nursing students at the Johns Hopkins University in Baltimore joined forces to address the media's disrespectful portrayal of nursing.

In 2009, the center was dissolved as a result of legal wrangling around record keeping and allegations of unpaid taxes. Sandy Summers then set up a new organization, called Truth About Nursing, a 501(c) (3) nonprofit organization that seeks to increase public understanding of the central, frontline role nurses play in modern health care, to promote more accurate, balanced, and frequent media portrayals of nurses, and increase the media's use of nurses as expert sources (Truth About Nursing, 2011c). "The Truth About Nursing's ultimate goal is to foster growth in the size and diversity of the nursing profession at a time of critical shortage, strengthen nursing practice, teaching and research, and improve the health care system" (Truth About Nursing, 2011c, para. 1).

Research Study Fuels the Controversy 24.2

Second-Graders' Image of Nurses

This unpublished study examined stereotypes held by 25 second-graders regarding "important" nursing roles and functions. In an effort to introduce students to nonhospital nursing roles, which students stated they already knew, a 30-minute slide show and discussion were held showing nurses actively engaged in less traditional nursing roles such as cardiac rehabilitation, primary care, flight nursing, education, management, and public health. In addition, nurse practitioners were introduced as primary care providers. Students were shown photos of nurses in all types of garb, except for white uniforms. Efforts were made to ensure ethnic and gender diversity in all presentation materials. At the conclusion of the presentation, students were asked to draw a picture of what they thought was the most exciting role that had been presented for nurses.

Source: Huston, C. (n.d.). *Nursing stereotypes ingrained by second grade*. Unpublished manuscript.

Study Findings

The caption on the first drawing was "the nurse is doing surgery on a real important disease." In the second, the nurse, with a red cross on her white uniform, was noted to be "rushing" into the hospital. In the third, the nurse, in her white starched cap, was making up a hospital bed.

In the fourth drawing, the nurse was giving a hospitalized patient a backrub. In another, a dour nurse, as denoted by a capital N on her starched white cap with a red cross on it, was entering a hospital nursery. In the sixth, a patient in a bed was hooked up to an intravenous line, expressing pain. The smiling nurse was walking away from him.

In the seventh drawing, the nurse was helping the child in the hospital bed, and it included a caption that the "nurse is in a rush." In another drawing, nurses were scurrying to patients in their hospital beds. Rushing, for nurses, seemed to be a recurrent theme.

In the eighth drawing, the most exciting role for a nurse was noted as transporting a cot from room to room. Similarly, another student noted that the most important thing a nurse did was to transport people to the operating room, and yet another student noted that transporting patients in wheelchairs to their cars was the most important thing that nurses did.

Several drawings included stern nurses in white uniforms and caps and with red crosses on their chests making patients take medicine that tasted bad. Others depicted nurses working in nurseries or teaching mothers how to care for a crying baby. Another depicted a flight nurse taking an injured patient to the hospital, and yet another showed a nurse, in a white uniform with a red cross on her chest and wearing a cap, taking blood pressures.

All of the nurses in the drawings were female and white. The overwhelming majority wore white uniforms and caps and had red crosses on their chests. All but one drawing depicted nurses in hospital settings. Many associated the nurse with pain or an unpleasant experience. Despite the educational intervention, these second-graders already held deeply ingrained stereotypes about nursing and nursing roles, which were resistant to change. This suggests that if stereotypes are this difficult to modify in second-graders, the challenges in changing the image of nursing with the greater public will likely be very difficult.

CONSEQUENCES OF INACCURATE OR NEGATIVE IMAGES

Inaccurate or negative public images of nursing have many consequences, particularly because these images influence the attitudes of patients, other health care providers, policy-makers, and politicians. They even influence how nurses think about themselves. They can also influence funding. When decision-makers don't understand the value of nursing, they don't fund it. Nursing residencies in the United States receive almost no support compared with physician residency programs. Perhaps even more critical is that negative attitudes about nursing might discourage capable prospective nurses, who will instead choose another career that offers greater appeal in stature, status, and salary.

Consider This Many nurses hold stereotypes about the profession to be true, just as the general public does.

Recruitment Challenges

As with other predominantly female professions, the literature suggests that many clients and their families undervalue nursing and do not understand what it is that nurses do that makes a difference in patient outcomes. Indeed, many nurses will honestly admit that they had little factual basis for what nursing would be like when they chose it as a profession. Instead, what drove them to become nurses were actually images that emphasized the caring, nurturing, and personal rewards associated with the profession.

Research by Price and McGillis Hall (2014) suggests that understanding how individuals come to know nursing as a career choice is of critical importance. Stereotypical imaging and messaging of the nursing profession shape nurses' expectations and perceptions of nursing as a career, which has implications for both recruitment and retention. Price and McGillis Hall conclude that strategies for future recruitment and socialization within the nursing and the health professions need to include contemporary and realistic imaging of both health professional roles and practice settings.

In an effort to recruit young people into the profession, the drug company Johnson & Johnson (J&J) began a series of television advertisements in 2002 as a part of its Campaign for Nursing's Future. Three new 30-second ads were released in 2005 and 2007, highlighting different aspects of nursing practice and promotion of diversity in nursing. New ads were released in 2011 and again in the last 2 years. Current ads are encompassing, and include a website dedicated to promoting men in nursing, with career resources as related reading that emphasize challenges faced by minority male nurses as well as the pride engendered as a result of being a nurse (Johnson & Johnson, 2015).

CHANGING NURSING'S IMAGE IN THE PUBLIC EYE

Changing nursing's image in the public eye will not be easy. Nor will there be a silver bullet. Instead, multiple strategies are needed, including active interaction with the media and restriction of the term *nurse* to licensed nurses. In addition, nurses must increase their efforts to publicly praise and value nursing in addition to emphasizing how nursing uniquely contributes to patients achieving their desired health outcomes. Finally, nurses will need to become even more involved in the political processes that shape their profession.

Accomplishing this will take time and resources, including the time, energy, and funding of coalitions, foundations, and professional nursing organizations. Perhaps most important, it will take a concerted effort by individual nurses that will come only by first recognizing that there is a need to take action and then by doing what is necessary to achieve that goal.

Finding a Voice in the Press

One of the most important strategies needed to change nursing's image is to change the image of nursing in the mind of the image makers. That means proactively seeking positive and accurate media exposure of what nursing really is and what nurses really do. This job cannot be left to professional nursing organizations or to the image makers. Nursing's contributions need to be recognized and proclaimed. Unfortunately, many nurses feel ill prepared or lack the self-confidence to interact with the media. Knowing how to interact with the media is not intuitive for most nurses. Media training should always be provided to give nurses the skills and self-confidence to be effective in this role. Tips for interacting with the media are shown in Box 24.3.

> **Consider This** Far too few nurses are both willing and appropriately trained to interact with the media.

Instead of being fearful of the media, nurses should view media as an opportunity to expose the difficulties encountered in the profession as well as more accurate stories about what nurses do and the difference they make in the lives of the populations they serve.

Nurses are uniquely qualified to speak with editors, reporters, and media producers on topics related to health care because they have a view from the frontlines and are able to localize national health care issues. Nurses are also well qualified to simplify medical gibberish, explain the latest health care research, and identify current trends. Nurses, then, must be taught the basic skills necessary to self-confidently interact with the media. Nurses must also never pass up the opportunity to work with the media and should always view the media as playing a critical role in changing nursing's image.

> **Consider This** Nurses are experts in health care. Their invisibility in the media is likely a result of nurses lacking the basic skills and self-confidence to get involved, not that the media does not want to talk to nurses.

BOX 24.3 Tips for Interacting With the Media

1. Be well informed about the topic.
2. Decide ahead of time what two to three key points you want to make and stay on track with the message.
3. Keep answers short, clear, and concise.
4. Stick to what you know and don't be pressured to answer questions you lack expertise in.
5. Talk in lay terms so that the public you want to reach understands your message.
6. Do not overestimate the reporter's expertise on the topic; be prepared to offer background information if necessary.
7. Remember that nothing is "off the record."
8. Be honest and friendly.
9. Respond immediately to media inquiries for interview since reporters are typically on short deadlines.
10. Be confident that you as a nurse are an expert on many issues consumers need and want to know.

Finally, nurses should recognize that media stereotypes are not limited to nonprofessional sources. Even advertisements in medical and nursing journals often include stereotypical and demeaning nursing images, with frequent depictions of nurses as dependent, passive minor figures on the health care scene. If nurses are not depicted accurately in their own trade publications, how can they expect representation in other types of media to be better?

Reclaiming the Title of "Nurse"

Another strategy needed to improve the image of nursing is to ensure that use of the term *nurse* is limited to licensed nurses. The International Council of Nurses (ICN) reaffirmed in 2012 that the term "nurse" "should be protected by law and applied to and used only by those legally authorized to practice the full scope of nursing" (ICN, 2012, para. 1). In addition, all state boards of nursing have passed legislation restricting unlicensed personnel from using the title of "nurse." Unfortunately, on a regular basis, nursing aides and attendants either intentionally or unintentionally misrepresent themselves as nurses.

With the increased use of unlicensed assistive personnel and cross-training, a blurring of titles, roles, and responsibilities has occurred among RNs, licensed vocational nurses, and unlicensed support staff. Nametags increasingly recognized all staff as "care partners" or "associates," and some hospitals went so far as to prohibit the listing of RN on a name tag. At the same time, a loss of differentiated uniforms further adds to the public's confusion about who is truly caring for them. In addition, the media frequently perpetuates the inappropriate use of the term "nurse" by referring to all nurse's aides, volunteers who do health-related work, and medical assistants as "nurses."

In addition, RNs often contribute to the confusion by how they introduce themselves to patients. Nurses are often very casual when introducing themselves to patients, rarely identifying their specific role as the leader of the health care team. Nor do they explain how the roles of other members of the health care team differ. This may be due in part to typical female role socialization, which encourages women not to promote themselves, or it may be part of a team-building effort. Either way, patients end up confused about who the leader of the team is or how their roles differ.

Jacobs-Summers and Jacobs-Summers (2011) urge nurses to project a professional image in all interactions. They suggest that when nurses meet patients, they introduce themselves as a nurse and include their surname as professionals do. This introduction should not be perceived as cold or formal; instead it demonstrates respect and pride in the profession.

Jacobs-Summers and Jacobs-Summers (2011) also encourage "nursing out loud." "This means describing more of what you're thinking while you're providing care, consistent with patient confidentiality and sensitivity. If you do, then patients, families, physician colleagues and others will get a better sense of your education and skill" (Jacobs-Summers & Jacobs-Summers, 2011, para. 5).

Dressing as Professionals

Nurses in this country began shedding their white uniforms in the 1960s as part of the anticonformist movement. As a result, the identity of the RN may be blurred. Whereas nursing caps and white starched uniforms were often impractical in caring for acutely ill patients, 30 years ago the public knew who the nurse was by the uniform he or she wore. Today, many patients are unable to tell the members of the health care team apart, a problem that has become worse as the result of widespread adoption of scrubs as work uniforms.

Some nurse leaders have suggested that a return to white uniforms would restore the public's perception of nursing's professionalism. Indeed, a study by Porr, Dawe, Lewis, Meadus, Snow, and Didham (2014) noted that white pantsuit uniforms scored higher for professionalism than uniforms with small print, bold print, or solid color, and most patients preferred that their nurses dress in white. Even more compelling were the findings by Wocial, Sego, Rager, Laubersheimer, and Everett (2014) that for nurses to communicate assurance, patients perceive they must first be clean, well groomed, and understated in overall appearance.

Nurses themselves, however, are split on the issue of whether uniforms are essential to maintaining professionalism in nursing. They argue that comfort and uniformity of dress are equally important and that uniforms are not a requirement for professional trust and respect.

Consider This Is it the white uniform that makes the professional, or is it the actions nurses take that define what a nurse is?

Positive Talk by Nurses About Nursing

Another strategy for improving the image of nursing is to change how nurses talk about nursing to others. Some nurses bad-mouth the profession and discourage young adults from considering nursing as a profession, yet go on to bemoan the current nurse shortage. The effect of these comments by nurses on the general public should not be underestimated in terms of their effect on the recruitment of young people into the profession.

The reality is that every nurse controls the image of nursing. Nursing, like any other profession, has strengths and weaknesses. It is important, however, that nurses enjoy their work, whatever it might be. Nurses should not stay in jobs that make them unhappy, because it demoralizes everyone around them. Whining and acting like a victim does little to improve the situation.

The bottom line is that nurses must be ambassadors for the profession and tell the public that nursing is an essential service with equal worth to other professions, that it can provide many services better than other health care disciplines, and that nursing is often more cost-effective than other disciplines. The public's demand for nursing likely rests on the demand nursing creates for itself in the public's eye.

Emphasizing the Uniqueness of Nursing

Another tactic nurses can use to improve nursing's image is not only to emphasize the profession's unique combination of "caring" and "curing" but also to underscore the depth and breadth of the scientific perspective that underlies its practice. Evidence-based practice and the application of best practice principles are an expectation for contemporary professional nursing practice. Nurses, then, must emphasize how clinical research and the use of current best evidence affect their decision-making and the care they provide.

In addition, newer research on nursing sensitivity and nursing outcomes is able to clarify what it is that nurses do that makes a difference in patient outcomes; there is increasing recognition that patients get better as a result of nursing interventions, not despite them.

Generally speaking, however, the public knows very little about the research base that drives high-quality, evidence-based practice, and it is nurses who are in the best position to tell them about it.

Participating in the Political Arena

The political process can influence nearly everything nurses do and every problem they confront each day. In addition, public opinion is often based on inaccurate images, and nursing is no exception. Participating in the political arena, then, becomes a powerful strategy for changing the public's image of nursing.

The reality, however, is that although the nursing profession has some strong professional organizations, only a small percentage of nurses are members of national nursing organizations. This limits the profession's ability to be a force in the political arena. In addition, many nurses know little about the political process or feel too overwhelmed by the daily demands of their job to become involved in addressing larger professional issues in the political arena. Some nurses just assume that the best interests of the profession are being guarded by some unknown force out there. Legislators wonder whether inactivity means simply not caring or not having an opinion. The result is that nurses are inadequately represented in the political arena, and another opportunity for nurses to be represented as knowledgeable, active participants in the health care system is lost.

Because the underlying causes of the profession's political inactivity are numerous, just as the strategies needed to address this issue are complex, it is discussed only briefly here. Instead, a separate chapter has been dedicated to more fully discuss the issue (see Chapter 23).

Conclusions

Public identity and image have been a struggle for nurses for at least 200 years. From a sociological perspective, conflicting stereotypes of nursing have not served the nursing profession well, and a disconnect exists between reality and public image. The greater public clearly does not fully understand what professional nursing is all about, and the nursing profession has done an inadequate job of correcting long-standing, historically inaccurate stereotypes.

The responsibility for changing nursing's image lies squarely on the shoulders of those who claim nursing as their profession. Until nurses are able to agree on the desired collective image and are willing to do what is necessary to both tell and show the public what that image is, little will change. Derogatory stereotypes are likely to continue to undermine public confidence in and respect for the professional nurse.

For Additional Discussion

1. Historically, images of physicians in the media have been more positive than those of nurses. Why? What factors have led to this difference?
2. Some nurses feel that no longer wearing white uniforms and caps has reduced the professionalism of nursing. Is how nurses dress an important part of public image? Would reverting to more traditional nursing attire improve nursing's public image?
3. Would you want your son or daughter to be a nurse? What have you told them about nursing that would either encourage them to enter the profession or discourage them from doing so?
4. Who are the best known nurses currently depicted in the media (radio, television, movies) you access on a regular basis? Do their characters represent nursing stereotypes that have been discussed in this chapter?
5. What do you believe to be the greatest restraining forces that discourage nurses from interacting with the media? Is media training the answer?
6. The contributions of J&J to improve the image of nursing and increase recruitment into the nursing profession are unparalleled. Why would a corporation such as J&J be interested in this pursuit? Why did such an initiative not originate with a professional nursing organization?
7. Are nurses confused about what shared image they want the public to have of their profession?

References

Amazon.com. (1996–2015). *Single dad, nurse bride* [Reader reviews]. Retrieved April 1, 2015, from http://www.amazon.com/Single-Nurse-Harlequin-Medical-Romance/dp/037319904X

American Association for the Advancement of Science. (2015). *Nurses need to counteract negative stereotypes of the profession in top YouTube hits.* Retrieved May 25, 2015, from http://www.eurekalert.org/pub_releases/2012-07/w-nnt071612.php

Campbell, L. (2013, October 28). *Nursing stereotypes: The good, the bad and the ugly.* Vancouver, BC: Association of Registered Nurses of British Columbia. Retrieved April 3, 2015, from http://www.arnbc.ca/blog/nursing-stereotypes-the-good-the-bad-and-the-ugly/

Center for Nursing Advocacy. (2008–2015). *Are nurses angels of mercy?* Retrieved April 1, 2015, from http://www.truthaboutnursing.org/faq/nf/angels.html

Ellman, L. (2006). *Doctors and nurses: A novel.* Retrieved May 26, 2015, from http://www.amazon.com/dp/1596911026/?tag=reviewsofbooks1-20&link_code=as3&creative=373489&camp=211189

Goodier, R. (2013). TV may reinforce stereotypes about men in nursing. Diversity Nursing Blog. Retrieved May 25, 2015, from http://blog.diversitynursing.com/blog/bid/152774/TV-may-reinforce-stereotypes-about-men-in-nursing

International Council of Nurses. (2012). *Position statement: Protection of the title "nurse."* Retrieved May 25, 2015, from http://www.icn.ch/images/stories/documents/publications/position_statements/B06_Protection_Title_Nurse.pdf

Jacobs-Summers, H., & Jacobs-Summers, S. (2011). *The image of nursing: It's in your hands.* Retrieved May 25, 2015, from http://www.nursingtimes.net/nursing-practice/clinical-specialisms/educators/the-image-of-nursing-its-in-your-hands/5024815.article

Johnson & Johnson. (2015). *Men in nursing.* Retrieved May 27, 2015, from http://www.discovernursing.com/men-in-nursing

Lovesick doctors and lovelorn nurses. (2007). *Nurse Ratched's Place.* Retrieved May 27, 2015, from http://nurse-ratcheds.blogspot.com/2007/11/lovesick-doctors-and-lovelorn-nurses.html

Merriam-Webster online dictionary. (2015). Image [Definition]. Retrieved April 1, 2015, from http://www.merriam-webster.com/dictionary/image

Nutty, A. (2015). Nurses top Gallup's "most ethical" poll for 15th year. *Alaska Nurse, 66*(1), 12.

Porr, C., Dawe, D., Lewis, N., Meadus, R. J., Snow, N., & Didham, P. (2014). Patient perception of contemporary nurse attire: A pilot study. *International Journal of Nursing Practice, 20*(2), 149–155. doi:10.1111/ijn.12160

Price, S. L., & McGillis Hall, L. (2014). The history of nurse imagery and the implications for recruitment: A discussion paper. *Journal of Advanced Nursing, 70*(7), 1502–1509. doi:10.1111/jan.12289

Procter & Gamble pulls offending ad. (2003). *Nursing, 33*(8), 35.

Riffkin, R. (2014). Americans rate nurses highest on honesty, ethical standards. *GALLUP.* Retrieved April 1, 2015, from http://www.gallup.com/poll/180260/americans-rate-nurses-highest-honesty-ethical-standards.aspx

Ten Hoeve, Y., Jansen, G., & Roodbol, P. (2014). The nursing profession: Public image, self-concept and professional identity. A discussion paper. *Journal of Advanced Nursing, 70*(2), 295–309. doi:10.1111/jan.12177

Truth About Nursing. (2007). *Getting fresher.* Retrieved May 27, 2015, from http://www.truthaboutnursing.org/news/2007/oct/06_dentyne.html

Truth About Nursing. (2008). *Let's "celebrate the ladies who give lollipops and band aids" with a Nurse Nancy bracelet!* Retrieved May 27, 2015, from http://www.truthaboutnursing.org/news/2008/mar/18_angela_moore.html

Truth About Nursing. (2011a). *News on nursing in the media. Heart attack grill: Successful protest in Las Vegas November 12!* Retrieved May 27, 2015, from http://www.truthaboutnursing.org/archives/2011/oct_nov_dec.html#nov

Truth About Nursing. (2011b). *News on nursing in the media. Understaffed: Fall 2011 TV review.* Retrieved May 25, 2015, from https://www.truthaboutnursing.org/news/2011/sep/fall_tv_preview.html

Truth About Nursing. (2011c). *Mission statement.* Retrieved May 25, 2015, from http://truthaboutnursing.org/about_us/mission_statement.html

Truth About Nursing. (2014a). *News on nursing in the media. All the costumes.* Retrieved May 25, 2015, from http://www.truthaboutnursing.org/

Truth About Nursing. (2014b). *Servanthood: Is Baylor ad praising its nurses as "servants" a problem?.* Retrieved May 25, 2015, from http://www.truthaboutnursing.org/news/2014/feb/baylor.html

Truth About Nursing. (2015, April 5). *News on nursing in the media: What goes up.* Retrieved May 25, 2015, from http://www.truthaboutnursing.org/

Wallen, A. S., Mor, S., & Devine, B. A. (2014). It's about respect: Gender-professional identity integration affects male nurses' job attitudes. *Psychology of Men & Masculinity, 15*(3), 305–312. doi:10.1037/a0033714

Wocial, L. D., Sego, K., Rager, C., Laubersheimer, S., & Everett, L. Q. (2014). Image is more than a uniform: The promise of assurance. *The Journal of Nursing Administration, 44*(5), 298–302. doi:10.1097/NNA.0000000000000070

25

Nursing, Policy, and Politics

Understanding the Connection: Nurses' Role in the Policy Process

Donna M. Nickitas and Sheila A. Burke

ADDITIONAL RESOURCES

Visit thePoint for additional helpful resources

- eBook
- Journal Articles
- WebLinks

CHAPTER OUTLINE

LEARNING OBJECTIVES

The learner will be able to:

1. Define the terms *politics* and *policy* and explore their relationship.
2. Differentiate among the problem stream, the political stream, and the policy stream in John Kingdon's three-stream model of policy development.
3. Identify nursing leaders who were pioneers in public policy, and describe their contributions in effecting social change.
4. Explore the relationships among social inequity, health disparities, and access to health care.
5. Describe strategies and approaches that enhance the integration of health policy into nursing education and practice.
6. Identify roles that nurses may undertake to help shape policies that address the social determinants.

INTRODUCTION

This chapter examines *the dynamic relationships of the nursing profession, policy, and politics* from an underlying assumption that nursing is a public good. For years, society has expressed appreciation and approval that the profession fulfills a critical role to advance the nation's health and health care (Institute of Medicine [IOM], 2011; Riffkin, 2014). Nurses have strong historical roots in advocacy and action, that include identifying how to best distribute resources to individuals, families, and populations (Lewenson & Nickitas, 2016). Nurses understand and are committed to improving care, demanding increased access, and providing greater efficiency and effectiveness that leads to better health and better health outcomes at lower costs. It is this commitment to advancing the nation's health that nursing has made to meet the demands for population health. Therefore, nurses at all levels of the profession—education, practice, and research—must understand and appreciate how they make crucial contributions to society (Kelly, Connor, Kun, & Salmon, 2008). The nursing profession is expected to protect, promote, and optimize health and well-being; prevent illness and injury; alleviate suffering through the diagnosis and treatment of human response; and advocate for the care of individuals, families, communities, and populations (American Nurses Association [ANA], 2010).

One important way for nurses to assume leadership roles and advance the nation's health is through involvement in the policy-making process (IOM, 2011). Nurses have been identified as having specific accountability to participate in supporting and realizing a vision for health care that is affordable, accessible, and of high quality (IOM, 2011). Because nurses are on the frontline of care delivery and have deep connections to patients, families, and communities, they are critical to safeguarding the health of the nation and ensuring that health care is accessible, safe, and of high quality. Nurses are well positioned to identify solutions to serious problems and have the capacity to be instrumental in implementing these solutions. When nurses work as full partners in the policy-making process, they achieve substantial improvements at the local, state, and national levels in both care delivery and health policy. To influence health policy, nursing professionals must be prepared to use the relevant knowledge and evidence needed to transform policy at all levels of the profession: practice, education, research, and leadership.

Consider This Professional nurses must work closely with Congress, federal agencies, and the health care system to advocate for nursing education and research funding to shape legislation impacting the profession.

For example, the Tri-Council is an alliance of four nursing organizations—the American Association of Colleges of Nursing [AACN], the ANA, the American Organization of Nurse Executives, and the National League of Nursing—each focused on leadership for nursing education, practice, and research (http://tricouncilfornursing.org/Home.php; Tri-Council for Nursing, 2015). Each organization has its own membership and mission, although they are bonded by common values, and meet regularly for the purpose of dialogue and consensus building to provide stewardship within the profession. These organizations represent the voice of nursing and collectively speak to the diverse interests of the profession, including the nursing work environment, health care legislation and policy, quality of health care, nursing education, practice, research, and leadership throughout the health care delivery system. In addition, the Tri-Council of Nursing has worked successfully to increase funding for Title VIII Workforce programs, National Institute for Nursing Research, and the National Health Service Corps.

PATIENT PROTECTION AND THE AFFORDABLE CARE ACT (PPACA)

On March 23, 2010, President Obama signed H.R. 3590, the Patient Protection and Affordable Care Act (hereafter called The Affordable Care Act). A week later, on March 30, 2010, the House and Senate both approved a package of fixes, H.R. 4872, the Health Care and Education Reconciliation Act of 2010. In reviewing the table of contents of the 974-page act, there are 10 major titles, and under each title, there are many subtitles, articles, and sections. Many of the health care reform activities over the next decade target new consumer protections, improving quality and controlling costs, increasing access to affordable care, and holding insurance companies accountable. Nurses have a role in ensuring better outcomes at lower costs. However, costs and coverage are only half the equation. "Nurses still have a responsibility to advocate for health care as a basic human right and for access to an affordable package of essential health

BOX 25.1 Key Features of the Affordable Care Act by Year

2010: A new **Patient's Bill of Rights** goes into effect, protecting consumers from the worst abuses of the insurance industry. Cost-free **preventive services** begin for many Americans.

2011: People with Medicare can get **key preventive services for free**, and also receive a **50% discount on brand-name drugs** in the Medicare "donut hole."

2012: Accountable Care Organizations and other programs help doctors and health care providers work together to deliver better care.

2013: Open enrollment in the Health Insurance Marketplace begins on October 1st.

2014: All Americans will have access to affordable health insurance options. The Marketplace allows individuals and small businesses to compare health plans on a level playing field. Middle- and low-income families will get tax credits that cover a significant portion of the cost of coverage, and the Medicaid program will be expanded to cover more low-income Americans. All together, these reforms mean that millions of people who were previously uninsured will gain coverage.

2015: Paying physicians based on value not volume. A new provision will tie physician payments to the quality of care they provide. Physicians will see their payments modified so that those who provide higher-value care will receive higher payments than those who provide lower-quality care. *Effective January 1, 2015.*

Source: http://health.gov/

services" (Nickitas, 2011, p. 57). For example, the ANA has advocated for decades to secure meaningful health care for all Americans (ANA, 2003). Since the passage of the Affordable Care Act, the ANA has and will continue to focus its efforts on the regulatory process to ensure that law is implemented as it was intended.

The US health care system has experienced considerable transformation since the passage of the Affordable Care Act (2010) to expand health insurance and advance the nation's health (Box 25.1). The law put into place comprehensive health insurance reforms that have been unfolding since 2010 (U.S. Department of Health and Human Services, 2010). However, there remain significant challenges still to be addressed, including an aging and increasingly diverse population, rising health care costs, expanding numbers of individuals living with chronic diseases, and a shortage of health care providers. One of the most critical challenges is addressing the resources required to provide the public with the access and quality care within this new health care environment. The United States continues to spend more money per capita on health care than any other country. In the United States, health care spending totals more than $8,000 per capita, amounting to an aggregate expenditure of more than $2 trillion, or 17% of the gross domestic product (GDP) (Centers for Medicare and Medicaid Services [CMS], 2012). The Centers for Medicare and Medicaid Services (CMS) estimate that American health spending will reach nearly $5 trillion, or 20% of GDP, by 2021. New analysis of Medicare spending from 2000 to 2011 found that in 2011, per capita spending increased with age, from $7,566 for beneficiaries age 70 to $16,145 at age 96, and then declined for even older beneficiaries (Neuman, Cubanski, & Damico, 2015). For health care costs to be contained and quality improved, real transformational change will require nurses on the frontline to understand how laws, regulations, and policies impact nursing education, training, and practice.

NURSING AND POLICY

All aspects of the nursing profession are affected by policy issues, including safety and quality, health care standards, educational requirements, and nursing workforce conditions (which include mandatory overtime, nurse-staffing, workplace incivility, and violence). Policy issues also include professional protections and requirements for nurses, for example, whistle-blowing, and the management of chemically impaired nurses. Indeed, nurses have been involved in shaping health and public policy for over a century. For example, many early nursing leaders and activists, including Florence Nightingale, Lillian Wald, and Lavinia Dock, addressed the social issues of their times from the perspective of the nursing profession. Nurses continue to this day to meet their social responsibility for initiating and supporting action to meet the health and social needs of the public.

It was professional advocacy and activism that created some of the earliest policy debates within nursing, including the requirements around the "training and education" of nurses. The 2011 IOM and the Robert Wood Johnson Foundation report, *The Future of Nursing, Leading Change, Advancing Health* (2011), called for nurses to be better prepared with requisite competencies, such as leadership, health policy, system improvements, research, evidence-based practice, and collaboration, to deliver high-quality care, as well as competency in specific content areas including population and community health, and geriatrics. The IOM *Future of Nursing* report (2011) represents a turning point for the nursing profession. It called for nurses to achieve higher levels of education and training to ensure delivery of safe, patient-centered care across health care settings. The report recognized that as the largest health care profession, nurses are central to remaking the US health care system so that all Americans have access to high-quality and cost-effective care. To achieve this, the report defined the following key recommendations:

- Nurses should practice to the full extent of their education and training.
- Nurses should achieve higher levels of education and training through an improved education system that promotes seamless academic progression.
- Nurses should be full partners, with physicians and other health care professionals, in redesigning health care in the United States.
- Effective workforce planning and policy-making require better data collection and an improved infrastructure (The Future of Nursing, [IOM, 2011]).

For nurses to practice to the fullest extent of their education and training, they must have both regulatory and legislative endorsement for entry into practice, licensure, and scope of practice activities. Since the report's publication, multiple initiatives have been launched to create the policy substance and structure for an improved education system to achieve higher levels of education and training for nurses. At this time, statewide coalitions and strategic consortiums are working together with state legislatures to adopt licensure laws that reflect new educational requirements for entry into practice and advanced practice parameters to ensure the protection of the public and remove barriers to practice.

Today, there are laws that define the scope of nursing practice and licensure as distinctly separate from medicine and inclusive of responsibilities independent of medicine (National Council of State Boards of Nursing [NCSBN], 2015). The NCSBN is an independent not-for-profit organization through which boards of nursing confer and develop approaches to address matters of common interest and concern that affect public health, safety, and welfare, including the development of nursing licensure examinations (https://www.ncsbn.org/about.htm). The members include the boards of nursing in the 50 states, the District of Columbia, and four US territories—American Samoa, Guam, Northern Mariana Islands, and the Virgin Islands.

To ensure the public continues to benefit from the care they receive, the NCSBN conducts innovative studies to evaluate safety and quality in nursing practice as well as in educational programs. For example, NCSBN conducted a landmark, national, multisite, longitudinal study of simulation use in prelicensure nursing programs throughout the country. Collaborating with learning institutions across the United States, this research study explored the role and outcomes of simulation in prelicensure clinical nursing education. "The results of this study provide substantial evidence that substituting high-quality simulation experiences for up to half of traditional clinical hours produces comparable end-of-program educational outcomes and new graduates that are ready for clinical practice" (Hayden, Smiley, Alexander, Kardong-Edgren, & Jeffries, 2014 , p. S3).

Consider This Nursing's involvement in policy and politics has influenced state Nurse Practice Acts that regulate nursing practice for patient safety and public protection.

Discussion Point

The responsibilities of a licensed nurse include knowledge of, and adherence to, the laws and rules that govern nursing as outlined in the Nurse Practice Act and regulations. Review the nursing laws and rules by locating your state practice act and regulations at https://www.ncsbn.org/nurse-practice-act.htm

Participating in shaping health and public policy is an essential part of the professional nursing role because policy shapes and directs the environment in which nurses provide care, and determines the scope of their responsibilities. Nurses' political involvement is an important personal and professional imperative that advances the nursing profession while also improving the public's health (Hall-Long, 2009). This chapter defines policy, explains the policy process, and the role of nurses in that policy process, and describes the relationship between the systems of policy and politics. The continuum of political engagement activities is discussed, and the roles in policy and politics that nurses participate in are examined. This chapter describes nursing leaders who have shaped public policy, traces nursing's involvement in key policy/political debates, and includes contemporary issues being debated today in the political arena such as health care reform. Because politics is part of every organization and a part of government at every level, the chapter describes the political skills essential for nurses to act on behalf of their profession, and to develop and shape the health care systems where the patients and public will receive their care.

Nurses can increase their influence in policy and make sure the contributions of nurses are visible through political advocacy and action (Lewenson & Nickitas, 2016). In 1999, the International Council of Nurses (ICN) announced its global vision for the 21st century, which declared, in part, that "our mission is to lead our societies to better health" (ICN, 2006). In a 2012 article on strengthening nursing's role in global policy, Benton states that "if nurses are to realize this vision, nurses must do more than care for patients and conduct research. They need to be actively involved in shaping health care policy" (Benton, 2012).

To become mobilized in nationwide coalitions where nurses are essential partners in providing care and promoting health, The Future of Nursing: Campaign for Action, a national initiative to implement the recommendations from the landmark IOM report *The Future of Nursing: Leading Change, Advancing Health* (2011), has developed 51 state coalitions to transform health and health care by engaging nurses to implement the recommendations from the report. The Future of Nursing: *Campaign for Action* seeks to promote healthier lives, supported by a system in which nurses are essential partners in providing care and promoting health. An initiative of American Association of Retired Persons and the Robert Wood Johnson Foundation, the campaign works with action coalitions in 50 states and the District of Columbia to implement the IOM's Future of Nursing recommendations. The vision is to ensure that everyone in America can live a healthier life. The campaign is coordinated by the Center to Champion Nursing in America, an initiative of American Association of Retired Persons (AARP), the AARP Foundation, and the Robert Wood Johnson Foundation.

> **Consider This** Learn more about how the campaign is helping shape the future of health and health care by visiting the national Campaign for Action website and get connected at www.CampaignforAction.org.

DEFINING POLITICS AND POLICY

It is essential to describe and differentiate the terms *policy* and *politics* and to clarify the relationship between them. The word *policy* is Greek in origin and is linked to citizenship (Politics, n.d.). In government, it comes from the relationship of citizens to one another in public (Aries, 2016). Government policy and programs often impact organizations and adjust delivery of health care services to assure greater equality in the distribution of goods and services. A broad definition describes policy as a deliberate system of principles to guide decisions and achieve rational outcomes. It often includes a statement of intent, and is implemented as a procedure or protocol, for example, that all students must be vaccinated against measles, mumps, and rubella prior to admission into the school system.

Public policy is a term used that describes government actions. Policy is enacted through government systems, such as in the United States where the three branches of government are the legislative, executive, and judicial systems. These branches of government have the authoritative capacity to make decisions or influence the actions, behaviors, or decisions of others. Each branch of government plays a vital role in the formulation and regulation of health policy.

It is important to ensure that nurses are connected to their representatives on Capitol Hill and remain involved with governmental agencies as they propose and enforce new laws. Professional organizations such as the ANA have special departments such as the Department of Governmental Affairs (GOVA) to amplify nurses' voices as policies are being created, fought for, and implemented. GOVA seeks to create long-lasting relationships with nurses and their representatives to influence governmental policy that creates a world where health services are accessible, of high quality, and include the nursing profession as an integral part.

Discussion Point

How does health policy connect to how care and treatment are provided at the institutional level and at the governmental level? What factors must be considered before policy development begins at both levels?

GOVERNMENTAL POLICY

At the federal level, the US Congress and the President make policy in three major areas: defense, domestic, and foreign. Health-related policies can be found in all three areas. Health-related *defense* policies include the types of health care the military and their families will receive. *Domestic* policy refers to policies such as the recent enactment of the 2010 Affordable Care Act, which was intended to be a comprehensive law aimed at protecting consumers, increasing access to care, promoting health, improving and refocusing the health care delivery system, and controlling costs. Health-related issues are a major part of *foreign* policy as well. Congress decides whether to assist other nations in preventing HIV/AIDS, in providing family planning and nutrition assistance to developing countries, or responding to emergent health issues such as the 2014 Ebola outbreak, which impacted global, regional, and military health policies. However, Congress cannot govern alone and must rely on its citizens to protect the nation's health. For example, the "Ebola epidemic, and its intrusion into the U.S. health care system, has brought nurses fully into the national conversation about how best to handle this potential public health care threat. For the overall good of the nation's health care system, nurses must stay engaged to ensure appropriate attention and training occurs not only for themselves but also for all health care workers and hospitals" (Nickitas, 2014, p. 218). Nursing's voice on Ebola and other public health policies is needed to inform the public, policy-makers, media, and other stakeholders.

Consider This Nurses serving in the military are affected by defense policy, nurses working to improve global health in developing countries are affected by foreign policy, and nurses working within the health care system anywhere in the United States are affected by domestic policy. The President and the Congress decide on the allocations of tax dollars to be spent on defense, foreign aid, and domestic health care issues. When more money is spent to fund one policy initiative, less is available for others, unless taxes are increased.

POLICIES AND VALUES

Policy involves the setting of goals and priorities by a society or an organization and the decisions about how and what resources should be used to achieve those goals. Thus, policies are often expressed as goals, programs, proposals, laws, and regulations that reflect the values and beliefs of those who develop the policies (Milstead, 2016). There are those occasions where policies may develop into moral dilemmas. This is because a policy relates to decisions about how to act toward others.

Policies developed by nurses have frequently demonstrated commitment to the value of assisting people to care for themselves despite their illness or disability, and this belief has distinguished nursing from other professions (Research Study Fuels the Controversy 25.1). Caring, whether it is for families, for patients, or for the environment, is a value central to nursing. Watson (2008) suggests that to help the current health care system retain its most precious resource—competent, caring professional nurses—a new generation of health professionals must ensure care and healing for the public, while learning about the value of serving others. For many years, caring had not generally been a value that received much attention from institutions and government policy-makers. Nurses had some success at the state and federal levels moving such a policy agenda forward; however, results at a national policy level had been limited. The importance of providing care within a context of caring has recently been receiving greater attention. More recently, the national standards for measurements of quality health care have been integrating the patient's perception of care. This has now been expanded to address the perceptions of quality and their relationship to person- and family-centered care: "The extent to which patients and their families are involved in making decisions and feel prepared to manage their conditions is critical to improving quality and reducing cost" (National Quality Forum, 2015). Commonwealth Fund research has shown that patient- and family-centered care that incorporates shared decision-making can reap potential health care savings of $9 billion over 10 years. Accordingly, the National Quality Strategy seeks to ensure person- and family-centered care across the health care landscape, and has outlined several goals to achieve this aim:

1. Improve patient, family, and caregiver experience of care related to quality, safety, and access across settings.
2. In partnership with patients, families, and caregivers—and using a shared decision-making process—develop culturally sensitive and understandable care plans.

Research Study Fuels the Controversy 25.1

Addressing Health Care Disparities in the Lesbian, Gay, Bisexual, and Transgender Population

The purpose of this recent review of the policies and literature regarding the health of the lesbian, gay, bisexual, and transgender (LGBT) population was to highlight the need for "long-overdue" attention to the significant health care disparities that plague these groups.

Source: Lim, F. A., Brown, D. V., & Justin, S. M. (2014). Addressing health care disparities in the lesbian, gay, bisexual, and transgender population: A review of best practices. *American Journal of Nursing, 114*(6), 24–34.

Study Findings

LGBT people are collectively considered to be a "priority population" in discussions of health care disparities. Such disparities are closely tied to sexual and social stigma. A major barrier to health equity lies in the failure of medical education to include the unique aspects of lesbian, gay, and bisexual health, and even less about transgender health, resulting in a shortage of providers who are culturally competent in and knowledgeable about LGBT health. Various intersecting and overlapping health inequities affect the diverse LGBT population. For example, HIV infection rates are disproportionately higher among men who have sex with men, with even higher rates for African American and Hispanic men and transgender individuals; gay men, lesbians, bisexuals, and transgender people experience higher rates of suicidal ideation and suicide attempts, depression, and life dissatisfaction; LGBT youth are disproportionately likely to be homeless, and once homeless, to experience more negative outcomes; and the prevalence of smoking and alcohol and drug use is higher in LGBT populations.

Lim and colleagues highlight many LGBT advocacy groups. They recommend the integration of knowledge and tools developed by these organizations and other researchers into medical and nursing education and practice. These include a list of top issues LGBT people should discuss with their health care providers; LGBT health care resources with links to websites such as the National Gay and Lesbian Task Force and videos like "To Treat Me, you Have to Know Who I Am: Welcoming Lesbian, Gay, Bisexual and Transgender (LGBT) Patients into Healthcare"; and Strategies to Promote Inclusive Patient- and Family-Centered Care. The authors conclude with a call to action to nurses. "As the largest group of direct patient care providers in this country," they write, "nurses are in an excellent position to 'bridge health [care] disparities and provide culturally sensitive care across the lifespan.'"

3. Enable patients and their families and caregivers to navigate, coordinate, and manage their care appropriately and effectively (http://www.qualityforum.org/Topics/Person-_and_Family-Centered_Care.aspx).

This represents a major shift as health care quality measures will not only determine whether care provided meets the technical accuracy and consistency with practice standards, but also address the quality of the health care experience.

Discussion Point

What values are reflected in state Nurse Practice Acts that address the scope of nursing practice for registered nurses (RNs) and advanced practice nurses? Do these values promote or restrict nursing practice or nursing licensure, credentialing, and reimbursement for services?

POLITICS

Definitions of *politics* stem from the original Greek meaning, which referred to the government of the city-state; the actions of a government, politician, or political party; the process by which communities make decisions and govern; or the managing of a state or government. Politics involves power and influence for key decision-making and requires significant investment in social capital. Politics is often described as the process of who gets to decide how limited resources are allocated and distributed.

In government, politics is an activity that is central to developing policy that protects the well-being of society. Although this chapter focuses on policy and politics as they relate to government, many of the principles are applicable to nongovernmental institutions and organizations as well. Therefore, nurses must understand how politics drives policy decisions and have the necessary skills and competencies to care for society, regardless of their institution or organizational affiliation. One way nurses can better understand politics is to first assess

BOX 25.2 Assessing Your Political Awareness and Activity

1. Are you a registered voter?
2. Are you affiliated with a political party (Republic, Democrat, or Independent)?
3. Did you vote in the last local or state primary election?
4. Did you vote in the most recent presidential election?
5. Did you vote in the last general election—local, state, and national?
6. Can you name your elected city, state, and national representatives?
7. Have you ever contacted any of these elected officials?
8. Have you every lobbied your elected officials about a personal or professional issue that was important to you?

their own political awareness and activity to express their participation in the political process (Box 25.2).

Consider This To lead change and be successful, nurses must understand the values and political issues at hand. Nurses who perform as advocates will

1. believe that they have the power and expertise to convince others for the need to change,
2. adapt themselves to handle the broader political value issues, and
3. learn to effectively mobilize their expert power and use strategic planning to influence key stakeholders for the needed change (Robertson & Middaugh, 2016).

Politics is a reality of all organized human activity; any group of two or more individuals has to establish how to make decisions that require common action and how to resolve conflicts. In fact, Kraft and Furlong (2010) suggest that politics involves how conflicts in society are identified and resolved in favor of one set of priorities or values over another. Because resources (money, time, and personnel) are limited or finite, choices must be made regarding their use. There is no perfect process for selecting optimum choices because whenever one valuable option is chosen, usually some other option must be left out. The challenge for policy analysts and political action is to understand how these choices are organized and which ones have the most influence and why.

For nurses to be effective advocates for others and to shape policy (and practice), they must develop and practice the necessary political acumen and skill. This requires the ability to understand another's values and position and to use that understanding to influence others to act. Nurses have expert knowledge in these practices since they are integral to the nursing process and are used to provide patient care. It is essential for nurses to understand and appreciate how the nursing process applies to the components of the political process. The skills that govern nursing practice provide a basis for nurses to direct toward political advocacy and action.

CONCEPTUALIZING POLITICS AND POLICY DEVELOPMENT

Although there are many models for conceptualizing politics and policy development, Kingdon's streams of policy development (Sabatier, 1999) provide a broad and comprehensive framework for assessing policy development and a continuum for political engagement.

Kingdon's Three Streams of Policy Development

John Kingdon posited that there are *three streams* that determine why some problems are chosen over others for policy development (Sabatier, 1999; Box 25.3). The three streams are the *problem stream*, the *policy stream*, and the *political stream*. These three streams often flow endlessly without converging, but when the streams come together, a window of opportunity opens to move an agenda, to legislate, or to regulate policy solutions to problems.

The *problem stream* includes what are defined as problems, indicators of a problem, and the social construction of problems. It also includes how problems come to the attention of policy-makers, such as in the form of causal stories or personal experiences. For example, the shooting that occurred in Newton, Connecticut, on December 14, 2012, in which 20 children and 6 adult staff members were killed, prompted renewed debate about gun control in the United States. Proposals included universal background check system, and Federal and State ban on sale and manufacture of certain types of automatic firearms and magazines with more than 10 rounds of ammunition (Steinhauer, 2013; Vigdor, 2013).

BOX 25.3 The Three Streams of John Kingdon's Streams

1. *Problem:* embodies the process of problem recognition
2. *Policy:* embodies the formulation and refining of policy proposals as responses to problem recognition
3. *Politics:* considers the associated benefits and costs to subgroups of the population and the degree of external pressure the legislator feels to take action

Another example of such a problem is the current nursing faculty shortage. According to the AACN report on *2013-2014 Enrollment and Graduations in Baccalaureate and Graduate Programs in Nursing,* US nursing schools turned away 78,089 qualified applicants from baccalaureate and graduate nursing programs in 2013 due to insufficient faculty, clinical sites, classroom space, clinical preceptors, and budget constraints (American Association of Colleges of Nursing [AACN], 2014a). Almost two thirds of the nursing schools responding to the survey pointed to faculty shortages as a reason for not accepting all qualified applicants into entry-level baccalaureate programs. To minimize the impact of faculty shortages on the nation's nursing shortage, the AACN is leveraging its resources to secure federal funding for faculty development programs, collect data on faculty vacancy rates, identify strategies to address the shortage, and focus media attention on this important issue (AACN, 2014b).

Kingdon's second stream is the *policy stream.* Ideas that are potential policy solutions are considered on the basis of their "technical feasibility and value acceptability" (Sabatier, 1999, p. 76). The reality is that policy-makers are presented with many problems, and it is impossible to address all of them. Policy-makers, then, are expected to set an agenda that reflects the values and issues on which to focus legislation or regulatory action. Because policy-makers want to be successful (for their own reelection and job security), most will avoid introducing legislative or regulatory proposals that are unlikely to pass and/or to be implemented. For example, legislation introduced in the first session of the 113th Congress included the Assault Weapons Ban (AWB) of 2013 and the Manchin-Toomey Amendment to expand background checks on gun purchases. Both were defeated in the Senate on April 17, 2013. However, three states in the union successfully passed gun legislation: New York enacted the Secure Ammunition and Firearms Enforcement (SAFE) Act, and Connecticut and Maryland both enacted new restrictions to their existing gun laws. Federal legislation to ban guns was defeated because Americans (and many special interest groups) advocated for the "right to bear arms" as protected by the Second Amendment of the US Constitution.

Consider This When support from the public, professional nursing, and consumer and hospital organizations came together to help fund the Nursing Education Act, it was because of the trust and value the public holds for the profession. In contrast, the ban on assault weapons met with opposition because of the change of national mood, the turnover of Congress and the White House to Republican rule, and opposition from the powerful interest group, the National Rifle Association.

The significance of *interest groups* as part of the political stream cannot be overestimated. Throughout American history, political ideological interest groups have shaped social change and policy decisions. Interest groups provide politicians with one of three resources essential for their success (ie, reelection). The first, and sometimes seemingly most important, is money; the second is the ability to mobilize voters; and the third is image. It is this image enhancement that may be most significant for nurses in terms of legislative interest. Clearly, having the support of nurses enhances a candidate's image. For more than 10 years, nurses have ranked as among the most highly trusted professions in public opinion polls. The evidence supports the general public impression that the endorsement of nurses demonstrates a candidate's integrity (Riffkin, 2014).

Consider This Nurses continue to outrank other professions in Gallup's annual Honesty and Ethics survey. Eighty-one percent of Americans say nurses have "very high" or "high" honesty and ethical standards, a significantly greater percentage than for the next highest-rated professions, military officers and pharmacists. Americans rate car salespeople, lobbyists, and members of Congress as having the lowest honesty and ethics, with the last two getting a majority of "low" or "very low" ratings (GALLUP, 2014).

Nursing is a profession of more than 3.1 million members nationally. When divided by 435 congressional districts nationally, there are approximately 5,000 RNs per congressional district who can and have mobilized voters. The power of the "nursing numbers" converts to votes that can make the difference in electing officials who support and endorse nursing's core values and positions.

A strong political stream, however, is not enough. Convergence of the three streams is required. Nursing and the professional organizations that represent nursing (interest groups) in the legislature at the state and federal levels, then, have repeatedly worked to achieve this degree of stream convergence in public policy decisions related to health care. For example, the Nurse-Family Partnership (NFP) is a community-based program in which nurses work with first-time low-income mothers or vulnerable mothers from pregnancy until the child turns 2 years old. The NFP has been estimated to save $9,118 per child and as much as $26,298 as a return to society, for a net return savings of $17,180—cost–benefit ratio reported as 2.88. However, the cost–benefit ratio of 5.70 was reported for mothers who were known to be at the highest risk (Karoly, Kilburn, & Cannon, 2005). As health care delivery shifts from fee-for-service models of care to a value-based model, nurses are well positioned to use clinical and administrative data to measure nursing care, the quality of that care, and patient satisfaction from that care (Nickitas, 2014, p. 106). The Nurse-Family Partnership has effectively harnessed the value of clinical and financial data to illustrate how nurses are tackling important health problems and rigorously evaluating them.

Consider This Nursing interest groups have seized upon the public's frustration with rising health care costs and promoted policies that emphasize the cost-effectiveness of advanced practice nurses (stream one—conditions, plus stream two—ideas/policies).

Analyzing Policy-Making and Professional Nursing

A more traditional approach to analyzing policy-making uses a systems-based model that considers policy-making in sequential stages. It is much like the nursing process: assess, plan, implement, evaluate, and assess again. In a policy system, a problem is identified and placed on the policy agenda; then developed, adopted, implemented, evaluated, and extended, modified, or terminated. The challenge of using a traditional systems model approach is that it fails to consider that the elected government's policy agenda rarely, if ever, reflects a consensus.

For example, in the last two election cycles, the country has become more and more divided along partisan lines and determined to have philosophical values determine how best to govern or what the government's role is on health policy as witnessed by the recent debates surrounding the Affordable Care Act 2010. Critics argue that the systems analysis of policy development leaves out the influence of interest groups, whether they are nursing organizations or health insurance companies.

In contrast, policy development, adoption and implementation, and politics are inextricably linked in Kingdon's model, and the political environment in which policy is formed is considered. Nursing can play a role in all three of Kingdon's policy streams that create windows of opportunity. Again, using the IOM report (2011), nurses are considered the agents who will transform the health care system, ensuring care is patient-centered, effective, safe, and affordable. This vision calls upon the entire nursing community to embrace this report as a blueprint for action, and requires each and every nurse to use evidence-based research and collaboration to improve health care. It also means working for and within a remodeled health care system that guarantees high-quality, patient-centered care.

Consider This According to the IOM's definition, patient-centered care is "providing care that is respectful of and responsive to individual patient preferences, needs, and values and ensuring that patient values guide all clinical decisions" (IOM, 2011, p. 6).

It is a core responsibility of the nursing profession to elevate public awareness about the quality of care or lack of access to care. All individuals and communities, but especially vulnerable populations, must have access to affordable health care and opportunities that promote their health and well-being. This will require full engagement of all nurses in improving the experience of care, improving the health of populations, and reducing per capita costs of health care (Berwick, Nolan, & Washington, 2008). The role of the nurse toward the fulfillment of the "Triple Aim" includes partnership with individuals and families, redesign of primary care, and population health management. This includes addressing the social determinants of health.

Social determinants of health, for example, age, level of education, socioeconomic status, and access to health care, have the greatest capacity to improve health of individuals and communities as well as reduce the local cost of health care. To truly capture the inclusion of social and behavioral determinants of health data, nurses must lobby their legislators and others to ensure the social determinants of health are captured and placed inside the Electronic Health Record.

Professional nursing organizations and consumers collectively can develop ideas and propose policies to solve problems of health care access, health and safety, or quality of care. Nursing professional organizations and interest groups like AARP can lobby and engage in political action to influence policy.

In all of these examples, nursing is acting as an interest group. The unique thing about nursing as an interest group is that when nurses advocate for nurses and nursing, patients and the public get better care. Political action is a key part of interest group action. Interest groups do more than support or oppose policies; they help to elect the policy-makers by engaging in grassroots campaign activity and raising money for campaigns.

Discussion Point

Nursing has the potential to hold a significant leadership position in policy and politics. At the national level, the profession is represented by the ANA, the AACN, National League for Nursing (NLN), National Students Nurses Association (NSNA), and many specialty organizations. What opportunities are available at the local, state, and national level for you to assume a leadership position?

POLICY-MAKING AND POLITICS: THE KEY TO INVOLVEMENT

Nursing's involvement in policy-making and politics must rise to the level of engagement. If nurses truly want to influence health care and improve quality, access, and value, they must engage the political process. For changes in health care reform to be fully realized, it will require nurses to envision themselves as leaders in the process and find others who will share and support their goals. Political engagement can be viewed along a continuum that extends from no engagement in politics to that of extreme activism. Individuals choose when and how much political engagement along the continuum they want throughout their lives in response to intrinsic and external motivators, time and energy resources, and situational opportunities and needs.

Consider This Political engagement is when individuals make things happen. From where you sit right now, identify three activities that you can make happen in school, in the community, and at home that can make a difference.

Political Advocacy

Nurses *who make things happen* fall into three categories: professionals, leaders, and political change agents. All three groups vote in every election and stay informed regarding issues affecting the health care system, and they speak out about working conditions and quality of care. They also participate in professional organizations, know who their local, state, and federal elected officials are, and communicate with them regarding issues of concern. Former ANA President, Karen Daley (2011) suggests there are a variety of ways that nurses can get involved and make a difference, including the following:

- Don't let policy happen "to you"—get involved in the policy committees at work and through state associations.
- Use your voice, experience, and expertise to help design and implement care environments and models. No one knows what patients want and need better than nurses do.
- Participate in workforce planning surveys and data-collection opportunities. Nurses must measure the value of what they do.
- Stay informed about and participate in the activities of a professional association. A few hours of voluntary time can make a big difference; remember there is strength in numbers.
- Embrace and act on the power of nursing expertise and wisdom.

Nursing Political Action Committees

In 1974, new laws were established allowing for contributions by Political Action Committees (PACs). Those laws limited the amount an individual could contribute to a campaign and allowed groups to contribute up to US$5,000 per election. Historically, nurses' political contributions have not compared to the contributions of physicians, nor do nurses' contributions approach the level of political contributions from the American Hospital Association (2014). ANA created the Nurses

Coalition for Action in Politics (N-CAP; the precursor of the ANA-PAC) to establish political power through the endorsement of candidates and political contributions.

The proliferation of nursing specialty organizations and unions all claiming to represent "nursing" may have unintentionally jeopardized the nursing profession's effectiveness in influencing elected officials since different nursing organizations bring different messages. Elected officials are unlikely to see how the goals of these organizations are related to each other. These officials tend to listen to those people they perceive as best positioned to help elect or reelect them, so whichever nursing organizations are most active in political campaigns through contributions and through grassroots activity (usually only important in an official's first few elections because of the power of incumbency) are the organizations that will be heard.

It is essential for all nurses to be involved in the organizations that represent nurses, especially those with PACs, because "money talks." Contributing to candidates that promote nursing's agenda to improve the quality of health care is important. The cost of campaigns has grown significantly, and it's a reality that it requires money to buy time in today's expanding media environment and conduct the social research that are now part of any elected official's career.

Nursing's future depends on nurses accepting their role in participating in policy. Without increased participation, nurses risk having their presence and concerns unrepresented. Nurses can be active members of nursing organizations that take political action; they can take on active roles in a political party and attend political meetings, forums, and rallies; they can help register people to vote; they can contribute and raise money for causes and campaigns through PACs. The ANA-PAC evaluates the voting records of incumbent candidates campaigning for reelection, and the ANA state constituents develop relationships with candidates running for open seats.

Song (2011) states,

> *ANA does not use dues dollars to support candidates. Rather, ANA-PAC raises money through the voluntary donations from member nurses across the country. These nurses understand the importance of having a seat at the table when Congress is discussing nursing issues, such as appropriate staffing, home health, and safe patient handling. ANA-PAC donates to candidates who work to implement healthy public policy for our profession.* (p. 15)

Discussion Point

Do all RNs benefit from the contributions and work of the members of the ANA who make monetary contributions to the ANA-PAC and help to elect "nurse-friendly" members of Congress?

Nurses naturally work to affect policy in the workplace, but often underestimate how their work and the environments in which they practice are controlled by the government (policy). Across the country, nurses require an increased awareness of how government decisions impact their practice and move to enter roles where they can participate in influencing change. Achieving this level of increased awareness requires that nurses examine their values and take action to become involved.

To become engaged in civic participation will mean that nurses will have to balance the care of patients with the concerns of health care policy. Find an organization that speaks to your professional and core values. Then investigate the organization's legislative and policy agenda, learn what legislations impact nurses or nursing. There are several places where information about federal legislation can be located.

Consider This

Thomas Website (http://thomas.loc.gov)

- Monitored by the Library of Congress
- Wealth of information available about the legislative process, including searches on bill status, public laws, House and Senate roll call votes, current activity in Congress

Senate (www.senate.gov) and House (www.house.gov) Websites

- Information about individual senators and representatives, committees, schedules, and search for legislation
- Members of Congress can be contacted directly from each of these sites

ANA Government Affairs Website (http://www.nursingworld.org/MainMenuCategories/Policy-Advocacy)

1. Contains legislation that has been identified as important to nurses and information about how nurses can contact their legislators to express concern and voice their opinion

National League for Nursing Website, the National League for Nursing's Public Policy Action Center (http://capwiz.com/nln/home)

1. Provides information about legislation affecting nursing and allows searches for elected officials using zip codes

To become better informed about current issues affecting nursing and health care, consult additional websites of professional organizations. Other ways for nurses to learn about and increase their influence in politics and health care policy are shown in Box 25.4. These include becoming involved in electing candidates nurses want to win. This requires that nurses take action to learn about candidates and their agendas. There is value in being strategic in selecting candidates to support. When nurses support candidates that have a good chance of being elected or with a history of advocating for health care topics nurses support, there is greater opportunity to influence policy. Nursing will benefit by managing its communication to avoid alienating elected officials involved with health care or social policies. One way to avoid eliciting negative responses from elected officials is for nursing (individually and as organizations) to present an evidence-based and objective approach to the issues, focusing on facts and not emotions. It is important for nurses to be aware that in elections where a candidate is an incumbent, the candidate will still need and value support. Activities nurses can undertake to support such a candidate include working with telephone or in-person outreach, fundraising, sending letters to the media, supporting the candidate in public forums, and either contributing funds personally or through engaging others to support the candidate.

Consider This Working together, speaking with one strong voice, nurses are a powerful political force.

Actions that nurses can take to increase their influence in the policy setting are also shown in Box 25.4. Again, becoming involved in a professional nursing organization and being informed head the list. Nurses have ready access to know the legislators who represent them. District office staff usually handles constituent case work dealing with local, state, or federal agencies. For example, if someone has a problem with the post office or is a veteran and cannot get benefits, they can seek help from their congressional representative's district office. The district Chief of Staff is often the only "policy person" in the district. The office in the Capitol deals with legislation and policy issues. Staff members are key in getting access to a legislator, so the politically astute nurse is polite and respectful in dealing with these individuals.

Finally, nurses who want to increase their influence in policy should write their legislative representatives regarding health care issues (Box 25.5). Letters should arrive before any proposed legislation is heard in committee because key decisions on proposed legislation are made in committee. Bills that have a financial impact are heard in a policy committee and a financial committee. Some bills are assigned to two or more committees. This is often a tactic used to defeat the bill before it comes to the floor. If your legislator is not on the committee, write to the Committee Chair at the committee office address. If you write to legislators who do not represent you (you do not reside in their district), however, they are unlikely to respond to your communications because you are not one of their constituents. It is a good idea to send a copy of the letter with a brief cover letter to your legislator urging his or her support when the bill comes to the floor (if bills pass out of committee, they go to the "floor" or the entire house of the legislature). If your legislator supports your position on legislation,

BOX 25.4 Actions Nurses Can Take to Increase Their Influence in Politics and Policy

To Influence Politics

- Be knowledgeable and get involved in campaigns (the earlier the better).
- Assist candidates in winning the endorsement of key organizations that you may be involved in, such as nursing organizations, parent–teacher organizations, and neighborhood organizations.

To Influence Policy

- Be a member of a nursing organization that influences policy at the local, state, and federal levels.
- Be informed. Subscribe to electronic Listservs of elected officials that you agree with and compare the records of your officials.
- Get to know your elected officials.
- Write lobbying letters.
- Write letters to the editor.
- Participate in coalitions of organizations.

BOX 25.5 Sample Lobbying Letter

[1]Lillian Wald, RN, BSN

Henry Street

New York, New York 00251

[2]The Honorable Harry Nemo

Member, U.S. House of Representatives

House Office Building

Washington DC, 20015

[3]RE: SUPPORT for HR 1435

[4]Dear Representative Nemo,

[5]I am a registered nurse, and I have worked in the area of home health care for over 5 years. In the past 2 years, more and more of the elderly patients I care for have had to be readmitted to the hospital shortly after being discharged from the hospital because they are not taking their prescribed medications.

As you know, H.R. 1435 would provide a guaranteed, affordable prescription drug benefit within the Medicare program. Currently, despite many drug coverage programs for seniors, many remain unaffordable.

[6]It will save costly hospitalizations to provide needed prescription drugs at affordable costs to seniors. Please support H.R. 1435 and please advise me of your current position on this bill.

Sincerely,

[7]Lillian Wald, RN, BSN

Legend

1. Include your address.
2. Use the proper form of address (most elected and appointed officials are addressed as "the Honorable").
3. State what the letter is regarding.
4. Use the office title in the salutation.
5. State your credentials and experience/belief/position.
6. Urge support/opposition, and *ask* for a response with the official's position.
7. Sign letter.

(Please be sure when signing your name to include RN after your name.)

send a thank you note! Thank you notes tell legislators that you are watching what they are doing.

Finally, nurse political change agents are nurses who use their nursing expertise to lobby elected and appointed officials on issues of concern to the profession; write letters to the editors of professional journals and newspapers (Box 25.6 for an example of a Letter to the Editor, which was sent to the editor of the *The New York Times* and published). The work of health and public policy cannot be done in isolation. Nurses must build and participate in coalitions, encourage the participation of other nurses, and mentor future leaders. Most importantly, nurses must use their political muscle to enact and implement policies that enhance access, affordable quality health care, including nursing care; seek appointments or assist other nurses and friends of nursing in securing appointments to governing boards in the public and private sectors; be active members of political parties; query candidates about their positions on health care and assist with fundraising for candidates that support nurses and nursing; seek elected and/or appointed office, and continue to identify themselves as an RN; work on staffs of elected/appointed officials; and extend their policy influence beyond the health system to the community and the globe.

NURSING LEADERS AS POLICY PIONEERS

Nursing has a long history of involvement in politics and policy development. There are numerous nursing

BOX 25.6 Letter to the Editor

Letter: When Doctors Humiliate Nurses

Published: May 14, 2015

Today, hospitals pride themselves on providing patient-centered care by a multidisciplinary team, a hallmark of their quality. When one team member bullies another, patient care suffers. As a nurse, I would not want my family member or my nursing student in a hospital where physicians demean and insult their nurse colleagues, thus hampering their ability to care.

A culture and a climate of respect and dignity not only win the day but also ensure patient safety and quality care. It's time physicians learned that nurses are on their team, poised to manage complex critical decisions and care for their patients. Please no bullying—It hurts.

Donna M. Nickitas

Old Greenwich, Conn., May 8, 2015

The writer is a nursing professor at Hunter College, Hunter-Bellevue School of Nursing.

leaders who served as pioneers in public policy formation in the early to mid-1900s. Only a few are presented here, as is the area of policy they were most noted for. Yet their stories are similar; all of them shared passion, courage, and perseverance. In addition, they all shared a commitment to collective strength. These same attributes are recognized in nursing policy activists today.

Lavinia Dock: Organizing Nurses for Social Awareness

At the 1904 ANA convention, Lavinia Dock, a founder of the ANA and the first to donate money to establish the *American Journal of Nursing* that same year, stated that it was essential that nurses exercise social awareness. As a result, delegates to the ANA convention that year considered social (policy) issues of the time, including child labor, women's suffrage, and sex education.

Lillian Wald: Public Health and Child Welfare

Lillian Wald, one of the founders of the ANA, exemplified involvement in social change, community leadership, and politics. She was born to a family of Jewish scholars and rabbis. She graduated from nursing school and entered Women's Medical College in New York to become a doctor. During her first year of medical school, she volunteered to teach hygiene to immigrant women attending a school program.

In 1893, she quit medical school with a classmate, Mary Brewster, and moved to New York's Lower East Side neighborhood to provide nursing care in the community. A friend and philanthropist, Jacob Schiff, and Solomon Loeb agreed to fund Wald and Brewster's purchase of a house to support their public health work. This house became the Henry Street Settlement and is considered the founding place for public health nursing. Neighbors came to the house for help with their health, housing, employment, and educational needs.

Wald was also concerned about the living conditions of the neighborhood and the lack of safe places for children to play. She helped found the Outdoor Recreation League, which worked to gain attention for the need for public parks and raised funds for what would become the first municipal playground in New York City.

Fortunately, Wald's concern for children at the time was shared by many wealthy charity leaders. During the 1890s, close to 250 new orphanages were incorporated. At the time, vast numbers of children were working under unsafe conditions in factories. Wald believed the government needed to protect children and that child labor should be abolished. In 1904, she participated in a meeting with President Theodore Roosevelt lobbying for the creation of a national Children's Bureau (Krain, n.d.). However, the powerful industrialist lobby made up of the wealthy factory owners who used child labor was successful in tabling the legislation through their lobbying and political support of legislators (Jewish Women's Archive, n.d.).

By 1909, Wald convinced the Metropolitan Life Insurance Company that business interests benefitted by protecting the health of employees, and the company began funding nurses from the Henry Street Settlement to care for sick employees of companies they insured. The Henry Street Visiting Nurses Society began with 10 nurses in 1893. By 1916, there were 250 nurses serving more than 1,300 patients a day in their homes.

Wald convinced the New York Board of Education to hire a nurse in 1902, and so began school nursing in the United States. Her lobbying work also led to a change in divorce laws so that abandoned spouses could sue for alimony, and she assisted the Women's Trade Union League in protecting women from "sweatshop working conditions" (National Association for Home Care and Hospice [NAHC], 2014, para. 6).

Margaret Sanger: Birth Control

One of the many nurses whose training included experience at the Henry Street Settlement was Margaret Sanger. Sanger witnessed maternal and infant mortality resulting from uncontrolled fertility in the neighborhoods of the Lower East Side of New York City. She cared for women suffering from self-induced abortions and was motivated to make birth control available to women. In 1912, she began writing a column on sex education titled "What Every Girl Should Know," but it was soon censored (Steinem, 2004).

In 1914, Sanger was indicted for disseminating contraceptive information. She jumped bail and fled to England. She returned to the United States and continued to promote access to birth control throughout her life. She opened a clinic in New York with her sister Ethel Byrne and was jailed, only being released after a hunger strike. She smuggled contraceptive diaphragms from Europe, and founded the National Committee on Federal Legislation for Birth Control and the American Birth Control League, which later became the Planned Parenthood Federation of America.

In 1965, after years of effort, the Supreme Court decision *Griswold v. Connecticut* made birth control legal for married couples. Sanger died shortly thereafter (Sanger, n.d.). Her ability to ultimately create changes in policy was a combination of her first bringing the public and policy-makers' attention to a compelling issue, the maternal and infant mortality caused by lack of spacing pregnancies and the related poverty and deprivation. She also supported her agenda by leveraging the other relevant societal conditions, which included the women's movement and women demanding that their rights include being able to control their pregnancies. Finally, policy change occurred with the legalization of birth control.

Martha Minerva Franklin: Segregation and Discrimination

Martha Minerva Franklin was another pioneering public policy nurse in the early 20th century. She founded the National Association of Colored Graduate Nurses (NACGN) in 1908 with the fundraising assistance of Lillian Wald and Lavonia Dock, who mailed letters to more than 1,000 nurses (ANA Hall of Fame: Martha Minerva Franklin, n.d.). The NACGN was formed because many states barred Black nurses from membership in state nurses associations. Segregation and discrimination kept nursing education and hospitals separate.

The NACGN was instrumental, however, in political lobbying efforts to integrate Black nurses into the armed services during World War II. In 1951, the NACGN merged with the ANA (Flanagan, 1976). Today, the National Black Nurses Association exists as one of more than 70 national nursing organizations, some organized around clinical issues, some relating to ethnicity, and some relating to religious beliefs.

NURSES AND SOCIAL CHANGE

Historically, nursing leaders have participated in many efforts to bring about social change. Nurse leaders in the early 20th century were integrally involved in passing socially focused legislation that outlawed child labor, supported the suffrage movement, and provided protection for women abandoned by their husbands.

Nursing was also at the forefront of and lent integrity to the civil rights movement. As a result of the civil rights movement, poll taxes and literacy tests were made illegal. In addition, politicians elected with the aid of newly enfranchised Blacks passed laws intended to eliminate discrimination based on race. Nursing was one of the first professions to eliminate segregation. However, educational opportunities remain out of reach for many students of color, and nursing's responsibility to ensure that the profession reflects the diversity of those entrusted to its care still requires much work.

Nursing did not formally participate in the "peace movement" against the Vietnam War, but some nursing leaders participated in the women's movement that emerged around that time. Nursing and teaching were professions almost exclusively made up of women, and employment ads at the time were separated for men and women.

In 1974, the ANA set up a special account to help pass the Equal Rights Amendment to the Constitution and also joined a national boycott and moved its convention to a state that had ratified the Amendment. The Amendment failed ratification by a sufficient number of states. The women's movement continued, and nursing and teaching were often used as examples of professions requiring a significant amount of knowledge and skill for which compensation fell far below male-dominated jobs requiring the same levels of knowledge and skill, or "comparable worth." Nursing became involved in working to establish comparable worth in employment settings during the 1970s. Many states passed "comparable worth laws" during the 1970s, supported by state nurses associations. During the 1980s and beyond, nurses at various places around the country went on strike to achieve wages of comparable worth. Nursing's involvement in the women's movement as its own interest group working in coalition with other women's interest groups strengthened that movement.

TWENTY-FIRST-CENTURY NURSING LEADERS: POLICY AND POLITICS

Mary Wakefield and the Nation's Health

Mary Wakefield, PhD, RN, was named administrator of the Health Resources and Services Administration (HRSA) by President Barack Obama on February 20, 2009. HRSA is an agency of the U.S. Department of Health and Human Services. HRSA seeks to close health care gaps for people who are uninsured, isolated, or medically vulnerable. Wakefield joined HRSA from the University of North Dakota (UND), where she was Associate Dean for Rural Health at the School of Medicine and Health Sciences. Wakefield had acquired expertise and insight working within state politics and Capitol Hill, and brought that to her post at HRSA.

In the 1990s, Wakefield served as Chief of Staff to North Dakota senators: Kent Conrad (D) and Quentin Burdick (D). Her extensive board experience and health care knowledge led to an elected position to the IOM. She served on the IOM committee that produced the landmark reports *To Err Is Human* and *Crossing the Quality Chasm*. She was co-chair of the IOM committee that produced the report *Health Professions Education*, and chaired the committee that produced the report *Quality Through Collaboration: Health Care in Rural America*.

Loretta Ford—First Pediatric Nurse Practitioner Model

Loretta C. Ford, Dean and Professor Emerita, School of Nursing, University of Rochester, is an internationally known nursing leader. She has devoted her professional life and career to practice, education, research, consultation and influencing health services, community health, and military nursing. Her studies on the nurse's expanded scope of practice in public health nursing led to the creation of the first pediatric nurse practitioner model of advanced practice at the University of Colorado Medical Center.

Ford is a visionary leader who saw the need to meld nursing education, practice, and research. She provided administrative leadership for a unification model in nursing at the University of Rochester Medical Center in the position of Dean of the School of Nursing and the Director of Nursing in the University's Strong Memorial Hospital. She has authored more than 100 publications on the history of the nurse practitioner, unification of practice, education and research, and issues in advanced nursing practice and health care. Currently, she consults and lectures on the historical development of the nurse practitioner and on issues in advanced nursing practice and health care policy.

Discussion Point

What can you do to help ensure nurses are able to use all of their knowledge, skills, and experience to better help patients?

Consider This The American Nurses Association (ANA) was selected to testify at key hearings on national health insurance, amplifying nursing's voice on television to households throughout the country in advocating for comprehensive health coverage, including nursing care in all settings for all Americans.

Conclusions

What would Lillian Wald do about health care coverage for children and access to health care? What would Minerva Franklin do about racial health inequalities? What would Florence Nightingale do to elevate nursing in the policy debates? So the question for today is "What should nursing say?" At a time when the country is deeply divided along party lines, nurses must voice their concerns and speak for the public they serve. Nurses are stakeholders in what happens in health care (access, insurance coverage, cost, research), in the workplace (quality, staffing levels, safety, scope of practice, autonomy, working conditions), in the economy (unemployment's effect on mental and physical health and access to care, funding for Medicare and Medicaid), in international trade issues (foreign nurse licensure, importation of less expensive prescription drugs), and in the environment (preventing illness caused by pollution). That is, nurses are directly affected by the outcome of countless policies that are enacted or regulated.

There are many levels of political involvement and many spheres in which nurses can be influential, both public and private. Nurses can influence policies in the workplace (both public and private) and the community (both public and private). The bottom line is that they must accept a responsibility to be involved in some way.

Pierce (2004) perhaps said it best:

> *As nurses, as voters, and as constituents, we must be a part of the solution. Our elected officials truly want to know what nurses think and it is our obligation as professionals and as citizens to let them know. Our patients and the American public trusts nurses and are counting on us to advocate on their behalf.* (p. 115)

For Additional Discussion

1. Are nongovernmental and governmental politics more alike than not? If not, how do they differ? If so, how are they alike?
2. Why do you believe nursing was the first profession to eliminate segregation?
3. What are the most significant nursing issues being debated in the policy arena?
4. With such limited membership in the ANA, will nurses ever have a political power base that is representative of the size of their voting block?
5. Why are so many nurses reluctant to become active in the political arena? Do they lack the skills to do so? The confidence? Do nurses perceive a lack of congruity between professional behavior and politics?
6. With the AMA typically being far better represented than the ANA in legislative lobbying, is nursing's risk of being dominated by medicine greater than ever?
7. How well informed are most legislators about contemporary health care and professional nursing issues?
8. What do you believe will be the next major policy issue affecting nursing to be debated in the political arena?

References

American Association of Colleges of Nursing. (2014a). *Nursing faculty shortage.* Retrieved from http://www.aacn.nche.edu/media-relations/fact-sheets/nursing-faculty-shortage

American Association of Colleges of Nursing. (2014b). *Standard data reports: 2013-2014 Enrollment and graduations in baccalaureate and graduate programs in nursing.* Retrieved from http://www.aacn.nche.edu/research-data/standard-data-reports

American Hospital Association. (2014). *The value of membership in the American Hospital Association.* Retrieved from http://www.aha.org/about/membership/value.shtml

American Nurses Association. (2003). *Nursing's agenda for the future.* Washington, DC: Author.

American Nurses Association. (2010). *Nursing's social policy statement.* Washington, DC: Author.

ANA Hall of Fame Inductee: Martha Minerva Franklin (n.d.). Retrieved from http://www.nursingworld.org/MarthaMinervaFranklin

Aries, N. (2016). To engage or not engage: Choices confronting nurses and other health professionals. In D. Nickitas, D. Middaugh, & N. Aries (Eds.). *Policy and politics for nurses and other health professionals* (pp. 16–33). Burlington, MA: Jones & Bartlett.

Benton, D. (2012, January 31). Advocating globally to shape policy and strengthen nursing's influence. *The Online Journal of Issues in Nursing, 17*(1), 5.

Berwick, D. M., Nolan, T. W., & Washington, J. (2008). The triple aim: Care, health, and cost. *Health Affairs, 27,* 759–769. doi:10.1377/hlthaff.27.3.759

Centers for Medicare & Medicaid Services. (2012). *National Health Expenditure Projections 2012–2022.* Retrieved from https://www.cms.gov/research-statistics-data-and-systems/statistics-trends-and-reports/nationalhealthexpenddata/downloads/proj2012.pdf

Daley, K. (2011). Lessons in leadership. *American Nurse, 43*(3), 3.

Flanagan, L. (1976). *One strong voice*. Kansas City, MO: American Nurses Association.

GALLUP. (2014). *Public rates nursing as most honest and ethical profession*. Retrieved from http://www.gallup.com/poll/9823/public-rates-nursing-most-honest-ethical-profession.aspx

Hall-Long, B. (2009). Nursing and public policy: A tool for excellence in education, practice, and research. *Nursing Outlook, 57*(2), 78-83.

Hayden, J. K., Smiley, R. A., Alexander, M., Kardong-Edgren, S., & Jeffries, P. R. (2014). The NCSBN National simulation study: A longitudinal, randomized, controlled study replacing clinical hours with simulation in prelicensure nursing education. *Journal of Nursing Regulation, 5*(2), S1–S44.

Institute of Medicine. (2011). *The future of nursing: Leading change, advancing health*. Washington, DC: National Academy of Sciences.

International Council of Nurses. (2006). *Code of ethics*. Retrieved from http://www.icn.ch/images/stories/documents/about/icncode_english.pdf

Jewish Women's Archive. (n.d.). *Women of valor: Lillian Wald*. Retrieved from http://jwa.org/womenofvalor/wald

Karoly, L. A., Kilburn, M. R., & Cannon, J. S. (2005). *Early childhood interventions: Proven results, future promise*. Santa Monica, CA: Rand Corporation.

Kelly, M. A., Connor, A., Kun, K. E., & Salmon, M. E. (2008). Social responsibility: Conceptualization and embodiment in a school of nursing. *International Journal of Nursing Education Scholarship, 5*(1), Article 28.

Kraft, M., & Furlong, S. (2010). *Public policy-politics, analysis, and alternatives* (3rd ed.). Washington, DC: CQ Press.

Krain, J. B. (n.d.). *Lillian Wald, American Jewish Success*. Retrieved from http://jwa.org/exhibits/wov/wald/lwbio.html

Lewenson, S. B., & Nickitas, D. M. (2016). Nursing's history of advocacy and action. In D. M. Nickitas, D. J. Middaugh, & N. Aries. *Policy and politics for nurses and other health professionals* (2nd ed., pp. 3–13). Burlington, MA: Jones & Bartlett.

Milstead, J. (2016). *Health policy and politics: A nurse's guide* (4th ed.). Burlington, MA: Jones & Bartlett.

National Association for Home Care and Hospice. (2014). *Happy Birthday Lillian D. Wald* Retrieved from http://www.nahc.org/mobile/happy-birthday-lillian-d-wald/

National Council of State Boards of Nursing. (2015). *About NCSBN*. Retrieved from https://www.ncsbn.org/about.htm

National Quality Forum. (2015). *Person-and family-centered care*. Retrieved from http://www.qualityforum.org/Topics/Person-_and_Family-Centered_Care.aspx

Neuman, P., Cubanski, J., & Damico, A. (2015). Medicare per capita spending by age and service: New data highlights oldest beneficiaries. *Health Affairs, 34*(2), 335–339.

Nickitas, D. (2011). Cost and coverage in turbulent times. *Nursing Economic$, 29*(2), 57–58.

Nickitas, D. (2014). When nurses speak, will the nation listen. *Nursing Economic$, 32*(6), 218–282.

Pierce, K. M. (2004). Insights and reflections of a congressional nurse detailee. *Policy, Politics & Nursing Practice, 5*(2), 113–115.

Politics. (n.d.). In *Online Dictionary of Social Sciences*. Retrieved September 18, 2008, from http://bitbucket.icaap.org/dict.pl

Riffkin, R. (2014). *Americans rate nurses highest on honesty, ethical standards*. Retrieved from http://www.gallup.com/poll/180260/americans-rate-nurses-highest-honesty-ethical-standards.aspx

Robertson, R., & Middaugh, D. (2016). Conclusions: A policy toolkit for healthcare providers and activists. In D. Nickitas, D. Middaugh, & N. Aries (Eds.), *Policy and politics for nurses and other health professionals* (pp. 39–22). Sudbury, MA: Jones & Bartlett.

Sabatier, P. A. (Ed.). (1999). *Theories of the policy process*. Boulder, CO: Westview.

Sanger, M. (n.d.). *Encyclopedia Britannica profiles: 300 women who changed the world*. Retrieved from http://search.eb.com/women/article-9065508

Song, A. (2011). Defining ANA-PAC's role in the political process. *American Nurse, 43*(3), 15.

Steinem, G. (2004). *Margaret Sanger*. Retrieved from http://www.time.com/time/time100/leaders/profile/sanger3.html

Steinhauer, J. (2013, January 24). Senator unveils bill to limit semiautomatic arms. *The New York Times*. Retrieved from http://www.nytimes.com/2013/01/25/us/politics/senator-unveils-bill-to-limit-semiautomatic-arms.html?_r=0

Tri-Council for Nursing. (2015). Retrieved from http://tricouncilfornursing.org/Position-Statements.php

U.S. Department of Health and Human Services. (2010, March 23). *Key features of the Affordable Care Act by year.* Retrieved from http://www.hhs.gov/healthcare/facts/timeline/timeline-text.html

Vidgor, N. (2013, January 24). State police: All 26 Newtown victims shot with assault rifle. *Connecticut Post (Hearts Media Service)*. Retrieved from http://www.ctpost.com/newtownshooting/article/State-Police-All-26-Newtown-victims-shot-with-4222299.php

Watson, J. (2008). Social justice and human caring: A model of caring science as a hopeful paradigm for moral justice and humanity. *Creative Nursing, 14*(2), 54–61.

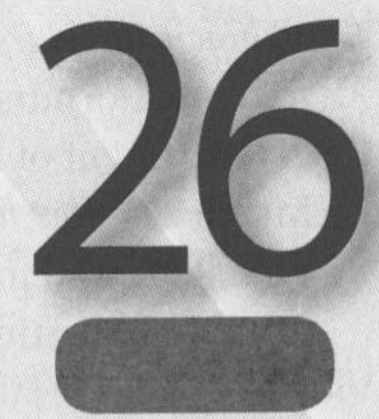

Professional Nursing Associations

Patricia E. Thompson and Cynthia Vlasich

ADDITIONAL RESOURCES

Visit thePoint for additional helpful resources

- eBook
- Journal Articles
- WebLinks

CHAPTER OUTLINE

Introduction

Types of Nursing Associations

Mission

Meeting the Mission

Choosing to Belong

Value to the Profession

Association Challenges

Sustainability

Resilience

Knowledge Dissemination

Leadership Development

Collaboration

Resource Management

Member Value

Research Opportunities

Conclusions

LEARNING OBJECTIVES

The learner will be able to:

1. Describe types of nursing associations and their value to members and the profession.
2. Explain the importance of nursing association missions.
3. Examine how nursing associations can strengthen their members' professional development across their careers.
4. Identify data an individual should access and review before selecting an association to join.
5. Identify challenges currently faced by nursing associations and possible solutions.
6. Explore the sustainability of nursing associations in the future.

INTRODUCTION

Nurses today have a choice in terms of what professional associations they will join. Each association will have a unique mission and vision, and offer different benefits to its members. They vary in focus from clinical specialty, academic development, scholarship, research, leadership, career advancement, to overall achievement.

Determining the associations that best meet the needs of each nurse is a personal decision and requires careful consideration, based on that nurse's individual career goals as well as expectations of association membership. However, it is critical for nurses to belong to and engage in associations, to enhance their own development and to advance the profession.

TYPES OF NURSING ASSOCIATIONS

A nursing association is typically a not-for-profit entity that exists to serve and represent its members, and meet the goals of the association based on its mission. The majority of organizations are based on individual membership; however, some organizations are association-membership based, such as the International Council of Nurses (ICN), which is a federation model. Other associations may be subsidiaries of a parent organization, such as the Association of Nurse Executives (AONE), which is a subsidiary of the American Hospital Association. Most associations, however, are autonomous.

An association's bylaws provide the governance structure through which that organization is led; incorporation laws within the country where the association is established provide the legal framework for its operation.

Consider This Bylaws govern an association and provide a list of the association's purposes, but most members never review them.

Nursing associations are usually supported by a governing board of directors, elected officers, and paid and/or volunteer staff. These positions provide opportunities for members to serve in leadership roles on the board and network with stakeholders across the association. No matter how an association is structured, the main goal of every membership-based association is to support its members and enable their success. Without members, associations would not exist. This goal, directly or indirectly, should be reflected in the association's mission, vision, and values.

MISSION

Each nursing association has an identified mission that sets it apart from other organizations and addresses its main purpose for existence. The association may also have identified a vision and values. The relationship between these is direct: the association mission is what the association does now, the association vision is what it hopes to become, and the association values are those specific beliefs that, with the mission and vision, guide the governing decisions of the association. The mission, vision, membership, and notable initiative of three professional associations in nursing (American Nurses Association, the Honor Society of Nursing, Sigma Theta Tau International [STTI], and the ICN) are compared in Boxes 26.1, 26.2, and 26.3.

Meeting the Mission

To effectively support and engage their members, associations must first understand who their members are and why they choose to belong. This process begins with analyzing the organization's member demographics and needs. Age, level of education, place(s) of employment, range of financial income, areas of interest/specialty, certification(s), career goals, and motivation to join are examples of demographic data that an association may collect.

Associations should also collect data from potential members who have chosen not to join; determining why they are not members, and their needs, is important in reviewing association benefits. For example, a recent survey by Wiley Publishing (2014) indicated that 24% of potential members declined due to cost, 15% did not join because they were not asked, and 12% did not know what associations were available to join. Data such as these provide excellent opportunities for associations to learn and grow.

Existing data demonstrate that people join associations for multiple reasons. They may want to shape the future of the profession, or enhance their careers. They may join to gain access to association journals and other information or continuing education that is available. They may believe in the association's mission and want to ensure it is achieved. Some join to enjoy the status of membership or because of the networking and mentoring available. Some join to celebrate and foster professional achievement, and some for the financial benefits of discounts and perks (Jacobs, 2014). Others join due to peer pressure or supervisor expectations.

BOX 26.1 American Nurses Association

The American Nurses Association (ANA) is the only full-service professional organization representing the interests of the nation's 3.1 million registered nurses (RNs) through its constituent and state nurses associations and its organizational affiliates. The ANA advances the nursing profession by fostering high standards of nursing practice, promoting the rights of nurses in the workplace, projecting a positive and realistic view of nursing, and by lobbying the Congress and regulatory agencies on health care issues affecting nurses and the public. It is headquartered in Silver Spring, Maryland, USA.

Mission Statement

Nurses advancing our profession to improve health for all.

Membership

Membership is open to RNs. ANA represents the interests of 3.1 million RNs through its constituent and state nurses associations and its organizational affiliates.

There are three types/levels of memberships available.

Organizational Affiliates—Specialty nursing organizations are allowed to hold organizational-level membership.

Notable Initiative

Health IT Initiatives

Health Information Technology (IT) enables health care providers to capture standardized data and use them to inform patient care and communicate across a range of clinical settings. Health IT also supports one of the strongest tenets of nursing—educating the patient and family.

ANA has launched and participated in several Health IT initiatives:

- Developing standardized nursing languages
- Nominating nurse leaders to federal Health IT committees and workgroups
- Developing position statements on Health IT initiatives, policy, and standards
- Participating in Health IT alliances, including the Alliance for Nursing Informatics, American Medical Informatics Association, and Healthcare Information and Management Systems Society
- Developing educational products that support the consumer eHealth campaign of the Office of the National Coordinator for Health IT
- Coordinating expert panel summit meetings to establish quality measurement models for inclusion in electronic health records

Subsidiaries

- American Nurses Credentialing Center (ANCC)
- American Nurses Foundation (ANF)
- American Academy of Nursing (AAN)

Website: http://www.nursingworld.org/

Source: American Nurses Association. (n.d.). Retrieved March 18, 2015, from http://www.ana.org

Associations must leverage their strengths and determine what they provide that is unique. Then, based on member assessments, associations must determine the scope and specific combination of services to meet their members' demands. They have a responsibility to determine member needs and appropriate delivery modalities for programs and services. This allows current and potential members to make informed decisions on which association(s) will best meet their needs.

Today most associations have members across multiple age ranges and at different points in their careers. Due to generational issues in how people work and what they expect both from their workplace and also from the associations they join, meeting the mission of the association means providing support for members across generations, career trajectories, with differing levels of experience and motivations to join. Many organizations create a menu of benefit options to address individual member needs.

BOX 26.2 The Honor Society of Nursing, Sigma Theta Tau International (STTI)

Sigma Theta Tau International (STTI) is a nursing association dedicated to creating a global community of nurses who use their knowledge, skills, and abilities to promote health, prevent disease, and advance the science and art of nursing. It supports the learning, knowledge, and professional development of nurses making a difference in global health by providing members with invaluable benefits and resources such as its in-house publishing division featuring award-winning books and esteemed scholarly journals, a unique open-access scholarly and clinical dissemination venue, continuing education opportunities, leadership institutes and academies, and international events. It was founded in 1922 and is headquartered in Indianapolis, Indiana, USA.

Mission Statement

The mission of the Honor Society of Nursing, STTI, is advancing world health and celebrating nursing excellence in scholarship, leadership, and service.

Vision

STTI's vision is to be the global organization of choice for nursing.

Membership

STTI has more than 135,000 active members around the world. Its members reside in more than 85 countries and participate in roughly 500 chapters at approximately 675 institutions of higher education.

STTI membership is by invitation to baccalaureate and graduate nursing students who demonstrate excellence in scholarship.

Nursing professionals exhibiting exceptional achievements in nursing, not previously inducted as nursing students, may seek to join STTI as a nurse leader.

Notable Initiative

Global Advisory Panel on the Future of Nursing

During the past decade, STTI, which holds special consultative status with the United Nations' ECOSOC (Economic and Social Council), has assumed an increasingly global role in advancing world health and promoting the nursing profession. Through the creation of Global Advisory Panel on the Future of Nursing (GAPFON) in 2014, STTI is partnering with global leaders to establish a voice and a vision for the future of nursing that will advance global health. GAPFON is hosting global regional meetings to identify priority health care issues. Recommendations from the meetings will result in implementation strategies and outcome measures for each priority (Klopper & Hill, 2015).

Subsidiaries

- STTI Foundation for Nursing
- The International Honor Society of Nursing Building Corporation
- Nursing Knowledge International (NKI)

Website: http://www.nursingsociety.org

Source: Sigma Theta Tau International. (n.d.). *About STTI*. Retrieved March 18, 2015, from http://www.nursingsociety.org/ABOUTUS/Pages/AboutUs.aspx

Different modalities are important to meet members' learning preferences and geographical locations. They include:

- Face-to-face programs and meetings
- Electronic mail, blogs, and communication boards
- Videoconferences, webinars, and other online options
- All forms of social media

Discussion Point

What strategies might be used to meet the needs of a geographically diverse membership?

For example, if association data indicate that a key motivator for membership is networking, then ensuring that rich opportunities to network one on one and with

BOX 26.3 International Council of Nurses

The International Council of Nurses (ICN) is a federation of more than 130 national nurses associations, representing more than 16 million nurses worldwide. Founded in 1899, ICN is the world's first and widest reaching international organization for health professionals. Operated by nurses and leading nurses internationally, ICN works to ensure quality nursing care for all, sound health policies globally, the advancement of nursing knowledge, and the presence worldwide of a respected nursing profession and a competent and satisfied nursing workforce. It is headquartered in Geneva, Switzerland.

Mission Statement

To represent nursing worldwide, advancing the profession and influencing health policy.

Vision (Strategic Intent)

To enhance the health of individuals, populations, and societies by

- championing the contribution and image of nurses worldwide
- advocating for nurses at all levels
- advancing the nursing profession
- influencing health, social, economic, and education policy

Membership

ICN is a federation of more than 130 national nurses' associations, representing millions of nurses worldwide. ICN works directly with these member associations on issues of importance to the nursing profession. There is no individual membership to ICN. Nurses who are part of their national nurses association are automatically part of ICN.

Notable Initiative

The Girl Child Education Fund (GCEF), a signature initiative of Florence Nightingale International Foundation (FNIF), supports the primary and secondary schooling of girls under the age of 18 in developing countries whose nurse parent or parents have died. Since the initiation of the program, 385 girls have been enrolled in the GCEF. The initiative is currently supporting 178 girls in Kenya, Swaziland, Uganda, and Zambia.

Foundations

- FNIF
- The International Council of Nurses Foundation (ICNF)

Website: http://www.icn.ch/

Source: International Council of Nurses. (2014, November 28). Retrieved March 18, 2015, from http://www.icn.ch

like interested groups should become a priority. To be responsive, that association might create networking activities at events and through online communities, and opportunities to collaborate on projects and programs that benefit not only the members involved with the actual work, but others in the profession.

CHOOSING TO BELONG

Nursing is a profession where association membership can provide great value. Many of the nurse leaders in our profession today have not only become known within the field of nursing through their involvement in professional associations, but have fine-honed their professional and leadership skills through such memberships.

Benefits vary based on the mission of the association, but they are all important for professional growth across the member's career. Examples include:

- Educational programs providing continuing education units on topics related to association mission with content focused on clinical practice, academics, leadership, scholarship, policy, and others
- Association journals providing current knowledge and updates
- Certification in specialty areas to demonstrate expertise and credibility

- Networking to connect and collaborate with experts in your area of interest
- Opportunities to identify mentors to assist the member with both short- and long-term goals related to career development
- Content related to developing knowledge and skills to be a mentor
- Awards and recognition such as research grants or travel stipends to present papers at conferences, or public recognition for outstanding accomplishments
- Discounts for goods or services, such as liability insurance, computers, or rental cars (Akans et al., 2013; Esmaeili, Deghan-Nayeri, & Negarandeh, 2013)

Discussion Point

Discuss how a mentor might advance your professional development, providing specific examples.

We all balance personal and professional demands and need to carefully weigh opportunities and obligations to ensure we maintain the blend needed for a healthy lifestyle and career. Association membership can assist with maintaining that personal/professional balance by providing the benefits listed above and many more—all in one place.

When considering which association(s) to join, it is important to review the benefits of the association based on a personal cost–benefit ratio. Each nurse must determine what they expect to gain from membership in any given association or a variety of associations, and in return, what they are willing to give in terms of membership dues and participation. Individuals must be able to analyze and determine the value to them of both tangible benefits and intangible benefits. Individuals should research various association options and analyze what each has to offer. In addition to culling through an association's website, they should call their membership offices to discuss the benefits of membership, and speak with colleagues about what they recommend. For example, if a membership association's annual dues are $100 and the benefits include free journal access, free continuing nursing education, and other tangible benefits, you have a direct cost–benefit ratio based on tangible value. One must then add the value of the intangible benefits, such as networking; the ability to meet and work with professional leaders within the association, to be mentored, to collaborate with others; and access to events or products. Based on that analysis, each individual can determine what the tangible and intangible cost–benefit ratio is, and thus the ultimate value, to them.

Many nursing colleagues choose to participate in two or more associations, gaining different value from each. Whether interests are focused at the local, state, provincial, national, regional, or global level, associations exist that can provide individuals with those opportunities.

Taking full advantage of the opportunities that association membership provides will be critical to attaining the full value of one's membership. The value of this experience will run parallel to the level of an individual's participation. Association membership can provide a wonderfully well-rounded and rich professional experience and greatly enhance one's career.

Discussion Point

Describe the factors important to you in deciding which nursing association(s) to join.

VALUE TO THE PROFESSION

Nursing associations exist to both support their members and address critical issues and challenges that face the profession and health care in general. Associations also need to engage their members effectively through offering professional education, networking, and mentoring opportunities. Many nursing associations, as a key part of their missions, have a goal to improve health care, either directly or indirectly. This work may be quite broad or focused in specific educational or clinical practice areas, and may be local, regional, national, and/or global in scope.

Each organization's support of the profession should be mission-specific and, depending on the organization, focus on one or more of the following:

- Policy, regulatory, and legislative support
  - Some associations exist to create, enact, and/or monitor compliance with professional practice laws and the standards created by various accrediting bodies. There are legal and voluntary standards that control the profession's work including

licensure at all levels of nursing practice. Various accreditation bodies exist to support education, quality, and credentialing regarding practice.

- Developing practice standards
  - The mission of many organizations, including those with a specialty focus, is to develop and promote quality and evidence-based practice standards. These expected professional performance levels are often included or indicated in regulatory statements and used as a benchmark any time a legal question arises regarding professional performance.
- Creating positive work environments
  - Working conditions are often addressed by various accrediting bodies that relate to education and practice settings. In addition, the missions of some organizations include collective bargaining, which is typically undertaken to support working conditions.

Discussion Point

Explain why practice standards need to be evidence-based.

Consider This Through maintaining professional values and standards, associations represent the profession to key stakeholders such as policy-makers and the public.

- Enhancing the profession
  - Professional associations are a voice for the profession to consumers, and to the policy-makers. They maintain professional values and standards, and support the profession through the opportunities they provide their members to grow and develop. Leadership opportunities to serve on boards, be involved on committees, and take action to move the organization and the profession forward in a positive way are often provided by professional associations.
  - Credentialing is another way organizations enhance the profession. It provides validity to knowledge and expertise for nurses in a particular area through assessment against established standards for that area.

Discussion Point

Some of the professional issues nursing associations address include scope of practice, quality and access to care, patient and nurse safety, and legislation that impacts practice. Select one of the above and explain the role of associations in addressing the issue. What other professional issues do nursing associations address?

ASSOCIATION CHALLENGES

Professional associations are charged to remain relevant, valuable, and significant to all their members, at a time when membership crosses not only multiple generations but also multiple cultures. Whether a national, regional, or international organization, the reality is we are a global community with members from different cultures. Effectively recognizing and understanding a variety of norms, standards, and protocols, as well as meeting different cultural expectations is required for global success.

With the often-noted differences in Baby Boomers, Gen Xers, and Millennials, providing value and significance to all these generational members is a daunting challenge. Whether they value career success, personal time, or the ability to design a customized career life that suits their individuality (Generational Differences Chart, 2015), each group has, in general, certain traits that, of course do not hold true for all members of that generation. So what does this mean for associations? It means the association must be flexible in programming and approach, and must offer a variety of options to provide value to different members.

As an association develops this menu of benefits, which may include programs, events, products, and services, each must be reviewed with keen attention to meeting the members' needs within both the mission and the resources of the organization.

Discussion Point

Discuss the challenges of meeting member needs across generations.

In addition to generational diversity, today many associations are responding to an increasingly global community due to expansion into multiple countries and regions. This growth broadens the traditional local chapter model to encompass state, province, country, and global regional models. This global diversity not only impacts how the organization must grow, but also brings additional complexity to meeting member needs, far beyond generational issues. Cultural diversity, combined with generational diversity, and the varying values that a rich cultural and generational membership mix provides, offers a unique opportunity and challenge for professional associations in meeting their members' needs.

Discussion Point

The practice of nursing differs greatly around the world. How do nursing associations bridge the chasm between different cultures, norms, and scopes of practice?

Associations should be strategic in planning for global expansion and recognizing the implications for the organization and membership. As organizations consider global growth, they must carefully scrutinize their organizational mission, intention, member demographics, and member demand, balanced against current and projected organizational resources to ensure they are positioned not only to initiate global growth, but also to achieve sustained, successful, and continued global expansion. As associations design the best multiple strategy approach to reach their members, the strategy must include a variety of modalities to facilitate participation across the globe.

Discussion Point

What are the benefits and challenges if a country-specific association decides to expand globally?

Members also value timely information about benefit opportunities, as well as how programs, events, products, and services are delivered. For example, an association may have an outstanding program; however, if it is not marketed effectively, and/or delivered in a manner that does not benefit the members, the program is of little value, and, indeed, can be detrimental if it leads to a disappointing experience for the members.

To that end, associations need to not only offer quality programs, but also market them effectively so that members recognize the value of the opportunities available for personal and professional growth. From a business construct, positioning the value of the association based on (1) features, (2) benefits, and (3) value, customized to differing membership audiences may be a highly effective messaging strategy.

Communication with members must be fluid, flexible, and varied. For example, some members will prefer communication via phone calls and tangible mailings, while others communicate primarily via email, text message, and social media.

Discussion Point

How have you changed the way you communicate with colleagues, family, and friends over the past 3 years? How do you prefer to communicate now versus 3 years ago?

Another strategic decision for associations to make is where to focus their resources and how to prioritize what professional issues to address. There are many nursing and health care issues, and it is easy for the board of an association to enthusiastically slip into a mode of wanting to solve them all. However, it is critical that the association board of directors ensures all initiatives relate to the mission, so the association stays within its legal parameters. The focus should also support the association vision, and uphold its values.

Discussion Point

Review missions of various professional nursing associations and determine which one(s) best meet your needs.

Consider This Nursing is the most trusted profession according to repeated Gallup poll results. And yet it is one of the least influential.

A major challenge faced by associations today is increasing their membership when current and potential members are careful in how they spend their money and time. Associations must develop strategies to demonstrate there is actual value in the dues a member pays and the time they volunteer. One strategy is to allow payment of dues over time. However, the most critical factor for members paying association dues is their ability to easily identify perceived personal value for their membership (Jacobs, 2014).

To address the demands of work, personal life, and other activities, associations need to help members recognize the many ways associations can save them time. For example, easy access to mentors and networks can facilitate the members' ability to reach career goals more quickly. Members can connect with experts to assist with practice, educational, leadership, and scholarship goals (Esmaeili et al., 2013; Jacobs, 2014).

Engaging members can also be a challenge, but is essential for the success of an association. For example, ensuring members are offered opportunities to lead and govern the organization is critical for most associations whose board, committee work, and program content are accomplished through member volunteers. Special emphasis should be placed on engaging new members immediately and often, as well as engaging all members in activities and programs that are meaningful to them will in turn develop long-term loyalty. Providing a diverse variety of rich opportunities for member volunteers can be one of the most powerful strengths of an association. If these opportunities effectively address cultural, gender, and generational diversity, they can assist the association in providing value to membership through engagement, and this will lead the organization to success with positive outcomes for everyone.

SUSTAINABILITY

The association that is nimble, designed to respond quickly and efficiently to new opportunities, able to divest itself of ineffective programs, and provides diverse, meaningful, and impactful programs and opportunities for its members is best poised for long-term success.

Resilience

As with any organization, associations that thrive in a culture of change are best suited to succeed. It is essential that organizations are flexible and able to adapt quickly for them to remain relevant. They must not only react to change, but must also be adept at predicting change. Nowhere is this more apparent than in professional associations. They must be responsive as well as responsible, be able to facilitate change as well as assist their members in successfully navigating through a changing environment.

Knowledge Dissemination

Professional knowledge is vast and growing daily. Analyzing and sharing fresh data in a way that is useful to members is a key value that organizations/associations provide and that members will continue to need in the future.

Leadership Development

Professional associations must have visionary leaders and highly competent staff to thrive. Associations also have a responsibility to help develop the next generation of nurse leaders both for the association and for the profession. They must create an environment to nurture and grow those nurse leaders. An association may barely survive or fully thrive depending on the knowledge and skill of its paid and volunteer leadership. Early identification, development, and mentoring of member leaders, who bring expertise and loyalty to leadership positions within the association, is vital both to current success and long-term sustainability.

Consider This The IOM report on the Future of Nursing addresses the need for more nursing leaders now and in the future. Professional associations provide knowledge, skills, and opportunities to develop as leaders.

Collaboration

Although some associations feel a competitive model of work is beneficial, those organizations that have similar missions can benefit in great measure through collaboration with each other. Collaboration can provide a collective voice, a respectful diversity of opinion, experts, and expertise, and strengthen results while minimizing resource outlay.

Consider This Collaboration among nursing associations to address key nursing and health care issues conserves resources and strengthens the voice of the profession.

Discussion Point

Is interprofessional collaboration important for nursing associations in addressing health care issues? Why?

No one association is as powerful individually as all are collectively. With that, are associations the appropriate venue for sustaining nursing in the future? The answer is a resounding YES. The benefit of collaboration has proven to be powerful; it can change practice, establish standards, enact laws, sustain workplace settings in which nurses can best succeed, and ensure an environment in which our students feel welcomed into the profession and safe.

Resource Management

The key for sustainability in the future is an infrastructure that includes adequate human and financial resources. Associations need to engage and maintain their members and volunteer leaders, as well as hire expert staff. These are the people who provide the vision, accomplish the work, and maintain the relevance of the organization. Associations need to develop a multisource revenue base. Relying mainly on dues for revenue will not result in sustainability (Research Study Fuels the Controversy 26.1). Nondues revenue from programs, products, and services is often used as part of a multisource revenue strategy. However, other options need to be explored. Collaborating with other associations for programming events conserves resources, as well as increases networking opportunities for members. In addition, associations that are going to be viable in the

Research Study Fuels the Controversy 26.1

Exploring the Future of Membership

The focus of this series of research studies was to assess association membership for the future. This was a multidisciplinary approach with grant funding provided by the ASAE Foundation to four different researchers to address changing characteristics of professional membership based on social and economic trends as they relate to level of involvement. Although addressing the same question, the methodology used by each researcher varied. One researcher used secondary data, one analyzed data from organizations that had creative and successful membership models, another completed detailed member interviews and used case studies, and the final researcher collected data through surveys, focus groups, and interviews.

Source: Barnes, J., & Nelson, J. (2014). Exploring the future of membership. *ASAE Foundation Research Series*, 1–18. Retrieved from https://mystuff.asaecenter.org/ebusiness/publications/publicationproduct?id=108025&CSURL=http%3A%2F%2Fwww%2Easaecenter%2Eorg%2FShop%2FBookstore%2Ecfm%3FQuery%3Dexploring%2Bthe%2Bfuture%2Bof%2Bmembership

Study Findings

The findings from the four research studies were presented in March 2014 at a conference attended by association leaders. Following the presentation, group discussions by conference participants focused on how the findings related to current membership concerns. In visioning the future of association membership, Barnes and Nelson (2014) noted that these discussions culminated in five themes:

- Membership in context: providing value to members where they are
- The impact of other decision-makers: engaging influencers to get new members
- Changing roles and responsibilities: the association position in the larger community
- Curation of information and data: a new opportunity for associations
- Removing barriers to change: tackling the obstacles preventing associations from getting better

This series of research studies simultaneously addressed a problem using different approaches and methodologies resulting in findings that have current applications for association membership as well as a blueprint for future strategies. These findings were then taken a step further by engaging key stakeholders at a conference to identify the implications and potential impact on their associations both now and in the future. This is an example of using the evidence from research to effect change.

future must have a strategy that includes building a reserve fund to survive when unexpected situations occur.

Member Value

The association that not only meets member needs but surpasses member expectations, now and in the future, positions itself for long-term sustainability. And those associations who provide such value that membership is seen as a necessity, not a choice, will flourish.

RESEARCH OPPORTUNITIES

The focus of professional associations is to meet the needs of members and nursing. Although there are examples and some qualitative data available, there is limited evidence to document the outcomes of association work. Therefore, more research needs to be conducted in this area. Below are some ideas that can be developed into studies:

- Survey members in board-level association positions to determine what motivated them to become engaged members.
- What are the characteristics of associations that will thrive in the future?
- Analyze outcomes of associations with a policy focus.
- Survey association executive officers to assess the future of associations.
- Is there a relationship between association membership and nurses in leadership roles?
- Does leadership in student nurse associations translate into membership in professional associations after graduation?
- How can associations address the needs of an increasingly diverse membership?
- What effect will the large number of retiring Baby Boomers have on association viability?

Conclusions

Nursing associations seek to elevate the practice of nursing, with the ultimate goal of supporting their members and improving the delivery of health care and health care outcomes. Every nurse can benefit personally and professionally from active membership in the organization(s) that best meet their needs. With visionary leadership and strong participation, associations advance our profession, locally, regionally, and globally.

For Additional Discussion

1. Determine the cost–benefit ratio for you to join a professional nursing association. Identify both the tangible and intangible benefits.
2. Explain how professional nursing associations enhance the nursing profession.
3. Discuss why effective marketing is key to a professional nursing association's success.
4. Explain how a professional nursing association should make decisions about which professional issues to address.
5. How can professional nursing associations help nursing become more influential?
6. How can collaboration benefit nursing associations and the profession?
7. How can professional nursing associations develop long-term loyalty from their members?
8. Identify key factors necessary for a professional nursing association to thrive.
9. "Resilience" is a popular term and is currently applied to many areas of health care. What does resilience really mean—in the broader framework of health care, as well as in your specific setting? Describe how a professional nursing association can develop and maintain resilience.
10. What professional nursing associations do you know most about? Least about?

(continued)

11. If you could provide recommendations or advice to any professional nursing association on how best to recruit and retain members, what would those recommendations/that advice be?
12. As you analyze your career goals and direction, which professional nursing associations would be best for you to affiliate with and become a leader of?
13. If you were launching a new professional nursing association, what would its mission be?
14. Of the various types of diversity, for example, culture, gender, age, socioeconomic status, etc., which do you feel would be most challenging for a professional nursing association to effectively address?

References

Akans, M., Harrington, M., McCash, J., Childs, A., Gripentrog, J., Cole, S., . . . Fuehr, P. (2013). Cultivating future nurse leaders with student nurses associations. *Nursing for Women's Health, 17*(4), 343–346. Retrieved from http://onlinelibrary.wiley.com/doi/10.1111/1751-486X.12054/epdf

Barnes, J., & Nelson, J. (2014). *Exploring the future of membership. ASAE Foundation Research Series,* 1–18). Retrieved from https://mystuff.asaecenter.org/ebusiness/publications/publicationproduct?id=108025&CSURL=http%3A%2F%2Fwww%2Easaecenter%2Eorg%2FShop%2FBookstore%2Ecfm%3FQuery%3Dexploring%2Bthe%2Bfuture%2Bof%2Bmembership

Esmaeili, M., Deghan-Nayeri, N., & Negarandeh, R. (2013). Factors impacting membership and non-membership in nursing associations: A qualitative study. *Nursing & Health Sciences, 15*(3), 265–272. Retrieved from http://onlinelibrary.wiley.com/doi/10.1111/nhs.12012/epdf

Generational differences chart. (2015, March 18). Retrieved from West Midland Family Center Website: http://www.wmfc.org/uploads/GenerationalDifferencesChart.pdf

Jacobs, S. (2014). *The art of membership: How to attract, retain, and cement member loyalty* (1st ed.). San Francisco, CA: Jossey-Bass.

Klopper, H. C., & Hill, M. (2015). Global Advisory Panel on the Future of Nursing (GAPFON) and global health. *Journal of Nursing Scholarship, 47*(1), 3–4.

Wiley Publishing. (2014). *Membership matters: Lessons from members and non-members* (pp. 1–8). Hoboken, NJ: Author.

Index

Note: Page numbers followed by *f*, *t* and *b* indicate figures, tables and boxes, respectively.

T

CCS1215